D1195767

Autism

AUTISM
Nature, Diagnosis, and Treatment

Edited by
GERALDINE DAWSON
University of Washington

Foreword by Eric Schopler

THE GUILFORD PRESS
New York   London

© 1989 The Guilford Press
A Division of Guilford Publications, Inc.
72 Spring Street, New York, NY 10012

Printed in the United States of America

Last digit is print number: 9 8 7 6 5 4 3 2 1

Library of Congress Cataloging-in-Publication Data

Autism: nature, diagnosis, and treatment / edited by Geraldine Dawson.
        p.   cm.
    Includes bibliographies and index.
    ISBN 0-89862-724-9
    1. Autism.   I. Dawson, Geraldine.
    [DNLM: 1. Autism.   2. Autism, Infantile.   3. Cognition.
    4. Language Development.   5. Psycholinguistics.   6. Social Behavior.
    WM 203.5 A9382]
    RC553.A88A87 1989
    616.89'82—dc 19
    DNLM/DLC
    for Library of Congress   88-16356
                                                                   CIP

To my parents
Frank Gates Dawson, Jr.
and
Beta Holmes Dale
who encouraged me to wonder and hope

Contributors

George M. Anderson, MD, Child Study Center and Children's Clinical Research Center, Yale University School of Medicine, New Haven, Connecticut

Magda Campbell, MD, Department of Psychiatry, New York University Medical Center, New York, New York

Eric Courchesne, PhD, Neuropsychology Research Laboratory, Children's Hospital Research Center, San Diego, California; Neurosciences Department, School of Medicine, University of California at San Diego, La Jolla, California

Geraldine Dawson, PhD, Psychology Department and Child Development and Mental Retardation Center, University of Washington, Seattle, Washington

Deborah Fein, PhD, Laboratory of Neuropsychology, Boston University School of Medicine, Boston, Massachusetts

R. Peter Hobson, MA, MB, BChir, MRCPsych, Department of Child and Adolescent Psychiatry, Institute of Psychiatry, London, England; MRC Developmental Psychology Project, London, England

Vanja A. Holm, MD, Child Development and Mental Retardation Center, University of Washington, Seattle, Washington

Jean Johnson, PhD, Speech and Hearing Center, University of California at Santa Barbara, Santa Barbara, California

Robert L. Koegel, PhD, Speech and Hearing Center, University of California at Santa Barbara, Santa Barbara, California

Arthur Lewy, MS, Psychology Department and Child Development and Mental Retardation Center, University of Washington, Seattle, Washington

Catherine Lord, PhD, Department of Pediatrics, University of Alberta/Glenrose Rehabilitation Hospital, Edmonton, Alberta, Canada

Joyce Magill, PhD, Department of Pediatrics, University of Alberta/Glenrose Rehabilitation Hospital, Edmonton, Alberta, Canada

Gary B. Mesibov, PhD, Division TEACCH, University of North Carolina at Chapel Hill, Chapel Hill, North Carolina

Robin S. Mitchell, MA, speech–language pathologist in private practice, St. Ives, New South Wales, Australia

Peter Mundy, PhD, Department of Psychiatry, Neuropsychiatric Institute, UCLA School of Medicine, Los Angeles, California

J. Gregory Olley, PhD, The Groden Center, Inc., Providence, Rhode Island

Edward M. Ornitz, MD, Department of Psychiatry and Brain Research Institute, UCLA School of Medicine, Los Angeles, California

Barry M. Prizant, PhD, Communication Disorders Department, Emma Pendleton Bradley Hospital, East Providence, Rhode Island; Division of Child and Adolescent Psychiatry, Brown University Program in Medicine, Providence, Rhode Island

Marian Sigman, PhD, Department of Psychiatry, Neuropsychiatric Institute, UCLA School of Medicine, Los Angeles, California

Elaine R. Silliman, PhD, Department of Communicology, University of South Florida, Tampa, Florida

Susan E. Stevenson, PhD, The Groden Center, Inc., Providence, Rhode Island

Helen Tager-Flusberg, PhD, Department of Psychology, University of Massachusetts at Boston, Boston, Massachusetts

Judy A. Ungerer, PhD, School of Behavioural Sciences, Macquarie University, Sydney, New South Wales, Australia

Mary E. Van Bourgondien, PhD, Division TEACCH, University of North Carolina at Chapel Hill, Chapel Hill, North Carolina

Christopher K. Varley, MD, Child Development and Mental Retardation Center, University of Washington, Seattle, Washington

Fred R. Volkmar, MD, Child Study Center and Children's Clinical Research Center, Yale University School of Medicine, New Haven, Connecticut

Lynn Waterhouse, PhD, Department of Linguistics, Trenton State College, Trenton, New Jersey

Amy M. Wetherby, PhD, Department of Communication Disorders, Florida State University, Tallahassee, Florida

Lorna Wing, MD, MRC Social Psychiatry Unit, Institute of Psychiatry, London, England

Foreword

This book, a new addition to the growing volume of autism research, stands as another important testimonial to the lasting significance of Leo Kanner's contribution. Almost half a century after Kanner first identified the complex set of characteristics known as the autism syndrome, this diagnostic category continues to generate productive research and improved methods of treatment. Like all exciting research at the frontier of knowledge, the autism classification has generated controversy over diagnostic criteria, measurements, boundaries, and uncertainties of etiology and treatment. Such disagreements and misunderstandings, reflected in some chapters of this volume, even surfaced at the 1988 meeting of the Autism Society of America, where a proposal was discussed (and dismissed) for removing autism from the next *Diagnostic and Statistical Manual of Mental Disorders* of the American Psychiatric Association. To the new student of autism, such controversy may give the erroneous impression that the definition of autism is lacking in reliability of diagnosis or in clinical validity. However, a more balanced perspective can be attained from a historical perspective, and in comparison with other classification categories for problems in the mental health field.

During the World War II era, when Kanner (1943) first discovered autism, many other diagnostic labels appeared at the same time, all referring to severely disturbed children. These included "atypical," "borderline psychotic," "symbiotic psychotic," and "schizophrenic," to name just a few of the better-known categories. Laufer and Gair (1969) cited over 20 such labels, all referring to similar children, but with no agreement among researchers as to how these different labels distinguished among children. Accordingly, these diagnostic categories have fallen into disuse. Autism, on the other hand, has not only remained but has been studied with empirical research methods and has contributed to our increasing, if incomplete, knowledge.

A similar relationship can be found between autism and the current labels published in the mental health taxonomy DSM-IIIR (revised third edition of the *Diagnostic and Statistical Manual of Mental Disorders*; American Psychiatric Association, 1987), far too many of which do not provide workable criteria for diagnoses. It is somewhat less taxing to see why autism permits such favorable comparison. The labels now obsolete had in common a primary basis in psychodynamic theory or hypothetical etiology; for example, symbiotic psychosis was predicated on a pathological closeness between mother and infant, while schizophrenia was thought to be the product of perplexity in parental communication. In other words, when labels are based on theories, be they psychodynamic or neurological, and are not confirmed by empirical reseach, such labels cannot adequately distinguish children and are likely to produce misleading directions for both study and treatment. Kanner's concept of infantile autism, on the other hand, was different in several respects. The children were described behaviorally, in clear and lucid prose. Case reports and their diagnostic criteria were, therefore, more easily translated into different languages and reported with consistency from one country to another. Moreover, Kanner's behavioral case description established a basis for employing empirical research on a scale not usually found in the area of mental health. I will briefly review how such research findings have produced specific modifications in the definition of autism and important improvements in treatment methods, permitting major changes in research directions—all under the rubric of autism.

During the past four decades, empirical research has demonstrated the following changes in the autism definition. In the past, Kanner and others believed that autism represented a single-cause disease process, most likely rooted in parental psychopathology (Bettelheim, 1967). Today it is widely accepted that autism is probably multiply determined. Moreover, it is also recognized that the child-rearing patterns of parents of autistic children are not significantly different from those of parents with "normal" children, with the exception that they have the additional stresses of raising a handicapped child (Cantwell & Baker, 1984).

Empirical findings have also clarified available demographic information. In the past, age of onset for autism was considered to be before 30 months. Subsequent studies have shown that onset can be later (Short & Schopler, 1988) and should be more accurately set at 36 months. This defining feature was dropped from DSM-IIIR.

In the past, mental retardation and autism were considered to be separate diagnostic categories. Autistic children were considered untestable with standard intelligence tests. Their unusual interests or peak skills, including musical and rote memory and number skills, were considered indicative of their normal or better intellectual potential. Today new instruments have shown that these children are testable (Mesibov, Schopler, Schaffer, & Landrus, 1988; Schopler & Reichler 1979). Moreover, it is widely recognized that autism and mental retardation can and do coexist.

The early definition of autism included the observation that autistic children had primarily well-to-do, highly educated parents. Later empirical studies showed that these observations were based on selection factors, and that such children exist in all racial and social groups. The factor of socioeconomic status was accordingly dropped from DSM-IIIR.

These new demographic data—higher age of onset, coexistence of mental retardation and autism, and lack of distinguishing family socioeconomic status—all had the effect of broadening the definition and increasing previous prevalence figures. Based on epidemiological studies, autism was first reported to occur in fewer than 5 of 10,000 children. More recently, prevalence rates were reported as higher than 15 in 10,000 (Wing, 1986).

This empirically based broadening of diagnostic criteria and the resulting overlap in the boundary areas have led some investigators to express concern about the validity of the syndrome. Unfortunately, such concern is often produced by the need of scientists for precision and specificity, rather than from rigorous concern for the problems under investigation as they arise in their natural environment. Problems of human development and adaptation are not so neat. They are usually the manifestation of complex factors, with a continuum in the frequency and intensity of the behaviors by which they are recognized.

Probably the most important effects of the empirical research tradition reflected in the autism syndrome are found in the areas of treatment and management. During the decades of the 1950s and 1960s, autism was considered to be an emotional disorder resulting from the child's withdrawal from pathological parenting. Treatment was either play therapy or removal from the family to residential treatment. Public school attendance was not an option usually available to such children. Today children with autism, like other handicapped children, are mandated by law to receive a public school education with individualized educational programs. Teachers and other professionals have access to methods of behavior management and appropriate educational structures. The children's learning can be fostered through special teaching curricula for social development and spontaneous communication (Watson, Schaffer, Lord, & Schopler, 1989).

If the empirical basis of the autism syndrome permitted important clarification in definition and treatment, it also produced some broader waves of research interest. These waves of interest have accelerated new knowledge by encouraging research across different disciplines and different centers and have also served an important heuristic function for the new student interested in autism research. They offer a reminder that progress in the behavioral sciences is not produced only by the specific hypothesis-driven research commitment required for many PhD dissertations and grant applications. The dilemma of the blind naturalists who, after their tactual examination of the elephant, defined it by either trunk, tail, or toe, can be avoided.

The movement between specific studies and broad waves of synthesis has occurred in several fundamental areas of research emphasis during the past several decades. First came a special interest in the autistic child's bizarre behavior. It obscured considerations of developmental delays and their biological correlates, and instead drew attention to parental pathology, widely assumed to cause disruption of the child's normal potential. The heterogeneity of the disturbing behaviors led clinicians to prefer the descriptor "childhood psychosis." This generic label readily accommodated the lack of distinction between explanatory theory and behavior represented by the many obsolete labels from the past. Likewise, distinction between autism and infantile psychosis was not clear. This confusing literature was first synthesized in Rimland's (1964) groundbreaking review. By evaluating the welter of published literature, using the rules of empirical evidence, he made a convincing case that the prevalent psychodynamic explanation for autism was misleading and without empirical support, and that causes were most likely to be found in biologically based deficits.

This formulation helped to inspire a new wave of autism research encompassing the areas of behavior, cognition, and language. Studies in this domain corrected Kanner's assertion that autistic children all had normal cognitive potential. These studies also showed that the majority of autistic children were mentally retarded as well. Their language problems involved delays not compensated for by gesture or mime; failure to respond to the communication of others; stereotyped repetition; pronoun reversal; and abnormalities of pitch, stress, rate, rhythm, and intonation. These studies were synthesized by Rutter (1978) and clearly documented the evidence for a cognitive deficit, as well as the large body of research supporting the classification of autism. At the same time, while it was recognized that many functions of cognition and social reciprocity overlapped with each other, the distinction between the two had not been formally studied.

The subsequent decade produced yet another wave of research interest in autism as an impairment of social interaction. Questions were raised as to how, and perhaps even whether, cognitive deficits give rise to abnormalities in social functions. Is it a problem in discriminating emotional cues? Is it an incapacity to take another person's point of view? Studies of these questions and related issues advanced the previously cited synthesis. They also provided the empirical underpinnings for the most recent update on the diagnosis and definition of autism (Rutter & Schopler, 1988). The material covered in Schopler and Mesibov's (1988) book reviews the most recent social-deficit focus, and also brings up to date the research basis for the autism diagnosis.

As more detailed information has become available on cognitive and social deficits in autism, and their relationship to each other, a new surge of interest is developing in the neurobiological correlates of these deficits. This current focus is very well represented by the chapters contributed to this volume. Through their interest in the neurobiological substrata, many of these authors help to bridge the interaction between cognitive and social deficits. By compiling these chapters, and also with her own research, Geraldine Dawson has provided valuable leadership to this exciting new direction. She has brought together a group that includes the new generation of investigators, some of whom bring new technologies and intriguing new research questions to the continuity of autism research. Here are just a few examples:

In what aspects of social interaction can the autistic child engage effectively? By what mechanisms does a deficiency in arousal modulation affect attention and emotional expression? If extensive Purkinje cell loss is demonstrated during early development, can early-onset cases be distinguished from late-onset cases through neuroanatomical examination? Can the autistic child's aversion to novel stimuli of normal intensity be localized to overactivation of right-hemisphere structures? Are autistic persons' attentional deficits related to stimulus characteristics such as social versus nonsocial, complexity, novelty, and predictability?

These and many other specific questions are raised by the studies reviewed in these chapters. They form the basis for new insights. They hold out the promise for new subgroups of autism with the hope for new treatment techniques not currently available. They foreshadow almost certainly a new synthesis of our knowledge.

Eric Schopler
Director, Division TEACCH
University of North Carolina at Chapel Hill

References

American Psychiatric Association. (1987). *Diagnostic and statistical manual of mental disorders* (3rd ed.—rev.). Washington, DC: Author.

Bettelheim, B. (1967). *The empty fortress: Infantile autism and the birth of the self.* New York: Free Press.

Cantwell, D. P., & Baker, L. (1984). Research concerning families of children with autism. In E. Schopler & G. B. Mesibov (Eds.), *The effects of autism on the family* (pp. 41–59). New York: Plenum.

Kanner, L. (1943). Autistic disturbance of affective contact. *Nervous Child, 2,* 217–250.

Laufer, M. W., & Gair, D. S. (1969). Childhood schizophrenia. In L. Bellak & L. Loeb (Eds.), *The schizophrenic syndrome.* New York: Grune & Stratton.

Mesibov, G. B., Schopler, E., Schaffer, B., & Landrus, R. (1988). *Individualized assessment and treatment for autistic and developmentally disabled children: Vol. 4. Adolescent and adult psychoeducational profile* (AAPEP). Austin, TX: Pro-Ed.

Rimland, B. (1964). *Infantile autism.* New York: Appleton-Century-Crofts.

Rutter, M. (1978). Diagnosis and definition of childhood autism. *Journal of Autism and Developmental Disorders. 8,* 139–161.

Rutter, M., & Schopler, E. (1988). *Autism and pervasive developmental disorders: Concepts and diagnostic issues.* In E. Schopler & G. B. Mesibov (Eds.), *Diagnosis and assessment in autism* (pp. 15–30). New York: Plenum.

Schopler, E., & Mesibov, G. B. (Eds.). (1988). *Diagnosis and assessment in autism.* New York: Plenum.

Schopler, E., & Reichler, R. J. (1979). *Individualized assessment and treatment for autistic and developmentally disabled children: Vol. 1. Psychoeducational profile.* Austin, TX: Pro-Ed.

Short, A., & Schopler, E. (1988). Factors relating to age of onset in autism. *Journal of Autism and Developmental Disorders.* 18(2), 207–216.

Watson, L., Schaffer, B., Lord, C., & Schopler, E. (1989). *Teaching spontaneous communication to autistic and developmentally handicapped children.* New York: Irvington.

Wing, L. (1986). *Children apart: Autistic children and their families.* Washington, DC: National Society for Autistic Children.

Preface

Someone saw Nasrudin searching for something on the ground.
"What are you looking for, Mulla?" he asked. "My key," said the Mulla.
So they both went down on their knees and looked for it.
After a time the other man asked: "Where exactly did you drop it?"
"In my own house."
"Then why are you looking here?"
"There is more light here than inside my own house."

            —Shah, 1972, p. 26

In science, Nasrudin's light, of course, is generated by current theories and technology. As scientists, we hope that as our theories expand and change focus, we cast a broader and more properly directed light on our subjects of study. In the field of autism, until recently, we have been very much like Nasrudin, casting a light in the wrong place, and concentrating it too narrowly. In the last decade, however, our theories have shifted their focus and, more importantly, have become broader, more comprehensive, and more integrative. These new theoretical perspectives have permitted more insight into the psychological nature of autism and have direct implications for its diagnosis and treatment. Another source of new light on autism has come from advances in technology, which have led to significant and previously impossible discoveries about the biological nature of autism. The purpose of this book is to share these exciting new perspectives and discoveries and reveal how they are shaping our understanding of the nature, diagnosis, and treatment of autism.

The book is divided into two sections. In Section I, models of the nature of autism are proposed from the perspectives of psychology and biology. In the first part of Section I, authors explore the complex interdependence of attentional, cognitive, linguistic, and socioemotional processing systems and how abnormalities of these systems bear upon the psychological world of the autistic person. In the second part of Section I, neurobiological perspectives on autism are offered and scrutinized. Authors reveal new research, based on the most sophisticated of available techniques for studying the brain, that can provide the necessary links between brain function and the primary features of autism—atypical language and social behavior. In Section II, clinical researchers introduce innovative methods for treating and diagnosing autism that are the outgrowth of much of the research presented in the first section of the book.

A recent development in the study of autism, and a principal theme of the book, is a renewed interest in a hypothesis that was advanced over 45 years ago by Leo Kanner, who was the first person to define autism as a clinical syndrome. In his classic 1943 paper describing 11 children with social difficulties and peculiar behavior, Kanner wrote: "these children have come into the world with innate inability to form the usual, biologically provided affective contact with people" (p. 250). After almost half a century of careful research, much of which was based on the assumption that autism primarily involved cognitive and linguistic impairments from which social difficulties arose, investigators now are interested in exploring Kanner's hypothesis from a scientific viewpoint. This interest was spurred by a critical insight recently grasped by several researchers—namely, that the core symptoms of autism (aberrations in social relationships, verbal and nonverbal communication, and symbolic thinking) have one important feature in common: These areas of functioning normally develop in the context of social interaction between a young infant and its caretaker. The logical extension of this insight is that a basic abnormality in autism may reside in the *social–affective* realm, rather than the strictly *cognitive* realm. Thus, the difficulty autistic individuals experience with the use of symbols (including language, gesture, and imaginary play), while having many cognitive ramifications throughout the lifespan, may be essentially social–affective in origin. Many developmental theorists have argued that the capacity to symbolize develops in a social context, from Piaget (1962), who believed that symbolic thought is derived from imitation of others, to Wolf and Gardner (1981), who posited that the ability to symbolize emerges from social play.

Given that a fundamental aspect of autism is a difficulty in forming social–affective relationships, we now may be able to direct our searchlight closer to the target by illuminating the nature of this basic difficulty, and considering how it would alter the cognitive, social, and linguistic development of individuals with autism.

These concerns are the focus of the first part of Section I of this book. In Chapter 1, by Peter Mundy and Marian Sigman, our commonly held notions about the essential nature of autism are questioned. These authors argue that the characterization of autistic persons as having a "pervasive lack of social responsiveness to others," a characterization found in most diagnostic manuals, is inaccurate. They propose, instead, that the social impairments of autistic persons are circumscribed, rather than pervasive, and support this claim with evidence from their own careful, seminal research on the social behavior of young autistic children.

In a highly integrative, groundbreaking piece of work, R. Peter Hobson provides us in Chapter 2 with a scholarly account of how Kanner's original formulation of autism, emphasizing disturbances of affective development, is both necessary and pivotal for our understanding of the syndrome. He unfolds a "theory of autism" in which he attempts to account for the unusual social and affective behavior of autistic individuals, as well as for their linguistic and cognitive characteristics.

In Chapter 3, Arthur Lewy and I examine the role of attention in explaining the socioemotional abnormalities of autistic individuals. In our model, neither affective nor perceptual–cognitive abnormalities are viewed as primary in autism; instead, we argue that the autistic individual's difficulty in arousal modulation directly influences the capacities to attend to and comprehend both social and nonsocial information, and, ultimately, to function adaptively in both of these spheres. We illustrate how therapies for autistic children can be designed that are sensitive to difficulties in arousal modulation and can positively influence the way in which these children respond to people.

In Chapter 4, Judy A. Ungerer grapples with a difficult, and important, conceptual issue in autism research: the distinction between primary, fundamental abnormalities and their secondary consequences. Making this distinction not only is helpful in uncovering the biological bases of autism, but also has considerable implications for treatment. Although it is possible that we may never "cure" autism in the sense of eliminating the primary cause of the disorder, a realistic and worthy goal of applied autism research is to devise therapies that ameliorate the secondary negative consequences of the primary abnormalities.

In the final chapter of this part of Section I, Helen Tager-Flusberg ponders the complex relationship between social and linguistic development in autistic children. She contends that, since human language is inseparable from social interaction, a wholistic view encompassing both of these domains is necessary to understand autism; she further proposes that a basic abnormality in autism exists at the intersection of language and socioemotional functioning.

What is apparent from the work presented in these chapters on the nature of autism is that we have moved away from explanations that posit a single abnormality, be it perceptual, cognitive, linguistic, or social, to explain autism. Our theories have become more encompassing and integrative, and take into account the complex interplay of different realms of functioning during an individual's development. I believe that, under this broader light, we are now in a better position to comprehend autism.

In the second part of Section I, the question of the nature of autism is addressed from a biological perspective. We are in an exciting, formative period of research on the neurobiology of autism, and, as these chapters demonstrate, advances in technology truly have begun to shed light on the syndrome. New research on the biological bases of normal social and emotional development is stimulating original thinking about the biology of autism. Indeed, today we take for granted that autism is a neurologically based syndrome, a notion that rests on solid empirical evidence rather than conjecture. Yet, only three decades ago, most researchers and clinicians assumed a psychogenic basis for autism. In this sense, we have come a great distance in our understanding, and, in large part, we have technology (combined with the investigative spirit of science) to thank for this progress.

Although it now is known that autism is caused by various factors and shows considerable variability in its biological and behavioral expression, the possibility that autistic individuals share certain unusual neurobiological characteristics continues to intrigue researchers. An obvious shift in our thinking is that we no longer are attempting to interpret autism in terms of an abnormality of one particular area of the brain. Most investigators now concur that autism involves both subcortical and cortical abnormalities and can be better interpreted from a dynamic brain-systems framework that considers the complicated interactions among many brain areas.

The chapters on biology begin with one by Eric Courchesne, who reports his recent discovery of specific cerebellar abnormalities in autistic individuals, a finding that may well prove to be among this decade's most important breakthroughs in our beginning grasp of the biology of autism. Courchesne considers the possible effects of abnormal cerebellar development on brain functioning and how these effects could be related to autistic symptoms.

In the next chapter, Arthur Lewy and I explore the reciprocal influences of subcortical and cortical abnormalities in autism and how they contribute to the cognitive and affective behavior of autistic individuals. Based on an integration of research on brain functioning in autism, including studies of autonomic responsivity and electrical brain recordings, we propose that autism involves an abnormality of the cortical–limbic–reticular system that mediates attention. We suggest ways in which an abnormally functioning attentional system could account for the unusual behavior of autistic persons.

Edward M. Ornitz, in Chapter 8, also argues for a central role of subcortical dysfunction in autism, an argument that rests on decades of his own careful research into subcortical functioning in autistic persons. He assumes that distorted sensory input at the subcortical level, when transmitted to higher centers, becomes distorted information, this being the basis of the deviant language and social communication. Ornitz describes a sophisticated neurological model of autism in which deviant attention to the environment is a central explanatory concept.

Next, Fred R. Volkmar and George M. Anderson peruse the existing studies on biochemical imbalances in autism and recommend future directions for research. Although no single neurochemical factor has yet been found that explains autism, reports of increased peripheral levels of serotonin, atypical levels of endogenous opioids, and various other fascinating, but unexplicated, biochemical imbalances in autistic individuals impel researchers in this area.

The second part of Section I concludes with a chapter on genetic influences in autism by Elaine R. Silliman, Magda Campbell, and Robin S. Mitchell. In addition to providing an up-to-date critical review of the research on genetic influences in autism, these authors introduce an innovative hypothesis regarding the possible connections among kinship, modes of language processing, and genetic influences.

In Section II, we turn our attention to the clinical issues of diagnosis and treatment. Lynn Waterhouse, Lorna Wing, and Deborah Fein have written a stimulating chapter in which they view autism as part of a spectrum of disorders involving abnormalities of social and language functioning. The implications of this interesting, but nevertheless controversial, point of view for defining and studying autism and related syndromes are discussed.

Two chapters on methods of facilitating language acquisition in autistic children are provided next. In both chapters, it is clear that language therapies for autistic children have changed dramatically in the last several years. Most importantly, it is now clear that language does not emerge as an isolated skill, but, rather, in the context of social interaction. This appreciation of the supportive role of social interaction in language development has significantly influenced our approaches to language therapy. Chapter 12, by Barry M. Prizant and Amy M. Wetherby, begins with a thoughtful examination of theories of normal language development and their roles in shaping our understanding of social-communicative behavior in autism. The authors describe how a socially based theory of language development can be used creatively to design language therapies for autistic children. In Chapter 13, Robert L. Koegel and Jean Johnson recognize the problem of motivation in autistic children. They point out that autistic children are sensitive to their failures to communicate, which can lead to frustration and apathy. While maintaining an objective behavioral methodology in their work, these authors embed their methods in naturalistic environments and ingeniously integrate them with motivational teaching techniques that are designed to promote feelings of efficacy, enjoyment, and spontaneous language use in autistic children.

We have only just begun to address the question of how to directly promote social development of autistic children. Since the prevailing view of the last few decades was that social abnormalities arose from difficulties in cognitive and linguistic processing, it made sense that the latter, rather than the former, sphere should be the target of intervention. Recently, however, researchers and clinicians have started to conceive of novel ways of directly promoting social development. So far, one of the most successful means of accomplishing this has been to use normally developing peers as therapists for children with autism. In Chapter 14, Catherine Lord and Joyce Magill carefully consider some of the methodological, theoretical, and practical issues that have arisen from studies of autistic children's interactions with peers. Because of its wide scope, this chapter will be valuable to both the researcher who studies peer interaction and the clinician who wishes to use peers as therapists.

In the next chapter, J. Gregory Olley and Susan E. Stevenson relate several new approaches to teaching social skills to very young autistic children. Now that public schools are legally mandated to provide early education for handicapped children, we are likely to see increasing numbers of preschool programs for young children with autism. Olley and Stevenson guide us through the practical and philosophical issues involved in designing early social skills programs for autistic children and highlight the educational components that hold most promise.

The other end of the age continuum, adolescence and adulthood in autism, is the topic of the chapter by Mary E. Van Bourgondien and Gary B. Mesibov. These authors are known for their pioneering efforts in diagnosing autism in later life, and in creating ways of helping older autistic people adaptively function in environments outside their parents' homes and institutions. In Chapter 16, they offer a useful, standardized method for diagnosing and assessing adolescent and adult persons with autism that can assist professionals in making informed and sensitive vocational and educational decisions.

Section II ends with a chapter by Vanja A. Holm and Christopher K. Varley, who provide a comprehensive review of our present knowledge of the usefulness of medications with autistic individuals. They include a balanced, state-of-the-art evaluation of fenfluramine, the drug treatment that has received the most attention in the last several years.

This preface began with a Sufi story about Nasrudin, who was looking for his key in a misdirected light. Unlike Nasrudin, we are not likely to find a single key to unlock the mysteries of a syndrome such as autism, in which profound difficulties in forming human relationships are caused by biological abnormalities. The complexities of human development do not lend themselves to a single solution. It is much more likely that we will discover and create a series of "keys" leading to diverse insights that must be related to one another. It is hoped that these insights will enhance our ability to assist, and form relationships with, these very special people who are autistic, and that, by this process, we will learn truths about ourselves.

Several people were instrumental in the writing and editing of this book and deserve acknowledgment. Sidney Segalowitz, Consulting Editor, and Seymour Weingarten, Editor-in-Chief of The Guilford Press, provided the initial encouragement to begin the book and valuable guidance throughout the process of its creation. Judith Grauman, Editorial Supervisor of The Guilford Press, expertly orchestrated the final editing and publishing phases of the book. Arthur Lewy and several other graduate students, Larry Galpert, Laura Grofer, Deborah Hill, and Heracles Panagiotides, critiqued many of the chapters and participated in numerous stimulating discussions of many of the ideas presented in the book. As always, I am grateful for the loving support, good humor, and patience of my husband, Joseph, and son, Christopher. Finally, I wish to acknowledge the many autistic persons and their families with whom I have worked, whose struggles and accomplishments are a source of inspiration for my life's work.

Geraldine Dawson

References

Kanner, L. (1943). Autistic disturbances of affective contact. *Nervous Child, 2*, 217–250.
Piaget, J. (1962). *Play, dreams, and imitation*. New York: Norton.
Shah, I. (Ed.). (1972). *The exploits of the incomparable Mulla Nasrudin*. New York: Dutton.
Wolf, D., & Gardner, H. (1981). On the structure of early symbolization. In R. Schiefelbusch & D. Bricker (Eds.), *Early language: Acquisition and intervention* (pp. 287–327). Baltimore: University Park Press.

Contents

I. PERSPECTIVES ON THE NATURE OF AUTISM

Social, Cognitive, and Language Development of Individuals with Autism

1. Specifying the Nature of the Social Impairment in Autism 3
   Peter Mundy and Marian Sigman
   Introduction: The Nature of Autism, 3
   Diagnostic Criteria and Social Responsiveness, 5
   Social Responsiveness and the Young Autistic Child, 6
   Defining the Social Deficits of Autistic Children, 9
   Summary, 17
   Acknowledgments, 18
   References, 18

2. Beyond Cognition: A Theory of Autism 22
   R. Peter Hobson
   Introduction, 22
   Foundations for Social and Cognitive Development, 24
   The Case of Autism, 32
   Conclusion: A Theory of Autism, 42
   Acknowledgments, 43
   References, 43

3. Arousal, Attention, and the Socioemotional Impairments of
   Individuals with Autism 49
   Geraldine Dawson and Arthur Lewy
   Attention in Normal Infants, 50
   Physiological Correlates of Attentional Deficits in Autism, 53
   Failure to Adequately Process Social Stimuli: A Function of
       Stimulus Predictability?, 56
   Socioemotional Development, 57
   Implications for Therapeutic Intervention with Autistic Children, 62
   Conclusion, 69
   Acknowledgments, 70
   References, 70

4. The Early Development of Autistic Children: Implications for
   Defining Primary Deficits   75
   Judy A. Ungerer
   Introduction, 75
   Approaches to Identifying Primary Deficits, 76
   Review of Research, 78
   Implications, 85
   References, 88

5. A Psycholinguistic Perspective on Language Development in the
   Autistic Child   92
   Helen Tager-Flusberg
   Introduction, 92
   The Nature of Language, 93
   The Foundations of Language, 95
   The Development of Phonology, 96
   Acquiring Words and Meanings, 98
   Grammatical Development, 101
   Acquiring Communicative Competence, 104
   The Language Deficit in Autism, 106
   The Developmental Process, 107
   The Relationship between Deficits in Language and Social-Emotional
       Development in Autism, 108
   Acknowledgments, 109
   References, 109

Neurobiological Issues in Autism: Research and Theory

6. Neuroanatomical Systems Involved in Infantile Autism:
   The Implications of Cerebellar Abnormalities   119
   Eric Courchesne
   Normal Cerebellar Anatomy, 120
   Normal Cerebellar Development, 121
   Evidence of Abnormal Cerebellar Development in Infantile Autism, 123
   Implications, 132
   Concluding Remarks, 140
   Acknowledgments, 140
   References, 141

7. Reciprocal Subcortical–Cortical Influences in Autism: The Role of
   Attentional Mechanisms   144
   Geraldine Dawson and Arthur Lewy
   Cortical Functioning in Autism: Research Findings, 145
   Subcortical Functioning in Autism: Research Findings, 158

Summary of Evidence on Brain Functioning in Autism, 161
Reciprocal Subcortical–Cortical Influences in Autism, 161
General Summary and Conclusion, 167
Acknowledgments, 168
References, 169

8. Autism at the Interface between Sensory and
   Information Processing   174
   Edward M. Ornitz
   The Autistic Behavioral Syndrome, 176
   Neurophysiological Investigation, 178
   Brain Stem Dysfunction Model of Autism, 183
   Neurophysiology of Neglect, 184
   Neurophysiology of Directed Attention, 186
   Deviant and Deficient Directed Attention in Autism, 188
   Neurophysiological Model for Dysfunction at the Interface between Sensory
        and Information Processing in Autism, 190
   Conclusions, 198
   Acknowledgments, 199
   References, 199

9. Neurochemical Perspectives on Infantile Autism   208
   Fred R. Volkmar and George M. Anderson
   Serotonin, 210
   Dopamine, 214
   Norepinephrine, 215
   Peptides, 217
   Other Compounds, 218
   Summary, 219
   Acknowledgments, 220
   References, 220

10. Genetic Influences in Autism and Assessment of Metalinguistic
    Performance in Siblings of Autistic Children   225
    Elaine R. Silliman, Magda Campbell, and Robin S. Mitchell
    Introduction: Genetic Issues in Autism, 226
    Overview of the Pertinent Literature: Twin and Sibling Studies, 228
    Metalinguistic Development and Its Assessment, 235
    Metalinguistic Awareness in Siblings of Autistic Children: Some
         Preliminary Evidence, 240
    Concluding Remarks, 250
    Acknowledgments, 252
    References, 252

II. NEW DIRECTIONS IN THE DIAGNOSIS AND TREATMENT OF INDIVIDUALS WITH AUTISM

11. Re-Evaluating the Syndrome of Autism in the Light of
Empirical Research   263
Lynn Waterhouse, Lorna Wing, and Deborah Fein
Introduction, 263
Problem 1: Fuzzy Boundaries, 265
Problem 2: Heterogeneity within Autistic Populations, 271
Problem 3: Brain–Behavior Links, 272
Problem 4: Finding Subgroups, 274
Problem 5: Social Impairment Features, 276
Problem 6: The Uniqueness of Each Case, 277
References, 278

12. Enhancing Language and Communication in Autism:
From Theory to Practice   282
Barry M. Prizant and Amy M. Wetherby
Introduction, 282
Types of Theories, 283
Implications for Communication Assessment and Enhancement, 292
Conclusions and Future Directions, 304
References, 304

13. Motivating Language Use in Autistic Children   310
Robert L. Koegel and Jean Johnson
Introduction, 310
The Importance of Motivation, 311
The Natural Language-Teaching Paradigm, 311
Effectiveness of the Paradigm, 319
Summary, 321
Acknowledgments, 321
References, 322

14. Methodological and Theoretical Issues in Studying Peer-Directed
Behavior and Autism   326
Catherine Lord and Joyce Magill
Issues in Studying Low-Frequency Behaviors, 327
The Concept of Intention, 333
Conclusions, 342
References, 343

15. Preschool Curriculum for Children with Autism:
    Addressing Early Social Skills   346
    J. Gregory Olley and Susan E. Stevenson
        What Is Meant by "Social Skills"?, 346
        What Is Meant by "Curriculum"?, 347
        Considerations in Developing a Social Skills Curriculum, 347
        Social Skills Curriculum Targets, 350
        Generalization, 356
        Curricula for Social Skills, 359
        Conclusion, 362
        References, 363

16. Diagnosis and Treatment of Adolescents and Adults with Autism   367
    Mary E. Van Bourgondien and Gary B. Mesibov
        Diagnosis, 367
        Assessment, 370
        Treatment Areas, 373
        Treatment Strategies, 376
        Treatment Issues, 377
        Summary and Conclusion, 382
        References, 383

17. Pharmacological Treatment of Autistic Children   386
    Vanja A. Holm and Christopher K. Varley
        Introduction, 386
        General Comments, 387
        Sedatives, 387
        Stimulants, 387
        Neuroleptics, 388
        Tricyclic Antidepressants, 389
        Fenfluramine, 389
        Opiate Antagonists, 395
        Vitamins and Diet, 396
        Anticonvulsants, 399
        Summary, 400
        References, 401

Index   405

Autism

SECTION I

Perspectives on the Nature of Autism

Social, Cognitive, and Language Development of Individuals with Autism

Specifying the Nature of the Social Impairment in Autism

PETER MUNDY

MARIAN SIGMAN

UCLA School of Medicine

INTRODUCTION: THE NATURE OF AUTISM

It does not take a great deal of experience with autistic children to be struck by the fundamental gaps in their social behavior. This complex disturbance in social behavior often makes the rearing and educating of these children very difficult. Yet the same disturbance in social behavior compels many researchers to attempt to delineate the nature of the disorder that afflicts these children. Scientific curiosity, it seems, is piqued by the notion that to understand what is deviant in the social phenotype of autistic children is to understand an important component of human nature (cf. Wing, 1976).

Kanner's Clinical Insight

Kanner (1943/1985) recognized the centrality of social deficits in his initial description of the syndrome of infantile autism. He suggested that the outstanding feature of autism is a disturbance of social development, characterized as "an inability [of autistic children] to relate themselves in the ordinary way to people and situations from the beginning of life" (p. 31). Kanner also suggested that autism is an endogenous form of psychopathology, brought about by a deficiency in the biological systems that regulate the ability of children to develop affective contact with others. Thus, Kanner initially believed that autistic children suffer from a biologically based disorder of affective systems that results in a profoundly disturbed pattern of social development.

Shifts in Theoretical Focus

At times in the past 40 years, theory and research on autism has shifted from both the biological and social-affective foci of Kanner's original clinical insight. Soon

after autism was accepted as a valid syndrome, theorists moved away from thinking of autism as an endogenous disorder. Several clinical theorists (e.g., Bettelheim, 1959) considered autism to be a negative emotional response to an inadequate caregiving environment. However, research results have failed to support
this environmental or psychogenic view of the etiology of autism (McAdoo &
DeMyer, 1978; Rimland, 1964; see also Donnellan, 1985).

In a second shift, the cognitive, perceptual, and linguistic disorders associated
with autism became the focus of theory and research (Hermelin & O'Connor,
1970; Ornitz & Ritvo, 1968; Rutter, 1968, 1978; Sigman & Ungerer, 1984b).
This shift may have occurred because research paradigms in cognitive and perceptual psychology and psycholinguistics were readily available (Hermelin, 1982). At
the same time, the idea re-emerged that the core disorders of autism are the result
of neurobiological deficits (Cohen, Caparulo, & Shaywitz, 1978/1985; Damasio
& Maurer, 1978). However, the social behavior of autistic children received relatively little attention during this period (Howlin, 1978). In part, the lack of emphasis on the social behavior of autistic children reflected the hypothesis that the
disorders of social communication in autism derive from a more basic disorder of
cognitive processes (e.g., Ricks & Wing, 1975; Rutter, 1978).

As is indicated in recent reviews and theoretical papers, research on the cognitive components of autistic behavioral disturbance remains a vital and useful
enterprise (Fein, Humes, Kaplan, Lucci, & Waterhouse, 1984; Prior, 1984). Currently, however, a shift in the literature is again discernible. In this, the social
and affective features of autism have become a focus for research and theory. This
shift is evident in recent reviews of the literature suggesting that the cognitive
deficits of autistic children are most pronounced in situations that demand the
processing of social and emotional cues (Rutter, 1983; Sigman, Ungerer, Mundy,
& Sherman, 1987). Researchers and clinicians are also attempting to define and
operationalize the social deficits of autism more precisely (Hobson, Chapter 2,
this volume; Mundy, Sigman, Ungerer, & Sherman, 1986; Volkmar, Cohen, &
Paul, 1986). Furthermore, research suggests that autism may be the result of a
disorder that primarily disrupts neurobiological processes specific to social and
emotional development (Deutsch, 1986; Panksepp, Siving, & Normansell, 1985).

Perhaps most indicative of the increasing interest in the social and affective
behavior of autism, though, is the growth in the size of the relevant literature. A
comparison of two reviews of social behavior in autistic children (Howlin, 1978,
1986) illustrates this growth. In 1978, Howlin required 7 pages and 39 citations
to do justice to this literature. By 1986, Howlin's coverage of the literature required 24 pages and 116 citations.

In some sense, then, the field has come full circle. The literature on autism
is expanding to include more research on the domains of behavior that Kanner
first suggested as central to the syndrome. This chapter presents a discussion of
research on the social behaviors of autistic children. However, so as not to dupli-
cate efforts, our goals are more circumscribed than those of recent reviews of
autistic social behavior (Dawson & Galpert, 1986; Hermelin, 1982; Howlin, 1986;

Olley, 1985). First, selected studies on the social capacities and interests of autistic children are reviewed. This section reflects our belief that in order to delineate the differences between the social behaviors of autistic children and normal children, the similarities in social behavior patterns must also be recognized. In the next section, we revert to the more traditional form and discuss areas of deficit in the social repertoire of autistic children. The studies to be reviewed focus on nonverbal communication, parent–child interaction, and affective expression in young autistic children. In the final major section, we discuss models of development that may help to explicate the nature of the social deficits of autistic children.

DIAGNOSTIC CRITERIA AND SOCIAL RESPONSIVENESS

The scarcity of empirical data on the social behavior of autistic children has impeded the development of accurate diagnostic descriptions of the social features of this syndrome. Current diagnostic systems do not go very far beyond broad qualitative descriptions. The diagnostic criteria of the *Diagnostic and Statistical Manual of Mental Disorders,* third edition (DSM-III; American Psychiatric Association, 1980) provide an example. The social deficit in autism is described as a "pervasive lack of responsiveness to other people" (p. 89). However, at least two well-documented findings make such a broad descriptive statement problematic.

Developmental Change in Social Behavior

First, the social deficits of autistic children do not appear to be of the same magnitude across development. The degree of social impairment appears most severe in the preschool years (ages 0–5), but often autistic children make some gains in social responsiveness in later years (Kanner, 1943/1985; Rutter, 1978).[1] Lord (1984), borrowing nomenclature from Wing and Gould (1979), has suggested that a transition from "aloof" to "passive but responsive" to "active but odd" social initiation frequently describes the social development of autistic children. Others have also shown that the social behaviors of autistic children differ across chronological age (CA) and/or developmental level (Goldfarb, 1974; Tonick, 1981; Wing, 1978).

Social Responsiveness in Structured Interactions

A second line of research indicates that autistic children are clearly responsive to others in situations where adults or peers actively engage them in social interac-

1. In part, it was the observation that the social deficits of autism change with development that led Rutter (1968) to consider cognitive rather than social deficits as the primary handicap of autism. However, although autistic social deficits change with age, they remain a significant handicap at all ages (Howlin, 1986).

tion (Clark & Rutter, 1981; Lord, 1984; McHale, 1983; Strain, Kerr, & Ragland, 1979). For example, Strain *et al.* (1979) reported that the positive social behaviors of four autistic children increased in response to peer-mediated social initiations. These positive social behaviors included cooperative responses such as sharing a toy, physical acts such as hugging or holding hands, and vocalizations to the peer that would tend to begin or maintain interactions. Similarly, McHale (1983) reported that autistic children exhibited less solitary and more cooperative play in response to the introduction of nonhandicapped peers[2] to a classroom over a 3-month period of observation. These studies are important because they demonstrate that autistic children are responsive to social stimulation. Moreover, these observations refute the hypothesis (Richer, 1976) that autistic children consistently avoid social interaction (see van Engeland, Bodnar, & Bolhuis, 1985, for additional data relevant to this issue).

Social Learning

Other, albeit more controversial, signs of social responsiveness are evident as well. At least two studies have demonstrated that social learning techniques constitute a viable educational method with autistic children (Charlop, Schreibman, & Tryon, 1983; Egel, Richman, & Koegel, 1981). Charlop *et al.* (1983) have reported that a small sample of low-functioning autistic children were taught receptive language skills by means of a peer modeling procedure. Aside from the potential intervention implications, these results are significant because they suggest that autistic children may be sufficiently observant of other people to learn from them.

SOCIAL RESPONSIVENESS AND THE YOUNG AUTISTIC CHILD

The data provided by the studies cited above indicate that broad statements about a "pervasive" lack of social responsiveness of autistic children do not adequately reflect the developmental and context-specific variation in social behavior exhibited by these children. However, these data were obtained predominantly from observations of school-age autistic children (i.e., older than 5 years of age). If the social deficits of autistic children are most pronounced early on, perhaps it is the very young autistic children who display little or no evidence of social relatedness. The data from several recent studies are pertinent with regard to this issue.

2. The issue of autistic children's response to peers is an important one for future research. It has been suggested that, although autistic social behavior improves with age in adult–child interactions, peer interactions remain the stage for the most evident social deficits of the autistic child (American Psychiatric Association, 1980; Howlin, 1986; Lord, 1984). However, in view of research suggesting that mental retardation is associated with deficits in peer-related social competence (Guralnick & Groom, 1985), it will be important for research to distinguish which elements of disturbed peer relatedness are specific to autism as opposed to a general manifestation of mental retardation.

Attachment

One method of examining the social responsiveness of young children is to employ an attachment paradigm. The concept of attachment in young children has been articulated by Bowlby and others (e.g., Bowlby, 1982; Bretherton & Waters, 1985). Evidence that young children have formed an attachment to a specific caregiver may be based on two kinds of observations. First, children may direct more social behavior to their caregivers than to other people. Second, children may demonstrate a distinct reaction to separations from and reunions with their caregiver (Ainsworth, Blehar, Waters, & Wall, 1978). In a study of 14 children aged 4 to 6, Sigman and Ungerer (1984a) reported that the autistic children exhibited significantly more proximity seeking to their caregivers than to a stranger, both in a free-play situation and after reunion with their caregivers following a 2-minute separation. During the caregiver situation, each child was alone with a stranger in a laboratory play room.

We felt that this finding was important enough to warrant replication. In a second study (Sigman, Mundy, Ungerer, & Sherman, 1987), 18 primarily nonverbal autistic children aged 4 to 6 were compared to samples of normal and mentally retarded children matched for mental age (MA) in an attachment paradigm. The results indicated that the autistic children, like the other groups, directed social behaviors (e.g., touches, looks, vocalizations, etc.) for significantly longer periods to caregivers than to strangers after a period of caregiver–child separation. Similarly, others have shown that the attachment behaviors of young autistic children, as defined in terms of response to caregiver separation, do not differ from those of children with pervasive developmental disorder or mental retardation (Shapiro, Sherman, Calamari, & Koch, 1985). These data replicate our previous finding that young autistic children exhibit patterns of behavior indicative of child–caregiver attachment. This is not to say that the quality of young autistic children's attachment to their caregivers is not disturbed. For example, clinical observation suggests that autistic children may not use positive affect in the expression of attachment as frequently as other children. However, these data do indicate that child–caregiver attachment is not completely absent among young autistic children.

Imitation of Autistic Children

Data from other researchers also indicate that social behaviors are observed even in the young autistic child. Two studies have demonstrated that young autistic children's awareness of others and social behaviors increase with a specific type of social stimulation. Tiegerman and Primavera (1984) report that imitation of autistic children's actions with objects led to an increase in these children's tendency to visually monitor the action of an adult. Data from Dawson and Adams (1984) go a step further. This study reports that imitation of autistic children led to an increase in social behaviors (e.g., eye contact, gesturing, touching, etc.) among the most socially aloof children. Like the findings for older children (e.g., Clark & Rutter, 1981), these findings illustrate the modifiable or context-specific variability of social behavior in young autistic children. To the extent that imitation presented the autistic children with a predictable pattern of adult behavior, these research results also support the suggestion that predictability may facilitate the behavioral competence of autistic children (Ferrara & Hill, 1980).

Mental Age and Social Responsiveness

Other important data on the social behaviors of young autistic children have been provided by Tonick (1981), who carried out a careful study of the social behaviors of high- and low-MA young autistic children. She reported that even the low-functioning autistic children displayed social initiations and responses to adults. These included eye contact, physical approaches, and nonverbal communicative gestures. Moreover, the high-functioning autistic children displayed higher frequencies of these behaviors, and both high- and low-functioning groups displayed an increase in social behavior when adults actively solicited social interaction.

Retrospective Data

On the basis of their recent data, Volkmar *et al.* (1986) have also questioned the validity of the DSM-III diagnostic criteria for the social deficits of autistic children. In a retrospective study, the parents of 50 autistic individuals were asked to rate the behavior of their children as they appeared before the age of 6. In approximately 40% of the cases, parents reported that their children, even when young, exhibited a variety of social behaviors, including cuddling, acceptance of affection, a responsive smile to mother, and an awareness of mother's absence. Thus, according to this study, even young autistic children exhibit some types of social behaviors.

Of course, for the most part, these studies only provide data on frequency counts of individual social acts. Autistic children may display observable frequencies of some types of social behavior, yet they may also display significant and observable disturbances in social competence. Nevertheless, broad descriptive statements suggesting that autistic children display little if any social responsiveness appear to be imprecise. This imprecision is widely recognized by clinicians, and undoubtedly played a role in current efforts to provide a more precise description of autistic social impairments (American Psychiatric Association, 1987). The success of these continuing efforts will hinge on the availability of new data on the specific types of social deficits autistic children display at different stages of development. In the next section, we discuss the contribution of studies on affective expression and nonverbal communication to defining the social deficits of young autistic children.

DEFINING THE SOCIAL DEFICITS OF AUTISTIC CHILDREN

If the diagnostic criteria for autistic social deficits are imprecise, how is it that diagnosticians seem able to discriminate autistic children from other children with developmental disorders? Perhaps clinicians rely on a "gut" feeling or general impression of how easy it is to relate to a child (Tonick, 1981). If so, what types of behaviors do clinicians interpret? Since many autistic children are nonverbal at the time of their initial diagnosis, clinicians must often interpret the nonverbal social behavior of these children. Two essential aspects of nonverbal social behavior in young children include the expression of affect and nonverbal communication. Not surprisingly, research on affective expression and nonverbal communication skills suggest that disturbances in these areas may be prominent features of the social deficits of nonverbal autistic children.

Studies of Affective Expression

Affect or emotion may be displayed by means of vocalization, facial expression, posture, and gesture. Ricks (1979) has examined the vocal expressiveness of non-verbal 3- to 5-year-old autistic children. In this study, autistic children and two comparison samples (nonverbal mentally retarded children and 8-month-old normal children) were presented with stimulus conditions designed to elicit four affective states: surprise, pleasure, frustration, and need/request. Recordings were made of the children's vocalizations in each situation. The results indicated that all the parents could reliably match the vocalizations of the normal and mentally retarded children with the correct affective state. However, parents of the normal and mentally retarded children could not identify their own children. Thus, the vocalizations of normal and mentally retarded children were specific to the eliciting situation and very similar across children. In the case of the autistic children, parents could identify their own child's vocalizations and correctly match them with the eliciting situations. However, these parents could not interpret the vocalizations of other autistic children. Contrary to the normal and mentally retarded children, the vocalizations of autistic children were expressive but idiosyncratic. That is, they carried meaning for their parents, but not for other adults.

A parallel finding with regard to facial expressions of 3- to 6-year-old autistic children has been presented by our own research group (Kasari, Yirmiya, Sigman, & Mundy, 1986). In this study, the facial expressions of eight autistic children were recorded during social interactions with an experimenter. Facial expression data on MA- and CA-matched mentally retarded children and MA-matched normal children were also obtained. The facial affect rating system developed by

Izard (1979) was used to identify 10 expressions: interest, enjoyment, surprise, sadness, anger, disgust, contempt, fear, shame, and discomfort/pain. In addition, combinations or blends of two or more of these expressions were also coded. The results indicated that autistic children displayed significantly more blends of facial expression. These blends included quite disparate affects, such as anger and enjoyment. Of course, we recognize the need to demonstrate this finding with larger samples of children. Nevertheless these data suggest that the clarity of the facial expression of young autistic children may be compromised by the presence of blends.

Similarly, Langdell (1981; cited in Hermelin, 1982) has reported a study in which autistic children were stimulated to display a "happy" or a "sad" face. The results indicated that raters of pictures of autistic facial expressions often found it difficult to determine whether a particular autistic expression was meant to convey a happy or a sad expression. Rater uncertainty was much less in evidence when judging the faces of control children.[3]

Evidence of a disturbance in the expression of affect among autistic children has been presented in several other studies. Attwood (1984; cited in Frith, 1984) compared a sample of autistic children (10 to 19 years old) to samples of Down syndrome children (10 to 19 years old) and normal children (3 to 6 years old). During peer interactions, the number of deictic gestures (attention directing), instrumental gestures (goal requesting), and expressive gestures (social-affective—e.g., embarrassment, consolation, etc.) displayed by each child was recorded. The results indicated that while the normal and Down syndrome children used all three types of gestures, the autistic children displayed deictic and instrumental gestures but did not show expressive gestures. Frith (1984) suggests that this expressive gestural deficit is the result of a limitation among autistic children in the capacity to recognize mental states in themselves and others.

Snow, Hertzig, and Shapiro (1986) have reported that 2- to 4-year-old autistic children displayed less positive affect in social interaction with adults than did an MA- and CA-matched sample of developmentally delayed children. Moreover, Snow *et al.* reported that when autistic children did display positive affect, they were less likely to display it to their social partners. This group effect on the focus of affective displays suggests that autistic and developmentally delayed children may differ in the communicative use of facial expressions.

Affect and Self-Recognition

Research on self-recognition in autistic children also provides data on the facial expression of affect. It has been suggested that an undifferentiated sense of self or an inability to distinguish between self and nonself is a cardinal feature of autism

---

3. Since the procedures here involved verbal instructions or imitation, it is not clear whether these results reflect a disturbance in the clarity of affective expression or an inability of the autistic children to comply with the task demands.

(Anthony, 1967; Creak, 1961; Ornitz & Ritvo, 1968). Contrary to this notion, Neuman and Hill (1978), using a paradigm developed by Gallup (1970), showed that a small sample of 5- to 11-year-old autistic children displayed evidence of visual self-recognition. In this paradigm, self-recognition is operationally defined as the ability to discriminate a change in one's mirror image. A small amount of rouge is placed on the end of the child's nose, and the child's response to his or her mirror image is observed. The child is expected to touch his or her nose or reflection, to smile, or to respond vocally if he or she recognizes the reflection and the change in the mirror image. Subsequently, other studies of autistic children have replicated this finding (Dawson & McKissick, 1984; Ferrari & Mathews, 1983; Spiker & Ricks, 1984).

Although the autistic children displayed evidence of self-recognition, Neuman and Hill (1978) noted that they did not display the same type of coy or self-conscious affect reported in similar studies of normal toddlers. Dawson and McKissick (1984) followed up on this anecdotal finding with a comparison of normal and autistic children. They found that the autistic children smiled as often at their mirror images as did the normal children (73% of the autistic children, 60% of the normal children). However, while coy behavior was occasionally seen in the normals (13%–27%), it was never observed in the autistic children. In contrast, Spiker and Ricks (1984) have reported that 79% of their sample of 51 autistic children displayed completely neutral affect throughout a mirror self-recognition procedure. These studies suggest that although autistic children do not display a deficit in visual self-recognition,[4] their affective response to mirror images differs from that of normal children. However, the studies cited above did not employ mentally retarded children as controls. Therefore, they do not address whether this difference in affective response to mirror images is specific to autism or a phenomenon also associated with mental retardation.

In collaboration with Judy Ungerer and Tracy Sherman we have directly addressed this issue. Eighteen 3- to 6-year-old autistic children were compared to MA-matched samples of normal and mentally retarded children on the mirror self-recognition procedure. Replicating previous research, there were no differences between the autistic children and the control groups on behaviors indicative of discrimination of self from mirror image. However, there were significant differences between the frequency of smiling at mirror images displayed across conditions by the autistic, mentally retarded, and normal groups (means = 1.5, 7.1, and 3.1 smiles, respectively). The autistic children were clearly different from the mentally retarded children as well as the normal children in the expression of affect to a mirror image.

The reader may notice that the details of the findings from studies using this paradigm are not consistent. Dawson and McKissick (1984) report smiling but no coy affect in an autistic sample; Spiker and Ricks (1984) report neutral affect in

---

4. However, recent research with a different paradigm suggests that autistic children may have difficulty with aspects of self-recognition (Waterhouse, 1987).

an autistic sample; and we report lower frequencies of smiling among autistic children when compared to normal and mentally retarded controls. Nevertheless, each of these studies suggests that the affective response of autistic children to their mirror images differs from the response of other children.

The data from the studies we have reviewed converge to suggest that autistic children display a disturbance in the vocal, gestural, and facial expression of affect. These data are important. Clear (i.e., reliably rated), discrete emotional expressions are displayed early in infancy (Izard, Heubner, Risser, McGinnes, & Dougherty, 1980). The signal value of clear emotional expressions provides the foundation for the earliest phase of social communication between child and caregiver (Adamson & Bakeman, 1982; see below). Therefore, a deficit in affective expression may be a primary disorder of autism. That is, a disorder of emotional expression may be one of the first social-developmental deficits to emerge in autistic children. Specific disorders in the development of nonverbal communication behaviors appears to be another type of social deficit to emerge early in the lives of autistic children.

Studies of Nonverbal Communication

The development of communication skills in the first 24 months of life in normal infants may be described in terms of three phases (Adamson & Bakeman, 1982). In the first phase (0–5 months), communication (if not all of social interaction) involves face-to-face exchanges of affective signals between an infant and the caregiver (Trevarthen, 1979). In contrast to this dyadic/affective phase, interactions in the second phase (6–18 months) are characterized by triadic exchanges (Bakeman & Adamson, 1984). These involve the child, the caregiver, and shared or coordinated attention with respect to some object of event that is external to the child–caregiver dyad. During this phase, the intentionality of the infant's communicative behavior becomes more apparent as the infant begins to use and respond to nonverbal acts (i.e., eye contact, direction of gaze, gestures such as pointing, and vocalizations) to refer to objects and events (Bates, Benigni, Bretherton, Camaioni, & Volterra, 1979; Rheingold, Hay, & West, 1976; Sugarman, 1984). In the third or locutionary phase (12–24 months), the child moves from reliance on gestures to the use and comprehension of words in communicating with his or her caregivers.

Herein, "nonverbal communication skills" refer to behaviors that develop during the second or triadic phase of communication development. At least three categories or functions of these behaviors have been described. "Affiliation" or "social interaction" behaviors involve the use of nonverbal behaviors or objects to elicit or maintain face-to-face interaction (e.g., reaching to another, taking turns with a ball). "Joint attention" or "indicating" behaviors involve the use of procedures (e.g., showing a toy) to coordinate attention between social partners in order to share an awareness of objects or events. "Regulation" or "requesting" behaviors involve the use of procedures (e.g., reaching to a toy) to gain another person's aid in obtaining objects or events (Bruner & Sherwood, 1983; Seibert, Hogan, & Mundy, 1982).

Elements of this tripartite taxonomy of nonverbal communication skills have been used in studies of autistic children. Wetherby and Prutting (1984) found that four autistic children exhibited nonverbal requests for objects, actions, and social routines, but did not engage in gestural acts simply to indicate or share an awareness of an object's existence or properties. Curcio (1978) has reported that gestural requests were observed among all 12 autistic children in his study, but none of these children exhibited indicating gestures. Furthermore, autistic children exhibit significantly fewer gestural indicating behaviors and are less responsive to adult indicating acts than are normal and language-delayed children (Loveland & Landry, 1986).

These studies suggest that the disordered social development of autistic children is characterized by stronger deficits in indicating skills than in affiliative or requesting skills. In each of the studies, though, psychometric data indicated that a majority of the autistic children were functioning in the mentally retarded range of intelligence. Greenwald and Leonard (1979) have shown that for mentally retarded children, the development of nonverbal indicating skills may lag behind the development of other nonverbal communication skills. It is not clear, then, whether a deficit in the development of joint attention skills is specific to autism or whether this deficit is a general concomitant of developmental disorder.

To address this issue, we compared eighteen 3- to 6-year-old autistic children to developmentally matched samples of young mentally retarded and normal children on measures of nonverbal affiliative, indicating, and requesting behaviors (Mundy *et al.*, 1986). A structured interaction with an experimenter was used to elicit behaviors in each of these categories. The results indicated that the autistic children displayed a pattern of strengths as well as weakness on the measures of social interaction and requesting behaviors. In contrast, the autistic children displayed only deficits in the production of indicating behaviors (i.e., showing, pointing, and referential looking or alternating looking between an active mechanical toy and eye contact with the experimenter). Moreover, the variables from within the indicating category best discriminated the autistic children from the other groups. The single best discriminant variable was referential looking. On the basis of this one behavior alone, 94.4% of the autistic children were correctly classified (group means for referential looks: autistic = 1.4, mentally retarded = 5.4, normal = 5.5). This deficit in eye contact was found only in the indicating category. A deficit was not observed on a similar social interaction variable, "eye contact after [being] tickled" (group means: autistic = 4.9, mentally retarded = 5.4, normal = 2.9). Nor was there a clearly autistic deficit on a similar requesting variable, "eye contact after toy is moved out of reach" (group means: autistic = 3.4, mentally retarded = 4.5, normal = 5.7). On this variable both the autistic and the mentally retarded children displayed eye contact less frequently than the normal children.

Deficits in indicating behaviors are not only displayed in the context of autistic children's interaction with an unfamiliar experimenter. In a study of the child–caregiver interactions of the same sample of autistic children, we found that these children did not show a general lack of social responsiveness to their caregivers when compared with mentally retarded and normal children. However, they did display the same specific deficit in nonverbal indicating behavior in the child–caregiver interaction as they had in the experimenter–child interaction (Sigman, Mundy, Sherman, & Ungerer, 1986).

It is of interest to note that the results of these studies appear to be inconsistent with Attwood's (1984; cited in Frith, 1984) finding that autistic individuals displayed deficits in expressive but not indicating (deictic) gestures. However, the children in Attwood's study were older (mean CA = 11.3 years) than the children in the studies of Wetherby and Prutting (1984), Loveland and Landry (1986), and our own. Perhaps developmentally younger autistic children display deficits in indicating skills, whereas more advanced children display deficits in affective/expressive but not deictic/gestural skills. To our knowledge, this hypothesis concerning developmental change in the social deficits of autistic children has not been addressed in the literature.

Nonverbal Communication, Affect, and Autistic Psychopathology

Data concerning the nonverbal communication deficits of autistic children have several implications. First, a quantitative deficiency in eye contact has long been associated with autism. Recently, though, it has been suggested that this deficiency may be qualitative rather than quantitative (Mirenda, Donnellan, & Yoder, 1983; Rutter, 1978). Our results (Mundy et al., 1986) agree with the latter position. These data indicate that autistic children display deficits in eye contact in some contexts but not others. They infrequently look to others (share attention) when presented with an interesting object. However, compared to control children, they do not display deficits in eye contact in response to being tickled or in response to the removal of an object.

More broadly, the results suggest that a deficit in the development of nonverbal indicating skills is a significant characteristic of preschool children who have received the diagnosis of autism. Understanding the psychological factors involved in this deficit may be revealing with regard to autism. One hypothesis we have explored is that the paucity of nonverbal indicating behavior displayed by young autistic children is related to deficits in symbolic/representational thinking in autistic children, which have previously been described (Ricks & Wing, 1975; Rutter, 1978; Sigman & Ungerer, 1984b). Representational thinking may be operationally defined in terms of a child's capacity to use one object to portray another object in play (e.g., using a sponge on a spoon to portray or represent food). We have found some evidence of an association between measures of symbolic/representational play skills and nonverbal indicating skills in young autistic children (Mundy, Sigman, Ungerer, & Sherman, 1987; Sigman & Mundy, 1987). However, these results were not so strong as to suggest that measures of indicating skills and symbolic skills index completely overlapping factors in autistic children. Moreover, multiple-regression analyses suggest that symbolic play and indicating skills have significant but independent paths of association with language development in young autistic children (Mundy *et al.*, 1987; Sigman & Mundy, 1987).

We interpret these results to indicate that the paucity of nonverbal indicating behaviors displayed by autistic children reflects an area of deficit that is, to some extent, independent of the deficit in symbolic skills displayed by these children. This conclusion is consistent with theory suggesting that the development of nonverbal indicating skills does not require the capacity for symbolic thought (Sugarman, 1984).

An alternative hypothesis may be derived from understanding the communicative function of indicating behaviors. The common function of such behaviors as pointing, showing, and referential eye contact seems to be to share the experience of an object or event with another person (cf. Rheingold *et al.*, 1976).[5] Theoretically, such a function demands the development of an adequate concept of others as agents who possess independent psychological states such as interest in objects (Werner & Kaplan, 1963). This interpretation places the development of indicating behaviors within a social-cognitive perspective. Does this mean that a deficit in nonverbal indicating skills reflects a cognitive (albeit social-cognitive) defect in autistic children? Perhaps, but what are the antecedents of such a defect?

The developmental model of Adamson and Bakeman (1982) suggests that face-to-face conveyance of affective signals precedes the development of nonverbal gestural communication. During this period, the conveyance of affective signals affords the infant the opportunity to develop an appreciation of the commonality of affective experience between self and other. Trevarthen (1979) refers to this developing sense of shared experience as "intersubjectivity." Werner and Kaplan (1963) suggest that this developmental period is characterized by the "primordial sharing situation," wherein interactions have the characteristic of "sharing experiences with others rather than communicating messages to others" (p. 42). Although not thoroughly defined, "communicating messages" seems to refer the use of conventional signals such as pointing or words to convey information from one person to another. Alternatively, "sharing experiences" refers to the capacity of the infant both to express varied emotional states and, more importantly, to respond in kind to emotions displayed by others. Klinnert, Campos, Sorce, Emde, and Svejda (1983) eloquently refer to this as the capacity of the infant to "resonate emotionally" to the expressions of others (p. 73). These authors conservatively estimate that this capacity is well developed in the normal infant by 5–7 months of age. Thus, the normal infant can directly share affective experiences with others very early in life. Furthermore, it may well be that the capacity to share

---

5. See Mundy *et al.* (1987) for contrasting descriptions of the functions of social interaction and requesting behaviors.

affective experience with others very early in life is necessary to the subsequent capacity to share the experience of an object or an event with another person (cf. Werner & Kaplan, 1963).

If this model of development is correct, we may view autistic children's deficits in nonverbal indicating skills, and the disturbance of social cognition inferred by these deficits, as the developmental sequelae of earlier-emerging deficits in the capacity to share common affective experiences with caregivers. As noted earlier, there is evidence indicating a disturbance in affective expression among autistic children. The work of Hobson (Chapter 2, this volume) also suggests that autistic children have difficulty interpreting affective signals. It is plausible that these affective disturbances, observed in older autistic children, reflect a deficit that also inhibits the young autistic child's capacity to "resonate emotionally" to the affect of others. Such an inability may severely retard the very young autistic child's ability to develop a sense of commonality between self or other. In a very real sense, then, the model we have briefly presented here is in keeping with Kanner's (1943/1985) original hypothesis that autistic children "come into the world with innate inability to form the usual, biologically provided affective contact with people" (p. 50).

Social Deficits and the Biological Hypothesis

We are not alone in speculating that Kanner's original hypothesis holds more than a grain of truth. Based on his extensive series of studies, Hobson (Chapter 2, this volume) argues that a deficit in the capacity to interpret emotional expressions is central to autistic psychopathology. Murray (1984) has also argued that a deficit in the capacity to regulate affect in relation to the affect and behavior of others may be at the core of autism. She goes on to suggest that this deficit may have a constitutional (biological) foundation, which may lead to the subsequent development of cognitive and linguistic deficits. Similarly, Fein, Pennington, Markowitz, Braverman, and Waterhouse (1986) have championed the hypothesis that autism is a neurological disorder that primarily affects social or affective development. Furthermore, these authors argue that this disorder is at least partially independent of the systems underlying the deficits in cognitive development displayed by autistic individuals. Consistent with this hypothesis, a biochemical model specific to the social deficits of autism has recently been presented (Panksepp, 1979; Panksepp *et al.*, 1985), but the evidence for this model is quite indirect. To the extent that this model has been tested directly in autistic individuals, the evidence is currently mixed (Deutsch, 1986).

In concluding this chapter, it is worth noting that the complexity of neuroanatomical and neurochemical systems makes the task of pinpointing the neurobiological substrate of autism an extremely difficult one. The difficulty of this task may also be exacerbated by a phenomenon referred to as the "primate isolation syndrome." Kraemer (1985) has recently reviewed evidence indicating that early social isolation may result in deficiencies in social behaviors among primates. Early isolation may affect both the neuroanatomical and neurochemical substrates of social behavior. Kraemer extrapolates from this literature to suggest that the neurobiological basis for different types of human psychopathology may involve a two-stage process. Disorders that occur early in development and disrupt early social interactions result in significant changes in early experience. These changes in experience may result in central nervous system (CNS) modifications related to social deprivation. Kraemer concludes by stating that "by the time significant psychopathological systems demand intervention later in life, some aspects of the disorder may be attributable to the primary process, but others may reflect behavioral and neurobiological aspects of the primate isolation syndrome" (p. 154).

Kraemer has presented this argument in the context of discussing schizophrenia and major affective disorder. However, his dual-process model may be even more pertinent to autism. Since it is likely that autism has a negatively impact on early interactions with others, it may well be that some of the variance observed in the social behaviors of autistic children reflects the extent to which there is an overlay of an "isolation syndrome" on the core developmental disorder that is autism. This is not to suggest that environmental deprivation per se produces an autistic-like pattern of behavior in children. However, it is important to acknowledge that isolation affects the development of the CNS, and that this may contribute an additional level of complexity to the already monumental task of identifying endogenous processes that result in autism.

Nevertheless, current research results direct us to think of the social and emotional deficits of autism as fundamental components of the disorder, not necessarily epiphenomena of cognitive dysfunction. Understanding both the behavioral and the neurobiological details of these social and emotional deficits remains a challenge for future clinical research on autism.

SUMMARY

This chapter has presented a discussion of recent developments in research on the nature of autistic social deficits. Although social deficits have been considered pathognomonic of autism since the initial description of the syndrome (Kanner, 1943/1985), it is only recently that social behavior has become a focus for clinical research in this area of psychopathology. Current research suggests that broad statements about a pervasive lack of social responsiveness among autistic children are inaccurate. Rather, autistic children appear to display some behaviors indicative of social responsiveness, social learning, and child–caregiver attachment. However, autistic children also display striking deficits in social behaviors. Developmentally, some of the earliest types of deficits seem to occur in affective expression and nonverbal communication. Understanding the nature of these deficits may provide important information regarding the nature and pathogenesis of autism.

Acknowledgments

This chapter was prepared with support from the Olive View Research and Education Institute, National Institute of Mental Health Grant No. MH 33815, and National Institute of Child Health and Human Development Grant No. HD 17662. We thank Connie Kasari, Nurit Yirmiya, and Fred Volkmar for their contributions to this chapter.

References

Adamson, L., & Bakeman, R. (1982). Affectivity and reference: Concepts, methods, and techniques in the study of communication development of 6- to 18-month-old infants. In T. Field & A. Fogel (Eds.), *Emotion and early interaction* (pp. 213–236). Hillsdale, NJ: Erlbaum.

Ainsworth, M. D. S., Blehar, M. C., Waters, E., & Wall, S. (1978). *Patterns of attachment: A psychological study of the strange situation.* Hillsdale, NJ: Erlbaum.

American Psychiatric Association. (1980). *Diagnostic and statistical manual of mental disorders* (3rd ed.). Washington, DC: Author.

American Psychiatric Association. (1987). *Diagnostic and statistical manual of mental disorders* (3rd ed.—rev.). Washington, DC: Author.

Anthony, E. J. (1967). Classification and categorization in child psychiatry. *International Journal of Psychiatry, 3,* 173–178.

Bakeman, R., & Adamson, L. B. (1984). Coordinating attention to people and objects in mother–infant and peer–infant interactions. *Child Development, 55,* 1278–1289.

Bates, E., Benigni, L., Bretherton, I., Camaioni, L., & Volterra, V. (1979). *The emergence of symbols: Cognition and communication in infancy.* New York: Academic Press.

Bettelheim, B. (1959). Joey: A "mechanical boy." *Scientific American, 200,* 116–127.

Bowlby, J. (1982). Attachment and loss: Retrospect and prospect. *American Journal of Orthopsychiatry, 52,* 664–678.

Bretherton, I., & Waters, E. (1985). Growing points of attachment theory and research. *Monographs of the Society for Research in Child Development, 50* (Serial No. 209).

Bruner, J., & Sherwood, V. (1983). Thought, language and interaction in infancy. In J. D. Call, E. Galenson, & R. L. Tyson (Eds.), *Frontiers of infant psychiatry* (pp. 38–55). New York: Basic Books.

Charlop, M. H., Schreibman, L., & Tryon, A. S. (1983). Learning through observation: The effects of peer modeling on acquisition and generalization in autistic children. *Journal of Abnormal Child Psychology, 11,* 355–366.

Clark, P., & Rutter, M. (1981). Autistic children's response to structure and to interpersonal demands. *Journal of Autism and Developmental Disorders, 11,* 201–217.

Cohen, D., Caparulo, B., & Shaywitz, B. (1985). Neurochemical and developmental models of childhood autism. In A. Donnellan (Ed.), *Classic readings in autism* (pp. 343–369). New York: Teachers College Press. (Original work published 1978)

Creak, M. (1961). Schizophrenic syndrome in childhood: A report of the working party. *British Medical Journal, ii,* 889–890.

Curcio, F. (1978). Sensorimotor functioning and communication in mute autistic children. *Journal of Autism and Childhood Schizophrenia, 2,* 264–287.

Damasio, A., & Maurer, R. (1978). A neurological model for childhood autism. *Archives of Neurology, 35,* 777–786.

Dawson, G., & Adams, A. (1984). Imitation and social responsiveness in autistic children. *Journal of Abnormal Child Psychology, 12,* 209–226.

Dawson, G., & Galpert, L. (1986). A developmental model for facilitating the social behavior of autistic children. In E. Schopler & G. Mesibov (Eds.), *Social behavior in autism* (pp. 237–256). New York: Plenum.

Dawson, G., & McKissick, F. (1984). Self-recognition in autistic children. *Journal of Autism and Developmental Disorders, 14,* 383–394.

Donnellan, A. (1985). Introduction. In A. Donnellan (Ed.), *Classic readings in autism* (pp. 1–10). New York: Teachers College Press.

Deutsch, S. (1986). Rational for the administration of opiate antagonists in treating infantile autism. *American Journal of Mental Deficiency, 90,* 631–635.

Egel, A., Richman, G., & Koegel, R. (1981). Normal peer models and autistic children's learning. *Journal of Applied Behavior Analysis, 14,* 3–12.

Fein, D., Humes, M., Kaplan, E., Lucci, D., & Waterhouse, L. (1984). The question of left hemisphere dysfunction in autistic children. *Psychological Bulletin, 95,* 258–281.

Fein, D., Pennington, B., Markowitz, P., Braverman, M., & Waterhouse, L. (1986). Toward a neuropsychological model of infantile autism: Are the social deficits primary? *Journal of the American Academy of Child Psychiatry, 25,* 198–212.

Ferrara, C., & Hill, S. (1980). The responsiveness of autistic children to the predictability of social and nonsocial toys. *Journal of Autism and Developmental Disorders, 10,* 51–57.

Ferrari, M., & Mathews, W. (1983). Self-recognition deficits in autism: Syndrome-specific or general developmental delay? *Journal of Autism and Developmental Disorders, 13,* 317–324.

Frith, D. (1984). *A new perspective in research on autism.* Paper presented at the Groupe de Travail sur les Aspects Cognitifs de l'Autism, Paris.

Gallup, G., Jr. (1970). Chimpanzees: Self-recognition. *Science, 167,* 86–87.

Greenwald, C., & Leonard, L. (1979). Communicative and sensorimotor development of Down's syndrome children. *American Journal of Mental Deficiency, 84,* 296–303.

Goldfarb, W. (1974). *Growth and change of schizophrenic children: A longitudinal study.* Washington, D.C.: V. H. Winston.

Guralnick, M., & Groom, J. (1985). Correlates of peer-related social competence of developmentally delayed preschool children. *American Journal of Mental Deficiency, 90,* 140–150.

Hermelin, B. (1982). Thoughts and feelings. *Australian Autism Review, 4,* 10–19.

Hermelin, B., & O'Connor, N. (1970). *Psychological experiments with autistic children.* Oxford: Pergamon Press.

Howlin, P. (1978). The assessment of social behavior. In M. Rutter & E. Schopler (Ed.), *Autism: A reappraisal of concepts and treatment* (pp. 63–69). New York: Plenum.

Howlin, P. (1986). An overview of social behavior in autism. In E. Schopler & G. Mesibov (Eds.), *Social behavior in autism* (pp. 103–131). New York: Plenum.

Izard, C. (1979). *The maximally discriminative facial movement coding system.* Newark: Instructional Resources Center, University of Delaware.

Izard, C., Huebner, R., Risser, D., McGinnes, G. & Dougherty, L. (1980). The young infant's ability to produce discrete emotion expressions. *Developmental Psychology, 16,* 132–140.

Kanner, L. (1985). Autistic disturbances of affective contact. In A. Donnellan (Ed.), *Classic readings in autism* (pp. 11–50). New York: Teachers College Press. (Original work published 1943)

Kasari, C., Yirmiya, N., Mundy, P. & Sigman, M. (1986, August) *Affect expressions: A comparison of autistic, MR, and normal children.* Paper presented at the annual meeting of the American Psychological Association, Washington, DC.

Klinnert, M., Campos, J., Sorce, J., Emde, R., & Svejda, M. (1983). Emotions as behavior regulators: Social Referencing in infancy. In R. Plutchnik & H. Kellerman (Eds.), *Emotion: Theory, research, and experience* (Vol. 2, pp. 57–86). New York: Academic Press.

Kraemer, G. (1985). Effects of differences in early social experience on primate neurobiological–behavioral development. In M. Reite & T. Field (Eds.), *The psychobiology of attachment and separation* (pp. 135–161). New York: Academic Press.

Lord, C. (1984). Development of peer relations in children with autism. In F. Morrison, C. Lord, & D. Keating (Eds.), *Applied developmental psychology* (Vol. 1, 166–230). New York: Academic Press.

Loveland, K., & Landry, S. (1986). Joint attention in autistic and language delayed children. *Journal of Autism and Developmental Disorders, 16,* 335–350.

McAdoo, W., and DeMyer, M. (1978). Personality characteristics of parents. In M. Rutter & E.

Schopler (Eds.), *Autism: A reappraisal of concepts and treatment* (pp. 251–267). New York: Plenum.

McHale, S. (1983). Social interactions of autistic and non-handicapped children during free play. *American Journal of Orthopsychiatry, 53,* 81–91.

Mirenda, P., Donnellan, A., & Yoder, D. (1983). Gaze behavior: A new look at an old problem. *Journal of Autism and Developmental Disorders, 13,* 397–409.

Mundy, P., Sigman, M., Ungerer, J., & Sherman, T. (1986). Defining the social deficits of autism: The contribution of nonverbal communication measures. *Journal of Child Psychology and Psychiatry, 27,* 657–669.

Mundy, P., Sigman, M., Ungerer, J., & Sherman, T. (1987). Play and nonverbal communication correlates of language development in autistic children. *Journal of Autism and Developmental Disabilities, 17,* 349–364.

Murray, L. (1984). *Emotional regulation of intersubjective encounters: Implications for the theory of autism.* Paper presented at the Groupe de Travail sur les Aspects Cognitifs de l'Autism, Paris.

Neuman, C., & Hill, S. (1978). Self-recognition and stimulus preference in autistic children. *Developmental Psychobiology, 11,* 571–578.

Olley, J. (1985). Social aspects of communication in children with autism. In E. Schopler & G. Mesibov (Eds.), *Communication problems in autism* (pp. 311–328). New York: Plenum.

Ornitz, E., & Ritvo, E. (1968). Perceptual inconstancy in early infantile autism. *Archives of General Psychiatry, 18,* 76–98.

Panksepp, J. (1979). A neurochemical theory of autism. *Trends in Neurosciences, 2,* 174–177.

Panksepp, J., Siving, S., & Normansell, L. (1985). Brain opioids and social emotions. In M. Reite & T. Field (Eds.), *The psychobiology of attachment and separation* (pp. 3–49). New York: Academic Press.

Prior, M. (1984). Developing concepts of childhood autism: The influence of experimental cognitive research. *Journal of Consulting and Clinical Psychology, 52,* 4–17.

Rheingold, H., Hay, D., & West, M. (1976). Sharing in the second year of life. *Child Development, 83,* 898–913.

Richer, J. (1976). The social avoidance behavior of autistic children. *Animal Behavior, 24,* 898–906.

Ricks, D. (1979). Making sense of experience to make sensible sounds. In M. Bullowa (Eds.), *Before speech: The beginning of interpersonal communication* (pp. 245–268). New York: Cambridge University Press.

Ricks, D., & Wing, L. (1975). Language, communication and the use of symbols. *Journal of Autism and Childhood Schizophrenia, 5,* 191–211.

Rimland, B. (1964). *Infantile autism.* New York: Appleton-Century-Crofts.

Rutter, M. (1968). Concepts of autism: A review of research. *Journal of Child Psychology and Psychiatry, 9,* 1–25.

Rutter, M. (1978). Diagnosis and definition. In M. Rutter & E. Schopler (Eds.), *Autism: A reappraisal of concepts and treatment.* (pp. 1–25). New York: Plenum.

Rutter, M. (1983). Cognitive deficits in the pathogenesis of autism. *Journal of Child Psychology and Psychiatry, 24,* 513–531.

Seibert, J., Hogan, A., & Mundy, P. (1982). Assessing interactional competencies. The Early Social-Communication Scales. *Infant Mental Health Journal, 3,* 244–259.

Shapiro, T., Sherman, M., Calamari, G., & Koch, D. (1985). *Attachment in autism and other developmental disorders.* Paper presented at the annual meeting of the American Academy of Child Psychiatry, San Antonio, TX.

Sigman, M., & Mundy, P. (1987). Symbolic processes in young autistic children. In D. Cicchetti (Ed.), *New directions in child development: Symbolic development in atypical children* (pp. 31–46). San Francisco: Jossey-Bass.

Sigman, M., Mundy, P., Sherman, T., & Ungerer, J. (1986). Social interactions of autistic, mentally retarded, and normal children and their caregivers. *Journal of Child Psychology and Psychiatry, 27,* 647–656.

Sigman, M., Mundy, P., Ungerer, J. & Sherman, T. (1987). *The development of social attachments in autistic children*. Paper presented at the biennial meeting of the Society for Research in Child Development, Baltimore.

Sigman, M., & Ungerer, J. (1984a). Attachment behaviors in autistic children. *Journal of Autism and Developmental Disorders, 14*, 231–244.

Sigman, M., & Ungerer, J. (1984b). Cognitive and language skills in autistic, mentally retarded, and normal children. *Developmental Psychology, 20*, 293–302.

Sigman, M., Ungerer, J., Mundy, P., & Sherman, T. (1987). Cognition in autistic children. In D. Cohen, A. Donnellan, & R. Paul (Eds.), *Handbook of autism and atypical developmental disorders* (pp. 103–120). New York: Wiley.

Snow, M., Hertzig, M., and Shapiro, T. (1986, October). *Affective expression in young autistic children*. Paper presented at the annual meeting of the American Academy of Child Psychiatry, Los Angeles.

Spiker, D., & Ricks, M. (1984).Visual self-recognition in autistic children: Developmental relationships. *Child Development, 55*, 214–225.

Strain, P., Kerr, M., & Ragland, E. (1979). Effects of peer-mediated social initiations and prompting/ reinforcement procedures on the social behavior of autistic children. *Journal of Autism and Developmental Disorders, 9*, 41–54.

Sugarman, S. (1984). The development of preverbal communication. In R. L. Schiefelbusch & J. Pickar (Eds.), *The acquisition of communicative competence* (pp. 23–67). Baltimore: University Park Press.

Tiegerman, E., & Primavera, L. (1984). Imitating the autistic child: Facilitating communicative gaze. *Journal of Autism and Developmental Disorders, 14*, 27–38.

Trevarthen, C. (1979).Communication and cooperation in early infancy: A description of primary intersubjectivity. In M. Bullowa (Eds.), *Before speech: The beginning of interpersonal communication* (pp. 321–347). New York: Cambridge University Press.

Tonick, I. (1981). *Social relatedness in autistic children*. Unpublished doctoral dissertation, University of Utah.

van Engeland, H., Bodnar, F., & Bolhuis, G. (1985). Some qualitative aspects of the social behavior of autistic children: An ethological approach. *Journal of Child Psychology and Psychiatry, 26*, 879–893.

Volkmar, F., Cohen, D., & Paul, R. (1986). An evaluation of DSM-III criteria for infantile autism. *Journal of the American Academy of Child Psychiatry, 25*, 190–197.

Waterhouse, L. (1987). *Self recognition and self reference in children with autistic spectrum disorder*. Paper presented at the biennial meeting of the Society for Research in Child Development, Baltimore.

Werner, H., & Kaplan, B. (1963). *Symbol formation*. New York: Wiley.

Wetherby, A., & Prutting, C. (1984). Profiles of communicative and cognitive–social abilities in autistic children. *Journal of Speech and Hearing Research, 27*, 364–377.

Wing, L. (1976). Kanner's syndrome: A historical perspective. In L. Wing (Ed.), *Early childhood autism* (pp. 3–14). Oxford: Pergamon Press.

Wing, L. (1978). Social, behavioral, and cognitive characteristics: An epidemiological approach. In M. Rutter & E. Schopler (Eds.), *Autism: A reappraisal of concepts and treatment* (pp. 27–46). New York: Plenum.

Wing, L., & Gould, J. (1979). Severe impairments of social interaction and associated abnormalities in children: Epidemiology and classification. *Journal of Autism and Developmental Disabilities, 9*, 11–29.

CHAPTER 2

Beyond Cognition
A Theory of Autism

R. PETER HOBSON
Institute of Psychiatry, London
MRC Developmental Psychology Project, London

In the beginning is relation.—Buber, 1958, p. 18

INTRODUCTION

Autistic children are profoundly impaired in their personal relations. These impairments are probably of a kind unique to autism. Autistic children also have a characteristic profile of disabilities in the realms of cognition, language, and play. It cannot be a coincidence that the one set of impairments is so intimately related to the other. A crucial issue for an understanding of the psychology of autism is the nature of the relationship between social and nonsocial facets of normal and autistic children's development.

In the present chapter, I attempt to indicate how, on a number of levels, autism should be counted a disorder of affective and social relations—and irreducibly so. In the course of my account, I suggest ways in which many but not all of autistic children's disabilities in cognition, language, and imaginative activity may stem from incapacities in "personal relatedness."

In certain important respects, the thesis I present is an elaboration of the early proposal of Kanner (1943), who concluded his original account of 11 children with "disturbances of affective contact" by suggesting that "these children have come into the world with innate inability to form the usual, biologically provided affective contact with people" (p. 250). Over the four decades that have passed since Kanner's paper, there has been surprisingly little theoretical or empirical work on the notion that autistic children's lack of affective contact with others may be basic to the nature of autism. Prior to the 1980s, and with a few exceptions (e.g., Ricks & Wing, 1975) those authors who argued for the centrality of perceptual or perceptual–motor (e.g., DeMyer, 1976; Schopler, 1965), linguistic (e.g., Churchill, 1972; Rutter, 1968), or cognitive (e.g., Hermelin & O'Connor, 1970; Rimland, 1964; Rutter, 1972) factors in the pathogenesis of autism

22

devoted relatively little attention to the affective dimension of the children's social relations, either as an explanatory factor or as an important aspect of the phenomena to be explained. This is all the more remarkable, given that most people are struck by the abnormal "feel" that is a unique quality of social contacts with autistic children. Psychodynamically oriented writers (e.g., Bettelheim, 1967; Mahler, 1968; Ruttenberg, 1971; Tustin, 1972) placed more emphasis on the significance of the child's affective experience, but were divided in their views on its nature and implications. Recent writings on autism have reflected a fresh concern with the importance of affective impairments (e.g., Fein, Pennington, Markowitz, Braverman, & Waterhouse, 1986; Hermelin & O'Connor, 1985; Hobson, 1982a). I adopt a position allied to that of Bosch (1970), and argue that Kanner's original formulation with its emphasis on disturbances of affective contact is necessary and indeed pivotal for our understanding of autism.

In fact, Kanner's account may be taken to imply the need for two distinct but complementary approaches to the social impairments of autistic children, and I follow each of these. The one approach accords with Kanner's suggestion that the study of autistic children "may help to furnish concrete criteria regarding the still diffuse notions about the constitutional components of emotional reactivity" (1943, p. 250). Here the emphasis is upon the individual child's contribution to the form of his or her social relations. The second approach focuses upon autistic children's impairments in affective contact *with others*. From this perspective, the essential matter is the nature of the relations that hold between an autistic child and one or more other individuals. The focus of interest is what happens or fails to happen within the dyad, and then between the child and others of the same cultural group. I develop the lines of Kanner's thinking in a way that may be summarized by the following set of proposals: (1) Autistic children lack such constitutional components of action and reaction as are necessary for the development of reciprocal personal relations with other people, relations which involve feelings. (2) Such personal relations are necessary for the "constitution of an own and common world" with others (Bosch, 1970, p. 115). (3) Autistic children's lack of participation in intersubjective social experience has two results which are especially important—namely, (a) a relative failure to recognize other people *as* people with their own feelings, thoughts, wishes, intentions, and so on; and (b) a severe impairment in the capacity to abstract and to feel and think symbolically. (4) The greater part of autistic children's characteristic cognitive and language disability may be seen to reflect either lower-order deficits that have a specially intimate relationship with affective and social development, and/or impairments in the social-dependent capacity to symbolize.

In the last 20 years, there has been considerable growth in knowledge about the psychological deficits of autistic children. Yet there remains the need for a conceptual framework to make sense of all that is known. Therefore, my principal aim in this chapter is to provide the outline of a psychological theory of autism. The theory entails an account of normal development in relation to which the development of autistic children starts to become intelligible. In accordance with this, the chapter falls into two contrasting parts. To begin with, I consider the implications of normal affective experience and communication for social, cognitive, and linguistic development. This establishes a base for what follows—namely, a reappraisal of a range of social and cognitive deficits in autism. Throughout this chapter, I use the word "he" to refer to an individual child, and the word "she" to refer to an adult caretaker, regardless of sex.

FOUNDATIONS FOR SOCIAL AND COGNITIVE DEVELOPMENT

Affect and Nonverbal Communication

It goes without saying that nonverbal communication between one individual and another is a subtle and complex affair. The extent to which a normal infant is "prewired" to manifest particular patterns of behavior, and to be sensitive to the bodily configurations, sounds, rhythms, actions, and movements of his caretakers, is a much-debated issue. There is not space here to review the evidence for biological constraints on the individual's expression of emotion and on his sensitivity toward the feelings of others (see, e.g., Chevalier-Skolnikoff, 1973; Darwin, 1872/1965; Ekman, 1982; Frijda, 1986; Izard, 1971). Much of this evidence seems to indicate that human beings have more or less innate patterns of facial, vocal, and possibly gestural expression of emotion, and probably an innate readiness to be sensitive to a range of such expressions in others. The expressions of emotion tend to occur in particular constellations, as infants soon recognize (Malatesta, 1981; Walker, 1982); infants and children manifest such expressions when confronted by particular kinds of environmental events (e.g., Charlesworth & Kreutzer, 1973; Ricks, 1975, 1979); and other individuals' responses to these expressions frequently take a form that includes coordinated feelings and propensities to action (e.g., Hoffman, 1975; Klinnert, Campos, Sorce, Emde, & Svejda, 1983; Simner, 1971).

Thus biologically based signals of emotion, and biologically based responsiveness (including emotional responsiveness) to those signals, constitute an important device for promoting interpersonal coordination. The effectiveness of this device depends upon a sufficiently regular association among the different expressions of particular emotions, and upon consistency in the ways these expressions relate to environmental events and to the individuals' propensities to particular forms of action. If it were frequently the case that children smiled broadly and then ran away, we should question the sense in which children's smiles were "smiles." In other words, a kind of intrapersonal coordination of expressions, common to all individuals, contributes to (and may be a precondition for) interpersonal coordination of feeling and action. And the observer may have a corresponding "receptive" intrapersonal coordination: One way we can evaluate a real smile or a happy vocalization or gesture is through the "feel" that each and all of these expressions gives us. The importance of interpersonal patterning of emotion-related behavior between infant and mother has been beautifully illustrated by

Murray and Trevarthen (1985). I note only that there are probably other, complementary modes of human preadaptation for reciprocal social exchanges (e.g., Dawson
& Galpert, 1986; Kaye, 1982; Stern, 1977).

At this point, it is pertinent to consider what we mean by "expressions of
emotion." The philosopher Stuart Hampshire (1960/1976) has emphasized that
there is a necessary connection between a person having a feeling such as anger,
and an inclination to behave in an identifiable manner—in this instance, to attack
or behave aggressively. Indeed, "posture, gesture, facial expression are often immediately legible by others, as signs of an inclination to behave in a specific way"
(Hampshire, 1960/1976, p. 75). Frijda (1986) has suggested that emotional expressions should be viewed as "relational behavior," in that they establish or alter a
relationship between the subject and some object by modifying the relationship
rather than the environment. Expressive behavior is not only largely innate and
preprogrammed, but also elicited by stimuli in a relatively crude fashion. Yet the
particular form of behavior is influenced by what is appropriate in the circumstances; in particular, it is directed toward or away from relevant objects. So in
certain respects, the capacity to produce and comprehend emotional expressions
should be considered alongside the capacity to produce and comprehend other
directed patterns of bodily action for which humans or animals are innately prepared.

One further point: Reference to an emotion involves reference to a quality of
relatedness which exists between the individual and the world as he construes it.
A person's feelings are about something or someone. This "aboutness" has been
termed "intensionality" (or "intentionality," or sometimes "Intentionality"), and
is perhaps a unique and essential characteristic of mental phenomena. Perceptions, thoughts, desires, and so on are unlike physical phenomena in having "reference to a content, direction toward an object" (Brentano, 1874/1973, p. 88).[1]

Knowledge of Persons

There is a perennial epistemological problem for which an understanding of personal relations holds the only solution: How does a person arrive at a "knowledge
of other minds"? That is, how does an individual come to understand the nature
of other persons, and to recognize that people have thoughts, wishes, feelings,
and so on (Hobson, 1982b, 1985)? On what basis is such knowledge constructed?

Among other philosophers, Ryle (1949), Wittgenstein (1953), Scheler (1954),
Merleau-Ponty (1962), and Hamlyn (1974) have reasoned against the idea that a
person infers the existence of other conscious human beings by applying analogy
from that individual's own case. The perception of other human beings is the
condition for, not the outcome of, the application of analogy, insofar as analogy

1. There is a philosophical dispute about the distinctions that should be drawn among the uses
and spellings of the concept or concepts of "intensionality" (see, e.g., Searle, 1979). I have bypassed
these issues, and for the purposes of this chapter I follow the spelling adopted by Russell (1984), except
when there is reason to cite other authors' preferred terms.

is applied at all. Hamlyn (1974) argued that a part of what is involved in having the concept of a person is that one should understand what it is to stand in personal relations with another person. This understanding must be based upon "natural reactions of persons to persons" (p. 5)—that is, upon biologically founded emotional attitudes and reactions to other people. Hamlyn stressed that reciprocal feelings can exist between one person and another, but not between persons and things: "Knowledge of others would then have for its foundation something like relations between the child and others based on feeling" (p. 32). It is important to observe that "personal relatedness" refers to a mode of relating, a personal attitude, not merely to the kind of being related to. As Macmurray (1961) and Polanyi (1965) have discussed, one can treat a person impersonally, and indeed one derives knowledge of persons as objects as well as knowledge of persons as persons.

The problem now becomes one of explicating such "natural reactions of persons to persons." These reactions arise on the basis of the experience of the individual's own body and his experience of the bodies of others. As Scheler (1954) has written, our knowledge of others' experiences "is given for us *in* expressive phenomena—again, not by inference, but directly, as a sort of primary 'perception'. It is *in* the blush that we perceive shame, *in* the laughter joy. . . . We can thus have insight into others, in so far as we treat their bodies as a *field of expression* for their experiences" (p. 10; similarly Wittgenstein, 1980). Merleau-Ponty (1962) stressed that a person does not understand the gestures of others by some act of intellect, some "cognitive operation," but rather through "the reciprocity of my intentions and the gestures of others, of my gestures and intentions discernible in the conduct of other people" (p. 185). Thus the child is situated in an intersubjective world before he comes to adopt a positive *vis-à-vis* that world (see also Habermas, 1970). As Merleau-Ponty (1964) took pains to point out, however, such a view does not imply that at an early age an infant knows the exact meaning of each of the emotional expressions of others. Rather, he must soon come to perceive an expression as such, even if he is wrong about its meaning. Macmurray (1961) concluded that the unit of personal existence is not the individual, but two persons in personal relation; like Merleau-Ponty (1962) and Buber (1958), among others, he went on to discuss how the self emerges from this primordial relatedness with others. Adult caregivers capitalize on the infant's potential for constructing a personal world, and contribute much to the final form that the "experienced world" takes (Newson, 1979). But if the infant were to lack the innate preparedness for bodily understanding of another's bodily expressions, adults would have limited opportunity to play their part in the generation and transmission of shared meanings.

Thus a child's knowledge of people is grounded in his personal, reciprocal, affectively charged relations with others. In anticipation of what is to follow, it is worth drawing attention to Macmurray's (1961) description of the "impersonal" relation with others, in which one person regards the other not as a person nor as an agent, but as an object possessing certain capacities and characteristics that make her useful. As Scheler (1954) commented, one may look at the face of a crying child as a merely physical object.

I now turn from matters that are manifestly "social-affective" in nature to consider two important aspects of cognitive function—namely, the capacities to abstract and symbolize.

The Capacity to Abstract

Bolton (1977) has offered a clear, concise resume of the phenomenological critique of the traditional theory of abstraction. According to this still prevalent theory, concepts are formed through a process in which the person recognizes similarities or identical elements in a set of objects. He thus abstracts those resemblances away from the other properties of the set of objects which are not relevant to the concept. Yet the perceiver himself may employ two or more concepts to refer to the same object; the same elements can be organized in many different ways, according to the point of view the person adopts. It is not simply that a person attends to and groups what is "given" to him, for he plays an active role in interpreting and structuring reality. The problem is to understand the ways in which the individual is active in "taking" reality, and by his own interests, feelings, and actions, determines those aspects of the world that are meaningful for him.

In order to generalize from one particular to another, and so to subsume certain particulars under a general category, the individual must already have some grasp of the general concept. There must be some intuition of the general in the perception of the particular—what Husserl (1901) called "ideational abstraction." And the way in which something comes to be regarded as an example of a type is through the links forged by an individual's intentions and points of view, including his feelings toward the things in question. Thus there are perceptual meanings, conceptual meanings, affective meanings, and so on. According to this account, there are two main determinants of the course of concept growth: the nature of the objects perceived by the subject, and the subject's intentions, purposes, and desires. A further source of the generality of a concept is agreement among individuals. Thus thinking is closely related to feeling and action, and later to social intercourse; correspondingly, it is possible to have several types of understanding of a concept, from the enactive to the contemplative.

In his writings on conceptual development, Werner (1948) too emphasized that abstraction is not a unitary function, but rather "a process that may be effected by different functions on quite different levels" (p. 234). Werner proposed that "the awareness of objects during early childhood depends essentially on the extent to which these objects can be responded to in motor–affective behavior" (p. 66). He drew comparisons between the primitive mental life of young children and that of animals. Animals live in a world of things-of-action, of which the "signal properties" are dependent upon the biological world of the particular animal (p. 62). For young children, too, it is their affective and motor behavior which impresses itself on the world of things: "Percepts are deeply conditioned by emotional and motor behavior" (p. 83). Although there is much that this account shares with that of Piaget (e.g., 1970/1972), who believed that an infant knows an object only to the extent that he acts upon it, Werner's emphasis on the affective dimension is crucial. For "such dynamization of things based on the fact that the objects are predominantly understood through the motor and affective attitude of the subject may lead to a particular type of perception. . . . I have proposed the term *physiognomic perception* for this mode of cognition in general" (Werner, 1948, p. 69). As Blocker (1969) has emphasized, the more sophisticated "geometrical–technical perception" is seen to arise out of the developmentally prior "physiognomic perception" as the child begins to acquire more self-reflective and analytic habits of thought.

Thus there are developmental changes in the process of abstraction itself. In primitive or concrete abstraction, things may be grouped according to the objects' "equal affective value" for the subject (Werner, 1948, p. 232), as well as by their perceptual similarity. Psychoanalytic writers (e.g., Ferenczi, 1913/1952) have also stressed the affective determinants of primitive and unconscious symbolism. In true conceptual abstraction, by contrast, "the quality (e.g., a color) common to all the elements involved is deliberately detached—mentally isolated, as it were— and the elements themselves appear only as visible exemplifications of the common quality" (Werner, 1948, p. 243). At the conceptual level, a person can shift his point of view in a purposeful grouping activity.

The Emergence of Symbols

How then does a child move from concrete to conceptual abstraction, from a world of things-of-action to one of objects-of-contemplation (Werner & Kaplan, 1963), from actions and feelings which are anchored to signals, to thought which is mediated by symbols?

Werner (1948) wrote that the individual who can achieve the higher (conceptual) form of abstraction is "one who can shift his point of view" (p. 240). It may be suggested that when a child becomes able to shift points of view in sufficiently diverse ways, at that stage he acquires the capacity to symbolize. To the extent that this is so, the issue becomes that of tracing what is involved in such a development, especially the psychological prerequisites for these emergent capacities.

I wish to advocate the view that a child comes to symbolize through a process that is essentially interpersonal in nature.[2] A paper by Russell (1984) takes us near

2. Geraldine Dawson (personal communication, October 1986; Dawson & Galpert, 1986) has drawn my attention to the work of Wolf and Gardner (1981), who provide an account of early symbolization which has some important points of correspondence with the outline presented here. Wolf and Gardner argue that a child's capacity to use "a set of understandings about the distinct situational roles that objects and persons can play in events" (p. 315) provides him with a critical point of entry into language and other modes of symbolization. The present account of the origins, development, and implications of the child's understanding of his own and others' orientations to the world might be reframed in terms of "role-structuring" as described by Wolf and Gardner.

to seeing how this may occur. Russell's argument pivots around the notion of intensionality: "What constitutes the intensional is the possibility of taking up different mental orientations to one element of reality, the linguistic face of which is a plurality of words applying to one object" (p. 60). The intensional aspects of a situation are those concerned with the subject's experiences, what he may take things *as* on this or on other occasions; the extensional aspects are concerned with the objective state of the world. Russell set himself the task of describing how the infant emerges from the primordial sharing situation described by Werner and Kaplan (1963), and in so doing develops the ability to understand and use language, especially to refer to things. What the infant needs to do is to dissociate his own consciousness from that of the adult. This the infant and caretaker achieve through "co-designation of extensions by intensions" (p. 57). Even before language, the infant can "refer" to the same objects through perception, action, and gesture. The same object may have different meanings for the child: There is intraindividual coreferentiality. At the same time, different adults will be referring in different ways to these same objects experienced by the child: There is interindividual coreference. In terms of language learning, the child now comes to grasp that he may call something by different names, just as he may refer to the different members of a class by the same name. All depends on the child's ability to recognize the different mental orientations that he and others may adopt toward the same object or state of affairs. Along with this recognition comes an awareness of how the world is distanced from the child's immediate (intensional) involvement with it. He comes to see the world objectively as well as subjectively.

From the remainder of Russell's account, I select two points for mention. First, Russell noted in passing that we should be impressed by how close children's intensions often are to adults' intensions. Second, he pointed out that different referential terms are employed in different contexts, and that the child has an opportunity to learn how different coreferential terms may be appropriate to reflect different mental orientations to reality.

Dore (1985) has emphasized that shared emotional experience provides the medium through which the infant–caretaker dyad negotiates its relationship. In Russell's terms, the mental orientation of both infant and caretaker is frequently, and perhaps predominantly, one of affective involvement (see also Murray & Trevarthen, 1985). The intraindividual coreference of both infant and caretaker often takes the form of co-occurring gaze, facial expression, gesture, body orientation, and so on, as typically each partner behaves in more than one modality. Interindividual coreference is often achieved through the adult's attunement to the infant's state (or vice versa), as described by Stern, Hofer, Haft, and Dore (1984). The partners also orient behaviorally to how each other references elements of their context. One result is just that described by Russell: The caretaker expresses and often conventionalizes the infant's state, and this enables the infant to make a connection between what he observes in and feels through the behavior of the other and his own initial experiences. There is interpersonal negotiation of meaning. For this, the experience of the dyad is central.

In keeping with this approach, Dore (1985) proposed that there are four major interacting phases in the emergence of word meaning, from the first phase of "proto-communicative signals," which are almost always accompanied by expressions of affect, to the final phase of "predicative syntagms," when the child produces one word about part of a situation for which he has other words that he might have chosen; he now presupposes shared knowledge of an aspect of context which could have been made explicit, but focuses on another.

Let me now draw the threads of the argument together. My intention is to trace the necessary prerequisites for the development of symbolism. One starting point is the way in which an infant apprehends his world. To be considered here are the forms of perception, action, and feeling that are formative in the organization of primitive mental life. I have emphasized that the earliest modes of abstracting may be encountered when the infant takes two or more things to be the same, at least in certain respects or for certain purposes. This sameness may be determined by the way different objects lend themselves to the infant's current actions, or evoke similar affective states or tendencies, through their perceptual properties. As Werner and Kaplan (1963), Piaget (Piaget & Inhelder, 1969), and others have emphasized, however, true symbolism is only achieved when the symbolizer recognizes the distinction between symbol and referent, such that the symbol stands for the referent and is not taken to be the referent. Development toward symbolism is promoted by the fact that not only does the infant reference different objects in the same ways, but he also references the same object in different ways. In addition, and crucially, his caretaker is both a special kind of referent herself, and before long the source of alternative ways of referencing a shared environment. The caretaker is special well before the child is able to symbolize, in that she both evokes and responds to patterns of perceptual, motor, and affective activity in the infant. The affective responsiveness between caretaker and infant, along with other kinds of attunement which are less recognizably affective in quality (such as certain imitative motor patterns), are especially important for the reason that the infant finds in and through his caretaker patterns of action and feeling in which he himself can participate. The infant's experience of noninferential empathy, and his discovery of the potential meaning of his actions through their completion by the other person, are the foundations for his dawning awareness of both separateness from and continuing relatedness to another individual. Finding his caretaker to be common to himself, yet in many ways separate, the infant comes to grasp that he can relate to the way his caretaker is relating to the world. The infant can feel with his caretaker's feeling, and yet recognize that the setting for the feeling is the caretaker's, not his own. Because infant and caretaker are naturally equipped to recognize what *is* at the focus of the other's attention—not least, what is the object of the other's feelings—the infant can come to learn (and be taught) the ways another person's mind may be oriented, even when this orientation currently differs from the infant's own. He can also act on his caretaker's capacity to act in the world.

Along with this development, and (I suggest) derived from it, the infant acquires the ability to relate to things as these relate to other things—in other words, to make the discovery that a sound, or a conventional gesture, or a physical object, can point to, reference, or stand for another. Among the factors that contribute to this development, the child's increased flexibility in adopting different orientations to whatever serves as a symbol is perhaps the most important, in that he can choose to take the symbol as standing for its referent even though he is quite clear about its own distinct characteristics. But there may be something further about the way a child's dawning awareness of symbolic relationships draws upon his grasp of the intensional relationship between a person and the world. His understanding that for a person, the meaning of an object has to do with the person's orientation to that object, may promote his understanding that the meaning of a symbol (for a person) has to do with the way the symbol can be oriented toward what it symbolizes. Once the child recognizes that a person is a being whose experiences are "about" things, he may then see how one object or event can also be "about" another. An individual who understands symbols is able to orient himself to a symbol in a way that encompasses the symbol's orientation to its referent. So just as the young child relates to the caretaker's relation to the world, he now comes to relate to one thing's symbolic relation to another. This ushers in a new phase of development, for the caretaker can now introduce novel symbolic meanings into the child's relations with his world. In addition, the primitive forms of taking one thing as another can undergo a formal transformation, so that affective modes of symbolism can continue to operate even when the objective properties of things are understood as such. Hence the symbolism of the dynamic unconscious.

Before turning to autism, I should like to acknowledge the theoretical contribution of Leslie (1987). Leslie has drawn attention to the connection between a child's developing "theory of mind" and his capacity for symbolic play. His suggestion that each of these phenomena reflects the child's "metarepresentational capacity" has contributed to the ideas presented here. This said, there are radical divergences between Leslie's view and my own. Leslie has considered the metarepresentational capacity to be essentially cognitive in nature and biologically determined (see also Frith, 1985). I believe that a child's understanding of persons— and I think it is misleading to call this a "theory of mind"—arises on the basis of relations that are affective–conative as well as cognitive in nature, and that a cognitively efficacious metarepresentational capacity stems from, rather than predisposes to, a dawning awareness of the intensional relations between other people and the world. I have tried to highlight some of the innately determined factors that contribute to the developmental process leading to this emergent capacity.

Thus, to work backwards: The development of mature forms of symbolizing activity—and of course there are many different kinds of symbols, not least within the realm of verbal language itself—depends upon the infant's experience of a world of shared feelings and patterns of activity with others, especially adults (see also Bates, 1979). This sharing can only occur when there is biologically based intraindividual coordination of patterns of perception, feeling, and action in both infant and caretaker. Symbols develop only when more primitive signals are effective in shaping feeling and action between infant and caretaker.

The account I have given is relevant for an understanding of the development of language, in relation not only to word meanings but also to language use. The importance of prelinguistic interpersonal coordination for the evolving patterns of language has been most eloquently stated by Bruner (e.g., 1975, 1978). I merely emphasize here that the "pragmatics" of language—the use of language in context (Bates, 1976)—reflects an individual's capacity to orient himself in diverse ways to both people and the nonpersonal world. An utterance will be appropriate only to the extent that the speaker has oriented himself to the nature of the listener, to the listener's orientation to the speaker, and to the relation of both speaker and listener to that which is being expressed or spoken about. In other words, an individual's proficiency in expressing and comprehending the pragmatic aspects of language is one index of his interpersonal role-taking capacities.

I have dwelt at length on matters of normal development. Only when we understand the nature of personal relatedness shall we understand the social disability of autistic children. And only when we understand what it means to abstract and symbolize, and to use language, can we come to understand these children's cognitive impairments. I now consider each aspect of the developmental account given above as it pertains to autistic children, and thereby arrive at a developmental theory of autism.

THE CASE OF AUTISM

Affect and Nonverbal Communication

There is abundant clinical description of autistic children's abnormalities in the expression of emotion, and in the ways they react or fail to react to expressions of emotion in others (see, e.g., Cohen, 1980; Kanner, 1943; Ricks & Wing, 1975; Rutter, 1985). Ricks and Wing (1975) suggested that in their facial expressions, for example, autistic children tend to show only the extremes of emotion, sometimes in ways that are inappropriate for their age and the social situation. Ricks (1975) demonstrated how in situations of requesting, frustration, greeting, and pleased surprise, young autistic children's vocalizations were highly idiosyncratic and quite unlike those of nonautistic children. In an experiment by Langdell (1981), judges rated autistic children's attempts to make happy and sad faces as poor. In an observational study by Attwood (1984), both autistic and nonautistic children were noted to display gestures in the course of their social interactions with peers, but the autistic children were exceptional in that they produced no gestural expressions of emotion. Therefore clinical and experimental studies are in agreement that facial expressions, gestures, and vocalizations expressive of emotion are probably abnormal and often idiosyncratic in autistic children. Although the evidence is not conclusive, it is nevertheless highly suggestive that such abnormality is manifested in autistic children of all ages and IQ levels, and is relatively independent of cognitive ability. Autistic children seem to lack the normal child's intraindividual coordination of affective expression and behavior. I have already emphasized the importance of this for the patterning of behavior and experience between child and adult, especially if they are to share feelings.

As I have also remarked earlier, there has been surprisingly little experimental investigation of autistic children's impairments in perceiving and reacting to, and in understanding, emotional expression in others. Langdell (1981) reported that relative to age- and IQ-matched nonautistic children, a group of young autistic children were less able to sort photographed faces into those that were "happy" and those that were "sad." We (Weeks & Hobson, 1987) reported a similar finding, *en passant*, and in our experiment autistic and same-age nonautistic retarded children were matched for verbal ability, so providing a more stringent test for the dissociation of such disability from intellectual impairment. This latter study involved a picture-sorting task in which subjects could sort photographs of the heads and faces of people according to their emotional expressions or the types of hats they were wearing. The principal finding was that the majority of nonautistic children sorted according to people's facial expressions before they sorted according to types of hats, but most autistic children gave priority to sorting by types of hats. By the end of the experiment, all 15 nonautistic children had sorted by emotional expressions without being told to do so, but only 6 of the 15 autistic children had done this, and 5 of the 15 autistic children failed to sort consistently by facial expressions even after explicit instruction. Thus it appears that facial expressions of emotion are less salient, and probably less discriminable, for autistic than for nonautistic children.

In order to capture some of the aliveness of faces and other emotional expressions, I (Hobson, 1982a, 1982b, 1986a) employed a videotape-and-picture technique to test whether autistic and matched normal and nonautistic retarded children could select an appropriate drawn or photographed facial expression of emotion to go with enacted gestures, vocalizations, or emotion-provoking situations. In an accompanying task, children were asked to judge comparable videotapes of four nonpersonal objects. The results were that neither autistic nor control subjects had difficulty in judging the appearances, sounds, and contexts of nonpersonal objects, but the autistic children were markedly less able to recognize which facial expression of emotion was the appropriate one to accompany a given gesture, vocalization, or context. Given that the children of both groups could recognize the different aspects of the nonpersonal objects, it remains to be established whether autistic children matched with nonautistic children for ability on the recognition of more subtle "thing-related" perceptual features would still show more impairment in emotion recognition than control subjects. Studies on this issue are currently in progress. There was also a question of whether the results might reflect autistic children's difficulties in judging faces per se. In a further experiment (Hobson, 1986b), groups of autistic and matched nonautistic retarded children were asked to choose drawings of emotionally expressive gestures to correspond with videotaped gestures, and then to match those drawings with videotaped faces and vocalizations. Again the autistic children were significantly impaired, even in choosing drawn gestures for vocalizations—a task in which facial expressions played no part. Autistic children appear to lack a readiness to perceive intraindividual coordination of affective expression in others. They seem not to recognize the "signal properties" of other people, nor to apprehend normally coherent patterns of feelings. One probable result is that they fail to participate in the coordinated patterns of feeling and action that usually occur between people. In particular, as Murray (1984) has noted, autistic children may lack appropriate regulation of affective states in relation to the behavior of others.

The above-described abnormality that reflects their expressive and/or receptive incapacities—that of imitation. For instance, Curcio (1978) and Dawson and Adams (1984) reported that autistic children were less adept on the Uzgiris–Hunt Gestural Imitation Scale, which tests for imitation of actions ranging from banging a hammer to wrinkling the nose, than they were on tests of the recognition of object permanence. Dawson and Adams (1984) noted that the children who were more able to imitate were also those who exhibited more social behavior. The upshot of these and other studies (e.g., DeMyer, 1975; Hammes & Langdell, 1981; Tubbs, 1966; Wing, 1969, 1971) is that there is plentiful evidence for autistic children's difficulties in imitating a diversity of actions, but they also have some abilities in this regard which may be susceptible to further development through sensitive intervention (Dawson & Galpert, 1986).

The above-described deficits in nonverbal communication appear to be basic to autism. I suggest how these impairments, which have both an individual and a social dimension, may underlie much of autistic children's cognitive and language disability. I begin by making brief reference to autistic children's limitations in explicitly social understanding.

Knowledge of Persons

If we wish to consider how much autistic children understand about the nature of other people, and to examine the way they have constructed or failed to construct a concept of persons (Hobson, 1983), we need to bear in mind the different forms of understanding that one person can have about another. I have addressed this issue earlier in the chapter. Clinical accounts reveal how patchy is the autistic child's knowledge, even sense, of other people (and see Tustin, 1981, for a psychodynamic perspective). This becomes particularly striking when an autistic individual is able to describe his own struggles to comprehend other human beings. Thus a patient described by Rutter (1983) complained that he couldn't "mind-read," and an autistic man of my acquaintance who had A levels (a rough American equivalent would be high advanced-placement test scores) in English and German could not grasp what a "friend" is. The autistic individual seems unable to fathom the nature of other people's relatedness to the world and to each other.

More recently, experimental evidence has begun to emerge that might begin to specify more exactly what autistic children do or do not understand of the experiences of others. One experiment (Hobson, 1984) provided evidence that they are relatively adept at inferring the visual–spatial perspectives of others. This indicates how there are aspects of the visually perceived world that autistic and nonautistic individuals share in common, so that autistic children do have some notion of what it means for others to "see." To contrast with this, an experiment by Baron-Cohen, Leslie, and Frith (1985) illustrated how autistic children may fail to understand or focus upon the "beliefs" of another being (in the form of a doll). In further studies, Baron-Cohen, Leslie, and Frith (1986) and I (Hobson, 1986b) have demonstrated how autistic children's lack of understanding of "Intentional" and emotion-related events may contrast with their grasp of other aspects of events involving people, perhaps especially events that children might learn to recognize by observing relatively stereotyped patterns of behavior "from the outside." Of course, what autistic children do or do not understand about people is of direct clinical relevance (Lord, 1984).

These clinical observations and experimental findings may be understood to reflect autistic children's restricted experience of personal relations. For autistic children seem to lack the bodily, especially affective, relatedness to other people on which a knowledge of persons is founded. This disability may extend to a limited recognition of others as agents, so they respond to the hand, not the person, acting on them (Kanner, 1943). They may acquire a largely impersonal knowledge of persons. For instance, one autistic child was heard to say of the crying of another, "He is making a funny noise." This is an uncanny echo of Scheler's (1954) remark, noted earlier, that one may look at the face of a crying child as a merely physical object.

Prima facie, such deficits seem to have only a tenuous relationship with such basic cognitive faculties as the capacities to abstract and symbolize. I have already argued that on the contrary, a normal child's conative–affective relations—specifically, his relations with other persons—have a direct bearing on the way his thinking develops. This argument is given added force when autistic children's cognitive development is taken into account. It is to this that I now turn.

The Capacities to Abstract and Symbolize

Hermelin and O'Connor concluded the 1970 summary of their work with the statement that "we regard the inability of autistic children to encode stimuli meaningfully as their basic cognitive deficit" (p. 129). These authors emphasized how autistic children tend to impose stimulus-independent, simple, rigid, and repetitive patterns on random as well as on structured, meaningful input. As Hermelin (personal communication, July 1984) has said, however, a number of the findings may be taken to exemplify not the causes but the results of an incapacity to think symbolically. Rutter (e.g., 1983) has interpreted the performance of autistic children on standardized IQ tests (e.g., Lockyer & Rutter, 1970) as indicative of a deficit in verbal sequencing and abstraction skills. Thus, one important level of explanation of autistic children's cognitive dysfunction is that which encompasses their difficulties with abstraction.

I suggest that this disability, although cognitive in many of its implications, is essentially affective–conative and/or social in origin, and is manifested in a variety of forms on successive developmental levels as autistic children mature. Early in development, it is reflected in their failure to connect aspects of experience and a delay in the emergence of symbolism; subsequently, it is evident in the children's rigid patterns of thinking, as seen (for example) in their language, play, and nonlinguistic cognitive performance. For the capacity to think abstractly and to symbolize is the primary source of creative, flexible thinking and imagination (Langer, 1957).

So what do we mean by autistic children's relative inability to abstract? As Klin (1986) has recently emphasized, the classic examination of an autistic individual's "concrete thinking" is that of Scheerer, Rothmann, and Goldstein (1945). Scheerer *et al.* reported that up to 15 years of age, their patient (L.) was "unable to define the properties of objects independent of ego-centered and situational use" (p. 9), so that the few words he could define were described in terms of how he could manipulate them (e.g., an envelope was "something that I put in with"). L. could neither grasp nor formulate similarities, differences, or absurdities, nor could he understand metaphor. When asked, "What would happen if you shot a person?", he replied, "He goes to the hospital" (p. 13; for similar examples, see Ricks & Wing, 1975; Wing, 1969, 1981). In addition, autistic children often fail to generalize the application of linguistic terms and nonlinguistic skills to further contexts in which those terms or skills would be appropriate (e.g., Kanner, 1943).

Scheerer *et al.* (1945) suggested that all of the examples given above and several other of L.'s deficits were attributable to an "impairment of abstract attitude" (p. 27). I believe that this formulation is highly apposite, suggesting as it does that the individual's attitude or mode of relating to the world is at the heart of the matter. For if autistic children do not have the inborn capacity to respond with those patterns of action and feeling that normally serve to connect one thing with another, and if moreover they fail to connect with other people and with others' relations to the world, then their attitude to their surroundings will remain anchored to particulars, lacking in depth, and often fixed in orientation.

Consider the way the autistic person is embedded in context. Scheerer *et al.* (1945) made an explicit link between L.'s "characteristic difficulty in shifting and rigidity" (p. 27), and that of cortically brain-damaged adults. But as Erard (1985) has argued, the concrete thinking of amnesic aphasic and indeed schizophrenic patients is not to be defined in terms of a failure to abstract from concrete *contents* of experience in the sense of individual, palpable, or perceptually given objects, but rather in terms of these patients' fixedness in immediate, unintegrated contexts of experience, often affectively determined. Such patients are overwhelmed by the immediate sensory–motor–affective experience of the moment, and are unable to sustain a frame of reference that transcends this single-minded perspective. Compared with this, the concrete thinking of autistic children seems to be in a class of its own.

First, Scheerer *et al.* (1945) noted that L. seemed to have particular difficulties in drawing analogies when abstract words (e.g., "sight," "difficult," "future") were presented in the words tested, and clinical descriptions such as that of Ricks and Wing (1975) may suggest that the concrete, perceptually given content *is* a significant feature in the thinking of autistic children. Thus one might contrast the schizophrenic patient who took the black color of doors to signify "dying," or another who saw the twisted legs of a table as meaning that the whole world was twisted (cited in Werner & Kaplan, 1963, p. 256), with the autistic child who, when asked if he had lost his tongue, anxiously started to search for it (Ricks & Wing, 1975, p. 210). In the former cases, the patients' associations were themselves emotionally charged and highly abstract, whereas in the latter case, the autistic child's emotional response resulted from but was not integral to his focus upon the perceptually given content of the metaphorical expression.

Second, it is not merely that autistic children are fixed for a time in one of many potential standpoints *vis-à-vis* a given situation, as is the case for other kinds of patients who think concretely: rather, there seem to be very few standpoints that they are ever able to adopt, and these are generally matter-of-fact in nature. Their rigidity is in many cases stable over long periods of time, apparently because they have few alternative perspectives to shift to. Although Scheerer *et al.* (1945) suggested that L. sometimes produced egocentric speech pertaining to subjective emotional experience, in most of the examples they cited it was L.'s nonemotional actions that seemed to determine the way he construed a given event or object. Weigl's (1941) description of concrete thinking applies very well to the autistic child, whose experience seems to reflect not only "a definite organization within a given unreflectively experienced sphere" (p. 32), but also the limited nature and range of his spheres of experience. Like other patients with concrete thinking, autistic children are limited in their ability to "construct a stable, categorical frame of reference that transcends the immediate context of experience" (Erard, 1985, p. 112), but in their case this context of experience is uniquely impoverished. Weigl (1941) suggested that we may better understand the processes of abstraction if we increase our knowledge of "those processes by means of which 'sorting according to *various* points of view' is accomplished" (p. 7), and it is to this that I now turn.

I have suggested that the autistic child's failure to integrate his experiences across a variety of times and settings is not the cause but the result of an impairment in abstract attitude. And in opposition to the view of Scheerer *et al.* (1945), I further suggest that the social impairments of autistic children are the cause rather than the result of this "intellectual" disability. According to Scheerer *et al.*, L.'s impairment in abstract attitude "underlies his lack of social awareness and of curiosity in people, his limited values, his inability to register or absorb anything of the socio-cultural and interhuman matrix around him, of all that has significance for a normal child" (p. 27). It is no doubt true that the incapacitating effects of an inability to abstract will extend to the person's social as well as nonsocial understanding. Yet I wish to argue that it is the autistic child's lack of affective and social awareness, together with his inability to register much of the human matrix around him, that determines his inability to abstract.

How does the normal child come to recognize and flexibly adopt various points of view? As I have already argued in the case of learning the meaning of words, he comes to relate to others' ways of relating to the world. In the case of language learning, he is thereby enabled to discover the appropriate use of words. This includes the use of "I" and "you," since he recognizes the relation of the speaker's use of "I" to the speaker's actions, feelings, and so on, and the speaker's use of "you" to the speaker's current relationship to the child as addressee (Charney, 1981). In the case of learning to adopt the abstract attitude, the child is introduced to the many ways in which others can take up attitudes to a shared world, and is induced to reflect on the variety of his own attitudes. These attitudes may apply to perceptual selectivities, conceptual groupings, affective responses, propensities to action, or many other aspects of relatedness. The shared world is also a multiply referenced world, once the child is aware of the intentions, thoughts, feelings, and so forth, of others and himself. Thus a feature of social intercoordination can become an intrapsychic capacity, in the manner Vygotsky (1962) described.

The situation is different for the autistic child. He does not have the normal child's affective responsiveness to features of the world, so he does not arrive at the usual affectively or conatively determined groupings. He is not attuned to his caretaker's expressions of affect, nor can she be attuned to his, for his own mode of relating to the world does not correspond with hers (recall Russell's [1984] point about the similarity of normal infants' and adults' intensional worlds). He does not reach the stage of recognizing the commonality between himself and others as persons, and so he does not come to relate to others' ways of relating to the world—especially to others' intensional relations—except in very limited ways. As a result, he is not introduced to the manifold ways of "taking" an object, and is rooted to a single, inflexible perspective. As a further result, he cannot grasp that one thing or event might have its own, quasi-intensional relation to other objects or events; he cannot take things as symbolic.

In relation to this, Ricks and Wing (1975) have provided a most valuable review of autistic children's impairments in a range of symbolizing activities. I confine myself here to a few observations on two areas of especial importance, those of symbolic play and language.

Symbolic Play

In an epidemiological study of mentally handicapped children, Wing, Gould, Yeates, and Brierley (1977) observed that children with a language comprehension mental age under 20 months did not demonstrate symbolic representational play which was flexible and varied in theme. Those children with no symbolic play, but with a mental age of over 20 months on nonverbal tasks, all manifested features of autism. In a further report, Wing and Gould (1979) described how there was a marked tendency for social impairments, repetitive stereotyped behavior, and an absence or abnormality of language and symbolic activities to occur together in "the triad of social and language impairment" (Wing, 1981). Nevertheless, in these and related studies (e.g., Riguet, Taylor, Benaroya, & Klein, 1981; Sigman & Ungerer, 1984; Ungerer & Sigman, 1981), it has been repeatedly noted that many autistic children do have at least some limited capacity to symbolize, but in such cases the quality of play seems to be sterile and ritualized (Wulff, 1985).

As I have already indicated, the "triad of social and language impairment" may best be understood in terms of a primary social-affective impairment which leads to deficits in symbolizing and to stereotyped behavior.

Language

I have argued that autistic children have impaired capacity for signal-dependent nonverbal communication, and that a relative inability to symbolize is one ultimate consequence of this. What of those autistic children who do achieve some recognition of the nature of symbols, and acquire receptive and expressive verbal abilities? I believe that those of the children's limitations that have constrained the development of language at all, and specifically their limited experience of a "coreferenced" world, are now reflected on a higher plane in the pattern of language they produce and comprehend. I shall give a few illustrations of what I mean.

A convenient place to start is with autistic children's performance on tests that are considered to evaluate language or language-related abilities. A number of studies (e.g., DeMyer, 1975; Lockyer & Rutter, 1970) have demonstrated that it is particularly on the Peabody Picture Vocabulary Test and those parts of the Wechsler Intelligence Scale for Children (WISC) that test general comprehension (e.g., "What is the thing to do when you cut your finger?" and "What is the thing to do if a boy much smaller than yourself starts to fight with you?"), vocabulary (e.g., "What does fur mean?"), and similarities (e.g., "In what way are a cat and mouse alike?") that autistic children show marked impairment, even in relation to matched receptive dysphasic children (Bartak, Rutter, & Cox, 1975), whereas on tests of digit span and information (e.g., "How many days in a week?") they are relatively less impaired. As both Gillies (1965) and Lockyer and Rutter (1970) observed, moreover, autistic children tend to find most difficulty on the Performance subtests of the WISC when they are asked to arrange a sequence of pictures so that they "tell a story"; and Tymchuk, Simmons, and Neafsey (1977) reported similar deficits on Picture Arrangement as well as on Comprehension in childhood psychotics with high verbal ability (see also Hermelin & Frith, 1971).

The question arises: What do these results signify? Among those autistic children who develop language, what can their specific profile of deficits tell us about what constrains their language development? I should like to suggest two ways in which one might approach such questions. The first is to consider the degree to which particular tests require a child to be able to address himself appropriately to the form of a question, and to the way in which the examiner intends the question, as well as to specific word meanings. A child must understand the speaker's (or implicit speaker's) meaning, as well as the question's meaning, if he is to give adequate responses to questions on similarities, or is to provide elaborate (i.e., multifaceted) replies to questions on vocabulary. The second, related approach is to consider the degree to which tests require the child to understand personal, social, and cultural meanings, and moreover to select the most relevant of these for a response to the particular orientation of the examiner and her questions. This is most obviously important for a child's responses to questions of so-called "general comprehension." The examples cited above illustrate how the comprehension tested is really not "general" at all, but is very much concerned with an understanding of conduct appropriate for social situations.

The point here is that it is only in part that these and other tests are tests of verbal ability; they are also tests of social understanding. The social understanding is not only one that applies to the meaning of certain words taken out of context, but more particularly it is an understanding of the ways in which context bears upon the meaning of words. When an autistic child is asked, "What is the thing to do when you cut your finger?", and he replies, "Bleed," he is unusual in the way he takes up the question and in what he supposes the question to be about. Only partly is he making a "verbal" mistake.

But what of autistic children's failures in tests of vocabulary, such as the Peabody Picture Vocabulary Test (Dunn, 1965)? The children's performance here is an index of their difficulty in learning words. Once again, I suggest that this difficulty results from limitations in their social understanding. For in order to learn words, a child needs to pick up those aspects of the world that are being "named" by another person in a variety of contexts. He needs to infer what the other person has in mind. As I have already discussed, a normal child is able to judge what is at the focus of another's interests, concerns, feelings, intentions, and so on, for two reasons: first, because there is a correspondence between the *kinds* of interests, concerns, and so forth, of the other and those of the child himself, so that the child is often correct in what he surmises to be in the other's mind; and second, because he is sensitive to direct and indirect cues from the other that serve to indicate what the speaker is focusing upon. Autistic children are at a severe disadvantage in both respects. It is not surprising that much of what they hear seems to lack the necessary anchorage in a perspective shared between adult and child for the adult's sounds to become the child's meaningful words (see also Lord, 1985).

In keeping with the argument already outlined, therefore, it may be suggested that autistic children's impaired verbal ability arises on the basis of their incomprehension of the nature of other human beings and their corresponding lack of coordinated reference with others. They are insufficiently primed to grasp what an adult is naming. All this is in addition to their relative failure to recognize and benefit from the flexibility and richness of the symbolic attitude.

Of course, the referential function of words is only one among many roles that words play. There are many different ways in which words are embedded in the patterns of conduct and "forms of life" of children and adults (Wittgenstein, 1953). Whether or not an autistic child grasps particular kinds of linguistic meaning will depend upon the degree to which he shares each kind of meaning with the people from whom he learns language. If this account is correct, one would expect that in certain conceptual or semantic domains, where there is congruence between the perspective of autistic and nonautistic individuals, autistic children might learn to use words in much the same way as do nonautistic children, whereas in other areas of life this would not be so. Accordingly, a map of the autistic child's abilities and limitations in the comprehension and production of semantic or syntactic forms might represent the domains in which he shares nonautistic individuals' "forms of life," and highlight those areas in which the autistic child's experience is markedly divergent from normal. As Bosch (1970) has argued, "it is in the language and through the language in particular that the success and failure of the constitution of the common and own worlds are most impressively revealed" (p. 61). Thus, in a well-controlled experiment on the conceptual basis for referential word meaning, Tager-Flusberg (1985) examined the range of referents to which autistic, nonautistic retarded, and normal children, matched for verbal mental age on the Peabody, applied particular words. All of the words referred to concrete objects—for example, kinds of birds, boats, food, or tools. The children's task was to indicate whether a pictured object was an instance of a particular word, or to select from an array of pictures those that belonged to the category named. The experiment was designed so that the ways in which children overextended and underextended the use of the words could be studied. The results were that the pattern of performance was the same in all three groups of children. In these semantic domains, therefore, autistic children at the same general level of vocabulary as nonautistic children were not applying idiosyncratic word meanings. There are two important qualifications to this conclusion, however. First, the range of meanings of the particular words under examination was limited: The children had to judge whether any pictured object was one of a class. It does not follow that the autistic children could recognize all kinds of meanings that even concrete objects such as boats or food might have for nonautistic children—for example, the meaning of boats as sources of recreation or livelihood, as vehicles used for discovery or warfare, as symbols of the female body, and so on. Second, the range of words was itself narrow, limited to what the author called "concrete objects." Even if we are conservative in drawing conclusions about the way in which knowledge of such meanings is organized in autistic children, these conclusions may not apply to other semantic domains. It is time that this was studied systematically. I shall only repeat a mention of autistic children's difficulties with personal pronouns, and the patient who could not understand the meaning of the word "friend." These phenomena may be understood in terms of the autistic person's failure to understand the nature of an "I" who exists in personal relation with a "you."

Finally, in recent years there has been increasing emphasis upon autistic children's "pragmatic" language disability (e.g., Baltaxe, 1977; Cromer, 1981; Fay & Schuler, 1980; Olley, 1985; Tager-Flusberg, 1981). For example, Baltaxe (1977) has provided a descriptive account of some ways in which the language of autistic adolescents illustrates their failure to observe speaker–hearer role relationships, to understand the rules of conduct that govern a dialogue, and to differentiate new and background information. In keeping with the view already outlined, it may be appropriate to consider such deficits as linguistic markers of an essentially social-cultural impairment—an impairment in adopting appropriate points of view or frames of reference—rather than an intrinsically "linguistic" disorder. I refer the reader to the relevant points made by Russell (1984) and Dore (1985), cited earlier in the chapter. It is also of note that autistic children who do understand means–ends relations may nevertheless fail to demonstrate those "pragmatic" actions that Bates (e.g., 1979) called "social tool use," especially in showing objects to others (Curcio, 1978), although general retardation may be a factor here (Lobato, Barrera, & Feldman, 1981). Even autistic children who reach the final stages of sensory–motor development often manifest impairments in symbolic play and language (Wetherby & Gaines, 1982; Wetherby & Prutting, 1984). Cognitive development appears to be insufficient for "pragmatic" and symbolic development. The development of an understanding of the nature of people may be crucial.

CONCLUSION: A THEORY OF AUTISM

The theory I have developed in this chapter is founded on the views of Kanner (1943) and Bosch (1970). Autistic children have a biologically based impairment of affective–conative relatedness with the environment, which has especially far-reaching implications for their social relations. The defining characteristic of autism is a uniquely severe disruption in the children's personal relatedness with others. They have a largely impersonal relation with other people.

From this starting point, we can move to other levels of explanation. What are the nature and origins of the impairments in personal relatedness? Autistic children seem to lack the coordination of sensory–motor–affective behavior and experience that is a usual feature of intraindividual as well as interindividual mental life. They lack the preparedness to respond to the "signal properties" of the world, and especially of other people, with coherent patterns of action and bodily expression. Neurologically, subcortical structures and especially the limbic system have an essential role in the genesis of such behavioral patterns, and it is probable that dysfunction of these structures is a common cause of autism (Damasio & Maurer, 1978). This need not always be the case, however. What is necessary is that, functionally, autistic children lack the modes of interpersonal coordination of action and feeling that are essential for personal contact. Thus severe receptive disabilities such as congenital blindness may predispose a child to autism (Keeler, 1958; Wing, 1969). But the "personal category" of experience and relatedness is a highly robust property of human psychology. Autism is a rare and profound disorder. For most autistic children, the deficit is at once productive and receptive.

The sensory–motor–affective impairment leads to abnormalities in the ways autistic children are active in "taking" reality. One result is that they fail to connect things with one another according to similarities in their experiences of each. For this reason, autistic children have deficits in the capacity to abstract, even on a primitive level. In addition, they are unable to participate in the affective life of others, and so to construct a knowledge of persons as persons. Lacking prereflective, biologically determined modes of intensionality, they fail to recognize not only the forms but also the objects of other people's feelings and sometimes actions. As a consequence of this, they are unable to grasp other people's mental orientations to reality, including their beliefs, wishes, thoughts, and so on.

So autistic children's inability to relate to other people as people includes a profound limitation in their capacity to relate to other people's modes of relating to the children themselves and to other aspects of the environment. Autistic children's relative inexperience of a world that is multiply referenced by others deprives them of the means to disengage from their immediate limited perspective and thereby to conceptualize in a flexible manner. One facet of this is their restricted grasp of the modes of relatedness that may apply between one thing or event and another, specifically the symbolic relation. As a result, autistic children suffer severe impairment in symbolic thinking and feeling. A further outcome is their disability in learning how to "mean" with words.

At the heart of this theory is the significance of autistic children's impaired affective relations with other people. The early work of Hermelin and O'Connor (1970) led the way in establishing that autistic children have specific cognitive deficits. In order to understand the nature of some of these deficits, and to arrive at a theory of autism, we need to reach beyond cognition.

Acknowledgments

I gratefully acknowledge my indebtedness to Beate Hermelin. I also thank Janet Ouston and Catherine Buckley.

References

Attwood, A. J. (1984). *The gestures of autistic children.* Unpublished doctoral dissertation, University of London.
Baltaxe, C. A. M. (1977). Pragmatic deficits in the language of autistic adolescents. *Journal of Pediatric Psychology, 2*(4), 176–180.

Baron-Cohen, S., Leslie, A. M. & Frith, U. (1985). Does the autistic child have a "theory of mind"? *Cognition, 21*, 37–46.

Baron-Cohen, S., Leslie, A. M. & Frith, U. (1986). Mechanical, behavioural and Intentional understanding of picture stories in autistic children. *British Journal of Developmental Psychology, 4*, 113–125.

Bartak, L., Rutter, M., & Cox, A. (1975). A comparative study of infantile autism and specific developmental receptive language disorder: I. The children. *British Journal of Psychiatry, 126*, 127–145.

Bates, E. (1976). Pragmatics and sociolinguistics in child language. In D. M. Morehead & A. E. Morehead (Eds.), *Normal and deficient child language* (pp. 411–463). Baltimore: University Park Press.

Bates, E. (1979). The emergence of symbols: Ontogeny and phylogeny. In W. A. Collins (Ed.), *Minnesota Symposium on Child Psychology: Vol. 12. Children's language and communication* (pp. 121–155). Hillsdale, NJ: Erlbaum.

Bettelheim, B. (1967). *The empty fortress.* New York: Free Press.

Blocker, H. (1969). Physiognomic perception. *Philosophy and Phenomenological Research, 29*, 377–390.

Bolton, N. (1977). *Concept formation.* Oxford: Pergamon Press.

Bosch, G. (1970). *Infantile autism* (D. Jordan & I. Jordan, Trans.). New York: Springer-Verlag.

Brentano, F. (1973). *Psychology from an empirical standpoint* (A. C. Rancurello, D. B. Terrell, & L. L. McAlister, Trans.). London: Routledge & Kegan Paul. (Original work published 1874)

Bruner, J. (1975). From communication to language—a psychological perspective. *Cognition, 3*(3), 255–287.

Bruner, J. (1978). Learning how to do things with words. In J. Bruner & A. Garton (Eds.), *Human growth and development* (pp. 62–84). Oxford: Clarendon Press.

Buber, M. (1958). *I and thou* (2nd ed., R. G. Smith, Trans.). Edinburgh: T. Clark & T. Clark.

Charlesworth, W. R., & Kreutzer, M. A. (1973). Facial expressions of infants and children. In P. Ekman (Ed.), *Darwin and facial expression.* New York: Academic Press.

Charney, R. (1981). Pronoun errors in autistic children: Support for a social explanation. *British Journal of Disorders of Communication, 15*(1), 39–43.

Chevalier-Skolnikoff, S. (1973). Facial expression of emotion in nonhuman primates. In P. Ekman (Ed.), *Darwin and facial expression* (pp. 11–89). New York: Academic Press.

Churchill, D. W. (1972). The relation of infantile autism and early childhood schizophrenia to developmental language disorders of childhood. *Journal of Autism and Childhood Schizophrenia, 2*, 182–197.

Cohen, D. J. (1980). The pathology of the self in primary childhood autism and Gilles de la Tourette syndrome. *Psychiatric Clinics of North America, 3*(3), 383–402.

Cromer, R. F. (1981). Developmental language disorders: Cognitive processes, semantics, pragmatics, phonology, and syntax. *Journal of Autism and Developmental Disorders, 11*(1), 57–74.

Curcio, F. (1978). Sensorimotor functioning and communication in mute autistic children. *Journal of Autism and Childhood Schizophrenia, 8*(3), 281–292.

Damasio, A. R., & Maurer, R. G. (1978). A neurological model for childhood autism. *Archives of Neurology, 35*, 777–786.

Darwin, C. (1965). *The expression of the emotions in man and animals.* Chicago: University of Chicago Press. (Original work published 1872)

Dawson, G., & Adams, A. (1984). Imitation and social responsiveness in autistic children. *Journal of Abnormal Child Psychology, 12*(2), 209–226.

Dawson, G., & Galpert, L. (1986). A developmental model for facilitating the social behavior of autistic children. In E. Schopler & G. Mesibov (Eds.), *Social problems in autism* (pp. 237–261). New York: Plenum.

DeMyer, M. K. (1975). The nature of the neuropsychological disability in autistic children. *Journal of Autism and Childhood Schizophrenia, 5*(2), 109–128.

DeMyer, M. K. (1976). Motor, perceptual–motor and intellectual disabilities of autistic children. In L. Wing (Ed.), *Early childhood autism* (2nd ed., pp. 169–193). Oxford: Pergamon Press.

Dore, J. (1985). Holophrases revisited: Their 'logical' development from dialog. In M. Barrett (Ed.), *Children's single-word speech* (pp. 23–58). Chichester, England: Wiley.

Dunn, L. M. (1965). *Expanded manual for the Peabody Picture Vocabulary Test*. Circle Pines, MN: American Guidance Service.

Ekman, P. (Ed.). (1982) *Emotion in the human face* (2nd ed.). Cambridge, England: Cambridge University Press.

Erard, R. E. (1985). Concrete thinking and the categorical attitude. In I. Fast (Ed.), *Event theory: A Piaget–Freud integration* (pp. 111–134). Hillsdale, NJ: Erlbaum.

Fay, W. H., & Schuler, A. L. (1980). *Emerging language in autistic children*. London: Edward Arnold.

Fein, D., Pennington, B., Markowitz, P., Braverman, M., & Waterhouse, L. (1986). Toward a neuropsychological model of infantile autism: Are the social deficits primary? *Journal of the American Academy of Child Psychiatry*, 25(2), 198–212.

Ferenczi, S. (1952). The ontogenesis of symbols. In *First contributions to psycho-analysis* (E. Jones, Trans.; pp. 276–281). London: Hogarth Press. (Original work published 1913).

Frijda, N. H. (1986). *The emotions*. New York: Cambridge University Press.

Frith, U. (1985). *A developmental model for autism*. Paper presented at Colloque International sur l'Autisme, Paris.

Gillies, S. (1965). Some abilities of psychotic children and subnormal controls. *Journal of Mental Deficiency Research*, 9, 89–101.

Habermas, J. (1970). Toward a theory of communicative competence. In H. P. Dreitzel (Ed.), *Recent sociology no. 2* (pp. 115–148). New York: Macmillan.

Hamlyn, D. W. (1974). Person-perception and our understanding of others. In T. Mischel (Ed.), *Understanding other persons* (pp. 1–36). Oxford: Blackwell.

Hammes, J. G. W., & Langdell, T. (1981). Precursors of symbol formation and childhood autism. *Journal of Autism and Developmental Disorders*, 11, 331–346.

Hampshire, S. (1976). Feeling and expression. In J. Glover (Ed.), *The philosophy of mind* (pp. 73–83). Oxford: Oxford University Press. (Original work published 1960)

Hermelin, B., & Frith, U. (1971). Psychological studies of childhood autism: Can autistic children make sense of what they see and hear? *Journal of Special Education*, 5, 1107–1117.

Hermelin, B., & O'Connor, N. (1970). *Psychological experiments with autistic children*. Oxford: Pergamon Press.

Hermelin, B., & O'Connor, N. (1985). Logico-affective states and non-verbal language. In E. Schopler & G. B. Mesibov (Eds.), *Communication problems in autism* (pp. 283–310). New York: Plenum.

Hobson, R. P. (1982a). The autistic children's concept of persons. In D. Park (Ed.), *Proceedings of the 1981 International Conference on Autism, Boston, U.S.A.* (pp. 97–102). Washington, DC: National Society for Children and Adults with Autism.

Hobson, R. P. (1982b, September). *The autistic child's knowledge of persons*. Paper presented at the conference of the Development Section of the British Psychological Society, Durham.

Hobson, R. P. (1983, May). *Origins of the personal relation, and the strange case of autism*. Paper presented at the meeting of the Association for Child Psychology and Psychiatry, London.

Hobson, R. P. (1984). Early childhood autism and the question of egocentrism. *Journal of Autism and Developmental Disorders*, 14(1), 85–104.

Hobson, R. P. (1985). Piaget: On the ways of knowing in childhood. In M. Rutter & L. Hersov (Eds.), *Child and adolescent psychiatry: Modern approaches* (pp. 191–203). Oxford: Blackwell.

Hobson, R. P. (1986a). The autistic child's appraisal of expressions of emotion. *Journal of Child Psychology and Psychiatry*, 27(3), 321–342.

Hobson, R. P. (1986b). The autistic child's appraisal of expressions of emotion: A further study. *Journal of Child Psychology and Psychiatry*, 27(5), 671–680.

Hoffman, M. L. (1975). Developmental synthesis of affect and cognition and its implications for altruistic motivation. *Developmental Psychology*, 11, 607–622.

Husserl, E. (1901). *Logische Untersuchungen* (Vol. 2). Halle, Germany: Niemeyer.

Izard, C. E. (1971). *The face of emotion*. New York: Appleton-Century-Crofts.

Kanner, L. (1943). Autistic disturbances of affective contact. *Nervous Child, 2,* 217–250.

Kaye, K. (1982). *The mental and social life of babies.* London: Methuen.

Keeler, W. R. (1958). Autistic patterns and affective communication in blind children with retrolental fibroplasia. In T. H. Hock & J. Zubin (Eds.), *Psychopathology of communication* (pp. 64–83). New York: Grune & Stratton.

Klin, A. (1986). *Infantile autism: Symptomatology, prognosis and epidemiology.* Unpublished manuscript, London School of Economics.

Klinnert, M. D., Campos, J. J., Sorce, J. F., Emde R. N., & Svejda, M. (1983). Emotions as behavior regulators: Social referencing in infancy. In R. Plutchik & H. Kellerman (Eds.), *Emotion: Theory, research and experience: Vol. 2. Emotions in early development* (pp. 57–86). New York: Academic Press.

Langdell, T. (1981). *Face perception: An approach to the study of autism.* Unpublished doctoral dissertation, University of London.

Langer, S. K. (1957). *Philosophy in a new key* (3rd ed.). Cambridge, MA: Harvard University Press.

Leslie, A. M. (1987). Pretense and representation: The origins of "theory of mind." *Psychological Review, 94*(4), 412–426.

Lobato, D., Barrera, R. D., & Feldman, R. S. (1981). Sensorimotor functioning and prelinguistic communication of severely and profoundly retarded individuals. *American Journal of Mental Deficiency, 85*(5), 489–496.

Lockyer, L., & Rutter, M. (1970). A five- to fifteen-year follow-up study of infantile psychosis: IV. Patterns of cognitive ability. *British Journal of Social and Clinical Psychology, 9,* 152–163.

Lord, C. (1984). The development of peer relations in children with autism. In F. J. Morrison, C. Lord, & D. P. Keating (Eds.), *Advances in applied developmental psychology* (pp. 165–229). New York: Academic Press.

Lord, C. (1985). Autism and the comprehension of language. In E. Schopler & G. Mesibov (Eds.), *Communication problems in autism* (pp. 257–281). New York: Plenum.

Macmurray, J. (1961). *Persons in relation.* London: Faber & Faber.

Mahler, M. S. (1968). *On human symbiosis and the vicissitudes of individuation.* New York: International Universities Press.

Malatesta, C. Z. (1981). Infant emotion and the vocal affect lexicon. *Motivation and Emotion, 5*(1), 1–23.

Merleau-Ponty, M. (1962). *Phenomenology of perception* (C. Smith, Trans.). London: Routledge & Kegan Paul.

Merleau-Ponty, M. (1964). The child's relations with others (W. Cobb, Trans.). In M. Merleau-Ponty, *The primacy of perception* (pp. 96–155). Evanston, IL: Northwestern University Press.

Murray, L. (1984). *Emotional regulation of intersubjective encounters: Implications for the theory of autism.* Paper presented at the Conference on Research in Autism, Paris.

Murray, L., & Trevarthen, C. (1985). Emotional regulation of interactions between two-month-olds and their mothers. In T. M. Field & N. A.Fox (Eds.), *Social perception in infants* (pp. 177–197). Norwood, NJ: Ablex.

Newson, J. (1979). The growth of shared understandings between infant and caregiver. In M. Bullowa (Ed.), *Before speech* (pp. 207–222). Cambridge, England: Cambridge University Press.

Olley, J. G. (1985). Social aspects of communication in children with autism. In E. Schopler & G. B. Mesibov (Eds.), *Communication problems in autism* (pp. 311–328). New York: Plenum.

Piaget, J. (1972). *The principles of genetic epistemology* (W. Mays, Trans.). London: Routledge & Kegan Paul. (Original work published 1970)

Piaget, J., & Inhelder, B. (1969). *The psychology of the child* (H. Weaver, Trans.). London: Routledge & Kegan Paul.

Polanyi, M. (1965). The structure of consciousness. *Brain, 88,* 799–810.

Ricks, D. M. (1975). Vocal communication in pre-verbal normal and autistic children. In N. O'Connor (Ed.), *Language, cognitive deficits, and retardation* (pp. 75–80). London: Butterworths.

Ricks, D. (1979). Making sense of experience to make sensible sounds. In M. Bullowa (Ed.), *Before speech* (pp. 245–268). Cambridge, England: Cambridge University Press.

Ricks, D. M., & Wing, L. (1975). Language, communication and the use of symbols in normal and autistic children. *Journal of Autism and Childhood Schizophrenia, 5*(3), 191–221.

Riguet, C. B., Taylor, N. D., Benaroya, S., & Klein, L. S. (1981). Symbolic play in autistic, Down's and normal children of equivalent mental age. *Journal of Autism and Developmental Disorders, 11*(4), 439–448.

Rimland, B. (1964). *Infantile autism.* New York: Appleton-Century-Crofts.

Russell, J. (1984). The subject–object division in language acquisition and ego development. *New Ideas in Psychology, 2,* 57–74.

Ruttenberg, B. A. A. (1971). A psychoanalytic understanding of infantile autism and its treatment. In D. W. Churchill, G. D. Alpern, & M. K. DeMyer (Eds.), *Infantile autism* (pp. 145–184). Springfield, IL: Charles C Thomas.

Rutter, M. (1968). Concepts of autism: A review of research. *Journal of Child Psychology and Psychiatry, 9,* 1–25.

Rutter, M. (1972). Childhood schizophrenia reconsidered. *Journal of Autism and Childhood Schizophrenia, 2,* 315–337.

Rutter, M. (1983). Cognitive deficits in the pathogenesis of autism. *Journal of Child Psychology and Psychiatry, 24*(4), 513–531.

Rutter, M. (1985). Infantile autism and other pervasive developmental disorders. In M. Rutter & L. Hersov (Eds.), *Child and adolescent psychiatry: Modern approaches* (pp. 545–566). Oxford: Blackwell.

Ryle, G. (1949). *The concept of mind.* Harmondsworth, England: Penguin.

Scheerer, M., Rothmann, E. & Goldstein, K. (1945). A case of "idiot savant": An experimental study of personality organization. *Psychological Monographs, 58,* 4(Whole No. 269), 1–63.

Scheler, M. (1954). *The nature of sympathy* (P. Heath, Trans.). London: Routledge & Kegan Paul.

Schopler, E. (1965). Early infantile autism and receptor processes. *Archives of General Psychiatry, 13,* 327–335.

Searle, J. R. (1979). What is an Intentional state? *Mind, 88*(349), 74–92.

Sigman, M., & Ungerer, J. A. (1984). Cognitive and language skills in autistic, mentally retarded, and normal children. *Developmental Psychology, 20,* 293–302.

Simner, M. L. (1971). Newborn's response to the cry of another infant. *Developmental Psychology, 5,* 136–150.

Stern, D. (1977). *The first relationship: Infant and mother.* Glasgow: Fontana/Open Books.

Stern, D., Hofer, L., Haft, W., & Dore, J. (1984). Affect attunement: The sharing of feeling states between mother and infant by means of inter-modal fluency. In T. Field & N. Fox (Eds.), *Social perception in infants* (pp. 249–268). Norwood, NJ: Ablex.

Tager-Flusberg, H. (1981). On the nature of linguistic functioning in early infantile autism. *Journal of Autism and Developmental Disorders, 11*(1), 45–56.

Tager-Flusberg, H. (1985). The conceptual basis for referential word meaning in children with autism. *Child Development, 56,* 1167–1178.

Tubbs, V. K. (1966). Types of linguistic disability in psychotic children. *Journal of Mental Deficiency Research, 10,* 230–240.

Tustin, F. (1972). *Autism and childhood psychosis.* London: Hogarth Press.

Tustin, F. (1981). *Autistic states in children.* London: Routledge & Kegan Paul.

Tymchuk, A. J., Simmons, J. Q., & Neafsey, S. (1977). Intellectual characteristics of adolescent childhood psychotics with high verbal ability. *Journal of Mental Deficiency Research, 21,* 133–138.

Ungerer, J. A., & Sigman, M. (1981). Symbolic play and language comprehension in autistic children. *Journal of the American Academy of Child Psychiatry, 20,* 318–337.

Vygotsky, L. S. (1962). *Thought and language* (E. Hanfmann & G. Vakar, Trans.). Cambridge, MA: MIT Press.

Walker, A. S. (1982). Intermodal perception of expressive behaviors by human infants. *Journal of Experimental Child Psychology, 33,* 514–535.

Weeks, S. J., & Hobson, R. P. (1987). The salience of facial expression for autistic children. *Journal of Child Psychology and Psychiatry, 28*(1), 137–152.

Weigl, E. (1941). On the psychology of so-called processes of abstraction (M. J. Rioch, Trans.). *Journal of Abnormal and Social Psychology, 36,* 3–33.

Werner, H. (1948). *Comparative psychology of mental development.* Chicago: Follett.

Werner, H., & Kaplan, B. (1963). *Symbol formation.* New York: Wiley.

Wetherby, A. M., & Gaines, B. H. (1982). Cognition and language development in autism. *Journal of Speech and Hearing Disorders, 47,* 63–70.

Wetherby, A. M., & Prutting, C. A. (1984). Profiles of communicative and cognitive–social abilities in autistic children. *Journal of Speech and Hearing Research, 27,* 364–377.

Wing, L. (1969). The handicaps of autistic children—a comparative study. *Journal of Child Psychology and Psychiatry, 10,* 1–40.

Wing, L. (1971). Perceptual and language development in autistic children: A comparative study. In M. Rutter (Ed.), *Infantile autism: Concepts, characteristics and treatment* (pp. 173–195). Edinburgh: Churchill Livingstone.

Wing, L. (1981). Language, social, and cognitive impairments in autism and severe mental retardation. *Journal of Autism and Developmental Disorders, 11*(1), 31–44.

Wing, L., & Gould, J. (1979). Severe impairments of social interaction and associated abnormalities in children: Epidemiology and classification. *Journal of Autism and Developmental Disorders, 9*(1), 11–29.

Wing, L., Gould, J., Yeates, S. R., & Brierly, L. M. (1977). Symbolic play in severely mentally retarded and in autistic children. *Journal of Child Psychology and Psychiatry, 18,* 167–178.

Wittgenstein, L. (1953). *Philosophical investigations* (G. E. M. Anscombe, Trans.). Oxford: Blackwell.

Wittgenstein, L. (1980). *Remarks on the philosophy of psychology* (Vol. 1, G. E. M. Anscombe, Trans.). Oxford: Blackwell.

Wolf, D., & Gardner, H. (1981). On the structure of early symbolization. In R. L. Schiefelbusch & D. D. Bricker (Eds.), *Early language: Acquisition and intervention* (pp. 287–327). Baltimore: University Park Press.

Wulff, S. B. (1985). The symbolic and object play of children with autism: A review. *Journal of Autism and Developmental Disorders, 15*(2), 139–148.

CHAPTER 3

Arousal, Attention, and the Socioemotional Impairments of Individuals with Autism

GERALDINE DAWSON
ARTHUR LEWY
University of Washington

It is well recognized that autistic children attend to their environments in unusual ways. Perhaps of most concern is their abnormal attention to people. In many instances, they appear oblivious to others and, despite bids for attention from those around them, fail to pay attention to them. In other instances, they may physically withdraw from people when approached. Along with these abnormal responses to people, unusual responses to objects are common. Autistic children often become fascinated with certain objects—a fascination that can lead to overly focused attention on the object, to the exclusion of the rest of the environment. The purpose of this chapter is to explore the nature and meaning of the unusual ways in which autistic children attend to and make meaning of their environments.

The idea that autistic children may have deficient arousal-modulating systems,[1] which influence how these children attend to their environments, was first discussed by Hutt, Hutt, Lee, and Ounsted (1964) and was later expanded upon by Ornitz and Ritvo (1968; see Ornitz, Chapter 8, this volume). Briefly, Hutt *et al.* proposed that the autistic child is in a chronic state of overarousal and that typical autistic behaviors, especially stereotypic, repetitive motor behaviors and behavioral withdrawal, function to reduce arousal. Ornitz and Ritvo modified this hypothesis to suggest that autism is characterized by fluctuations between states of over- and underarousal, resulting in a failure to modulate sensory intake adequately and an unstable perceptual experience. According to Ornitz and Ritvo, the child's sensitivity and attention to stimuli fluctuate and depend on whether the child is in a state of over- or underarousal.

Although both Hutt *et al.*'s and Ornitz and Ritvo's theories help explain the functional significance of repetitive motor behavior and some of the unusual attentional sensitivities of autistic children, at least two important questions have

---

1. Lacey (1967) has argued convincingly against a unidimensional concept of arousal. In this chapter, the term "arousal" refers to the complex *patterns* of cardiovascular, respiratory, and central nervous system (CNS) changes that accompany different states of responsivity to external stimuli.

not been adequately addressed by either theory. First, neither theory has fully explained the uneven developmental profile found in autism. It is well known that autistic persons often show great variability in skill levels across different functional domains; typically, language (verbal and nonverbal) and social skills are very impaired, whereas visual–spatial skills and object concepts are relatively unimpaired (e.g., Dawson, 1983; Dawson & Adams, 1984). Second, it remains to be explained why the autistic person's deficiencies in arousal modulation and attention result in specific difficulties in developing social relationships, and why the social deficits take the form that they do. The purpose of this chapter is to address these questions and to provide a beginning theoretical framework and some testable hypotheses regarding the relationships among the autistic child's arousal level, attentional deficits, developmental profile, and impaired socioemotional development. We begin with a brief review of the physiological correlates of attention in normal infants. The concept of "optimal stimulation" is introduced, and its relationship to attention is discussed. A review of research on the physiological correlates of attention in autistic children follows. We then offer hypotheses regarding the role of deficiencies in arousal modulation in the autistic child's attention to, and understanding of, social and nonsocial information and their implications for social and emotional development in autism. Finally, we describe how therapies for autistic children can be designed to be sensitive to difficulties in arousal modulation and can alter the way in which these children attend to social stimuli. Data on the effectiveness of one such therapeutic method, imitative play, are presented.

ATTENTION IN NORMAL INFANTS

Young infants normally show an early attentional preference for social stimuli. Beginning with an initial visual preference for contours and movement (Haith, 1966; Karmel, Hoffman, & Fegy, 1974; Kessen, Haith, & Salapatek, 1970; Wickelgren, 1969), young normal infants quickly develop greater interest in animate than inanimate objects (Carpenter, 1974; Field, 1979b; Sherrod, 1979), as evidenced by prolonged visual attention to social stimuli. This visual interest in social stimuli is important to parents, who readily respond to their infant's gaze by providing stimulation in the form of facial expressions, vocalizations, rocking, and so on. Parents' sensitivity to their infant's gaze patterns is apparent from their tendency to reduce stimulation when their infant looks away (Stern, 1971). Thus, gaze behavior serves a regulatory function in early infant–caretaker interactions, allowing the young infant to modulate arousal levels by controlling the amount of social stimulation (Brazelton, 1982).

Physiological Correlates of Attention

The infant's initial visual orientation to social stimuli and the sustained attention that occurs during social interaction are accompanied by predictable physiological changes associated with arousal. These changes involve the cardiovascular, respiratory, and central nervous systems (Brock, Rothbart, & Derryberry, 1986; Porges, 1976; Sroufe & Waters, 1976). To explain these physiological changes, Porges (1976, 1984) suggests a two-component model of attention. The first component, termed the "reactive component," consists of an individual's initial involuntary reaction to external stimuli, and is determined by such stimulus characteristics as intensity, novelty, and unpredictability. The second component consists of voluntary, sustained attention toward an external stimulus and is determined by ideational or symbolic qualities attributed to the stimulus. Each of these components is discussed separately.

The reactive component, or "orienting response," has been carefully described by Sokolov (1963) and Graham (Graham & Clifton, 1966; Graham & Jackson, 1970). The orienting response typically is elicited by stimuli that are of mild intensity and slightly discrepant from the individual's expectation. Behaviorally, the orienting response involves turning toward the stimulus of interest and suppressing bodily movement, presumably in order to reduce background noise and increase auditory and visual acuity. Physiological changes include pupil dilation, electroencephalographic (EEG) desynchronization, increased electrodermal activity, suppression of respiratory frequency, decreased peripheral blood flow, and an initial slowing of heart rate. There exists a developmental shift in the stimuli that are maximally effective for eliciting an orienting response, from simple to more complex. In newborns, the most effective acoustic stimulus may be the simple sine wave (Graham, Anthony, & Zeigler, 1983). The orienting response in newborns is similar to that of adults, except that it tends to occur more slowly and last longer.

The orienting response can be distinguished from the "aversive response" (also referred to as a "defensive response"), which typically is elicited by intense and/or painful stimuli. The aversive response is characterized by heart rate acceleration and, unlike the orienting response, fails to habituate when the noxious stimulus is presented repeatedly (Graham & Jackson, 1970).

Several authors have suggested that these two basic initial responses to stimuli reflect two arousal systems (e.g., Routtenberg, 1968; Sokolov, 1963). The first, evoked by novel stimuli of mild to moderate intensity, serves to enhance optimal conditions for the perception of the stimulus. The second, evoked by noxious stimuli of high intensity, serves to limit the effects of the stimulus on the organism. Lacey and Lacey (1970) proposed that the directional heart rate changes that accompany the orienting and aversive responses are directly related to changes in the organism's sensory threshold. They argue that attention to the environment (intake) is associated with heart rate decrease, whereas inattention (rejection) to the external environment is associated with heart rate increase. On the whole, studies have supported Lacey and Lacey's general model regarding the relationship between arousal, as indexed by heart rate, and efficiency of information processing (see Coles, 1983, for a recent review).

Recall that there exist two components to Porges's model of attention, and that the second component involves sustained, voluntary attention that is characterized by tonic physiological changes. Specifically, it has been demonstrated (e.g., Porges & Raskin, 1969) that, during sustained attentional tasks, subjects respond with a significant reduction in heart rate and heart rate variability (the time between successive heart beats becomes more constant), and an inhibition of respiratory activity. In a recent study of 6-month-old infants (Linnemeyer & Porges, 1986), it was found that individual differences in spontaneous baseline heart rate variability were correlated with two measures of visual recognition memory. Furthermore, heart rate decelerated in response to a visual stimulus during familiarization and recognition trials only for the infants who performed well on the visual recognition memory task. Thus, even in infancy, these physiological indices are correlated with measures of information processing.

Optimal Level of Stimulation

The fact that arousal state and efficacy of information processing are related to characteristics of the stimulus (e.g., intensity and novelty) suggests that there are optimal levels of stimulation. The idea that all organisms have a biologically determined optimal level of stimulation has been discussed by Hebb (1955), Schneirla (1959), Berlyne (1960), and others. According to Schneirla (1959), "Intensity of stimulation basically determines the direction of reaction with respect to the source, and thereby exerts a selective effect on what conditions generally affect the organism. Low intensities of stimulation tend to evoke approach reactions, high intensities withdrawal reactions with reference to the source" (p. 3). He continued, "The conclusion seems warranted that in neonate mammals generally these early biphasic processes of a physiological order, aroused according to stimulus magnitude, furnish a basis for individual perceptual, motivational, and emotional development" (p. 31).

Whereas Schneirla emphasized stimulus magnitude or intensity, Berlyne (1960) suggested that affective connotations, complexity, novelty, degree of predictability, and incongruity are important stimulus characteristics that determine optimal levels of stimulation. Zentall and Zentall (1983) have described a homeostatic model in which it is proposed that organisms will work to regulate the level of stimulus input and thereby optimize the level of arousal. Like Hutt, Lee, and Ounsted (1965), Zentall and Zentall (1983) used this model to explain the motor stereotypies of autistic children by suggesting that these behaviors function homeostatically to regulate level of stimulus input, thereby reducing high levels of arousal for autistic children.

Field (1982) used an optimal stimulation framework to explain the frequent and correlated negative affective behavior, gaze aversion, and elevated heart rate levels of preterm infants. She suggested that preterm infants may have lower thresholds and narrower ranges of responsivity to stimulation than normal infants. This poses a more difficult task for their parents, who must provide finely tuned amounts and intensities of stimulation. According to Field's (1982) "activation band model," attention and positive affect during social interaction may occur within a range of activation that has as its lower limit an attention threshold and as its upper limit an aversion threshold. If stimulation and/or responsivity exceed moderate levels, the upper limits of the activation band are approached, at which point the infant will exhibit an inattentive response (and, in some cases, aversion and distress). The range of activation is influenced by development factors, the infant's rest–activity and arousal cycles, and innate individual differences in threshold levels.

PHYSIOLOGICAL CORRELATES OF ATTENTIONAL DEFICITS IN AUTISM

The research on physiological correlates of attention in autism is fraught with the usual methodological difficulties that are too often found in other studies of autistic children. These include imprecise diagnostic criteria, lack of appropriate control groups, and failure to consider developmental changes in autistic individuals. With respect to the third issue, it is quite possible that, like cognitive and social abnormalities, physiological abnormalities attenuate as the autistic child develops, so that in the older child they are only evident under stressful conditions. Persisting behavioral and physiological abnormalities may reflect either primary deficiencies or the secondary influences of these primary deficiencies on subsequent biological and behavioral development. The variability found in samples of autistic individuals and the discrepancies among studies can be explained in many cases by considering the variability in developmental levels of subjects within and across studies. The attentional responses of a preschool-age, socially withdrawn, nonverbal autistic child to a repetitive auditory stimulus cannot be meaningfully equated to those of an adolescent who is "active but odd" (Wing & Gould, 1979) in his or her social interactions and who is capable of a fairly high degree of verbal comprehension and expression. And yet most of the available studies tend to average responses from subjects who vary in developmental level to this extreme degree.

Despite these methodological difficulties, there is fairly clear psychophysiological evidence of abnormalities of attention in autistic children. Several studies of cardiovascular responses to the presentation of novel stimuli suggest that autistic individuals have an abnormal orienting response. Findings include accelerations in heart rate, reductions in rate of habituation (Palkowitz & Wiesenfeld, 1980), a failure to habituate (James & Barry, 1980), and a failure to reinstate to novelty when habituation occurs (Bernal & Miller, 1971). James and Barry (1980) also report a failure to habituate for respiratory responses to novel stimuli. Studies of electrodermal responses to novel, repetitive stimuli have yielded less consistent findings with regard to specific types of abnormalities. However, most authors reported some abnormality, including reduced response to the first trials (Bernal & Miller, 1971; van Engeland, 1984); reduced or absent habituation (Stevens &

Gruzelier, 1984); and higher mean levels of skin conductance, which was accompanied by greater intraindividual variability (Palkowitz & Wiesenfeld, 1980). Based on the available research, it is quite likely that autistic children often fail to show the adaptive orienting response to novel stimuli that is associated with sensory intake and processing. The evidence thus far suggests that novel stimuli may elicit an aversive response (characterized by slow or absent habituation), which is associated with sensory rejection.

The failure to adequately process novel stimuli by autistic individuals is also supported by studies of cortical event-related potentials, which have demonstrated that a reduced P3 wave, normally associated with the processing of unexpected, novel stimuli, is reduced in autistic individuals (e.g., Courchesne, Kilman, Galambos, & Lincoln, 1984; Courchesne, Lincoln, Kilman, & Galambos, 1985; Dawson, Finley, Phillips, Galpert, & Lewy, in press; Dawson & Lewy, Chapter 7, this volume; Novick, Vaughan, Kurtzberg, & Simson, 1980).

In contrast to the relatively large number of studies that have investigated autistic individuals' responses to discrete, novel stimuli, there exists little research on physiological responses during complex tasks involving sustained attention. This type of research was attempted by Cohen and Johnson (1977) and Kootz and Cohen (1981). However, the tasks presented were too difficult for most of the autistic subjects, and the data were inconclusive. Hutt, Forrest, and Richer (1975) found significantly higher levels of spontaneous heart rate variability in autistic children as compared to normal children, which decreased when the children engaged in a simple, repetitive task. Several other studies of spontaneous heart rate measured in a variety of environmental conditions have also found that autistic children exhibit both greater heart rate variability and significantly elevated heart rates, as compared to normal children. These findings suggest that at least some children may have chronically high levels of autonomic activity (Cohen & Johnson, 1977; Kootz & Cohen, 1981; Kootz, Marinelli, & Cohen, 1982; Hutt et al., 1975). Kootz et al. (1982) found that lower-functioning autistic children were more likely to exhibit increased heart rate in response to changes in the environment than higher-functioning autistic children.

Hutt et al. (1965) demonstrated that autistic children showed high levels of desynchronized EEG indicative of increased arousal, which attenuated after bouts of motor stereotypies. Like Zentall and Zentall (1983), Hutt and his coworkers interpreted these findings according to a feedback model in which behavioral responses (in this case, motor stereotypies) function to regulate the level of stimulus input and arousal. Attempts to find empirical corroboration for this original work have yielded mixed results (Clark & Rutter, 1981; Hermelin & O'Connor, 1970; Hutt et al., 1975; Ornitz, Brown, Sorosky, Ritvo, & Dietrich, 1970; Sroufe, Steucher, & Stutzer, 1973). In one study (Hermelin & O'Connor, 1970) that attempted, but failed, to replicate Hutt et al.'s (1965) results, the investigators tested only those subjects who showed high levels of alpha frequency in their pretest EEG recordings, and thus selected out subjects with potentially high levels of EEG desynchronization. Unfortunately, these investigators also confounded stimulus complexity with time in the experimental environment; degree of familiarity with the environment is likely to be a critical factor in determining the arousal state of a child. Carefully controlled research on the relationship between cortical and autonomic indices of arousal and both spontaneous and task-related behavior of autistic children is needed.

It is very likely that optimal levels of stimulation will vary across autistic persons as a function of developmental level, degree of familiarity with the situation, and biologically based individual differences, including the severity of autistic disorder. Studies have shown that autistic children may increase their self-stimulatory behavior (which may reflect arousal level) in response to certain unfamiliar aspects of a situation (e.g., the therapist) but not others (e.g., the learning task), and that frequency of stereotypies as a function of environmental stimulation may depend on the developmental level of the child (Frankel, Freeman, Ritvo, & Pardo, 1978). It is also possible that autistic children may cope with overstimulating stimuli in different ways. They may use gaze aversion, social withdrawal, incessant questioning, and ritualistic behavior, as well as motor stereotypies. Clinical observations suggest that motor stereotypies can serve many functions for autistic children, including seeking social attention. Thus, although it should be possible to determine when a given child is likely to exhibit motor stereotypies, this pattern is likely to be idiosyncratic, rather than applicable to all children with autism.

The study of physiological indices of arousal is further complicated by two factors. First, since physiological measures of arousal, such as EEG desynchronization and heart rate, correlate poorly with one another in normal individuals (Lacey, 1967), we should not expect these different measures to yield consistent results across studies for autistic children. A more reasonable approach may be to look for *patterns* of physiological responses among such measures. Second, if the homeostatic model is correct in proposing that organisms will work to optimize levels of arousal by modulating the level of stimulation (Zentall & Zentall, 1983), then measures of physiological arousal may deviate from normal levels only prior to behavioral compensation. As Kinsbourne (1987) has recently argued, an organism biased toward overarousal may also be unstable, permitting arousal levels to swing to both maladaptive extremes as compensatory mechanisms come into play. Thus, it may be necessary to study an individual over time in a variety of situations to detect patterns of physiological arousal in response to changes in the natural environment.

To summarize the available research to this point, autistic individuals often fail to exhibit a normal, adaptive orienting response to a variety of stimuli. Experimental studies of the electrodermal, respiratory, and heart rate orienting responses in autistic children most often find absent or reduced habituation, consistent with an aversive response to novelty and reduced stimulus intake. Adequate studies of physiological correlates of attention in more complex, sustained attention tasks are lacking. In studies of spontaneous autonomic and cortical activity in autistic individuals, indices of arousal have often been found to be high in autistic children. Although some studies report negative findings, lower-than-normal values on measures of autonomic and cortical arousal have not been reported. Although the research is by no means conclusive, the findings thus far, taken together, suggest that many autistic individuals have chronically high levels of arousal. Attempts to find predictable relationships between or among environmental complexity, physiological measures of arousal, and autistic behaviors (e.g., motor stereotypies) have not always succeeded. Since level of arousal is likely to be influenced by developmental level, environmental conditions, and severity of the disorder, both intra- and interindividual variability in physiological and behavioral indices of arousal in autistic persons are to be expected. Future studies that carefully control for subject variables, such as developmental level and degree of autistic impairment, and that assess individuals in a variety of conditions differing in complexity and familiarity may yield a better understanding of the complex relationship between levels of physiological arousal and behavior in autism.

FAILURE TO ADEQUATELY PROCESS SOCIAL STIMULI: A FUNCTION OF STIMULUS PREDICTABILITY?

A crucial question is how the autistic child's deficits in arousal modulation and attention may selectively affect social and linguistic processing, while allowing for adequate processing of many aspects of nonsocial information. Based on theory (Berlyne, 1960) as well as experimental evidence (Graham *et al.*, 1983), it is clear that normal individuals respond most readily to stimuli that are slightly discrepant from expectations and are mildly to moderately novel. Indeed, such stimulus characteristics are necessary to elicit an orienting response. Highly predictable stimuli fail to elicit orienting, and highly intense or unpredictable stimuli lead to aversive responses. Studies of the orienting response in autistic children suggest that these children may have lower-than-normal thresholds for aversion to stimuli that are unpredictable and novel. If so, one would expect that their ranges of optimal stimulation would be narrower than those of normal individuals.

The possibility that this narrow range of optimal stimulation may have selective effects on the processing of social information[2] is suggested when one considers the basic differences between objects and people as sources of information (see Gelman & Spelke, 1981). First, whereas objects are primarily characterized by their physical properties, which are *determinate*, people are characterized by their actions, intentions, motives, and feelings, all of which are often *indeterminate*. Second, whereas objects cannot respond with independent action, so that what they do *can be predicted* by the characteristics of the object and the actions

2. Throughout this chapter, we use the term "social" to refer to all forms of stimulation usually provided by people, including spoken language, gestures, facial expressions, and so on.

on them, people act in turn and deliver communications that are *not fully pre-dictable*. Thus, not only do objects and people provide information of differing levels of complexity, but, perhaps more importantly, the information they provide differs in degree of novelty and predictability. We propose that it is the complex, novel, and unpredictable nature of people that makes them overstimulating for children with autism, who may have a decreased ability to process information of this nature because of their low aversion thresholds. Ferrara and Hill's (1980) research on autistic children's responsivity to complexity and predictability in toys provides some support for this hypothesis. In their study, social and nonsocial toys were presented in situations that either allowed the children to predict, or pre-vented the children from predicting, their appearances. It was found that autistic children's behavior was seriously disrupted if they could not predict the sequences of environmental stimuli, but that their responsiveness to environmental stimuli increased when events were predictable. In contrast, developmentally matched normal children were relatively little affected by predictability. Furthermore, the two groups of children differed in their responsiveness to toy characteristics. The normal group manipulated and looked at the complex toys more than the simple toys, regardless of their social–nonsocial features. For autistic children, increased toy complexity resulted in reduced manipulation time, regardless of whether the toy was social or nonsocial. When both types of toys were of low complexity, autistic children both manipulated and looked at the social toys more than the nonsocial toys.

The autistic child's need for predictability has been noted in numerous clin-ical accounts, and has been demonstrated in experimental studies as well (e.g., Schopler, Brehm, Kinsbourne, & Reichler, 1971). Moreover, in contrast to many symptoms of autism, which disappear or attenuate with development, the need for a highly structured and routine (in other words, predictable) environment per-sists for autistic persons of all ages and functioning levels. Thus, on the basis of its salience and persistence, one finds evidence for the notion that the need for predictability is basic to the autistic syndrome.

SOCIOEMOTIONAL DEVELOPMENT

In the preceding section, we have argued that deficiencies in arousal modulation may selectively affect attention to, and processing of, social information. It has been suggested that, because of their low aversion thresholds, autistic individuals may have a decreased ability to process social information because of its complex, novel, and unpredictable nature. In this section, we propose three pathways by which the autistic child's hypothesized low aversion threshold for novelty and unpredictability may distort socioemotional development: in the early formation of attachments to people, in the expression of emotions, and in the interpersonal coordination of affective expression.

Attachment

Recent views of attachment have stressed both psychological and physiological processes. Based on their studies of the behavioral and physiological responses of infant rhesus monkeys during separation and reunion with their mothers and peers, Reite and Capitanio (1985) have argued that "attachment in fact represents a neurobiologically based and mediated biobehavioral system, one of whose major functions is to promote the development and regulation (or modulation) of psychobiological synchrony between organisms'" (p. 224). Field (1985) has elaborated on this position by proposing that "attachment might be viewed as a relationship that develops between two or more organisms as their behavioral and physiological systems become attuned to each other. Each partner provides meaningful stimulation for the other and has a modulating influence on the other's arousal level" (p. 415). The data supporting this position, which are quite substantial (see Field, 1985, for a review), come from physiological and behavioral studies of human infants, children, and adults and nonhuman primates during periods of separation and reunion with caretakers and peers and during periods of exploration and play. Following Field's argument, mothers provide both stimulation and arousal-modulating functions during their interactions with their infants, thus helping their infants to maintain an optimal level of arousal for exploration and play. Furthermore, the arousal-modulating properties of the mother are suggested to be one of the major maternal qualities that promote the early infant's attachment to her. Quality of attachment is believed to be a joint function of the infant's level of arousal and mother's efficacy in modulating arousal.

What are the implications for this view of development of attachment for understanding autism? If we are correct in suggesting that, because of biologically based deficiencies, social stimulation often exceeds optimal levels for the autistic child (thus failing to provide the reinforcing arousal-modulating function), one might expect major disruptions in the establishment of an attachment bond. There is evidence that autistic children seek more proximity to their caregivers than to a stranger (Sigman, Mundy, Ungerer, & Sherman, 1987; Sigman & Ungerer, 1984), suggesting that attachment is not completely absent. However, differential proximity seeking reflects only a primitive level of attachment, and, based on clinical observations, there is good reason to believe that attachment is disturbed (or at least delayed) in autism. It is possible that seeking more proximity to a parent as opposed to a stranger may be a function of the parent's ability to provide highly ritualized, and thus familiar and predictable, forms of social interaction. In our own clinical work, we find ourselves being readily shaped by the autistic child's responses (e.g., gaze aversion, turning and walking away, and distress) to provide highly routine and ritualized forms of social stimulation. This shaping is likely to facilitate our forming positive relationships with autistic children, who may find this type of interaction more optimally stimulating and thus more reinforcing.

Based on this line of reasoning, one would predict that the frequency of social withdrawal and inattentiveness would vary as a function of familiarity with the social partner. The more familiar the child is with the social partner, the more predictable and less overstimulating the partner's behavior may be for the child. This prediction is borne out by recent studies of the influence of familiarity on the behavior of autistic children. Lord and Magill (Chapter 14, this volume) found that, in a day camp situation, autistic children showed significant increases in social interaction with their peers over time—increases that were independent of whether the autistic children had had previous experience in a day camp situation. Interestingly, it has been reported that echolalic speech and self-stimulatory behavior of autistic children occurred significantly more often with an unfamiliar therapist than with a familiar one (Charlop, 1986; Runco, Charlop, & Schreibman, 1986).

Affective Expression and Interpersonal Coordination

As described above, an individual's response to a stimulus (i.e., whether that stimulus will elicit approach or withdrawal) is influenced by stimulus characteristics, such as intensity, predictability, and novelty, and by individual differences in optimal levels of stimulation. The observation that normal infants typically attend to social stimulation and respond with positive affective responses such as interest and smiling (Sroufe & Waters, 1976) suggests that this type of stimulation is optimally arousing for most infants.

In contrast, autistic children may fail to attend to social stimuli or respond with negative affective reactions, which suggests that their optimal range of stimulation may be much narrower than normal. In a study of emotional expressions of autistic children in social interaction with adults, Snow, Hertzig, and Shapiro (1986) found that 2- to 4-year-old autistic children displayed less positive affect in social interaction than did developmentally delayed children matched for mental and chronological age. Furthermore, Snow *et al.* reported that when autistic children did display positive affect, they were less likely to display it to their social partners. Yirmiya, Kasari, Mundy, and Sigman (1987) found that, compared to developmentally matched mentally retarded children, autistic children spent significantly more time displaying discrete negative affective expressions in a situation found to be pleasurable by other children of a similar developmental level. In an observational study of preschool-age autistic children and their mothers, we (Dawson, Galpert, Hill, & Spencer, 1988) found that although developmentally matched autistic and normal children were equally likely to exhibit smiles during play with their mothers, autistic children were significantly less likely to combine their smiles with sustained gaze toward their mothers. Taken together, the results of these three studies suggest that the autistic child's early emotional development may be distorted by a failure to sustain attention to social stimuli and, possibly, by a tendency to experience less positive affect and more negative affect in social situations.

If the hypothesized links between and among social stimulation, physiological measures of arousal, attention, and affect are supported by data from future studies, we may be a step closer to clarifying Kanner's (1943) original position that autistic children "come into the world with innate inability to form the usual, biologically provided affective contact with people" (p. 250). Indeed, the capacity of the young infant to "resonate emotionally" (Klinnert, Campos, Sorce, Emde, & Svejda, 1983, p. 73) to the affective expressions of its caretaker may depend upon the young infant's and the caretaker's having similar affective responses to mutual social stimulation. Interpersonal coordination of affective expression (termed "affective attunement" by Stern, Hofer, Haft, & Dore, 1985) would be difficult to achieve if each person in the relationship had very different attentional and emotional responses to the relationship itself. Normally, the mother's and infant's mutual interest and pleasure in each other's smiling and vocalizations ensure that they will often experience shared feeling states. However, the failure of the autistic child to respond with similar interest and pleasure to the mother's affective displays undoubtedly will interfere with their ability to have a shared affective experience, thus greatly hampering the development of interpersonal coordination of affective expression.

Furthermore, since much of the early process of socialization of emotion takes place within the context of sustained, mutually pleasurable face-to-face interactions, the autistic child will miss an important opportunity for learning about emotions. Here we examine only one of these early interactional patterns, that of the mother imitating her infant's facial expressions and vocalizations. We have chosen this early interactional pattern because it is one of the earliest and most common forms of interaction between a mother and her young infant (Papousek & Papousek, 1979), and because of its central role in the socialization of emotion (Malatesta & Izard, 1984)

Maternal imitation normally elicits visual orientation and interest on the part of the young infant. It is believed to serve the functions of facilitating early turn-taking behavior (Stern, 1974), helping the infant develop a sense of "self related to other" (Baldwin, 1899/1973), and possibly enhancing the development of infant imitation (Francis, Self, & Noble, 1981). Malatesta and Izard (1984) propose, moreover, that visually mediated feedback—specifically, maternal imitation of the infant's facial expressions—is necessary for the continued articulation and modulation of emotional expressions. In a study by Malatesta and Haviland (1982), mothers showed low frequencies of imitation of negative affect and a preponderance of imitation of positive affect. Thus, mothers tend to selectively imitate positive affect, as well as prototypic emotion expressions, which may facilitate the infant's articulation of emotional expressions. Furthermore, maternal imitation, in the form of matching facial expressions, may promote the development of an association between visual images of facial expressions and feeling states, as the mirroring of emotional expressions permits simultaneity in the viewing and experiencing of affect (Malatesta & Izard, 1984).

The influence of autistic children's hypothesized low aversion threshold to social stimulation, including maternal imitation, on their early emotional development may be similar to what has been found in the early interactional patterns of preterm infants and their mothers. As stated earlier, preterm infants are less able to tolerate normal levels of social stimulation and tend to exhibit more negative affect and gaze aversion during face-to-face interactions. Malatesta, Grigoryev, Lamb, Albin, and Culver (1986) found that, compared to mothers of normal infants, mothers of preterm infants displayed significantly less imitation of the infants' facial expressions. Moreover, higher rates of maternal contingent responding to infant affect predicted enhanced positivity (increased rates of joy, interest, and surprise expressions) on the part of the preterm infants, suggesting that the mothers' imitative behavior was shaping the emotional responses of their young infants.

If the early interactional pattern of maternal imitation is similarly disrupted in autistic children, but in a more extreme and persisting manner, it follows that autistic children would show less positive affect (as reported above), and that facial expressions of emotion would be less well articulated. Kasari, Yirmiya, Sigman, and Mundy (1986) found that autistic children displayed significantly more blends of facial expressions, and suggested that the clarity of the facial expressions of young autistic children may be compromised by the presence of blends. Langdell (1981) reported that raters of pictures of autistic children's facial expressions often found it difficult to interpret their expressions. These findings suggest that autistic children have less well-articulated facial expressions, which may reflect the influences of the lack of socialization of emotion in autism rather than primary expressive impairments per se.

Summary

We propose that the autistic child's failure to establish affective contact with others, as originally noted by Kanner (1943) is, at least in part, the result of a low aversion threshold for social stimulation. When the threshold is exceeded, the child may become inattentive and, possibly, express negative affect. Social stimuli may be particularly arousing, and therefore may be most likely to exceed the child's lower aversion threshold because of their unpredictable and complex nature. In contrast, nonsocial stimuli, which often provide predictable and less complex information, may be more easily assimilable and may even have an arousal-reducing function for children with autism.

Since the formation of attachment bonds may depend, in part, on the ability of the attachment figure to modulate arousal and to provide optimal levels of stimulation, the autistic child's tendency to experience aversion and negative affect when his or her caretaker provides social stimulation may significantly disrupt the attachment process.

Interpersonal coordination of affect may depend on the infant's innate, or early-developing, capacity to sustain attention to social stimuli and to have affective responses of interest and pleasure to social stimulation that are similar to those of his or her caretaker. The autistic child's failure to have responses to social stimulation that are both generally positive and similar in nature to the caretaker's may interfere with development of the ability to "resonate emotionally" to the affective expressions of others. Finally, it is suggested that, since early socialization of emotion depends on the mutual enjoyment of face-to-face interaction by the mother and infant, the young autistic child will fail to receive the benefits of these interactions, which include an increased ability to articulate, modulate, and eventually represent emotions.

IMPLICATIONS FOR THERAPEUTIC INTERVENTION WITH AUTISTIC CHILDREN

Imitative Play with Autistic Children

We have been studying the beneficial effects of using certain interactive strategies for facilitating the social attention of autistic children. In this section, we consider how this intervention approach may address the autistic child's particular sensitivities to social stimulation.

It has been well documented that autistic children tend not to imitate either body movements or facial expressions of others (e.g., Curcio, 1978; Dawson & Adams, 1984). In an attempt to facilitate imitative and social behavior, we (Dawson & Adams, 1984) examined the effects of imitating autistic children's behavior on the children's social attentiveness. The major inspiration for these initial efforts was Piaget's (1962) description of an early stage of imitation, in which the young infant responds with increased attentiveness and motor activity to the imitations of others. We found that imitating the autistic children's behavior did, in fact, significantly increase attentiveness on the part of the children (as measured by the duration of gaze toward the experimenter), as well as general social responsiveness (as measured by touching, gaze, vocalizations, and gestures). The imitative strategy also had a positive influence on the children's toy play, which became significantly less perseverative (as measured by the number of different toys played with and the number of different schemes used). These effects also have been reported by Tiegerman and Primavera (1981, 1984), who found that, compared to a noncontingent interactional strategy, imitation of autistic children significantly increased gaze toward the experimenter and exploratory play with objects.

Why should imitative play be facilitative of social attention in autistic children? Part of the answer, discussed at length elsewhere (Dawson & Galpert, 1986), may be that this interactional strategy is appropriate for the developmental capabilities of young autistic children. In a study of the imitative abilities of preschool-age autistic children (Dawson & Adams, 1984), we found these children to be functioning at very early levels in their imitative abilities (many were at the 1- to 4-month level). One of the primary means by which parents normally interact with their young infants is imitation of their behavior, including vocalizations and facial expressions. Thus, by adopting an early interactive strategy, we may be providing a social environment that is developmentally appropriate and meaningful to the autistic child.

Although this developmental interpretation may provide part of the explanation for why imitation is an effective strategy for children with autism, another part of the explanation may be that this strategy is sensitive to the autistic child's narrow range of optimal stimulation. Imitation of the child's behavior provides a highly predictable response to the child. The response was made even more predictable in our study, since we reliably imitated virtually every behavior of each child; in natural parent–infant interactions, parental imitation is much less systematic. In our study, the experimenter's response was identical to that of the child. Thus, we speculate that the information-processing demands were minimized; the child already had a visual and kinesthetic representation of the experimenter's behavior in short-term memory when the experimenter performed the behavior. Furthermore, the child could easily regulate the amount of stimulation by varying the frequency and intensity of his or her own actions.

This explanation for why imitative play may be facilitative of social attention in children with autism is supported by a study carried out by Field (1977, 1979a) with preterm infants, who often exhibit high levels of gaze aversion and negative affect. Field found that preterm infants become more attentive when their mothers systematically imitated their infants' behavior than during spontaneous interactions. Corresponding decreases were noted in tonic heart rate. When mothers were asked to keep their infants' attention using their typical modes of interaction, the general level of the mothers' activity increased, as did the infants' gaze aversion and heart rate. It would be useful to examine physiological measures of arousal along with behavioral measures of attention (gaze) and affect during spontaneous and imitative interaction sessions with autistic children. It then could be determined whether imitative play serves to reduce arousal for autistic children and whether these reductions are accompanied by positive influences on social attention.

The imitation strategy may be especially beneficial for autistic children, since it simplifies, exaggerates, and distills many important features of early social interactions. Simultaneous imitation with identical toys provides a highly salient and predictable contingent response for the child, and thereby may facilitate a sense of social effectiveness (Lamb, 1981). The imitative strategy puts the child in the role of the initiator, which may be important for autistic children, who typically fail to initiate social interaction. As mentioned earlier, imitation provides an opportunity for the experience of shared communication and mutuality between the child and others, promotes imitation on the part of the child, and may enhance self-awareness.

We consider imitation to be only one example of many possible interactive strategies that may promote social responsiveness in autistic individuals. Imitative play, as described here, is a very early form of interaction, and therefore is perhaps most appropriate for use with children who are functioning at early developmental levels (i.e., below 1 year). We suggest that imitative play used in this way may provide a foundation for establishing social interest and play—a foundation that can be built upon with more sophisticated forms of social interaction, such as games that require turn taking and rule-governed behavior.

An Intervention Study Using Maternal Imitation

Encouraged by the possible therapeutic value of imitative play with autistic children, we (Dawson & Galpert, 1987) recently explored the effects of this method when used by mothers of autistic children at home over a 2-week period. Fifteen autistic children, 2 to 6 years of age, and their mothers participated in this study. During each dyad's first visit to the laboratory, the mother was given three toys and instructed to play with her child however she chose (Free Play 1). Next, a set of identical toys was introduced. After the mother had been coached briefly in imitating her child, she was instructed to imitate her child's toy play, body movements, and vocalizations for approximately the same period of time (Imitation 1). The mother was then given the two sets of identical toys and instructed to perform the imitative procedure for 20 minutes each day for the next 2 weeks. After 2 weeks, the mother and child returned to the laboratory for a repeat of a free play and two imitation conditions. First, the free-play session (Free Play 2) was carried

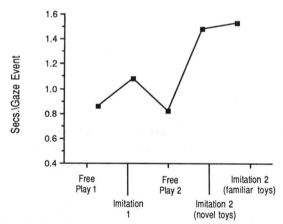

FIGURE 3-1. Mean duration of gaze at mother's face (average number of seconds per gaze) for 15 autistic children during each of five conditions: (1) free play with mother, pre-2-week intervention (Free Play 1); (2) mother imitates child's play, pre-2-week intervention (Imitation 1); (3) free play with mother, post-2-week intervention (Free Play 2); (4) mother imitates child's play with unfamiliar toys, post-2-week intervention (Imitation 2 [novel toys]); and (5) mother imitates child's play with familiar toys, post-2-week intervention (Imitation 2 [familiar toys]). From *Mothers' Use of Imitative Play for Facilitating Eye Contact and Toy Play in Autistic Children* by G. Dawson and L. Galpert, 1987, paper presented at the biennial meeting of the Society for Research in Child Development, Baltimore. Reprinted by permission of the authors.

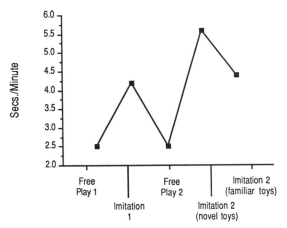

FIGURE 3-2. Total duration of gaze toward mother's face (divided by the number of minutes spent in each condition, which varied slightly across children) for 15 autistic children duirng each of the five conditions described for Figure 3-1. From *Mothers' Use of Imitative Play for Facilitating Eye Contact and Toy Play in Autistic Children* by G. Dawson and L. Galpert, 1987, paper presented at the biennial meeting of the Society for Research in Child Development, Baltimore. Reprinted by permission of the authors.

out, using a novel set of toys. Next, a set of identical toys was introduced, and an imitation session was carried out (Imitation 2 [novel toys]). The purpose of using a novel set of toys was to assess whether the intervention effects generalized to unfamiliar stimuli. Finally, another imitation session was carried out with the original, familiar toys (Imitation 2 [familiar toys]).

All sessions were videotaped. The following child social behaviors were coded for all five conditions: looking at mother's face, looking at mother's actions with toys, vocalizations, and positive and negative affect. In addition, number of toy changes and number of different play schemes were coded for the imitation conditions. We chose not to code children's toy play during the free-play conditions, because the mothers tended to structure the play highly in these conditions, making it difficult to obtain an independent measure of the children's use of toys.

The first question to be addressed was whether the children showed immediate increases in attention to mother and other social behaviors in the imitation conditions as compared to the free-play conditions (Free Play 1 vs. Imitation 1, and Free Play 2 [novel toys] vs. Imitation 2 [novel toys]). For both comparisons, increases were found in the average duration of gaze, as well as in the total duration of gaze, toward mother's face. These data are displayed in Figures 3-1 and 3-2. In addition, decreases in the amount of time spent looking at mother's actions with toys were found in the imitation conditions as compared to the free-play conditions. These data are shown in Figures 3-3 and 3-4. Only limited support for a positive influence on vocalizations was found (a nonsignificant trend toward increased vocalizations during Imitation 1 as compared to Free Play 1). Signifi-

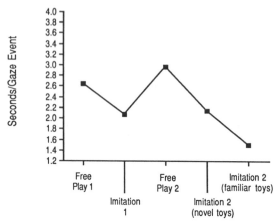

FIGURE 3-3.   Mean duration of gaze at mother's actions with toys (average number of seconds per gaze) for 15 autistic children during each of the five conditions described for Figure 3-1. From *Mothers' Use of Imitative Play for Facilitating Eye Contact and Toy Play in Autistic Children* by G. Dawson and L. Galpert, 1987, paper presented at the biennial meeting of the Society for Research in Child Development, Baltimore. Reprinted by permission of the authors.

cant changes in child's affect as a function of condition were not found. It was noted that not all mothers imitated vocalizations; it would be of interest to evaluate the effects of maternal imitation on vocalizations and affect in a study in which mothers are asked to focus more systematically on these behaviors.

The question of whether there were cumulative increases in gaze at mother's face and exploratory toy play as a result of the 2-week intervention was investigated in two comparisons. First, the pre- and postintervention imitation conditions using the familiar set of toys (Imitation 1 vs. Imitation 2 [familiar toys]) were compared. Second, to determine whether the effects generalized to a novel set of toys, we compared the preintervention imitation conditions (Imitation 1) with the postervention imitation condition using novel toys (Imitation 2 [novel toys]). For both comparisons, significant cumulative increases in average duration of gaze at mother's face were found, which can be seen in Figure 3-1. As can be seen in Figure 3-2, increases in total duration of gaze at mother's face were also found, but this did not reach statistical significance (a nonsignificant trend was found for one comparison). Significant decreases in the total duration of gaze at mother's actions with toys were found for both comparisons. These data are shown in Figures 3-3 and 3-4. These findings suggest that the effect of the imitative therapy specifically increased *social* attentiveness. That is, the children were not simply finding their mothers' contingent actions with toys to be more interesting. Instead, it appears that, since they were focusing more on the mothers' faces and less on their toy play, the intervention was facilitating social attentiveness.

Finally we found some support for our earlier finding of a positive effect of imitation on exploratory toy play by the children. When the preintervention imitation condition was compared with the postintervention imitation condition with novel toys, significant increases in the number of toy changes and number of different play schemes were found. When the preintervention imitation condition was compared with the postintervention imitation condition with familiar toys, a nonsignificant trend toward increased number of toy changes was found. These data are displayed in Figures 3-5 and 3-6.

Interestingly, the imitation intervention did not have an effect on the *frequency* of gaze toward the mother. Rather, it was found that gazes tended to be of longer duration. During the free-play conditions, the autistic children were looking at their mothers' faces with the same frequency as during the imitation conditions, but the looks were of a brief duration. These data are consistent with our data from the observational study of smiling during snack time with mothers (Dawson *et al.*, 1988), described above, in which it was found that, compared to developmentally matched normal children, autistic children's smiles were more likely to be accompanied by either no eye contact or transient eye contact (i.e., eye contacts of very brief duration). These findings suggest that an autistic child may be interested in the mother, as evidenced by frequent looks at her face, but that the gaze may be difficult to sustain, perhaps due to the overstimulating consequences of interacting with the mother.

In our clinical work, we have been experimenting with other forms of imitation. One form is "alternating imitation," in which the therapist or parent waits until the child has completed a behavior before imitating him or her. This, of course, is necessary for imitating vocalizations. Another form is "modifying imi-

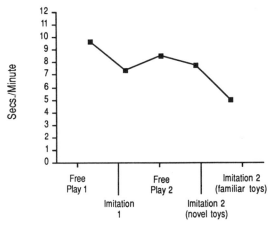

FIGURE 3-4. Total duration of gaze toward mother's actions with toys (divided by the number of minutes spent in each condition, which varied slightly across children) for 15 autistic children during each of the five conditions described for Figure 3-1. From *Mothers' Use of Imitative Play for Facilitating Eye Contact and Toy Play in Autistic Children* by G. Dawson and L. Galpert, 1987, paper presented at the biennial meeting of the Society for Research in Child Development, Baltimore. Reprinted by permission of the authors.

tation" (Kaye, 1979), in which the therapist or parent responds contingently with a dissimilar response. Research on maternal imitation with normal infants indicates that modifying imitation by mothers tends to increase in frequency after about 6 months of age (Kaye, 1979). The potential usefulness of imitating autistic children's facial expressions also warrants further study.

In clinical practice, sensitivity to the child's cues that suggest overstimulation, such as inattention, negative affect, motor stereotypies, and repetitive behaviors (vocal or motor), may help the therapist to gauge whether his or her behavior is optimally stimulating for the child. Increased sensitivity to the child's natural arousal cycles, both during the day and within a therapeutic session, may also be helpful.

Summary

Studies of spontaneous interactions between autistic children and their caregivers suggest that autistic children do show an interest in others, which is evident in their frequent gazes toward their mothers and proximity seeking. However, they may have difficulty sustaining their attention to others and exhibit higher frequencies of negative affect expressions during interaction because of a hypothesized low aversion threshold for social stimulation. We now have empirical evidence that autistic children's attention to others can be increased by sensitive interactive

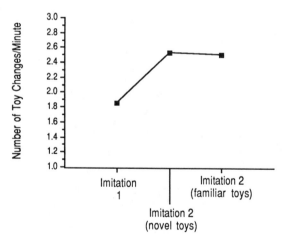

FIGURE 3-5.   Mean number of changes from one toy to another (per minute) shown by 15 autistic children during each of three conditions: (1) mother imitates child's play, pre-2-week intervention (Imitation 1); (2) mother imitates child's play with unfamiliar toys, post-2-week intervention (Imitation 2 [novel toys]); and (3) mother imitates child's play with familiar toys, post-2-week intervention (Imitation 2 [familiar toys]). From *Mothers' Use of Imitative Play for Facilitating Eye Contact and Toy Play in Autistic Children* by G. Dawson and L. Galpert, 1987, paper presented at the biennial meeting of the Society for Research in Child Development, Baltimore. Reprinted by permission of the authors.

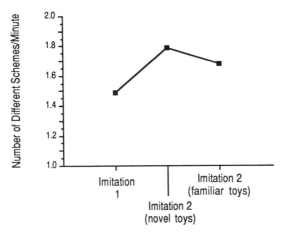

FIGURE 3-6. Mean number of different play schemes used per minute by 15 autistic children during each of the three conditions described for Figure 3-5. From *Mothers' Use of Imitative Play for Facilitating Eye Contact and Toy Play in Autistic Children* by G. Dawson and L. Galpert, 1987, paper presented at the biennial meeting of the Society for Research in Child Development, Baltimore. Reprinted by permission of the authors.

strategies that provide simplified, predictable, and highly contingent responses and allow the children to control and regulate the amount of stimulation. The question of why these strategies are effective is still a matter of speculation. We offer a psychophysiological explanation for why autistic children may be more attentive to their social partners during certain kinds of interactions, such as imitative play; we also describe a number of testable hypotheses that focus on the possible relationships between autistic children's deficits in arousal modulation, and their attention and affective responses to social stimulation.

CONCLUSION

In this chapter, we describe a model for understanding the nature and implications of the unusual ways in which autistic children attend to their environments. We propose that autistic children's deficiencies in arousal modulation, attention to social and nonsocial stimuli, and socioemotional impairments are closely linked. In this model, neither affective nor perceptual–cognitive impairments are viewed as primary in autism; instead, we argue that the autistic child's deficiencies in arousal modulation will directly influence his or her attention to and processing of both social and nonsocial information, as well as affective expression. Our studies of imitative play have demonstrated that autistic children's attention to social stimuli can be influenced by changing the nature of the social stimuli (from more complex and variable to more simple and predictable). These findings suggest that the key to understanding autistic children's attentional deficits lies not in the distinction between social and nonsocial stimuli per se, but rather between the very different types of information usually provided by social and nonsocial stimuli.

We readily admit that the model we have described is speculative. However, it is our hope that the ideas presented here will stimulate much-needed research that focuses on the links between and among physiological arousal, attention, and the cognitive and affective impairments of individuals with autism.

Acknowledgments

We wish to thank Larry Galpert, John Gottman, Mark Greenberg, and Deborah Hill for their critical feedback on earlier versions of this chapter. This work was supported in part by a grant from the John D. and Catherine T. MacArthur Foundation awarded to Geraldine Dawson.

References

Baldwin, J. M. (1973). *Social and ethical interpretations in mental development.* New York: Arno Press. (Original work published 1899)

Berlyne, D. E. (1960). *Conflict, arousal and curiosity.* New York: McGraw-Hill.

Bernal, M. E., & Miller, W. H. (1971). Electrodermal and cardiac responses of schizophrenic children to sensory stimuli. *Psychophysiology, 7,* 155–168.

Brazelton, T. B. (1982). Joint regulation of neonate–parent behavior. In E. F. Tronick (Ed.), *Social interchange in infancy: Affect, cognition and communication.* Baltimore: University Park Press.

Brock, S. E., Rothbart, M. K., & Derryberry, D. (1986). Heart-rate deceleration and smiling in 3-month-old infants. *Infant Behavior and Development, 9,* 403–414.

Carpenter, G. (1974). Visual regard of moving and stationary faces in early infancy. *Merrill–Palmer Quarterly, 20,* 181–194.

Charlop, M. H. (1986). Setting effects on the occurrence of autistic children's immediate echolalia. *Journal of Autism and Developmental Disorders, 16,* 473–483.

Clark, P., & Rutter, M. (1981). Autistic children's responses to structure and to interpersonal demands. *Journal of Autism and Developmental Disorders, 11*(2), 201–217.

Cohen, D. J., & Johnson, W. T. (1977). Cardiovascular correlates of attention in normal and psychiatrically disturbed children. *Archives of General Psychiatry, 34,* 561–567.

Coles, M. G. H. (1983). Situational determinants and psychological significance of heart rate change. In A. Gale & J. A. Edwards (Eds.), *Physiological correlates of human behavior* (Vol. 2). New York: Academic Press.

Courchesne, E., Kilman, B. A., Galambos, R., & Lincoln, A. J. (1984). Autism: Processing of novel auditory information assessed by event-related brain potentials. *Electroencephalography and Clinical Neurophysiology, 59,* 238–248.

Courchesne, E., Lincoln, A. J., Kilman, B. A., & Galambos, R. (1985). Event-related brain potential correlates of the processing of novel visual and auditory information in autism. *Journal of Autism and Developmental Disorders, 15,* 55–75.

Curcio, F. (1978). Sensorimotor functioning in mute autistic children. *Journal of Autism and Childhood Schizophrenia, 8,* 281–292.

Dawson, G. (1983). Lateralized brain dysfunction in autism: Evidence from the Halstead–Reitan Neuropsychological Battery. *Journal of Autism and Developmental Disorders, 13,* 269–286.

Dawson, G., & Adams, A. (1984). Imitation and social responsiveness in autistic children. *Journal of Abnormal Child Psychology*, 12, 209–225.

Dawson, G., Finley, C., Phillips, S., Galpert, L., & Lewy, A. (in press). Reduced P3 amplitude of the event-related brain potential: Its relationship to language ability in autism. *Journal of Autism and Developmental Disorders*.

Dawson, G., & Galpert, L. (1986). A developmental model for facilitating the social behavior of autistic children. In E. Schopler & G. Mesibov (Eds.), *Social behavior in autism*. New York: Plenum.

Dawson, G., & Galpert, L. (1987). *Mothers' use of imitative play for facilitating eye contact and toy play in autistic children*. Paper presented at the biennial meeting of the Society for Research in Child Development, Baltimore.

Dawson, G., Galpert, L., Hill, D., & Spencer, A. (1988). *Affective exchanges between autistic children and their mothers*. Paper presented at the 1988 International Conference on Infant Studies, Washington, DC.

Ferrara, C., & Hill, S., (1980). The responsiveness of autistic children to the predictability of social and nonsocial toys. *Journal of Autism and Developmental Disorders*, 10, 51–57.

Field, T. (1977). Effect of early separation, interactive deficits and experimental manipulations on infant–mother face-to-face interaction. *Child Development*, 48, 731–771.

Field, T. (1979a). Interaction patterns of high-risk and normal infants. In R. Field, A. Sostek, S. Goldberg, & H. H. Schuman (Eds.) *Infants born at risk*. New York: Spectrum.

Field, T. (1979b). Visual and cardiac responses to animate and inanimate faces by young and preterm infants. *Child Development*, 50, 188–194.

Field, T. (1982). Affective displays of high-risk infants during early interactions. In T. Field & A. Fogel (Eds.), *Emotion and early interaction*. Hillsdale, NJ: Erlbaum.

Field, T. (1985). Attachment as psychobiological attunement: Being on the same wavelength. In M. Reite & T. Field (Eds.), *The psychobiology of attachment and separation*. New York: Academic Press.

Francis, P. L., Self, P. A., & Noble, C. A. (1981). *Maternal imitation of their newborn infants: Momma see, Momma do*. Paper presented at the biennial meeting of the Society for Research in Child Development, Boston.

Frankel, F., Freeman, B. J., Ritvo, E. & Pardo, R. (1978). The effect of environmental stimulation upon the stereotyped behavior of autistic children. *Journal of Autism and Childhood Schizophrenia*, 8(4), 389–394.

Gelman, R., & Spelke, E. (1981). The development of thoughts about animate and inanimate objects: Implications for research on social cognition. In J. H. Flavell & L. Ross (Eds.), *Social cognitive development*. Cambridge, England: Cambridge University Press.

Graham, F. K., Anthony, B. J., & Zeigler, B. L. (1983). The orienting response and developmental processes. In D. Siddle (Ed.), *Orienting and habituation: Perspectives in human research*. New York: Wiley.

Graham, F. K., & Clifton, R. K. (1966). Heart rate changes as a component of the orienting response. *Psychological Bulletin*, 65, 305–320.

Graham, F. K., & Jackson, J. C. (1970). Arousal systems and infant heart rate responses. In H. W. Reese & L. P. Lipsitt (Eds.), *Advances in child development and behavior* (Vol. 5). New York: Academic Press.

Haith, M. M. (1966). Response of the human newborn to visual movement. *Journal of Experimental Child Psychology*, 3, 235–243.

Hebb, D. O. (1955). Drives and the CNS. *Psychological Review*, 9, 243–252.

Hermelin, B., & O'Connor, N. (1970). *Psychological experiments with autistic children*. Oxford: Pergamon Press.

Hutt, S. J., Forrest, S. J., & Richer, J. (1975). Cardiac arrhythmia and behavior in autistic children. *Acta Psychiatrica Scandinavica*, 51, 361–372.

Hutt, S. J., Hutt, C., Lee, D., & Ounsted, C. (1964). Arousal and childhood autism, *Nature*, 204, 908–909.

Hutt, S. J., Hutt, C., Lee, D., & Ounsted, C. (1965). A behavioral and electroencephalographic study of autistic children. *Journal of Psychiatric Research*, 181–197.

James, A., & Barry, R. J. (1980). Respiratory and vascular responses to simple visual stimuli in autistics, retardates and normals. *Psychophysiology*, 17, 541–547.

Kanner, L. (1943). Autistic disturbances of affective contact. *The Nervous Child*, 2, 217–250.

Karmel, B., Hoffman, R., & Fegy, M. (1974). Processing of contour information by human infant evidenced by pattern dependent evoked potentials. *Child Development*, 45, 39–48.

Kasari, C., Yirmiya, N., Mundy, P., & Sigman, M. (1986). *Affect expressions: A comparison of autistic, MR, and normal children*. Paper presented at the annual meeting of the American Psychological Association, Washington, DC.

Kaye, K. (1979). Thickening thin data: The maternal role in developing communication and language. In M. Bullowa (Ed.), *Before speech*. Cambridge, England: Cambridge University Press.

Kessen, W., Haith, M., & Salapatek, P. (1970). Human infancy: A bibliography and guide. In P. Mussen (Ed.), *Carmichael's manual of child psychology* (Vol. 1). New York: Wiley.

Kinsbourne, M. (1987). Cerebral–brainstem relations in infantile autism. In E. Schopler & G. Mesibov (Eds.), *Neurobiological issues in autism*. New York: Plenum.

Klinnert, M., Campos, J., Sorce, J., Emde, R., & Svejda, M. (1983). Emotions as behavior regulators: Social referencing in infancy. In R. Plutchnik & H. Kellerman (Eds.), *Emotion: Theory, research, and experience* (Vol. 2). New York: Academic Press.

Kootz, J. P., & Cohen, D. J. (1981). Modulation of sensory intake in autistic children: Cardiovascular and behavioral indices. *Journal of the American Academy of Child Psychiatry*, 20, 692–701.

Kootz, J. P., Marinelli, B., & Cohen, D. J. (1982). Modulation of response to environmental stimulation in autistic children. *Journal of Autism and Developmental Disorders*, 12, 185–193.

Lacey, J. I. (1967). Somatic response in patterning and stress: Some revisions of activation theory. In M. H. Appley and R. Trumbull (Eds.), *Psychological stress: Issues in research*. New York: Appleton-Century-Crofts.

Lacey, J. I., & Lacey, B. C. (1970). Some autonomic–central nervous system interrelationships. In P. Black (Eds.), *Physiological correlates of emotion*. New York: Academic Press.

Lamb, M. E. (1981). The development of social expectations in the first year of life. In M. E. Lamb & L. R. Sherrod (Eds.), *Infant social cognition: Empirical and theoretical considerations*. Hillsdale, NJ: Erlbaum.

Langdell, T. (1981). *Face perception: An approach to the study of autism*. Unpublished doctoral dissertation, University of London.

Linnemeyer, S. A., & Porges, S. W. (1986). Recognition memory and cardiac vagal tone in 6-month old infants. *Infant Behavior and Development*, 9, 43–56.

Malatesta, C. Z., Grigoryev, P., Lamb, C., Albin, M., & Culver, C. (1986). Emotion socialization and expressive development in preterm and full-term infants. *Child Development*, 57, 316–330.

Malatesta, C. Z., & Haviland, J. M. (1982). Learning display rules: The socialization of emotion expression in infancy. *Child Development*, 53, 991–1003.

Malatesta, C. Z., & Izard, C. E. (1984). The ontogenesis of human social signals: From the biological imperative to symbol utilization. In N. Fox & R. Davidson (Eds.), *The psychobiology of affective development*. Hillsdale, NJ: Erlbaum.

Novick, B., Vaughn, H. G., Jr., Kurtzberg, D., & Simson, R. (1980). An electrophysiological indication of auditory processing defects in autism. *Psychiatry Research*, 3, 107–114.

Ornitz, E. M., Brown, M. B., Sorosky, A. R., Ritvo, E. R., & Dietrich, L. (1970). Environmental modification of autistic behavior. *Archives of General Psychiatry*, 22, 560–565.

Ornitz, E. M., & Ritvo, E. R. (1968). Perceptual inconstancy in early infantile autism. *Archives of General Psychiatry*, 18, 76–98.

Palkowitz, R. W., & Wiesenfeld, A. R. (1980). Differential autonomic responses of autistic and normal children. *Journal of Autism and Developmental Disorders*, 10, 347–360.

Papousek, H., & Papousek, M. (1979). Early ontogeny of human social interaction: Its biological roots and social dimensions. In M. von Cranach, K. Foppa, W. Lepenies, & D. Ploog (Eds.), *Human ethology: Claims and limits of a new discipline*. Cambridge, England: Cambridge University Press.

Piaget, J. (1962). *Play, dreams, and imitation*. New York: Norton.

Porges, S. (1976). Peripheral and neurochemical parallels of psychopathology: A psychophysiological model relating autonomic imbalance to hyperactivity, psychopathy, and autism. In H. W. Reese (Ed.), *Advances in child development and behavior* (Vol. 2). New York: Academic Press.

Porges, S. W. (1984). Physiologic correlates of attention: A core process underlying learning disorders. *Pediatric Clinics of North America, 31*, 371–385.

Porges, S. W., & Raskin, D. C. (1969). Respiratory and heart-rate components of attention. *Journal of Experimental Psychology, 81*, 497–503.

Reite, M., & Capitanio, J. P. (1985). On the nature of social separation and social attachment. In M. Reite & T. Field (Eds.), *The psychobiology of attachment and separation*. New York: Academic Press.

Routtenberg, A. (1968). The two arousal hypothesis: Reticular formation and limbic system. *Psychological Review, 75*, 51–80.

Runco, M. A., Charlop, M. H., & Schreibman, L. (1986). The occurrence of autistic children's self-stimulation as a function of familiar versus unfamiliar stimulus conditions. *Journal of Autism and Developmental Disorders, 16*(1), 31–44.

Schneirla, T. C. (1959). An evolutionary and developmental theory of biphasic processes underlying approach and withdrawal. In M. R. Jones (Ed.), *Nebraska Symposium on Motivation* (Vol. 7). Lincoln: University of Nebraska Press.

Schopler, E., Brehm, S., Kinsbourne, M., & Reichler, R. J. (1971). Effect of treatment structure on development in autistic children. *Archives of General Psychiatry, 24*, 415–421.

Sherrod, L. (1979). Social cognition in infancy: Attention to the human face. *Infant Behavior and Development, 2*, 279–294.

Sigman, M., Mundy, P., Ungerer, J., & Sherman, T. (1987). *The development of social attachments in autistic children*. Paper presented at the biennial meeting of the Society for Research in Child Development, Baltimore.

Sigman, M., & Ungerer, J. (1984). Attachment behaviors in autistic children. *Journal of Autism and Developmental Disorders, 14*, 231–244.

Snow, M., Hertzig, J., & Shapiro. T. (1986). *Affective expression in young autistic children*. Paper presented at the annual meeting of the American Academy of Child Psychiatry, Los Angeles.

Sokolov, E. N. (1963). *Perception and the conditioned reflex*. New York: Macmillan.

Sroufe, A. L., Stuecher, H. U., & Stutzer, W. (1973). The functional significance of autistic behaviors for the psychotic child. *Journal of Abnormal Child Psychology, 1*(3), 225–240.

Sroufe, A. L., & Waters, E. (1976). The ontogenesis of smiling and laughter: A perspective on the organization of development in infancy. *Psychological Review, 83*, 173–187.

Stern, D. N. (1971). A micro-analysis of mother–infant interaction: Behavior regulating social conduct between a mother and her 3½ month old twins. *Journal of the American Academy of Child Psychiatry, 10*, 501–517.

Stern, D. N. (1974). The goal and structure of mother–infant play. *Journal of the American Academy of Child Psychiatry, 13*, 402–421.

Stern, D. N., Hofer, L., Haft, W., & Dore, J. (1985). Affect attunement: The sharing of feeling states between mother and infant by means of inter-model fluency. In T. M. Field & N. A. Fox (Eds.), *Social perception in infants*. Norwood, NJ: Ablex.

Stevens, S., & Gruzelier, J. (1984). Electrodermal activity to auditory stimuli in autistic, retarded, and normal children. *Journal of Autism and Developmental Disorders, 14*, 245–260.

Tiegerman, E., & Primavera, L. (1981). Object manipulation: An interactional strategy with autistic children. *Journal of Autism and Developmental Disorders, 11*, 427–438.

Tiegerman, E., & Primavera, L. (1984). Imitating the autistic child: Facilitating communicative gaze behavior. *Journal of Autism and Developmental Disorders, 14*, 27–38.

van Engeland, H. (1984). The electrodermal orienting response to auditive stimuli in autistic children, normal children, mentally retarded children, and child psychiatric patients. *Journal of Autism and Developmental Disorders, 14,* 261–279.

Wickelgren, L. (1969). Ocular response of human newborns to intermittent visual movement. *Journal of Experimental Child Psychology, 8,* 469–482.

Wing, L., & Gould, J. (1979). Severe impairments of social interaction and associated abnormalities in children: Epidemiology and classification. *Journal of Autism and Developmental Disorders, 9,* 11–29.

Yirmiya, N., Kasari, C., Mundy, P., & Sigman, M. (1987). *Facial expressions of emotion: Are autistic children different from normal and mentally retarded children?* Paper presented at the biennial meeting of the Society for Research in Child Development, Baltimore.

Zentall, S. S., & Zentall, T. R. (1983). Optimal stimulation: A model of disordered activity and performance in normal and deviant children. *Psychological Bulletin, 94,* 446–471.

CHAPTER 4

The Early Development of Autistic Children
Implications for Defining Primary Deficits

JUDY A. UNGERER
Macquarie University

INTRODUCTION

Since Kanner (1943) first described the syndrome of infantile autism, researchers have struggled to identify an etiology for the disorder. This has not been an easy task, since probable biological causes (e.g., genetic transmission and central nervous system infection) have been found in only some cases, and knowledge of these causes has done little to clarify the neuropsychological basis of the disorder.

Attempts to identify the underlying neuropsychological disturbance in infantile autism have been hindered by the difficulty in differentiating primary and secondary deficits. Not all the functional deficits of autistic children are likely to be primary, in the sense of being direct manifestations of the core, underlying disturbance. Rather, many of the deficits may be either secondary consequences of more primary problems or a function of the general retardation in development frequently (but not necessarily) associated with autism. Differentiating between primary and secondary deficits is essential, because it is the primary deficits that are more likely to provide information about the neuropsychological basis of the disorder.

The importance of differentiating between primary and secondary deficits can be seen more easily in disorders with physical sequelae. For example, in anorexia nervosa, a primary deficit or symptom is the failure to maintain an adequate body weight (American Psychiatric Association, 1980). A secondary deficit is amenorrhea. Secondary deficits appear as a consequence of primary deficits, and thus the primary deficits are what directly reflect the underlying physical and/or psychological disturbance. A second example is alcohol dependence, which has as a primary deficit a pathological pattern of alcohol use (American Psychiatric Association, 1980). A secondary deficit that emerges as a consequence of the primary drinking problem is cirrhosis of the liver. Differentiation between primary and secondary deficits is critical to understanding the basic disturbance in any disorder. It also may have important implications for the focus of treatment, since the amelioration of a disorder may only occur when primary deficits are reduced. Removal of secondary deficits may improve a person's overall condition, but is likely to have little effect on the underlying disturbance.

Theories concerning which of the autistic child's deficits are primary have varied over the years. Kanner's (1943) original description of the disorder emphasized the inability to establish normal social relationships as primary, but later researchers did not always agree with this viewpoint. For example, Wing (1976) wrote in the foreword to a book of collected papers on autism: "The present authors all regard early childhood autism and related conditions as resulting from a *basic disturbance of cognitive development*, the effects of which include abnormalities of language and communication and a variety of *secondary behavioral and emotional problems*" (p. xi, italics added). Thus, Wing and her colleagues considered the abnormalities in social relationships a secondary outcome of the disturbances in cognitive development. Children who are unable to communicate normally with others are, as a consequence, hindered in their development of social-emotional relationships, and show abnormalities in this domain as well. More recently, the focus of the discussion of primary deficit has returned to the social sphere (Fein, Pennington, Markowitz, Braverman, & Waterhouse, 1986; Hobson, 1983b).

The purpose of this chapter is to review current research on behavioral deficits in infantile autism, with the goal of determining the implications of this research for identifying primary deficits. Since primary deficits are likely to be observed early in the development of autistic children, the focus of the review is on studies investigating skills known to appear in normal children in the first 2 years of life. This is the period of development known in Piagetian theory as the sensory–motor stage, and the development of sensory–motor skills is emphasized. However, the scope of the chapter is broader and includes recent work on early social concepts in autistic children. The chapter ends with a presentation of current approaches to defining the primary deficits in infantile autism that have been strongly influenced by the research on early-developing skills.

APPROACHES TO IDENTIFYING PRIMARY DEFICITS

The deficits found among autistic children are varied and complex, and the determination of which deficits are primary has been difficult to establish. Two different approaches to the problem can be found in the literature. The first involves defining criteria for labeling deficits as primary, whereas the second involves studying particular subgroups of autistic individuals. As an example of the first approach, Rutter (1983) has suggested criteria for identifying primary deficits that include being present in all cases, remaining relatively stable over time, and having prognostic significance. Rutter has used these criteria to argue for the primacy of cognitive deficits in autism that involve language, coding, sequencing, and abstraction skills; however, these same criteria can be used to support arguments for the primacy of social deficits as well (Fein *et al.*, 1986).

A second approach to identifying primary deficits involves the study of subgroups of autistic individuals who are believed to manifest autism in a relatively pure form. For example, Prior (1979) has argued for studying normally intelligent autistic individuals in order to control for the influence of developmental level on performance. However, since 70%–80% of autistic individuals are also mentally retarded, this approach could lead to a failure to understand the autistic syndrome as it is manifested in most individuals. In particular, an understanding of possible interactive relations between developmental level and autistic features would be lost. An alternative approach, which maintains access to the full range of autistic individuals, is to control for developmental factors by using control groups matched for mental age. In addition, matching for chronological age as well as mental age is generally recommended, since biological/maturational factors may have significant effects on performance in some domains (James & Barry, 1981). Skills that are dependent on brain maturation (e.g., performance on cerebral lateralization tasks) and skills that may be strongly influenced by physical maturation (e.g., social interactions with adults and peers) are best studied using controls matched for mental and chronological age.

A second subgroup of autistic individuals that has more recently become a focus of study in the search for primary deficits is young children, typically in the preschool age range. The rationale for studying young autistic children has been the belief that primary deficits are most likely to appear in their purest form early in development. Deficits that are identified in older age groups may not be primary, but rather may develop as a secondary consequence of earlier appearing problems. For example, it is possible to argue that language deficits in autistic children are a secondary consequence of the failure during infancy to establish normal social relationships, which are believed to underlie the development of verbal communication skills (Werner & Kaplan, 1963). It is important to note that such arguments for labeling deficits as primary or secondary are strongly influenced by our knowledge of the relationships among skills in normal development. However, development in clinical groups may proceed differently, with skills such as language and social interaction showing greater dissociation, as is seen in children with aphasic disorders. The study of young autistic children may provide some important insights into the nature of primary deficits, but these ultimately must be evaluated within the context of information from other autistic groups.

In the remainder of this chapter, the results of research aimed at identifying deficits in young autistic children are reviewed. This work has brought a change in emphasis in our understanding of the nature of the autistic disorder, and with it a sense that we are closer to identifying deficits that are truly primary. Whereas studies of older autistic children have focused on describing cognitive and language deficits, studies of younger children have increasingly moved toward emphasizing the social aspects of the disorder. This is in part a response to a general trend in research on both clinical and normal populations to study the social and emotional components of development. However, it is also a change in emphasis that is forced by the age group of children under study. Development in the early years is strongly influenced by the social context in which it occurs, and it is difficult to classify achievements as strictly, or even predominantly, cognitive or social in nature. For example, the development of symbolic play in the second year of life has generally been regarded as a significant cognitive achievement. However, the earliest forms of symbolic play are based on the imitation of other persons, and this emphasizes the importance of the social context for symbolic play development.

What becomes clear in the study of young children is that cognitive, social, and affective functioning are inextricably intertwined, and division of skills into separate domains of development may be inaccurate and misleading. At the very least, it is necessary to recognize the importance of interactions across developmental domains in the early years. This is not a trivial matter, because whether we conceptualize deficits as being cognitive, social, or some interaction of the two will influence our ability to recognize relations among deficits, and thereby our ability to identify those that are truly primary.

REVIEW OF RESEARCH

The sensory–motor period in normal children spans the age range from birth to approximately 2 years. During this age period the infant undergoes dramatic changes in its cognitive, social, and emotional functioning. The infant's behavior at birth is dominated by simple reflex schemes and reactions to immediately present events. By age 2, the infant has an extensive knowledge of objects, people, and events in its environment, and is capable of mental problem solving, imitation of past events, symbolic play, and communication via gestures and language. The infant also has a rudimentary concept of the self, as well as the ability to express a complex range of emotions and to understand and sympathize with the emotional expressions of others. The achievements of the sensory–motor period are broad, and many aspects of this development have been studied in autistic children. This review emphasizes those studies most relevant to understanding the primary deficits of the autistic syndrome.

Object Concepts

Piaget's (1952) theory of cognitive development and related research have provided a description of the normal infant's understanding of objects during the sensory–motor period. At birth, infants are thought to be unable to differentiate between their own actions and the objects to which their actions are directed. Gradually during the first year of life, they come to differentiate between themselves and objects, to attribute some degree of permanence to absent objects, and to manipulate and combine objects to solve problems and achieve desired ends. During the second year, these skills become elaborated through the development of the ability to form and manipulate mental representations of objects and to form object categories. A mature understanding of object permanence is achieved with the ability to mentally represent absent objects, and with problem solving that is accomplished mentally rather than being restricted to the trial-and-error manipulation of real objects.

Piaget (1952) has described the infant's developing object knowledge in a succession of six stages during the sensory–motor period. Although there is disagreement over the actual age of achievement of the six sensory–motor stages (Gibson & White, 1978; Moore & Meltzoff, 1978) and the nature of the changes in the infant's understanding (Bower, 1974; Uzgiris, 1976), empirical studies have largely validated the behavioral observations of Piaget regarding the infant's developing object knowledge. The longitudinal progression reported by Piaget with his own children has been supported in controlled studies (Decarie, 1967; Escalona & Corman, 1969; Kopp, Sigman, & Parmelee, 1974; Uzgiris & Hunt, 1975), although individual infants do occasionally show some minor regressions in the order of sensory–motor attainments in test situations (Kopp, Sigman, & Parmelee, 1973, 1974).

The development of sensory–motor object concepts in autistic children has received considerable attention in the research literature. Early studies reported conflicting findings, with some researchers demonstrating sophisticated object concepts at sensory–motor stage 5 or 6 (Curcio, 1978; Serafica, 1971) and others reporting autistic children to be arrested at stage 4 of sensorimotor development, with only rudimentary object permanence and problem-solving skills (Bettelheim, 1967; Christ, 1977).

However, more recent research using formal scales of sensory–motor development (Casati & Lezine, 1968; Uzgiris & Hunt, 1975) has consistently found no differences in the sensory–motor object concepts of autistic and mental-age-matched mentally retarded and normal children (Dawson & Adams, 1984; Lancy & Goldstein, 1982; Sigman & Ungerer, 1981, 1984b). Autistic children appear to have the same capacity for mental problem solving and representation of absent objects as mentally retarded and normal children of comparable mental age.

The development of object concepts in autistic children also shows no delay in the area of category knowledge. We (Ungerer & Sigman, 1987) observed the spontaneous object-sorting behavior of a group of young autistic children with mental ages ranging from 1½ to 3 years. Category knowledge was inferred from the tendency to pick up same-category objects in succession and to form spatially separate groupings of same-category objects. The autistic children were found to be comparable to mental-age-matched retarded and normal children in their ability to form different shape and color perceptual categories and functional categories (e.g., animals, food, furniture, and vehicles).

Symbolic Play

One of the most significant accomplishments of the sensory–motor period in normal children is the development of symbolic play. As with the development of sensory–motor object concepts, symbolic play is an important manifestation of the young child's early representational skills. Research on play with objects in normal children indicates that qualitative, age-related changes in play appear to underlie the emergence of symbolic play at approximately 20 months of age. Prior to 9 months of age, play is characterized by the simple manipulation of objects, which includes close visual and tactual inspection of single objects along with mouthing, waving, banging, and other exploratory acts. At 8 to 9 months, play advances to the relational use of objects in combination—for example, using one object to push another. A few months later, stacking objects and using objects as containers are observed. At 12 months, infants begin to play with objects in a functionally appropriate or conventional way. Between 12 and 22 months of age, mature symbolic play gradually emerges and is marked at the end of the second year by the child's ability to treat representations of animate objects (e.g., dolls and stuffed animals) as if they could initiate their own actions, to transform objects by using one object as if it were another different object, and to create totally imaginary objects through the use of gesture and language (Inhelder, Lezine, Sinclair, & Stambak, 1972; Nicolich, 1977; Piaget, 1962; Sinclair, 1970; Ungerer, Zelazo, Kearsley, & O'Leary, 1981).

Studies of play behavior in autistic children have shown clear differences between autistic and mental-age-matched retarded and normal groups, particularly in the area of symbolic play (Riguet, Taylor, Benaroya, & Klein, 1981; Wing, Gould, Yeates, & Brierly, 1977). In our own research, we have demonstrated symbolic play deficits in both highly structured play interactions and in free play settings. In our first study (Sigman & Ungerer, 1984b; Ungerer & Sigman, 1981), the play behaviors of 16 young autistic children were compared to those shown by 16 mental-age- and chronological-age-matched retarded children and 16 mental-age-matched normal children. In general, the results from both structured and free-play assessments indicated that the autistic children were similar to the mentally retarded and normal groups in the simple manipulation of objects and in relational play. However, their functional object use and symbolic play were consistently less mature. In a free-play setting, the autistic children spent less time than the control groups engaged in functional play, and in both structured and free-play settings their spontaneous functional and symbolic play were less diverse. In the structured setting, the diversity of the autistic children's functional play could be increased with the support of verbal prompts and modeling, but their symbolic play remained less varied.

The play assessments were repeated with a new sample of 18 autistic children and matched mentally retarded and normal controls, and similar findings emerged (Mundy, Sigman, Ungerer, & Sherman, 1987). When the diversity of functional and symbolic play acts was compared for the three new groups, the autistic children showed fewer functional and symbolic play acts than the other children in both the structured and free-play settings, but only the group differences in symbolic play in the structured setting were statistically significant. In addition, the symbolic play behavior that most clearly differentiated the three groups was the ability to use a doll as an independent agent of action. Mentally retarded and normal children were able to attribute animate characteristics to dolls, whereas autistic children rarely performed this play behavior.

Imitation

Imitation has been accorded an important role in the cognitive and social development of the infant during the sensory–motor period. From a cognitive perspective, imitation is significant in the development of representational thought, particularly in the area of symbolic play. The earliest manifestations of symbolic play, which appear at 12 months of age, involve imitation of conventional uses of objects (e.g., drinking from a cup or eating from a spoon). Imitation is also of cognitive significance as a means children use for understanding puzzling events (Uzgiris, 1981). Imitation facilitates learning and enables children to check the accuracy of their understanding. At a later age these functions are performed mentally in thought.

Piaget (1962) has identified stages in the development of imitation that correspond to his six general stages of sensory–motor development. In Piaget's theory, imitation during the first few months of life is restricted to actions already in the child's behavioral repertoire, and progresses by the end of the second year to include the imitation of novel acts and the deferred imitation of absent models. Although there is some debate over the age at which imitation can first be observed, with some studies reporting imitation of facial expressions and finger and hand movements in neonates (Abravanel & Sigafoos, 1984; Field, Woodson, Greenberg, & Cohen, 1982; Meltzoff & Moore, 1977), Piaget's description of the development of imitation has been substantiated in other work (Uzgiris & Hunt, 1975).

In more recent years, the role of imitation in social development has received considerable emphasis. Observations of interactions between caregivers and infants stress the importance of mutual imitation in sustaining social interaction, in enhancing the infant's understanding of body schema, and in providing a sense of mutuality and shared experience (Stern, 1977; Uzgiris, 1981). Thus, imitation within the context of early social interaction may contribute to the development of later self-awareness and to the understanding of the relationship between self and others in terms of shared physical, cognitive, and emotional experience.

Research on imitation skills in autistic children has consistently shown marked delays in both vocal and gestural domains, although some imitation of body movements and actions with objects has been described (Curcio, 1978; Dawson & Adams, 1984; DeMyer *et al.*, 1972; Hammes & Landgell, 1981). We (Sigman

& Ungerer, 1984b) have reported significantly lower levels of performance for vocal and gestural imitation than for object permanence skills in autistic children ranging in age from 2 to 6 years. Dawson and Adams (1984) reported similar discrepancies between the development of imitation and object permanence in a comparable sample of young autistic children. Moreover, Dawson and Adams (1984) noted a correlation between the children's ability to imitate and other aspects of their social behavior, including levels of social responsiveness, free play, and language, but not their object permanence skills. A relation between imitation skills and social relatedness has also been reported by Wing and Gould (1979). Of interest is the observation that autistic children who have acquired some imitation skills are able to apply these skills to learn new behaviors in peer modeling contexts (Charlop, Schreibman, & Tryon, 1983). Thus, imitation appears to be associated with both social responsiveness and social learning in autistic children.

Knowledge of Self and Other Persons

Among the most important concepts acquired by normal children during the sensory–motor period are a sense of self and of other persons, and a basic understanding of self–other relationships. This knowledge has its roots in the earliest interactions between the infant and its caregivers and continues to be elaborated through a variety of experiences over the course of the infant's life. Among the earliest forms of self–other knowledge achieved during the sensory–motor period is a differentiation of self from others. Self–other differentiation is thought to derive from the infant's reciprocal interactions with other persons (Lewis & Brooks-Gunn, 1979). In their earliest forms, these interactions consist of the caregiver's contingent responses to the infant's cry signals, visual regard, and social smiles. The infant's role in these interactions is later elaborated through the use of communicative gestures (e.g., pointing) and language. Reciprocal interactions are thought to assist the infant in differentiating self from other because they provide the infant with a sense of competence and control over the social environment. They may also facilitate the development of a physical schema for the self, since interactions always involve the other person's relating to the infant's specific location in space (Lewis & Brooks-Gunn, 1979).

In addition to learning to differentiate self from other, infants during the sensory–motor period develop the capacity for visual self-recognition. Research on normal children indicates that the development of visual self-recognition is a gradual process that is first manifested at 9 to 12 months of age and is well established by the end of the second year (Lewis & Brooks-Gunn, 1979). When self-recognition first appears, it is based on action as well as physical features, since self-recognition is restricted to images that directly reflect the infant's own movements (e.g., mirror images and immediate-playback video representations). By 15 to 18 months of age, self-recognition based on an awareness of physical features alone is observed. Infants show recognition of static images such as photographs, and they show an awareness of distortions in their facial features. If a spot of rouge is placed on an infant's nose, the infant will touch the spot when looking at its mirror image. Self-conscious or coy responses to mirror images and the verbal labeling of images are also observed in the 15- to 18-month period. Between 18 and 21 months, self-recognition across a wide range of representative modes is clearly established, and personal pronouns begin to be used. Thus, self-recognition when it first appears is dependent on both physical features and action. At about 15 months, and certainly by 21 months of age, feature recognition, independent of action, accounts for self-recognition (Lewis & Brooks-Gunn, 1979).

During the sensory–motor period, the infant not only learns to recognize itself, but also learns to recognize and differentiate among other persons in its environment. The knowledge that the infant acquires of others during this period takes several forms. First, infants learn to differentiate between familiar others and strangers in the first few months of life. Studies have shown differentiation of mother and stranger and father and stranger by infants as young as 3 months of age (Banks & Wolfson, 1967; Bronson, 1972; Brooks-Gunn & Lewis, 1979; Lamb, 1976). In addition, infants by 6 months of age are able to differentiate among people of different ages, possibly through the use of facial configuration and height cues (Brooks & Lewis, 1976; Fagan, 1972). Differential responding to others on the basis of gender cues has also been demonstrated (Fagan, 1972; Kagan & Lewis, 1965; Lewis & Brooks, 1974).

The infant's knowledge of self and other is not restricted to observable physical features, but also extends to the understanding of internal mental states. Infants during the sensory–motor period provide evidence of understanding that a focus of attention between self and other can be shared when they point, show, or make eye contact with others while holding an object or watching an interesting event. This knowledge of joint attention is a more abstract form of person knowledge than the other types of knowledge considered up to this point, since it cannot be derived primarily from an appreciation of external perceptual cues. Rather, it entails a knowledge of similarities between internal states that may be facilitated by perceptual cues, such as direction of eye gaze, but cannot be fully derived from them. In normal children, an understanding of joint attention is well established by 2 years of age and is thought to have its roots in the reciprocal interactions of caregivers and infants in the earliest months of life. Interactions involving joint attention are considered important for promoting the child's understanding of relationships between the self and others, and for the development of conversational skills, the normal functional use of language, and possibly the acquisition of terms such as personal pronouns (Loveland & Landry, 1985).

In summary, during the first 2 years of life, normal infants acquire considerable knowledge about the self and other persons. As noted above, they learn to recognize visual representations of themselves in photographs and mirrors, and to differentiate among other persons on the basis of familiarity, age, and gender cues. Although most of what infants learn about others is based on perceptual information, some more abstract knowledge of internal mental states also is acquired.

An example of the latter is the awareness that attention to objects and events can be shared with another. Theorists argue that the development of knowledge about the self and others has its foundation in the reciprocal social interactions of infants and their caregivers. It is within these social exchanges that the earliest understanding of persons and human relationships is formed.

What kinds of knowledge of self and other persons do we find among young autistic children? There is little information, other than anecdotes from case studies, on the development of reciprocal social interactions between autistic infants and their caregivers. The information that is available, however, suggests that development in this area is both deviant and delayed. In the first year of life, autistic infants may fail to show an anticipatory posture or put out their arms to be picked up as normal infants do (Rutter, 1983). Later, reciprocal games such as "peekaboo," imitative behavior, and communicative gestures such as "bye-bye" or pointing may fail to appear (Park, 1986). Given the hypothesized importance of early reciprocal interactions for later social development in normal children, the deviant behavior of autistic infants is noteworthy.

Consistent with these reports are the results of a limited number of studies looking at reciprocal social interactions between caregivers and somewhat older autistic children. Ricks (1975) reported that the vocal signals of autistic children may be idiosyncratic and unintelligible except to caregivers who have had extensive experience in learning to decipher their children's verbal cues. Furthermore, we (Mundy, Sigman, Ungerer, & Sherman, 1986) observed deficits in autistic children in a range of behaviors critical for successful social interactions. These included taking turns and using eye contact and pointing to request objects out of reach. However, more direct requests for aid that did not entail directing an adult's attention to a distant object, such as combining eye contact to an adult with reaching for or giving an object, were not deficient. These results are consistent with the notion that autistic children understand adults as agents who can facilitate their interactions with the environment, but have difficulty grasping that adults can also share their focus of attention.

In contrast to the majority of studies on reciprocal social interactions which show deficits in autistic children, research on visual self-recognition indicates more normal behavior. Using as an index of self-recognition a child's response to a mark on his or her nose as observed in a mirror reflection, autistic children have been reported to show touching of the mark on their noses (and hence self-recognition) at the same developmental level as normal children. However, they failed to show the coy, silly, or self-conscious behavior that is sometimes observed in normal groups (Dawson & McKissick, 1984; Ferrari & Matthews, 1983; Neuman & Hill, 1978; Ungerer, Mundy, Sigman, & Sherman, 1988).

The autistic child's ability to recognize and differentiate among other persons has been explored in several studies. Young autistic children have been shown to respond differentially to familiar caregivers and strangers following brief separations (Sigman & Ungerer, 1984a), and their understanding of people as permanent objects is comparable to that observed in mentally retarded and normal groups

(Sigman & Mundy, 1987). However, their ability to identify emotional cues in others and to differentiate among others on the basis of age cues appears to be impaired (Hobson, 1983a, 1983b). The difficulty does not seem to be one of impaired perception, since autistic children are well able to differentiate among faces of different people and to detect changes in facial cues (Langdell, 1978; Sigman, Ungerer, Mundy, & Sherman, 1987). Rather, the difficulty lies in the autistic children's failure to extract social meaning from the range of social and emotional cues provided by others and to use this social meaning to organize their world (Rutter, 1983). Autistic children have difficulty understanding abstract relationships between self and other that cannot be derived primarily from perceptual cues.

Thus, autistic children's knowledge of the self and other persons does not appear to be delayed when the concepts to be derived are based primarily on external perceptual cues. Their knowledge of people as physical objects is comparable to that observed in mentally retarded and normal groups. However, when the knowledge to be acquired is tied to those properties of people that clearly differentiate them from nonsocial, physical objects, such as the fact that people can think and feel (Gelman & Spelke, 1981), clear deficits among autistic children are observed.

IMPLICATIONS

Studies of early functioning in autistic children have been consistent in demonstrating an unevenness in development, with specific areas of deficit coexisting with relatively normal areas of functioning. Sensory–motor object knowledge, including object permanence and means–ends skills, is not delayed beyond what would be expected from the autistic child's general level of retardation, and therefore does not constitute a specific area of deficit. Following a similar developmental pattern are the abilities to form object categories, to engage in spatial-relational object play, and to acquire basic concepts of the self and other persons (e.g., visual self-recognition, person permanence, and an understanding of others as agents of action capable of facilitating the autistic child's interaction with the object world). In contrast, specific areas of deficit that have repeatedly been identified include symbolic play, vocal and gestural communication, imitation, and more abstract concepts of persons (e.g., the notion of shared attention, empathy, and the meaning of facial and affective expressions). In each case, development in these areas of deficit is clearly delayed beyond what would be expected from an assessment of the autistic child's general level of retardation. Comparisons of the performance of autistic children with that of mentally retarded children consistently show poorer functioning in the autistic groups. The use of the term "specific area of deficit" should not be interpreted to mean that these skills are never acquired by autistic children. Rather, it means that the development of these skills is always extremely delayed, although they may eventually appear in some form among the more able children.

The consistency with which the specific areas of deficit have been identified by different researchers is heartening, but the significance of these deficits for identifying the neuropsychological basis of autism is still unclear. However, a consistent trend in the interpretation of these findings is emerging that is leading to a clear change in emphasis in our understanding of the deficits associated with autism. Previous attempts to define primary deficits in autistic children emphasized the cognitive, perceptual, and language delays associated with the disorder. In contrast, the current trend is to emphasize the social deficits of autism as primary. This social emphasis has taken two forms: (1) attempts to define the known areas of deficit in social terms, and (2) attempts to postulate underlying social processes whose disruption could conceivably cause the range of deficits observed in autistic children.

Social interpretations of known deficit areas have been proposed by several researchers. Hermelin (1982; see also Hermelin & O'Connor, 1985) has suggested that the primary deficit in autism involves "impairments in a genetically pre-programmed innate communication system, which in humans includes a non-verbal branch serving the expression of feelings, as well as a verbal one which has evolved for expressing primarily observations and thoughts" (p. 17). Hermelin notes that such a deficit would result in profound cognitive impairments, as well as severe emotional and social impairments. However, details as to how these impairments might arise are not given. Hermelin's approach to describing the language, gestural, and emotional deficits in autism stresses their communicative function, and thus is clearly social in emphasis. These areas of functioning are not deficient because of impairments in shared underlying cognitive skills, but rather because of impairments in a shared social-communicative function.

In a recent review paper, Rutter (1983) has also emphasized the importance of social deficits in infantile autism. He proposes that the autistic child's social abnormalities, and, in particular, deficits in reciprocal social interaction, derive from an impaired ability to process stimuli that carry emotional or social meaning, such as facial expressions and gestures expressing emotional states. The ability to understand and generate such expressive behavior is considered critical for the smooth regulation of social interaction with others. Rutter does not, however, go so far as to conclude that this deficit is the primary cause of the autistic child's deviant development. On the contrary, he has refrained from identifying a single, primary deficit, and rather has grouped the deficit in the processing of social stimuli with other cognitive deficits thought to underlie the autistic syndrome, including deficits in language, sequencing, abstraction, and coding skills.

Finally, our work (Sigman *et al.*, 1987) also underscores the social nature of the early-appearing deficits in autistic children. Our extensive research on the functioning of young autistic children has provided much of the evidence for the specific areas of developmental strength and deficit reviewed earlier in this chapter. Focusing on the deficits in symbolic play with dolls and joint attention identified in our work, we have concluded that young autistic children have particular difficulties in acquiring knowledge of others and an awareness of self. In addition, we (Ungerer & Sigman, 1981) have noted that the deficits observed in symbolic play and language may derive from an impairment in the social-communicative function of these skills, since both play and language are used by children as a means of sharing their experiences with others. Werner and Kaplan's (1963) theory of symbolic development underscores this association by proposing that the development of verbal and gestural symbols derives from a common social core involving communicative interaction between the infant and the caregiver.

Although we (Sigman *et al.*, 1987) have identified social factors that may underlie the deficits observed in autistic children, there are limits to this approach. It is often as easy to identify cognitive factors that may underlie deficits as it is to identify social ones. For example, symbolic play and language both involve the cognitive ability to generate symbols and to learn the system of rules regulating the form of their expression, whereas symbolic play and joint attention are thought to reflect the cognitive ability to form second-order representations (Frith, 1984; Leslie, 1984). Whether a cognitive or social perspective is most valid for defining the primary deficits in autism is not readily apparent. We (Mundy *et al.*, 1986) also note that tasks thought to share a common social core are not always as highly intercorrelated as might be expected. The absence of robust correlations among deficits does not negate the possibility of a common social core, but it does emphasize two things: (1) The many differences that exist among deficits may make it difficult to identify commonalities that are also present; and (2) relations among deficits are dynamic, and the nature of the similarities and differences that are observed may vary with the developmental level of the child.

The study of relations among deficits in autistic children can only provide limited information about the underlying nature of the disorder. To get closer to an understanding of autism, it is necessary to identify the developmental processes that underlie the observed deficits. The work of Hobson (1983b; see also Chapter 2, this volume) approaches this problem from a social-affective perspective. Hobson proposes that the acquisition of knowledge about persons and things social is dependent on the individual's ability to engage in a quality of personal relatedness with others, which has as its basis affective or empathic responsiveness to other people. Without the ability to engage in this form of personal relatedness, the individual's potential for acquiring social knowledge is severely restricted. Within this context, autism is considered to involve "a profound disruption in the biologically-based capacity for a quality of 'personal relatedness' with others" (1983b, p. 23) which has far-reaching implications for the development of the autistic child's thought, feeling, language, self-awareness, and much else besides.

Hobson's proposal—that the child's knowledge of self and other persons derives from empathic interactions with others—provides a mechanism for understanding the profound deficits that characterize the autistic syndrome. Whether this explanation or some related social mechanism is most successful in defining the underlying cause of autism remains for further research to establish. However,

the trend of current thinking is clear. Combined with recent attempts to conceptualize the autistic child's known deficits in social terms, the conclusion is readily
drawn that a disruption in social-affective development must be considered a *primary* deficit in autism. Whether this social-affective deficit is the single underlying cause of autism is, however, not so easily established. As noted earlier in this
chapter, social, affective, and cognitive development are inextricably intertwined,
particularly in the early childhood years, and any attempt to define early social
deficits or social-affective developmental mechanisms will quickly call forth cognitive counterparts. The early onset of the autistic disorder and the dynamic nature of development also increase the probability that different systems will be
affected. Behavioral observations of autistic children may never bring us closer to
an answer to this problem. However, they can direct the search for biological
"cause" to consider the role of neuropsychological systems governing social and
affective development (Fein *et al.*, 1986). In this way, they will have exerted an
important influence on our attempts to identify the essential nature and underlying cause of the autistic syndrome.

References

Abravanel, E., & Sigafoos, A. (1984). Exploring the presence of imitation during infancy. *Child Development, 55,* 381–392.
American Psychiatric Association. (1980). *Diagnostic and statistical manual of mental disorders* (3rd ed.). Washington, DC: Author.
Banks, J., & Wolfson, J. (1967, April). *Differential cardiac response of infants to mother and stranger.* Paper presented at the meeting of the Eastern Psychological Association, Boston.
Bettelheim, B. (1967). *The empty fortress: Infantile autism and the birth of the self.* New York: Free Press.
Bower, T. (1974). *Development in infancy.* San Francisco: W. H. Freeman.
Bronson, G. (1972). Infants' reactions to unfamiliar persons and novel objects. *Monographs of the Society for Research in Child Development, 47*(3, Serial No. 148).
Brooks, J., & Lewis, M. (1976). Infants' responses to strangers: Midget, adult and child. *Child Development, 47,* 323–332.
Brooks-Gunn, J., & Lewis, M. (1979). Early social knowledge: The development of knowledge about others. In H. McGurk (Ed.), *Childhood social development.* London: Methuen.
Casati, I., & Lezine, I. (1968). *Les étapes de l'intelligence sensorimotrice.* Paris: Les Editions de Centre de Psychologie Appliquée.
Charlop, M., Schreibman, L., & Tryon, A. (1983). Learning through observation: The effects of peer modeling on acquisition and generalization in autistic children. *Journal of Abnormal Child Psychology, 11,* 355–366.
Christ, A. (1977). *Factors affecting the cognitive assessment of psychotic children arrested at the senso-rimotor stage of development.* Paper presented at the meeting of the American Academy of Child Psychiatry, Toronto.
Curcio, F. (1978). Sensorimotor functioning and communication in mute autistic children. *Journal of Autism and Childhood Schizophrenia, 8,* 281–292.
Dawson, G., & Adams, A. (1984). Imitation and social responsiveness in autistic children. *Journal of Abnormal Child Psychology, 12,* 209–226.
Dawson, G., & McKissick, F. (1984). Self-recognition in autistic children. *Journal of Autism and Developmental Disorders, 14,* 383–394.

Decarie, T. G. (1967). *Intelligence and affectivity in early childhood*. New York: International Universities Press.

DeMyer, M., Alpern, G., Barton, S., DeMyer, W., Churchill, D., Hingtgen, J., Bryson, C., Pontius, W., & Kimberlin, C. (1972). Imitation in autistic, early schizophrenic, and non-psychotic subnormal children. *Journal of Autism and Childhood Schizophrenia, 2,* 264–287.

Escalona, S., & Corman, H. (1969). *Albert Einstein Scales of Sensorimotor Development*. Unpublished manuscript.

Fagan, J. (1972). Infants' recognition memory for faces. *Journal of Experimental Child Psychology, 14,* 453–476.

Fein, D., Pennington, B., Markowitz, P., Braverman, M., & Waterhouse, L. (1986). Toward a neuropsychological model of infantile autism: Are the social deficits primary? *Journal of the American Academy of Child Psychiatry, 25,* 198–212.

Ferrari, M., & Matthews, W. (1983). Self-recognition deficits in autism: Syndrome-specific or general developmental delay? *Journal of Autism and Developmental Disorders, 13,* 317–324.

Field, T., Woodson, R., Greenberg, R., & Cohen, D. (1982). Discrimination and imitation of facial expression by neonates. *Science, 218,* 179–181.

Frith, U. (1984). A new perspective in research on autism. In Association pour la Recherche sur l'Autisme et les Psychoses Infantiles (Ed.), *Contributions à la recherche scientifique sur l'autisme: Aspects cognitifs*. Paris: Editor.

Gelman, R., & Spelke, E. (1981). The development of thoughts about animate and inanimate objects: Implications for research on social cognition. In J. Flavell & L. Ross (Eds.) *Social cognitive development*. Cambridge, England: Cambridge University Press.

Gibson, E. J., & White, S. J. (1978). C'est moi. *Contemporary Psychology, 23,* 609–611.

Hammes, J., & Langdell, T. (1981). Precursors of symbol formation and childhood autism. *Journal of Autism and Developmental Disorders, 11,* 331–346.

Hermelin, B. (1982). Thoughts and feelings. *Australian Autism Review, 4,* 10–19.

Hermelin, B., & O'Connor, N. (1985). *Logico-affective states and non-verbal language*. Unpublished manuscript.

Hobson, R. P. (1983a). The autistic child's recognition of age-related features of people, animals, and things. *British Journal of Developmental Psychology, 1,* 343–352.

Hobson, R. P. (1983b). *Origins of the personal relation, and the unique case of autism*. Paper presented at the meeting of the Association for Child Psychology and Psychiatry, London.

Inhelder, B., Lezine, I., Sinclair, H., & Stambak, M. (1972). Les débuts de la fonction symbolique. *Archives de Psychologie, 41,* 187–243.

James, A., & Barry, R. (1981). General maturational lag as an essential correlate of early-onset psychosis. *Journal of Autism and Developmental Disabilities, 11,* 271–283.

Kagan, J., & Lewis, M. (1965). Studies of attention in the human infant. *Merrill–Palmer Quarterly, 11,* 95–127.

Kanner, L. (1943). Autistic disturbances of affective contact. *The Nervous Child, 2,* 217–250.

Kopp, C., Sigman, M., & Parmelee, A. (1973). Ordinality and sensory–motor series. *Child Development, 44,* 821.

Kopp, C., Sigman, M., & Parmelee, A. (1974). Longitudinal study of sensorimotor development. *Developmental Psychology, 10,* 687–695.

Lamb, M. (Ed.). (1976). *The role of the father in child development*. New York: Wiley.

Lancy, D., & Goldstein, G. (1982). The use of nonverbal Piagetian tasks to assess the cognitive development of autistic children. *Child Development, 53,* 1233–1241.

Langdell, T. (1978). Recognition of faces: An approach to the study of autism. *Journal of Child Psychology and Psychiatry, 19,* 255–268.

Leslie, A. M. (1984). Pretend play and representation in infancy: A cognitive approach. In Association pour la Recherche sur l'Autisme et les Psychoses Infantiles (Ed.), *Contributions à la recherche scientifique sur l'autisme: Aspects cognitifs*. Paris: Editor.

Lewis, M. & Brooks, J. (1974). Self, other and fear: Infants' reactions to people. In M. Lewis & L. Rosenblum (Eds.), *The origins of fear: The origins of behavior* (Vol. 2). New York: Wiley.

Lewis, M., & Brooks-Gunn, J. (1979). *Social cognition and the acquisition of self*. New York: Plenum.

Loveland, K., & Landry, S. (1985, April). *Joint attention and language in autism and developmental language delay.* Paper presented at the biennial meeting of the Society for Research in Child Development, Toronto.

Meltzoff, A., & Moore, M. (1977). Imitation of facial and manual gestures by human neonates. *Science, 198,* 75–78.

Moore, M., & Meltzoff, A. (1978). Object permanence, imitation, and language development: Toward a neoPiagetian perspective of cognitive and communicative development. In F. D. Minifie & L. L. Lloyd (Eds.), *Communicative and cognitive abilities: Early behavioral assessment.* Baltimore: University Park Press.

Mundy, P., Sigman, M., Ungerer, J., & Sherman, T. (1986). Defining the social deficits of autism: The contribution of non-verbal communication measures. *Journal of Child Psychology and Psychiatry, 27,* 657–669.

Mundy, P., Sigman, M., Ungerer, J., & Sherman, T. (1987). Nonverbal communication and play correlates of language development in autistic children. *Journal of Autism and Developmental Disorders, 17*(3), 349–364.

Neuman, C., & Hill, S. (1978). Self-recognition and stimulus preference in autistic children. *Developmental Psychobiology, 11,* 571–578.

Nicolich, L. (1977). Beyond sensorimotor intelligence. *Merrill–Palmer Quarterly, 23,* 89–99.

Park, C. (1986). Social growth in autism: A parent's perspective. In E. Schopler & G. Mesibov (Eds.), *Social behavior in autism.* New York: Plenum.

Piaget, J. (1952). *The origins of intelligence in children.* New York: Norton.

Piaget, J. (1962). *Play, dreams and imitation.* New York: Norton.

Prior, M. (1979). Cognitive abilities and disabilities in infantile autism: A review. *Journal of Abnormal Child Psychology, 7,* 357–380.

Ricks, D. (1975). Vocal communication in pre-verbal normal and autistic children. In N. O'Connor (Ed.), *Language, cognitive deficits and retardation.* London: Butterworths.

Riguet, C., Taylor, N., Benaroya, S., & Klein, L. (1981). Symbolic play in autistic, Down's, and normal children of equivalent mental age. *Journal of Autism and Developmental Disorders, 11,* 439–448.

Rutter, M. (1983). Cognitive deficits in the pathogenesis of autism. *Journal of Child Psychology and Psychiatry, 24,* 513–531.

Serafica, F. (1971). Object concepts in deviant children. *American Journal of Orthopsychiatry, 41,* 473–482.

Sigman, M., & Mundy, P. (1987). Symbolic processes in young autistic children. In D. Cicchetti (Ed.), *New directions in child development: Symbolic development in atypical children.* San Francisco: Jossey-Bass.

Sigman, M., & Ungerer, J. (1981). Sensorimotor skills and language comprehension in autistic children. *Journal of Abnormal Child Psychology, 9,* 149–165.

Sigman, M., & Ungerer, J. (1984a). Attachment behaviors in autistic children. *Journal of Autism and Developmental Disorders, 14,* 231–244.

Sigman, M., & Ungerer, J. (1984b). Cognitive and language skills in autistic, mentally retarded, and normal children. *Developmental Psychology, 20,* 293–302.

Sigman, M., Ungerer, J., Mundy, P., & Sherman, T. (1987). Cognition in autistic children. In D. Cohen, A. Donnellan, & R. Paul (Eds.), *Handbook of autism and atypical developmental disorders.* Silver Springs, MD: V. H. Winston.

Sinclair, H. (1970). The transition from sensory–motor behavior to symbolic activity. *Interchange, 1,* 119–125.

Stern, D. (1977). *The first relationship: Infant and mother.* Cambridge, MA: Harvard University Press.

Ungerer, J., Mundy, P., Sigman, M., & Sherman, T. (1988). *Mirror response, self-recognition, and affect in autistic children.* Manuscript in preparation.

Ungerer, J., & Sigman, M. (1981). Symbolic play and language comprehension in autistic children. *Journal of the American Academy of Child Psychiatry, 20,* 318–337.

Ungerer, J., & Sigman, M. (1987). Categorization skills and receptive language development in autistic children. *Journal of Autism and Developmental Disorders, 17,* 3–16.

Ungerer, J., Zelazo, P., Kearsley, R., & O'Leary, K. (1981). Developmental changes in the representation of objects in symbolic play from 18 to 34 months of age. *Child Development, 52,* 186–195.

Uzgiris, I. (1976). Organization of sensorimotor intelligence. In M. Lewis (Ed.), *Origins of intelligence.* New York: Plenum.

Uzgiris, I. (1981). Two functions of imitation during infancy. *International Journal of Behavioral Development, 4,* 1–12.

Uzgiris, I., & Hunt, J. M. (1975). *Assessment in infancy.* Urbana: University of Illinois Press.

Werner, H., & Kaplan, B. (1963). *Symbol formation.* New York: Wiley.

Wing, L. (Ed.). (1976). *Early childhood autism.* Oxford: Pergamon Press.

Wing, L, & Gould, J. (1979). Severe impairments of social interaction and associated abnormalities in children: Epidemiology and classification. *Journal of Autism and Developmental Disorders, 9,* 11–29.

Wing, L., Gould, J., Yeates, S., & Brierly, L. (1977). Symbolic play in severely mentally retarded and in autistic children. *Journal of Child Psychology and Psychiatry, 18,* 167–178.

CHAPTER 5

A Psycholinguistic Perspective on Language Development in the Autistic Child

HELEN TAGER-FLUSBERG
University of Massachusetts at Boston

INTRODUCTION

Since Kanner (1943) first described the characteristics of autistic children more than 40 years ago, there has been considerable controversy over the nature of the language and communication deficits and their role in the definition of the syndrome. One view (e.g., Bettelheim, 1967; Boucher, 1976b; Waterhouse & Fein, 1982) is that the language deficits are simply the product of other critical aspects of the syndrome, but are not important for understanding autism. The opposite view is that the language deficits are primary, placing autism at the more disordered extreme of the continuum of developmental aphasia (e.g., Churchill, 1972; Rutter, Bartak, & Newman, 1971). Although there is general agreement that no autistic child, however verbal, speaks or communicates in age-appropriate ways, and that language impairment is a criterial symptom of autism, there is still little agreement about the nature of the language deficits specific to this pervasive developmental disorder.

Three related issues have been raised at various times in the literature. First, to what extent is language merely delayed or truly deviant in the autistic child? This question focuses on the nature of the language disorder and how it might be defined in relation to normally developing language, and also to language disorders in other impaired populations. Second, when language is acquired, are the developmental processes similar to or different from those reported for normally developing children? Because of the paucity of longitudinal data, there are few studies relevant to this central issue. And third, are language deficits among the primary aspects of the syndrome, or are they secondary to the social-emotional aspects of the disorder? There are, as noted above, broad differences of opinion of this issue; yet, as we shall see, one must consider the definition of language in order to address it in any meaningful way.

Although there has been considerable controversy on all these points, much of the argument has taken place on the basis of very little documented evidence. There have been few relevant studies yielding sufficient data to decide any one of these issues. The richest data on language development come from studies of spontaneous speech; however, those studies of autistic language have relied on very small samples, and data have not always been collected under optimal conditions. Furthermore, research on language and communication in the autistic child has lagged behind the rapidly growing literature in developmental psycholinguistics; thus there has been too little reliance on sophisticated linguistic analyses. More serious problems emerge when no attempt is made to compare autistic children's language to that of either normal children or mentally retarded children. There are descriptive clinical reports of certain autistic errors that turn out to be prevalent in normally developing language. For example, Wing (1969) noted a number of so-called "abnormalities" of language in a group of verbal autistic children, including the omission of prepositions, conjunctions, pronouns, and so forth. These omissions yield what is called, in the psycholinguistic literature, "telegraphic speech" (e.g., "Go walk shops"), and they are typical in normally developing 2-year-olds (cf. Brown, 1973).

In this chapter, I review current knowledge in the field with respect to the issues outlined above, relying as much as possible on more recent studies that have avoided some of the problems outlined here. Many of these studies have used higher-functioning autistic children, in part because they have some spontaneous language, and in part because they will provide more information about the deficits specific to autism (cf. Prior, 1979; Rutter, 1983); therefore, I focus the review on this portion of the autistic population. It is crucially important to understand the place of language deficits within the syndrome, both because language is a key prognostic factor (Rutter, Greenfield, & Lockyer, 1967), and because such an understanding will lead to the development of improved therapeutic programs. In order to address the role of language in autism, it is necessary to consider the nature of language itself, and its relation to cognitive and social-emotional functioning within the child. Therefore, I begin with a discussion of these issues and then move on to a critical review of the development of language in autistic children, with special emphasis on the similarities and differences among autistic, retarded, and normally developing children. Finally, I return to consider how recent findings can help answer some of the controversies outlined here.

THE NATURE OF LANGUAGE

Language is a complex and multifaceted system. It can be analyzed at a number of distinct levels: the speech sounds, which combine to create words or morphemes that carry meaning, which in turn combine according to grammatical rules to form sentences. Studies of language and language acquisition up until a decade ago focused exclusively on understanding these phonological, semantic, and syntactic components and their interrelationships. More recently, there has been a shift in emphasis toward the communicative uses, or "pragmatics," of language. Studies of the uses of language in interpersonal communication—for a

variety of discourses, for narration, instruction, and storytelling, and so forth—
have enriched the fields of linguistics and psycholinguistics considerably.

Research in developmental psycholinguistics has demonstrated the strong interrelationships among these various strands of language in the normally developing child. For example, Schwartz and Leonard (1979) found that phonological
factors partially determined early words produced by very young children. Semantic factors have been shown to influence the acquisition of a variety of syntactic
rules (e.g., de Villiers, 1980; Maratsos, Kuczaj, Fox, & Chalkley, 1979) and morphological rules (e.g., Bloom, Lifter, & Hafitz, 1980). Thus, for example, Maratsos *et al.* (1979) found that young children first understand passive sentences
with verbs describing actions but cannot understand passive sentences with non-
actional verbs. This suggests that semantic classes of verbs constrain early passive-
sentence development. In a similar vein, Bloom *et al.* (1980) showed that children's earliest uses of past-tense morphology were restricted to verbs that denote
perfective aspect—that is, for events that have a clear result and denote completion. And pragmatic functions and syntactic forms influence each other in a variety of ways in development (e.g., de Villiers & de Villiers, 1981; Maratsos, 1976;
Tager-Flusberg, de Villiers, & Hakuta, 1982).

The interrelationships among the different components of language and aspects of cognitive and social-emotional development have also been the focus of
much psycholinguistic research (see de Villiers & de Villiers, 1986, for a recent
review). In the normally developing child, one finds strong connections among
cognitive functioning, social interaction, and language and communication, such
that, in normal development, language is inextricably linked to these other developmental systems, and these distinct aspects of development are in close synchrony with one another.

Elsewhere (Tager-Flusberg, 1988), I have argued that language disorders are
characterized in part by the breakdown in these developmental synchronies. This
is particularly the case in autism in which asynchronies in development are quite
pervasive: Even in higher-functioning autistic children, language is severely delayed relative to their overall cognitive level, while social and affective development are profoundly impaired at all levels. In Down syndrome, there is a different
profile of asynchrony: Cognitive and social development remain closely linked
(Cicchetti & Sroufe, 1976), while language is more seriously delayed (Beeghly &
Cicchetti, 1986; Rondal, 1978). These asynchronies provide distinct developmental profiles leading to specific differences in language development. For example,
this kind of analysis predicts that because social-emotional functioning is severely
impaired in autism, the communicative aspects of language (e.g., pragmatic functioning, conversational ability, and discourse style) will be more impaired in autistic children than in children with Down syndrome, and in comparison to other
aspects of their linguistic functioning. Within this framework, it is clear that the
entire developmental picture must be considered in order to understand the language deficits of the autistic child.

THE FOUNDATIONS OF LANGUAGE

During the first year of life, normal children do not speak or understand language; however, it is at this time that the groundwork is laid for the development of the speech sound system and for the communicative uses of language. Research has shown that at 1 month infants are capable of discriminating various speech sounds in the same way adults do (see Aslin, Pisoni, & Jusczyk, 1983, for a review), suggesting that these perceptual abilities are innate. As infants get older, they gradually lose the ability to discriminate categories that are not functional in their own language, showing that experience later modifies the innate ability (Trehub, 1976).

Babies begin producing different speech sounds at around 5 months, when they start babbling. At about 10 months, babbling becomes increasingly more complex as the infant includes a variety of stress and intonational patterns, often called "jargon babbling." Although the role of babbling in language development has not been clearly established, Oller (1980) and Stark (1986) have suggested that it reflects the maturation of the central nervous system and articulatory structures and is relevant to the infant's developing phonological abilities.

In the normal child, listening to and producing speech sounds often take place while interacting with an adult. Much of the research in this area has focused on mother–child interaction, which takes place in the context of the developing affective relationship. As early as 3 months, infants engage in eye-to-eye contact with their mothers and usually speech and vocalizations accompany these "gaze couplings" (Jaffe, Stern, & Perry, 1973; Lewis & Freedle, 1973; Snow, 1977). Thus, from the start, the social niche of language is clearly established for the baby through nonverbal and vocal interactions with the mother (Clarke-Stewart, 1973).

Very little is known about the life of the autistic child during the first year. Generally researchers must rely on retrospective parental reports, which may be biased once a parent is aware of a child's developmental disorder. Nevertheless, some parents do report that it was difficult to maintain eye contact or engage in interaction with their autistic babies (Stern, 1971). The autistic infant's preference for being alone, which has often been noted, would reduce that infant's opportunities for early social contact. There are no clear data available on the autistic infant's interest in speech or babbling, but at the least, we know that for some autistic children the social context for language is not clearly established. Furthermore, the role of language in forming affective relationships may be impaired even when the autistic child does begin developing attachments.

In normal infants, the ability to communicate a variety of messages—through cries, for example—also begins early. Mothers of infants are able to differentiate cries signalling different needs, with very little experience. In contrast, Ricks and Wing (1976) have reported that mothers of autistic children sometimes found it difficult to interpret their babies' needs, and in a controlled study Ricks (1975) found that older preverbal autistic children had idiosyncratic means of conveying different needs. These problems with early communication may make it significantly harder for the autistic child to develop the means for "intentional communication," which normally begins at about 9 months. Bruner and his colleagues (Bruner, 1978; Ratner & Bruner, 1978) have argued that mother–infant game playing (e.g., "peekaboo" or "patty-cake") also plays a significant role in helping to establish intentional communication, but autistic infants are less likely to be interested in these kinds of activities.

Bates (1979) has found that preverbal normally developing children use two types of communicative functions in interactions with adults: "protodeclaratives," which are used to establish joint attention on an object and are often accompanied by a pointing gesture; and "protoimperatives" (or "instrumentals," in Halliday's [1975] scheme), which are used when the child wants something from the adult. There is strong evidence from Curcio (1978) that although nonverbal autistic children do use protoimperatives, protodeclaratives are generally absent even when the children do have the requisite cognitive skills. Thus, at least some preverbal autistic children are capable of intentional communication, but they do not have the complete range of communicative functions available to them. Mundy and Sigman's review (Chapter 1, this volume) of the literature on problems in joint attention in autistic children suggests that this area of deficit may be linked to the paucity of protodeclaratives in preverbal autistic communication. The importance of prelinguistic development was demonstrated in Sugarman's (1984) training study with an autistic child, in which she showed that preverbal intentional communication was functionally prerequisite to the emergence of language in that child.

From this review of the prelinguistic period of language development, we may conclude that autistic children differ from normally developing children and mentally retarded children (cf. Beeghly & Cicchetti, 1986) in their interest in establishing eye contact, maintaining gaze coupling, establishing joint attention, using pointing gestures, and using protoimperative communicative functions. This set of behaviors lies at the intersection of language and social development, and may be among the first signs of developmental disorder in the autistic child. This suggests that from the beginning, the core problems in autism are a function of combined, interrelated deficits in social-affective and linguistic-communicative functioning.

THE DEVELOPMENT OF PHONOLOGY

During the transition from prespeech babbling to speech, the normal infant begins to use "protowords"—invented or derived forms used in specific situations (Menn, 1976)—alongside regular and jargon babbling. At the next phase, children begin to master the pronunciation of the words they are learning. Their successive attempts show regular patterns, although there is individual variation in the rules and strategies that children use in acquiring the phonological rule system of their language.

Both clinical reports (e.g., Eisenberg, 1956) and controlled studies (Bartolucci & Pierce, 1977; Bartolucci, Pierce, Streiner, & Eppel, 1976; Boucher, 1976a) find that verbal autistic children do not show serious problems in articulation. Error patterns among autistic subjects are similar to those in matched retarded children, and mirror those cited in the literature on phonological development in normal children. Reviews of this literature have concluded that autistic children do not show deficits (though perhaps they are delayed; cf. Bartak, Rutter, & Cox, 1975) in phonological development (Paul, 1987; Tager-Flusberg, 1981a). In other words, the *pattern* of phonological development, including the order of emergence of classes of speech sounds, the systematic errors made, and so forth, is the same in autistic and normally developing children; however, the entire process begins later and proceeds at a slower rate in autistic children.

But in addition to accurate articulation of phonemes and the acquisition of a phonological rule system, speech production involves the appropriate use of stress, intonation, and other prosodic features. Less attention has been paid in the psycholinguistic literature to the development of these aspects of nonsegmental phonology, though their importance is becoming increasingly recognized (Crystal, 1986). In speech, prosody plays a central role, interacting with syntax, semantics, and pragmatics; in fact, it can only be understood in relation to these other aspects of language (Crystal, 1975). For example, prosody can mark grammatical distinctions; it is used to convey nuances of meaning; it is critical for expressing differences between types of speech acts and other pragmatic functions. Prosody also is intimately related to the communication of affect and attitude (Frick, 1985), generally interacting with nonverbal aspects of social interaction. Recent work (see van der Hulst & Smith, 1985; Waugh & van Schooneveld, 1980) has begun to delineate these wide-ranging linguistic and nonlinguistic functions of prosodic aspects of language, though an integrated theoretical perspective is still lacking.

Within the first year, the normal child's vocalizations have prosodic patterns that resemble those of the child's language environment (e.g., Boysson-Bardies, de Sagart, & Durand, 1984). Once language begins developing, children use clearly determined and systematic prosodic "envelopes" (Bruner, 1975; Dore, 1975), so that by the end of the second year children have mastered the use of prosody to convey various pragmatic functions, as well as social and affective information (Furrow, 1984). Specific control over tone patterns, pitch variation, and timing appropriate to the language being acquired continues developing throughout the preschool years (Allen, 1983; Weeks, 1971), but it is not until children reach the age of puberty that they have full mastery of rhythm and stress, which are important for syntactic and semantic interpretation (Atkinson-King, 1973; Myers & Myers, 1983). Thus research to date has emphasized the early acquisition of the social, pragmatic, and affective aspects of the prosodic system. In contrast, those components of intonation that interact with other parts of the linguistic system show more gradual development.

From the earliest studies of the language of autistic children (cf. Kanner, 1946), deficits in prosody have been noted to be among the most striking and consistent features of the disorder. Descriptions of the speech of autistic children include atypical patterns of speech quality, loudness, rhythm, stress, and intonation (e.g., Goldfarb, Braunstein, & Lorge, 1956; Pronovost, Wakstein, & Wakstein, 1966). One significant finding in long-term follow-up studies of autistic children is that despite marked improvement in other aspects of language functioning, deficits in prosody persist through adolescence (Kanner, 1971; Rutter *et al.*, 1967; Simmons & Baltaxe, 1975) and even adulthood (Ornitz & Ritvo, 1976). Thus there appears to be little developmental change in prosodic impairments in autism.

Baltaxe and Simmons (1985) have reviewed recent empirical literature on how autistic children process a variety of prosodic features. Studies of perception of features such as stress (Frankel, Simmons, & Richey, 1987; Frith, 1969) suggest that at least some autistic children can perceive prosodic cues, and certainly their ability to imitate speech accurately supports these findings (Paccia & Curcio, 1982). It would be interesting to explore whether autistic children can interpret social or affective meanings conveyed by prosodic information; however, no studies to date have focused on these issues.

Studies of autistic children's use of prosody suggest that they may not be globally impaired (Baltaxe & Simmons, 1985), although wide individual differences have been found among autistic subjects. Autistic children were found to be able to mark primary sentence stress, which is syntactically determined, at a level comparable to that of normal and aphasic control subjects (Baltaxe & Guthrie, 1987); however, they were less successful at using contrastive stress (Baltaxe, 1984), which usually marks pragmatic or lexical distinctions. Research on the hemispheric representation of prosodic aspects of speech suggest that syntactically relevant aspects of prosody are primarily controlled by the left hemisphere, whereas pragmatic and social-emotional aspects of prosody are primarily controlled by the right hemisphere (see Etcoff, 1986, and Foldi, Cicone, & Gardner, 1983, for reviews). Although significantly more work needs to be done clarifying how autistic children's prosodic deficits may reflect possible neurological impairments and how they interact with linguistic, pragmatic, and social-emotional functioning, the fact that the degree of prosodic dysfunction is unrelated to general language ability and remains a pervasive problem over time suggests that prosody may provide important clues into the nature of the core deficits in autism.

ACQUIRING WORDS AND MEANINGS

Early development of words and their meanings is guided primarily by conceptual development (Clark, 1974; Nelson, 1974). Some have argued that as language begins to emerge around the first birthday, words may be used in highly limited idiosyncratic ways; for example, a child may call his or her own highchair "chair," but may not use the term to label other chairs. This period soon gives way to the use of words to label categories, though typically words are both overextended and underextended in meaning (e.g., Anglin, 1977). Lexical development proceeds very rapidly in the toddler and preschool years, with only limited exposure needed for new words to be acquired (Carey & Bartlett, 1978). In the early school years, systematic reorganizations take place in the child's lexicon as new semantic relations and fields are established and consolidated (Bowerman, 1978). Beyond this point, children continue to develop more complex ways of dealing with words—for example, analogies, definitions, and metaphor, which require the perception of relationships within and across semantic fields.

Kanner's early observations of autistic children's "metaphorical" language, especially their use of irrelevant words in which conventional meaning was ignored, suggest that autistic children have particular difficulty with linguistic meaning. A number of researchers have hypothesized that autism involves a primary cognitive deficit in semantics (Fay & Schuler, 1980; Hermelin & O'Connor, 1970; Menyuk, 1978; Schwartz, 1981; Simmons & Baltaxe, 1975; Tager-Flusberg, 1981a); however, the hypothesis rests on evidence based on autistic subjects' failure to use relational meaning in memory (Hermelin & O'Connor, 1967), learning (Schmidt, 1976), or language comprehension experiments (Tager-Flusberg, 1981b). In other words, the research shows that autistic children consistently fail to use meaning in cognitive processing tasks, but the studies do not distinguish whether the subjects fail because they lack the underlying conceptual or linguistic/semantic categories, or because they cannot use what they have acquired.

Descriptions of autistic children with minimal linguistic capacities typically note that the few words or phrases that may have been acquired are used in very limited contexts (Kanner, 1946; Simon, 1975). Their use of words in this way is perhaps similar to very young normal children's first use of words, suggesting that for these children words are not yet based on conceptual categories. It represents an initial stage of lexical development in which these autistic children remain for a prolonged period.

Menyuk (1978) and Fay and Schuler (1980) have hypothesized that autism involves a fundamental deficit in acquiring basic conceptual knowledge that underlies meaning. Although this may be true for lower-functioning autistic children who have only a few words that are used idiosyncratically, such a profound conceptual deficit appears to be related more to intellectual functioning than to autism itself. Thus low-functioning autistic and nonautistic mentally retarded children show similar patterns of deficit in this area. On the other hand, recent research with higher-functioning verbal autistic children has demonstrated that, like matched normal and moderate or mildly mentally retarded children, they have little difficulty in organizing conceptual knowledge for categories of concrete objects (Tager-Flusberg, 1985a; Ungerer & Sigman, 1987); in representing word meanings, at least for nouns (Tager-Flusberg, 1985b); or in naming abilities (Tager-Flusberg, 1986b). These studies demonstrate that autism does not involve a deficit in conceptual or semantic representation. Thus recent evidence suggests that the semantic deficit in autistic children is restricted to their inability to *use* meaning in higher-level processing of information (Tager-Flusberg, 1986c), not in the acquisition of conceptual categories or meaning per se.

But meanings associated with concrete objects may be acquired and represented in ways quite different from other types of meanings, particularly relational meanings, as noted by Menyuk and Quill (1985). These authors suggest that autistic children may have greater difficulty acquiring and using appropriately words that are intrinsically relational, such as verbs, prepositions, and relational adjectives, which do not map directly onto simple perceptually based categories as nouns do (see also Hobson, Chapter 2, this volume). There are no studies that have directly examined autistic children's comprehension and use of these kinds of terms in isolation, compared to matched retarded children. Studies of comprehension beyond the single word (which is the way to tap relational meaning) do find that autistic children have significantly more problems than matched controls (Cantwell, Baker, & Rutter, 1978; Lord, 1985; Paccia & Curcio, 1982; Prior & Hall, 1979; Tager-Flusberg, 1981b). One cannot, however, distinguish what the source of the autistic child's comprehension difficulty is; it may be with relational meaning, or with the syntactic or pragmatic contexts in which the relational terms are embedded.

In an ongoing longitudinal study of language acquisition in a group of higher-functioning autistic children, we have examined their use of relational terms in spontaneous speech protocols (Tager-Flusberg, Calkins, Nolin, Anderson, & Chadwick-Dias, 1987). Samples of spontaneous speech were collected in each child's home every 2 months, while the child played with his or her mother. These visits were audio- and videotaped, and complete transcripts were later prepared from the tapes. We have data from nine autistic children who have been followed for periods ranging from 6 to 30 months. In addition, we have similar data from six Down syndrome children who are matched in age and language level to a subgroup of the autistic children. Although this study is still in progress, we have begun to examine certain aspects of the children's language that bear on important issues in the current literature. In our analysis of the children's use of different word classes (nouns, verbs, adjectives, etc.), we found no significant differences between the distributions from the language samples of the autistic and Down syndrome children. Furthermore, there were no significant errors made that would suggest that these words were being used in aberrant ways by the autistic children, but we did find that the autistic children used a significantly smaller range of terms within each category than the Down syndrome children did. These data suggest that there is no fundamental deficit in relational meaning, though further research on the topic is clearly needed.

We have little idea about how autistic children develop word meaning beyond the 4-year-old level. Do they undergo semantic reorganizations in the way normal children do? Do they have fundamental difficulty with abstract meanings, metaphor, analogy, and other types of word play? These questions will need to be examined in the language of older, higher-functioning children before we have a clear understanding of semantic representation and possible deficit in autistic individuals.

GRAMMATICAL DEVELOPMENT

By the time normally developing children reach the age of 2, they are beginning to put words together to form simple sentences. Gradually over the next few years, their sentences grow from two-word utterances expressing a limited range of meanings, to longer and longer utterances in which a virtually unlimited variety of complex meanings can be expressed using the full range of syntactic structures available in the language. The average length of children's sentences grows gradually, as measured by "mean length of utterance" (MLU), the most useful measure of grammatical development in normal and language-impaired children (Brown, 1973; Miller, 1981). The order of emergence of different grammatical structures and morphemes is quite predictable, though rates of development may vary considerably from one child to the next. It is not until middle childhood that normally developing children have mastered the full range of syntactic structures (e.g., complements, relative clauses, embedded "wh-" questions) in both comprehension and production.

Most recent reviews of the literature on grammatical functioning in autistic children have concluded that autism does not involve a fundamental problem with syntax (see Paul, 1987; Swisher & Demetras, 1985; Tager-Flusberg, 1981a, 1985c). This conclusion is based largely on the studies by Bartolucci and his colleagues (Pierce & Bartolucci, 1977) and Cantwell *et al.* (1978), both of which relied on cross-sectional samples of spontaneous speech. These studies found that autistic children did not develop anomalous syntax or use bizarre grammatical constructions. Their subjects showed appropriate variations in sentence length and complexity, and the grammatical rule systems of autistic children, like those of matched retarded and normal children, were rule-governed.

Since Cunningham's (1966) seminal work, there have been no longitudinal studies that could critically assess whether the same developmental path is followed by autistic and normally developing children. Simon (1975), for example, argues that autistic children do *not* develop normally. She claims that they do not show the gradual growth in MLU, the use of two-word "telegraphic" utterances, or the same order of emergence of syntactic structures that are the hallmarks of normally developing syntax. Simon's evidence comes from her analysis of autistic children's excessive reliance on echolalia, or imitated speech, which suggests that they do not analyze what they hear or say. Echolalia is one of the distinguishing characteristics of autistic speech and is especially pronounced in those children who have not acquired much functional language. Does echolalia reflect a different developmental pattern of grammatical development?

Both Schuler (1979) and Prizant (1983; Schuler & Prizant, 1985) find that echolalia serves important communicative functions for autistic children, but they argue that it represents a wholistic rather than an analytical approach to language development, as Simon suggested. Their studies, though, have relied on cross-sectional samples of autistic language that cannot, by definition, provide information about developmental patterns. In our longitudinal study of autistic children's language, we have focused on the role of echolalia in language acquisition by comparing within children over time the structures used in spontaneous versus imitated and other types of "formulaic" language, including routines, partial imitations, and repetitive word combinations (Calkins & Tager-Flusberg, 1986). We confirmed that, compared to Down syndrome and normal children matched on language level (MLU), the autistic children used significantly more formulaic language. However, contrary to the predictions of Simon, Schuler, and Prizant, the autistic children, like the control children, used more advanced grammatical structures in their spontaneous than in their formulaic speech. Thus, at the least, higher-functioning autistic children who do acquire functional language echo structures that they already have available in their linguistic repertoire, and in this respect follow a developmental path similar to that of normally developing and other language-delayed children.

We examined MLU patterns for our sample of autistic children to see whether they showed similarities to other children in their growth function, and indeed they did (Tager-Flusberg, 1986a). Using more detailed methods of analysis, we also found that, contrary to Simon's claims, the autistic children showed the same order of emergence across a wide range of syntactic structures. Differences did occur among the groups of children in the frequency with which specific structures were used: The autistic children consistently used a narrower range and more limited variety of grammatical structures, compared to either the Down syndrome or normal children with whom they were matched for MLU. These findings parallel those reported on word meaning. Development of grammar does not appear deviant in children with autism; however, they show significantly more restricted uses of those grammatical structures that are available to them.

Studies of language in autistic children have also focused on the acquisition of grammatical morphology, those closed-class noun phrase and verb phrase words and affixes (e.g., articles, prepositions, verb endings, auxiliaries) that develop gradually in the preschool years (cf. the study of 14 English morphemes by Brown, 1973). The findings from these studies have not been consistent. Fein and Waterhouse (1979) reported no special problems with morphology in their autistic sample, whereas Bartolucci and his colleagues (Bartolucci, Pierce, & Streiner, 1980) and Howlin (1984) did find significant differences in their autistic subjects, which Bartolucci et al. attribute to semantic difficulties with deictic categories. None of these studies was longitudinal in design, and all relied on relatively small language samples, which provided few contexts for the use of at least some of the morphemes in question. These limitations make it difficult to conclude whether there are significant problems in morpheme acquisition.

We have begun to look at the development of grammatical morphology in our longitudinal autistic sample. Because none of our subjects has reached the point of full mastery on all the morphemes, we can only compare order of emergence and developmental patterns. Thus far, our autistic sample looks quite similar to the Down syndrome and normal matched controls on both these analyses. However, for all three groups, across the morphemes we do find wide individual variability that makes it difficult to discern potential group differences. Another approach is to focus on one aspect of morphology and then look in detail at its development across time in the different groups of children. We have chosen to study in this way the acquisition of the past tense, which is marked by "-ed" for regular verbs and by a variety of irregular forms for many common English verbs (Tager-Flusberg & Baumberger, 1987). Both Bartolucci *et al.* (1980) and Howlin (1984) found that autistic children had greater difficulty marking the past tense than did their control groups. Across all examples of verbs that required past-tense marking, the autistic subjects looked similar to the normal and Down syndrome children. However, we also found that autistic children tended to repeat the same verb many times and to use fewer different verbs, or less variety, than the other children. When we examined past-tense usage only on different verbs, not counting repeated uses of the same verb, then significant differences between our subject groups emerged. Across a range of verbs, then, autistic children are less likely to mark past tense than are control groups, confirming the findings of Bartolucci *et al.* (1980) and Howlin (1984).

In trying to understand why autistic children are more deficient in the use of the past tense, we found that unlike the other groups in our study, the autistic children did not closely monitor their mothers' use of particular verbs in the past tense; instead, they spoke about different events and used the past tense, in a more limited way, with different verbs. We also found that in certain types of discourse contexts autistic children failed to use the past tense, whereas in others they were appropriate in their tense usage. Thus, for example, in conversations centering on the ongoing activity, the autistic children were equivalent to the control children in using the past tense to describe activities that had taken place. In contrast, if they were narrating an event that had happened outside the context of the ongoing activity, such as what had happened at school, then the autistic children were more likely to use the present tense, inappropriately. We interpret this as a failure to have learned the social convention of narrating events in the past tense. (Note that in some dialects it is appropriate to narrate stories and events in the present tense, although this was not typical for the families in our study.) These explanations of the sources of difficulty in using the past-tense morphology for the autistic children differ from that presented by Bartolucci and his colleagues. Our detailed longitudinal analysis suggests that differences emerge in the ways that autistic children use tense and aspect to mark semantic distinctions that they have acquired, not in the acquisition of the semantic categories themselves.

Thus far, studies on grammatical development in autistic children confirm the view that autism does not involve a specific deficit in acquiring either syntactic structure or grammatical morphology. Moreover, autistic children apparently follow the same developmental path in acquiring linguistic forms, despite their heavy reliance on formulaic speech. Higher-functioning autistic children develop the ability to express themselves using a variety of linguistic forms, though they generally rely on a more limited range in their conversations. Significant differences between autistic and mentally retarded or normal children do emerge when one looks at the ways in which the children use the linguistic forms that they have acquired.

ACQUIRING COMMUNICATIVE COMPETENCE

There has been a consistent theme running through the previous sections on the development of language in autistic children. The acquisition of the phonological system, of words and their meanings, or of grammatical forms does not reveal any fundamental problem specific to autism. However, again and again, recent detailed analyses of autistic language reveal that there are differences in the ways in which language is used by autistic children. Frequencies of usage in words and structures are different; prosodic cues are not used normally; there is an overreliance on formulaic speech; and the social conventions of specific forms are not used. These findings all point to a fundamental difference in the ways in which autistic children use language to communicate with others.

Earlier in the chapter, I have noted that even in the prelinguistic period autistic children do not have the full range of nonverbal communicative functions available to them. Since psycholinguistic studies of normal children began focusing on the acquisition of pragmatics (cf. Bates, 1976), there has been a proliferation of research on pragmatic functioning in autistic children. In general, the emphasis has been on identifying an area of fundamental linguistic deficit (Tager-Flusberg, 1981a)—a hypothesis that originated in some of Kanner's early observations (Kanner, 1943). Studies that have focused on verbal autistic children have highlighted a variety of pragmatic deficits, including the paucity of language used to request or share information (Ball, 1978; Hurtig, Ensrud, & Tomblin, 1982; Mermelstein, 1983; Paul & Cohen, 1984; Shapiro, Fish, & Ginsberg, 1972), nonsocialized language (Cunningham, 1968), problems with speaker–listener relations (Baltaxe, 1977), difficulties in initiating and maintaining topics in conversation (Tager-Flusberg, 1982), and problems in conversational turn-taking (Fay & Schuler, 1980; Paccia-Cooper, Curcio, & Sacharko, 1981).

Other researchers, most notably Prizant (1983; Prizant & Duchan, 1981; Prizant & Rydell, 1984) and Wetherby (Wetherby, 1986; Wetherby & Prizant, 1985; Wetherby & Prutting, 1984), have preferred to emphasize the spared communicative abilities that are evident in autistic children's language. They note that autistic children can use language to communicate a range of primitive functions, which Wetherby (1986) divides into "nonsocial" (to achieve environmental ends, such as a desired object or action) and "social" (to attract or direct attention to self, object, or event). Wetherby (1986) argues that whereas normal children acquire all these functions simultaneously in the prelinguistic period, autistic children acquire the same range of functions, but more slowly and sequentially; social functions are a relatively late achievement, not fully evident until the autistic child does have some language. Wetherby acknowledges that her developmental model rests only on data from the early stages, though it is implicit in her model that verbal autistic children do eventually achieve a wide range of communicative competence.

Fewer studies have examined the range of functions communicated by autistic children who have reached the later stages of language acquisition. In our longitudinal study of autistic and Down syndrome children, we selected the acquisition of a particular structure, negation, and examined its development in form, meaning, and function (Tager-Flusberg & Keenan, 1987). We analyzed, from the transcripts of children at various stages of language development, all utterances that expressed negation. The development of both form and meaning demonstrated similarities among the groups of children matched on language level (MLU), though as one might predict, there were significant frequency differences. In contrast, dramatic group differences emerged in our analysis of the development of pragmatic function. Children normally use negation to respond, to emphasize, to question, to inform, to correct, and to control. Whereas normal children at the earliest stages of language development already had the full range of these functions available to them, this was not true for the impaired groups. Down syndrome children were more like the normals; however, only when they could use three- or four-word utterances were they able to inform and ask questions with an embedded negative. The profile of development for the autistic children was quite distinct from that for the other two groups. Like the other groups, autistic children developed early the capacity to respond to, emphasize, and control or correct their own behavior. In contrast, examples of negative utterances used to inform others and to control or correct the behavior of others were completely absent from the language of children still in the process of development. In the more advanced children, examples of these pragmatic functions did finally appear, but only in very limited ways.

This study highlights a number of issues. Although autistic children may occasionally use language to achieve some social end, such uses are infrequent and odd, even in linguistically advanced, higher-functioning autistic individuals. What is most striking about the language of autistic children is the developmental asynchrony between form and function (Mermelstein, 1983; Tager-Flusberg, 1981a, 1988). This study, focusing on a single linguistic construction, clearly demonstrates this asynchrony. The most pervasive aspect of autistic children's language disorder lies in their problems with communication.

But the findings from this study also suggest that certain types of communicative functions are less available to autistic children than others, and a simple distinction between "nonsocial" and "social" does not explain the particular pattern of results that we found. Some social functions were used—for example, responding, usually to a question posed by the mother. The functions that were least used, and were the latest to develop, all involved some kind of influence on the mother—informing her about something, correcting her, or controlling her behavior. The problem that autistic children have is in realizing that they are able to have an effect on another person. Why should this be so? In a recent landmark paper, Baron-Cohen, Leslie, and Frith (1985) propose that the essential deficit in autism is a lack of a "theory of mind" (cf. Premack & Woodruff, 1978). Their main thesis is that autistic children have a unique difficulty in understanding other people's beliefs, desires, knowledge, or internal states. The findings from our study on the developmental pragmatics of negation fit well with this hypothesis. The common element in all the communicative functions with which autistic children have difficulty is that they require an understanding that one can add to the knowledge of or influence the behavior of another. Although Baron-Cohen et al. (1985) have used their cognitive theory of autism to explain the particular social and symbolic play deficits that are characteristic of the syndrome, the theory explains the unique pattern of linguistic pragmatic deficits identified in this study, and in the other studies cited above.

THE LANGUAGE DEFICIT IN AUTISM

Autistic children have great difficulty with language and communication. Language problems are, of course, a cardinal feature of the syndrome, and this selective review of the literature confirms clinical intuition. One striking feature of language deficit in autism is that even when language does develop in higher-functioning children, language ability lags considerably behind nonverbal cognitive functioning. We have not even begun to address why almost half the population of autistic children never acquire functional language (cf. Paul, 1987). Before we come to any real understanding about the nature of the language deficit in autism, and its role in the etiology of the disorder, psycholinguistic research will need to focus on this neglected population.

Nevertheless, the studies that have been done with verbal autistic children suggest that we can define the language deficit in the following way. From the earliest stages in communicative development, autistic children show profound problems with key aspects of intentional communication, especially those that are exclusively social-interactive, such as establishing joint attention, informing, and initiating. This deficit continues to pervade the autistic child's communicative behavior once language begins to be established. The grammatical structures used, the lexicon that develops, and the meanings conveyed in the child's language all reflect this fundamental communicative deficit, though the forms themselves are not aberrant. This latter finding reflects the fact that the linguistic system itself is highly constrained (Tager-Flusberg, 1986a).

The key characteristic of language in autism is the asynchrony between form and function—between syntactic and lexical aspects of the language that are typically in advance of many aspects of pragmatic functioning. A parallel asynchrony may exist in autistic children's more advanced productive abilities compared to their comprehension (cf. Lord, 1985; Menyuk & Quill, 1985); however, the findings suggesting this may have resulted from differences in the ways in which production and comprehension are assessed. Production is typically assessed in naturalistic settings, whereas comprehension requires a more artificial context that adversely influences an autistic child's performance.

This profile of language in autism contrasts with that of the normally developing child, in that normal language development is defined as synchronous and there are close interrelationships among the individual strands that make up the linguistic system. Other language-impaired populations will also be characterized by delay and asynchrony (Tager-Flusberg, 1988), though in different disorders the asynchrony will take on different forms. Thus, for example, research on Down syndrome suggests that in this mentally retarded population children typically have more advanced lexical and conversational skills, and less advanced syntactic and morphological skills (Rondal, 1987). Other retarded populations do not necessarily show this profile of language asynchrony.

THE DEVELOPMENTAL PROCESS

Among the major questions that have been raised with respect to language acquisition in autistic children is whether autistic children follow the same developmental pathway as normal children do, and whether the acquisition processes are the same. There have been few longitudinal studies designed to address these questions directly; nevertheless, recent research does provide us with some clues into the ways in which autistic children acquire language.

In normal children, the course of language development is guided by prelinguistic accomplishments in intentional communication, motivated by both social and nonsocial goals. This is clearly not the case for autistic children, who, instead, can be viewed as acquiring language despite their deficits in at least some aspects of intentional communication. This difference suggests that there may indeed be different patterns of language development, though the literature on autism suggests that deficits in intentional communication selectively impair developments in speech acts and communicative competence.

The work of Wetherby (1986) offers an important perspective on how the process of pragmatic development is different in autistic children. Her account of the sequential acquisition of first nonsocial and then social communication in autistic children contrasts strikingly with the normal simultaneous pattern of development in this domain. Our study on negation (Tager-Flusberg & Keenan, 1987) provides direct support for her model, though we claim that there are certain aspects of communicative competence that autistic children never achieve, especially the ability to communicate about the beliefs, ideas, and intentions of other people.

In the area of syntax, there are different views on the developmental processes involved in autistic children. Prizant (1983) has argued, based on Peters's (1977,

1983) work, that there are two different approaches to language acquisition—"gestalt" and "analytic"—that in fact lie on a continuum. The first is characterized by heavy reliance on formulaic language (including imitations and routines) that remains unanalyzed for some time, and is thus more advanced than the child's rule system can generate. The second is characterized by steady, gradual growth in MLU and little use of formulaic language. Although most of the developmental psycholinguistic research has focused on analytic language learners, there are normal children who show the gestalt profile.

Autistic children clearly fall at the gestalt end of the continuum. Prizant argues that autistic children typically are gestalt language learners; he defines "gestalt" not simply as a style of learning, but as involving different developmental pathways in acquiring linguistic structures. Our own work (Calkins & Tager-Flusberg, 1986; Tager-Flusberg, 1986a) on the role of formulaic language in the process of grammatical rule learning offers a different perspective: Although autistic children indeed have a pronounced gestalt language profile, we view this as a reflection of communicative style, rather than an alternative means for acquiring language. We argue that the evidence available is more consistent with the view that the process of grammatical development is the same in autistic, retarded, and normal children. Clearly, more work needs to be done in this area before the question about how autistic children develop language is fully settled.

THE RELATIONSHIP BETWEEN DEFICITS IN LANGUAGE AND SOCIAL-EMOTIONAL DEVELOPMENT IN AUTISM

I have opened this chapter with the debate over the role of language deficits in defining the syndrome of autism. Are language deficits primary, or secondary to other core problems in the area of social-emotional functioning? The phrasing of this question and the way the debate has been argued in the literature both presuppose that one can package different aspects of psychological functioning into separate parcels. Although to a certain extent one can differentiate between, for example, social interaction and emotional experience, or language and cognition, in other respects they may be indivisible from each other. Viewing psychological components as independent categories may provide us with viable research strategies, as it would be impossible to make significant advances if we were to study development exclusively in a wholistic fashion. On the other hand, we run the risk of losing sight of the broader picture when we divide a child up into our convenient packages.

The picture of language and communicative development in autism that has been given here demands a broader perspective in order to discern the nature of the psychological deficit that is at the core of the syndrome. At a basic level, human language is inseparable from social interaction, which is why children raised in isolation do not acquire any language (cf. Curtiss, 1977). Before language develops, one can interact socially in very meaningful ways; likewise, once language has been acquired, communication is possible without social interaction. But in the course of development, the two are inextricably linked: Language itself reflects the individual's social relationships, and social interaction and understanding are themselves significantly influenced and advanced through the medium of language.

In autism, there is a fundamental deficit at the intersection of language and social-emotional functioning. Autistic children's language and communicative patterns reflect their failure to understand the nature of another person—in other words, their failure to develop a theory of mind (Baron-Cohen et al., 1985). Their social interactive behaviors are clearly enhanced by the acquisition of language, and certainly in some older, higher-functioning autistic individuals, language comes to dominate their social relationships (perhaps to an excessive degree). By studying the content of autistic children's language—as we began doing in the study of negation (Tager-Flusberg & Keenan, 1987)—we will gain new insights into the ways in which autistic people view their world, especially their social world.

In this view of autistic deficits, both the language and the social problems are criterial features of the disorder. Put another way, the core deficit in autism lies at the nexus between social-emotional and language-communicative functioning. This provides a descriptive account of autism without answering whether this social-communicative dysfunction is derived from more primary deficits, though Baron-Cohen et al. (1985) propose that a cognitive deficit, in the development of second-order mental representations, is actually at the heart of the disorder. Instead of maintaining our current approach of studying the individual psychological components of the autistic child, future progress in delineating the core deficit in autism will come from understanding more about the interrelationships among the different components of psychological functioning, especially at the intersection between social interaction and language development.

Acknowledgments

Preparation of this chapter was supported by a grant from the National Institute of Child Health and Human Development (No. RO1 HD 18833) and by a Social and Behavioral Sciences Research Grant (No. 12-181) from the March of Dimes Research Foundation.

References

Allen, G. D. (1983). Linguistic experience modifies lexical stress perception. *Journal of Child Language, 10*, 535–549.

Anglin, J. (1977). *Word, object, and conceptual development.* New York: Norton.

Aslin, R. N., Pisoni, D. B., & Jusczyk, P. W. (1983). Auditory development and speech development in infancy. In M. M. Haith & J. J. Campos (Eds.), *Handbook of child psychology: Vol. 2. Infancy and developmental psychobiology* (pp. 573–687). New York: Wiley.

Atkinson-King, K. (1973). Children's acquisition of phonological stress contrasts. *UCLA Working Papers in Phonetics, 25,* 1–28.

Ball, J. (1978). *A pragmatic analysis of autistic children's language with respect to aphasic and normal language development.* Unpublished doctoral dissertation, Melbourne University.

Baltaxe, C. A. M. (1977). Pragmatic deficits in the language of autistic adolescents. *Journal of Pediatric Psychology, 2,* 176–180.

Baltaxe, C. A. M. (1984). The use of contrastive stress in normal, aphasic, and autistic children. *Journal of Speech and Hearing Research, 27,* 97–105.

Baltaxe, C. A. M., & Guthrie, D. (1987). The use of primary sentence stress by normal, aphasic, and autistic children. *Journal of Autism and Developmental Disorders, 17,* 255–271.

Baltaxe, C. A. M., & Simmons, J. Q. (1985). Prosodic development in normal and autistic children. In E. Schopler & G. Mesibov (Eds.), *Communication problems in autism* (pp. 95–125). New York: Plenum.

Baron-Cohen, S., Leslie, A. M., & Frith, U. (1985). Does the autistic child have a "theory of mind"? *Cognition, 21,* 37–46.

Bartak, L., Rutter, M., & Cox, A. (1975). A comparative study of infantile autism and specific developmental receptive language disorder: I. The children. *British Journal of Psychiatry, 126,* 127–145.

Bartolucci, G., & Pierce, S. J. (1977). A preliminary comparison of phonological development in autistic, normal, and mentally retarded subjects. *British Journal of Disorders of Communication, 12,* 134–147.

Bartolucci, G., Pierce, S. J., & Streiner, D. (1980). Cross-sectional studies of grammatical morphemes in autistic and mentally retarded children. *Journal of Autism and Developmental Disorders, 10,* 39–50.

Bartolucci, G., Pierce, S. J., Streiner, D., & Eppel, P. T. (1976). Phonological investigation of verbal autistic and mentally retarded subjects. *Journal of Autism and Childhood Schizophrenia, 6,* 303–316.

Bates, E. (1976). *Language and context: The acquisition of pragmatics.* New York: Academic Press.

Bates, E. (1979). *The emergence of symbols: Cognition and communication in infancy.* New York: Academic Press.

Beeghly, M., & Cicchetti, D. (1986, October). *Early language development in children with Down syndrome: A longitudinal study.* Paper presented at the Eleventh Annual Boston University Conference on Language Development, Boston.

Bettelheim, B. (1967). *The empty fortress: Infantile autism and the birth of self.* New York: Free Press.

Bloom, L., Lifter, K., & Hafitz, J. (1980). Semantics of verbs and the development of verb inflection in child language. *Language, 56,* 386–412.

Boucher, J. (1976a). Articulation in early childhood autism. *Journal of Autism and Childhood Schizophrenia, 6,* 297–302.

Boucher, J. (1976b). Is autism primarily a language disorder? *British Journal of Disorders of Communication, 11,* 135–143.

Bowerman, M. (1978). Systemizing semantic knowledge: Changes over time in the child's organization of word meaning. *Child Development, 49,* 977–987.

Boysson-Bardies, B., de Sagart, L., & Durand, C. (1984). Discernable differences in the babbling of infants according to target language. *Journal of Child Language, 11,* 1–15.

Brown, R. (1973). *A first language.* Cambridge, MA: Harvard University Press.

Bruner, J. (1975). The ontogenesis of speech acts. *Journal of Child Language, 2,* 1–19.

Bruner, J. (1978). From communication to language: A psychological perspective. In I. Markova (Ed.), *The social context of language* (pp. 36–64). London: Wiley.

Calkins, S., & Tager-Flusberg, H. (1986, August). *A comparison of echolalic and spontaneous speech in autistic and Down syndrome children.* Paper presented at the annual meeting of the American Psychological Association, Washington, DC.

Cantwell, D., Baker, L., & Rutter, M. (1978). A comparative study of infantile autism and specific developmental receptive language disorder: IV. Analysis of syntax and language function. *Journal of Child Psychology and Psychiatry, 19,* 351–362.

Carey, S., & Bartlett, E. (1978). Acquiring a single new word. *Papers and Reports on Child Language Development, 15,* 17–29.

Churchill, D. (1972). The relation of infantile autism and early childhood schizophrenia to developmental language disorders of childhood. *Journal of Autism and Childhood Schizophrenia, 2,* 182–197.

Cicchetti, D., & Sroufe, A. L. (1976). The relationship between affective and cognitive development in Down's syndrome infants. *Child Development, 47,* 920–929.

Clark, E. V. (1974). Some aspects of the conceptual basis for first language acquisition. In R. L. Schiefelbusch & L. L. Lloyd (Eds.), *Language perspectives: Acquisition, retardation and intervention* (pp. 105–128). Baltimore: University Park Press.

Clarke-Stewart, K. A. (1973). Interactions between mothers and their young children: Characteristics and consequences. *Monographs of the Society for Research in Child Development, 38* (6–7, Serial No. 153).

Crystal, D. (1975). *The English tone of voice.* London: Edward Arnold.

Crystal, D. (1986). Prosodic development. In P. Fletcher & M. Garman (Eds.), *Language acquisition* (2nd ed., pp. 174–197). Cambridge, England: Cambridge University Press.

Cunningham, M. A. (1966). A five year study of the language of an autistic child, *Journal of Child Psychology and Psychiatry, 7,* 143–154.

Cunningham, M. A. (1968). A comparison of the language of psychotic and non-psychotic children who are mentally retarded. *Journal of Child Psychology and Psychiatry, 9,* 229–244.

Curcio, F. (1978). Sensorimotor functioning and communication in mute autistic children. *Journal of Autism and Childhood Schizophrenia, 8,* 281–292.

Curtiss, S. (1977). *Genie: A psycholinguistic study of a modern-day "wild child."* New York: Academic Press.

de Villiers, J. G. (1980). The process of rule learning in child speech: A new look. In K. E. Nelson (Ed.), *Children's language* (Vol. 2, pp. 1–40). New York: Gardner Press.

de Villiers, J. G., & de Villiers, P. A. (1981). Semantics and syntax in the first two years: The output of the form and function and the form and function of the input. In F. D. Minifie & L. L. Lloyd (Eds.), *Communicative and cognitive abilities: Early behavioral assessment* (pp. 309–348). Baltimore: University Park Press.

de Villiers, J. G., & de Villiers, P. A. (1986). The acquisition of English. In D. I. Slobin (Ed.), *Cross-linguistic study of language acquisition* (pp. 27–139). Hillsdale, NJ: Erlbaum.

Dore, J. (1975). Holophrases, speech acts, and language universals. *Journal of Child Language, 2,* 21–40.

Eisenberg, L. (1956). The autistic child in adolescence. *American Journal of Psychiatry, 112,* 607–612.

Etcoff, N. L. (1986). The neuropsychology of emotional expression. In G. Goldstein & R. E. Tarter (Eds.), *Advances in clinical neuropsychology* (Vol. 3, pp. 127–179). New York: Plenum.

Fay, W., & Schuler, A. L. (1980). *Emerging language in autistic children.* Baltimore: University Park Press.

Fein, D., & Waterhouse, L. (1979, February). *Autism is not a disorder of language.* Paper presented at the meeting of the New England Child Language Association, Boston.

Foldi, N. S., Cicone, M., & Gardner, H. (1983). Pragmatic aspects of communication in brain-damaged patients. In S. J. Segalowitz (Ed.), *Language functions and brain organization* (pp. 51–86). New York: Academic Press.

Frankel, F., Simmons, J. Q. & Richey, V. E. (1987). Reward value of prosodic features of language for autistic, mentally retarded and normal children. *Journal of Autism and Developmental Disorders, 17,* 103–113.

Frick, R. W. (1985). Communicating emotion: The role of prosodic features. *Psychological Bulletin, 97,* 412–429.

Frith, U. A. (1969). Emphasis and recall in normal and autistic children. *Language and Speech, 12,* 29–38.

Furrow, D. (1984). Young children's use of prosody. *Journal of Child Language, 11,* 203–213.

Goldfarb, W., Braunstein, P., & Lorge, I. (1956). A study of speech patterns in a group of schizophrenic children. *American Journal of Orthopsychiatry, 26,* 544–555.

Halliday, M. A. K. (1975). *Learning how to mean: Explorations in the development of language.* London: Edward Arnold.

Hermelin, B., & O'Connor, N. (1967). Remembering of words by psychotic and subnormal children. *British Journal of Psychology, 58,* 213–218.

Hermelin, B., & O'Connor, N. (1970). *Psychological experiments with autistic children.* Oxford: Pergamon Press.

Howlin, P. (1984). The acquisition of grammatical morphemes in autistic children: A critique and replication of the findings of Bartolucci, Pierce, and Streiner, 1980. *Journal of Autism and Developmental Disorders, 14,* 127–136.

Hurtig, R., Ensrud, S., & Tomblin, J. B. (1982). The communicative function of question production in autistic children. *Journal of Autism and Developmental Disorders, 12,* 57–69.

Jaffe, J., Stern, D., & Perry, C. (1973). "Conversational" coupling of gaze behavior in prelinguistic human development. *Journal of Psycholinguistic Research, 2,* 321–330.

Kanner, L. (1943). Autistic disturbances of affective contact. *The Nervous Child, 2,* 217–250.

Kanner, L. (1946). Irrelevant and metaphorical language in early infantile autism. *American Journal of Psychiatry, 103,* 242–246.

Kanner, L. (1971). Follow-up study of eleven autistic children, originally reported in 1943. *Journal of Autism and Childhood Schizophrenia, 2,* 119–145.

Lewis, M., & Freedle, R. (1973). Mother–infant dyad: The cradle of meaning. In P. Pliner, L. Karames, & T. Alloway (Eds.), *Communication and affect, language and thought* (pp. 167–194). New York: Academic Press.

Lord, C. (1985). Autism and the comprehension of language. In E. Schopler & G. Mesibov (Eds.), *Communication problems in autism* (pp. 257–281). New York: Plenum.

Maratsos, M. P. (1976). *The use of definite and indefinite reference in young children.* Cambridge, England: Cambridge University Press.

Maratsos, M. P., Kuczaj, S. A., Fox, D. E. C., & Chalkley, M. A. (1979). Some empirical studies in the acquisition of transformational relations: Passives, negatives and the past tense. In W. A. Collins (Ed.), *Children's language and communication* (pp. 1–45). Hillsdale, NJ: Erlbaum.

Menn, L. (1976). *Patttern, control, and contrast in beginning speech: A case study in the acquisition of word form and function.* Unpublished doctoral dissertation, University of Illinois.

Menyuk, P. (1978). Language: What's wrong and why. In M. Rutter & E. Schopler (Eds.), *Autism: A reappraisal of concepts and treatment* (pp. 105–116). New York: Plenum.

Menyuk, P., & Quill, K. (1985). Semantic problems in autistic children. In E. Schopler & G. Mesibov (Eds.), *Communication problems in autism* (pp. 127–145). New York: Plenum.

Mermelstein, R. (1983, October). *The relationship between syntactic and pragmatic development in autistic, retarded, and normal children.* Paper presented at the Eighth Annual Boston University Conference on Language Development, Boston.

Miller, J. (1981). *Assessing language production in children: Experimental procedures.* Baltimore: University Park Press.

Myers, F. L., & Myers, R. W. (1983). Perception of stress contrasts in semantic and nonsemantic contexts by children. *Journal of Psycholinguistic Research, 12,* 227–238.

Nelson, K. (1974). Concept, word and sentence: Interrelations in acquisition and development. *Psychological Review, 81,* 267–284.

Oller, D. K. (1980). The emergence of the sounds of speech in infancy. In G. H. Yeni-Komshian, J. F. Kavanagh, & C. A. Ferguson (Eds.), *Child phonology: Vol. 1. Production* (pp. 93–112). New York: Academic Press.

Ornitz, E. M., & Ritvo, E. R. (1976). The syndrome of autism: A critical review. *American Journal of Psychiatry, 133*, 609–622.

Paccia, J., & Curcio, F. (1982). Language processing and forms of immediate echolalia in autistic children. *Journal of Speech and Hearing Research, 25*, 42–47.

Paccia-Cooper, J., Curcio, F., & Sacharko, G. (1981, October). *A comparison of discourse features in normal and autistic language.* Paper presented at the Sixth Annual Boston University Conference on Language Development, Boston.

Paul, R. (1987). Communication. In D. J. Cohen & A. M. Donnellan (Eds.), *Handbook of autism and pervasive developmental disorders* (pp. 61–84). New York: Wiley.

Paul, R., & Cohen, D. J. (1984). Responses to contingent queries in adults with mental retardation and pervasive developmental disorders. *Applied Psycholinguistics, 5*, 349–357.

Peters, A. M. (1977). Language learning strategies: Does the whole equal the sum of the parts? *Language, 53*, 560–573.

Peters, A. M. (1983). *The units of language acquisition.* Cambridge, England: Cambridge University Press.

Pierce, S. J., & Bartolucci, G. (1977). A syntactic investigation of verbal autistic, mentally retarded and normal children. *Journal of Autism and Childhood Schizophrenia, 7*, 121–134.

Premack, D., & Woodruff, G. (1978). Does the chimpanzee have a "theory of mind"? *Behavior and Brain Sciences, 4*, 515–526.

Prior, M. R. (1979). Cognitive abilities and disabilities in infantile autism: A review. *Journal of Abnormal Child Psychology, 7*, 357–380.

Prior, M. R., & Hall, L. C. (1979). Comprehension of transitive and intransitive phrases by autistic, mentally retarded and normal children. *Journal of Communication Disorders, 12*, 103–111.

Prizant, B. M. (1983). Language acquisition and communicative behavior in autism: Toward an understanding of the "whole" of it. *Journal of Speech and Hearing Disorders, 48*, 296–307.

Prizant, B. M., & Duchan, J. F. (1981). The functions of immediate echolalia in autistic children. *Journal of Speech and Hearing Disorders, 46*, 241–249.

Prizant, B. M., & Rydell, P. (1984). An analysis of the functions of delayed echolalia in autistic children. *Journal of Speech and Hearing Research, 27*, 183–192.

Pronovost, W., Wakstein, M., & Wakstein, P. (1966). A longitudinal study of the speech behavior and language comprehension of fourteen children diagnosed atypical or autistic. *Exceptional Children, 33*, 19–26.

Ratner, N. K., & Bruner, J. S. (1978). Games, social exchange and the acquisition of language. *Journal of Child Language, 5*, 391–401.

Ricks, D. M. (1975). Vocal communication in preverbal normal and autistic children. In N. O'Connor (Ed.), *Language, cognitive deficits, and retardation* (pp. 75–80). London: Butterworths.

Ricks, D. M., & Wing, L. (1976). Language, communication, and the use of symbols. In L. Wing (Ed.), *Early childhood autism: Clinical, educational, and social aspects* (2nd ed., pp. 93–134). New York: Pergamon Press.

Rondal, J. A. (1978). Developmental sentence scoring procedure and the delay–difference question in language development of Down's syndrome children. *Mental Retardation, 16*, 169–171.

Rondal, J. A. (1987). Down syndrome. In K. Mogford & D. Bishop (Eds.), *Language development in exceptional circumstances* (pp. 49–73). London: Churchill Livingstone.

Rutter, M. (1983). Cognitive deficits in the pathogenesis of autism. *Journal of Child Psychology and Psychiatry, 24*, 513–531.

Rutter, M., Bartak, L., & Newman, S. (1971). Autism—a central disorder of cognition and language? In M. Rutter (Ed.), *Autism: Concepts, characteristics, and treatment* (pp. 63–102). London: Churchill Livingstone.

Rutter, M., Greenfield, D., & Lockyer, L. (1967). A five to fifteen year follow up study of infantile psychosis: II. Social and behavioral outcome. *British Journal of Psychiatry, 113*, 1183–1199.

Schmidt, J. (1976). *Relations between paired-associate learning and utterance patterns in children with echolalia.* Unpublished doctoral dissertation, Boston University School of Education.

Schwartz, R. G., & Leonard, L. B. (1979, October). *Do children pick and choose? An examination of phonological selection and avoidance in early lexical acquisition.* Paper presented at the Fourth Annual Boston University Conference on Language Development, Boston.

Schuler, A. L. (1979). Echolalia: Issues and clinical applications. *Journal of Speech and Hearing Disorders, 44,* 411–434.

Schuler, A. L., & Prizant, B. M. (1985). Echolalia. In E. Schopler & G. Mesibov (Eds.), *Communication problems in autism* (pp. 163–184). New York: Plenum.

Schwartz, S. (1981). Language disabilities in infantile autism: A brief review and comment. *Applied Psycholinguistics, 2,* 25–31.

Shapiro, T., Fish, B., & Ginsberg, G. L. (1972). The speech of a schizophrenic child from two to six. *American Journal of Psychiatry, 128,* 1408–1414.

Simmons, J. Q., & Baltaxe, C. A. M. (1975). Language patterns of adolescent autistics. *Journal of Autism and Childhood Schizophrenia, 5,* 333–351.

Simon, N. (1975). Echolalic speech in childhood autism. *Archives of General Psychiatry, 32,* 1439–1446.

Snow, C. (1977). The development of conversation between mothers and babies. *Journal of Child Language, 4,* 1–22.

Stark, R. E. (1986). Prespeech segmental feature development. In P. Fletcher & M. Garman (Eds.), *Language acquisition* (2nd ed., pp. 149–173). New York: Cambridge University Press.

Stern, D. N. (1971). A micro-analysis of mother–infant interaction. *Journal of the American Academy of Child Psychiatry, 10,* 501–517.

Sugarman, S. (1984). The development of preverbal communication: Its contribution and limits in promoting the development of language. In R. L. Schiefelbusch & J. Pickar (Eds.), *The acquisition of communicative competence* (pp. 23–67). Baltimore: University Park Press.

Swisher, L., & Demetras, M. J. (1985). The expressive language characteristics of autistic children compared with mentally retarded or specific language-impaired children. In E. Schopler & G. Mesibov (Eds.), *Communication problems in autism* (pp. 147–162). New York: Plenum.

Tager-Flusberg, H. (1981a). On the nature of linguistic functioning in early infantile autism. *Journal of Autism and Developmental Disorders, 11,* 45–54.

Tager-Flusberg, H. (1981b). Sentence comprehension in autistic children. *Applied Psycholinguistics, 2,* 5–24.

Tager-Flusberg, H. (1982). Pragmatic development and its implications for social interaction in autistic children. In D. Park (Ed.), *Proceedings of the International Symposium for Research in Autism* (pp. 103–108). Washington, DC: National Society for Autistic Children.

Tager-Flusberg, H. (1985a). Basic level and superordinate level categorization in autistic, mentally retarded and normal children. *Journal of Experimental Child Psychology, 40,* 450–469.

Tager-Flusberg, H. (1985b). The conceptual basis for referential word meaning in children with autism. *Child Development, 56,* 1167–1178.

Tager-Flusberg, H. (1985c). Psycholinguistic approaches to language and communication in autism. In E. Schopler & G. Mesibov (Eds.), *Communication problems in autism* (pp. 69–87). New York: Plenum Press.

Tager-Flusberg, H. (1986a, October). *Constraints on the process of grammatical development: Evidence from autistic and Down syndrome children.* Paper presented at the Eleventh Annual Boston University Conference on Language Development, Boston.

Tager-Flusberg, H. (1986b). Constraints on the representation of word meaning: Evidence from autistic and mentally retarded children. In S. Kuczaj & M. Barrett (Eds.), *The development of word meaning* (pp. 139–166). New York: Springer-Verlag.

Tager-Flusberg, H. (1986c). The semantic deficit hypothesis of autistic children's language. *Australian Journal of Human Communication Disorders, 14,* 51–58.

Tager-Flusberg, H. (1988). On the nature of a language acquisition disorder: The example of autism. In F. Kessel (Ed.), *The development of language and language researchers: Essays presented to Roger Brown* (pp. 249–267). Hillsdale, NJ: Erlbaum.

Tager-Flusberg, H., & Baumberger, T. (1987). *The acquisition of past tense morphology in autistic, Down syndrome and normal children.* Unpublished manuscript, University of Massachusetts at Boston.

Tager-Flusberg, H., Calkins, S., Nolin, T. L., Anderson, M. J., Chadwick-Dias, A. M. (1987). A *longitudinal study of language acquisition in autistic and Down syndrome children.* Unpublished manuscript, University of Massachusetts at Boston.

Tager-Flusberg, H., de Villiers, J. G., & Hakuta, K. (1982). The development of sentence coordination. In S. A. Kuczaj (Ed.), *Language development: Syntax and semantics* (pp. 201–243). Hillsdale, NJ: Erlbaum.

Tager-Flusberg, H., & Keenan, T. L. (May 1987). *The acquisition of negation in autistic and Down syndrome children.* Paper presented at the Symposium for Research on Child Language Disorders, Madison, WI.

Trehub, S. E. (1976). The discrimination of foreign speech contrasts by infants and children. *Child Development, 47,* 466–472.

Ungerer, J. A., & Sigman, M. (1987). Categorization skills and receptive language development in autistic children. *Journal of Autism and Developmental Disorders, 17,* 3–16.

van der Hulst, H., & Smith, N. (1985). *Advances in non-linear phonology.* Dordrecht, The Netherlands: Foris.

Waterhouse, L., & Fein, D. (1982). Language skills in developmentally disabled children. *Brain and Language, 15,* 307–333.

Waugh, L., & van Schooneveld, C. (1980). *The melody of language: Intonation and prosody.* Baltimore: University Park Press.

Weeks, T. (1971). Speech registers in young children. *Child Development, 42,* 1119–1131.

Wetherby, A. M. (1986). Ontongeny of communication functions in autism. *Journal of Autism and Developmental Disorders, 16,* 295–316.

Wetherby, A. M., & Prizant, B. M. (1985). Intentional communicative behavior of children with autism: Theoretical and practical issues. *Australian Journal of Human Communication Disorders, 13,* 21–59.

Wetherby, A. M., & Prutting, C. (1984). Profiles of communicative and cognitive–social abilities in autistic children. *Journal of Speech and Hearing Research, 27,* 364–377.

Wing, L. (1969). The handicaps of autistic children: A comparative study. *Journal of Child Psychology and Psychiatry, 10,* 1–40.

Neurobiological Issues in Autism:
Research and Theory

Neuroanatomical Systems Involved in Infantile Autism
The Implications of Cerebellar Abnormalities

ERIC COURCHESNE

Children's Hospital Research Center, San Diego
University of California at San Diego

The neurobiological substrate of infantile autism is unknown, as is its etiology. In the 20 years following Kanner's (1943) original description, research focused on psychogenic explanations of autism, even though Kanner (1943) had initially concluded it was a biological disorder. It was not until Rimland (1964) presented the first neurobiological explanation of autism and a review of evidence from twin studies that research began to focus on the biology of autism. Rimland's (1964) original theory was that autism is a cognitive disorder and the result of malfunctioning of systems within the brain stem that regulate arousal, attention, and orienting to environmentally important information. Biochemical, neurophysiological, and psychophysiological evidence supports the possibility that numerous systems within the brain stem do not function properly in autism.

There is, however, only meager evidence regarding the anatomy of the brain stem in autism. The brain stem has been examined in only two reports on autism (Bauman & Kemper, 1985; Williams, Hauser, Purpura, DeLong, & Swisher, 1980), and the only abnormality reported was in a single postmortem case in which there was a reduced size in the neurons of the inferior olive, which is a major source of input to the cerebellum (Bauman & Kemper, 1985). Instead, the majority of neuroanatomical studies of autism have focused on hippocampus, cerebral cortex, and the lateral ventricles. Although the ventricles may be enlarged in some autistic people, the enlargement is not distinctive of autism and may occur at any time during childhood and adulthood. Postmortem neuropathology studies and the most recent *in vivo* computerized tomography (CT) studies have found no convincing evidence of significant abnormalities in the cerebral cortex in autism (Bauman & Kemper, 1985; Creasey *et al.*, 1986; Prior, Tress, Hoffman, & Boldt, 1984; Williams *et al.*, 1980). Although CT scan studies have not found clear evidence of hippocampal abnormality, Bauman and Kemper (1985) reported that neurons in the hippocampus were abnormal in one autopsy case.

The paper by Williams *et al.* (1980) was the first report of Purkinje cell loss in autism; this loss was the only subcortical neuropathological finding (they also studied cortex, hippocampus, thalamus, and brain stem). In their single-case post-mortem study, Bauman and Kemper (1985) reported Purkinje and granule cell loss in the neocerebellum. In a recent report on four postmortem cases, Ritvo *et al.* (1986) confirmed these earlier reports of Purkinje cell loss; they did not eval-uate granule cells or other brain structures. Purkinje cell loss may occur at any time during childhood and adulthood and is not necessarily indicative of pathol-ogy beginning early in development. Also, Purkinje cell loss may be secondary to seizure disorder and medications used to control it, and several of the postmortem cases had such confounding seizure disorders and history of medication use.

Nonetheless, we were intrigued by the implications of Purkinje and granule cell loss. In a preliminary formulation, I (Courchesne, 1985, 1987) suggested that if such cell loss could be shown to occur early in development, then it could play a part in producing some of the behavioral and biochemical abnormalities seen in autism, as well as producing the abnormal neurophysiology of autism that has recently been described (Courchesne, Kilman, Galambos, & Lincoln, 1984; Courchesne, Lincoln, Kilman, & Galambos, 1985; Courchesne, Lincoln, Yeung-Courchesne, Elmasian, & Grillon, 1989). Specifically, since Purkinje cells serve as inhibitory modulators of the action of cerebellar nuclei, extensive Purkinje cell loss could result in abnormal neurophysiological activity in these cerebellar nu-clei. Abnormal output from these nuclei could affect systems mediating attention, intentional motor behavior, emotional behavior, ocular–vestibular functioning, dopaminergic activity, and serotonergic activity, because they have direct and in-direct connections with systems mediating these functions (e.g., pontine, mesen-cephalic, and thalamic levels of the reticular activating system; basal ganglia and ventral lateral and ventral medial thalamus; vestibular nuclei; and raphe magnus and raphe pontis nuclei). Abnormalities in each of these domains (i.e., attention, motor behavior, emotion, nystagmus, dopamine levels, and serotonin levels) have been noted in autism.

We have recently obtained evidence suggesting that early in development there may be extensive cell loss in neocerebellar cortex (Courchesne, Hesselink, Jernigan, & Yeung-Courchesne, 1987; Courchesne, Yeung-Courchesne, Press, Hesselink, & Jernigan, 1988). Before describing this evidence, I briefly describe some aspects of normal cerebellar anatomy and development.

NORMAL CEREBELLAR ANATOMY

The cerebellum in composed of the vermis, which is a narrow structure in the midline, and the right and left cerebellar hemispheres, which are large lobes on either side of the vermis (Figure 6-1). Like the cerebral cortex, cerebellar cortex is a thin layer of gray matter (neurons) covering the entire surface of cerebellar vermis and hemispheres, and white matter (axons) underlies this layer of cere-bellar cortex. At the center or core of the cerebellum lie several nuclei—the fastigial, interpositus, and dentate nuclei. The arrangement can be likened to an

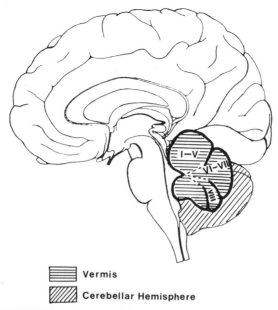

Vermis

Cerebellar Hemisphere

FIGURE 6-1. Diagram of the midline view of the human brain.

apple with its outer layer of skin, underlying white matter, and clusters of seeds at its core. Figure 6-2 shows this three-part arrangement in the vermal region of the cerebellum. Of the several types of cells in cerebellar cortex, two prominent ones are Purkinje and granule cells. There are roughly 15 million Purkinje cells and 50 billion granule cells, with the latter figure being comparable to the total number of cells in *cerebral* cortex. The basic neuronal circuitry of the cerebellum is shown schematically in Figure 6-3. Several neuronal systems outside of the cerebellum project to both deep cerebellar nuclei and to cerebellar cortex. The only output from cerebellar cortex is from Purkinje cells. They inhibit neurons in the deep cerebellar nuclei. These nuclei, in turn, project to numerous neural systems outside of the cerebellum (Figure 6-4; further details mentioned below).

NORMAL CEREBELLAR DEVELOPMENT

Neurogenesis of Purkinje cells occurs during the end of the first trimester; after neurogenesis, these cells migrate to what will become the cortical surface of the cerebellum (Rakic & Sidman, 1970). Neurogenesis and migration of granule cells occurs from the second trimester through early postnatal life in humans. From the time of Purkinje cell neurogenesis to birth, the circumference of the human cerebellar vermis increases in size by more than 50-fold, and by 2-fold in the first postnatal year (Figure 6-5). Figure 6-6 is a schematic depiction of the develop-

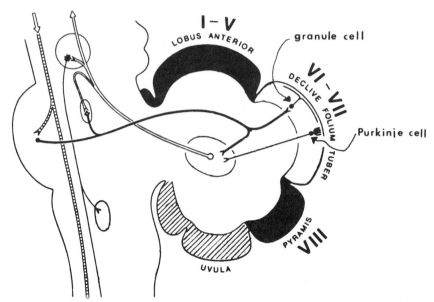

FIGURE 6-2.   Diagram of the midline view of the cerebellar vermis and brain stem of the human brain. Schematic representation shows the lobules of the vermis; mossy fiber pathways project to granule cells in cerebellar cortex; granule cells connect to the Purkinje cells in cortex; Purkinje cells project from cortex to deep cerebellar nuclei; and, finally, neurons project from deep cerebellar nuclei to brain stem and thalamic systems. Adapted from *The Human Central Nervous System* by R. Nieuwenhuys, J. Voogd, and C. van Huijzen, 1981, Berlin: Springer-Verlag. Copyright 1981 by Springer-Verlag. Adapted by permission.

mental increase in the thickness of cerebellar cortex, and Figure 6-7 shows the developmental increase in the size of the cerebellar vermis of the rat during early postnatal life.

The timing of development differs from region to region in the cerebellum. For example, in the rat, Purkinje cells in anterior vermis differ from those in posterior vermis in the site of neurogenesis and in the timing of neurogenesis and migration (Altman & Bayer, 1985). There are also regional differences in granule cell genesis and migration (Figure 6-8). Vermal lobules I–V, IX, and X develop earlier than vermal lobules VI, VII, and VIII. Moreover, granule cell genesis and migration develop earlier in the depth of vermal fissures than on the outer surface of vermal lobules. Similarly, morphological maturation of Purkinje cells (e.g., loss of neurites on the cell body and full expansion of dendritic trees) in the deep fissures precedes maturation of those on the outer folial surfaces. In sum, one can imagine cerebellar development to be analogous to the growth of a tree: The main branches appear first and then expand and grow outward, with the surface being younger than the deep main branches; some branches grow more quickly than others.

EVIDENCE OF ABNORMAL CEREBELLAR DEVELOPMENT IN
INFANTILE AUTISM

In a recent single-case report of a young man with the classic, "Kanner syndrome" form of autism, we found magnetic resonance imaging (MRI) evidence of diminished development or "hypoplasia" of neocerebellar vermal lobules VI and VII (i.e., declive, folium, and tuber); these lobules were 44% smaller than normal

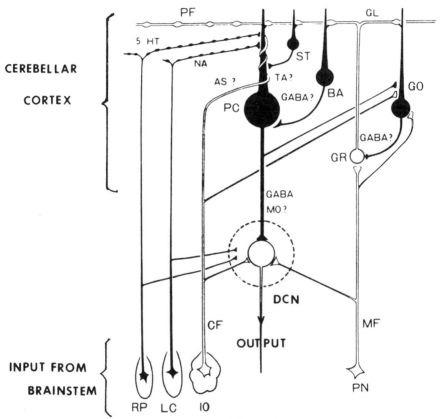

FIGURE 6-3. Basic neuronal circuitry of the cerebellum and putative neurotransmitters in the cerebellum. PC, Purkinje cell; GO, Golgi cell; BA, basket cell; ST, stellate cell; GR, granule cell; PF, parallel fiber; MF, mossy fiber; CF, climbing fiber; DCN, deep cerebellar nuclear cell; PN, precerebellar neuron that issues mossy fibers; IO, inferior olive; LC, locus ceruleus; RP, raphe nuclei. Inhibitory neurons and synapses are black-filled, and excitatory ones have been left unfilled. Candidates for neurotransmitter substances are indicated for some synapses. Question mark indicates that criteria for identification have not yet been fulfilled. GL, glutamate; AS, aspartate; TA, taurine; MO, motilin; NA, noradrenalin; 5-HT, serotonin; GABA, gamma-aminobutyric acid. Adapted from *The Cerebellum and Neural Control* by M. Ito, 1984, New York: Raven Press. Copyright 1984 by Raven Press. Adapted by permission.

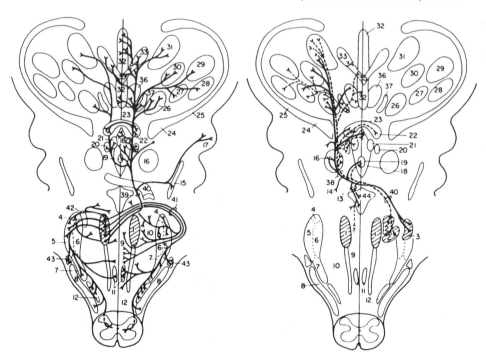

FIGURE 6-4. Diagram of the efferent connections of the cerebellar nuclei. Left: Fastigial nucleus. Right: Interpositus and lateral cerebellar nuclei. 1, fastigial nucleus; 2, nucleus interpositus anterior; 2', nucleus interpositus posterior; 3, lateral (dentate) nucleus; 4, superior vestibular nucleus; 5, lateral vestibular nucleus; 6, medial vestibular nucleus; 7, inferior (descending) vestibular nucleus; 8, lateral reticular nucleus; 9, medial bulbar reticular formation; 10, lateral bulbar reticular formation; 11, perihypoglossal nuclei; 12, nucleus parasolitarius; 13, descending limb of the brachium conjunctivum; 14, pontine reticular formation; 15, lateral lemniscal nucleus; 16, red nucleus; 17, superior colliculus; 18, periaqueductal gray; 19, Edinger–Westphal's nucleus; 20, interstitial nucleus; 21, nucleus of Darkschewitsch; 22, posterior commissure nucleus; 23, posterior commissure; 24, Forel's field; 25, reticular nucleus; 26, center median nucleus; 27, ventral posteromedial nucleus; 28, ventral posterolateral nucleus; 29, lateral posterior nucleus; 30, ventral lateral nucleus; 31, ventral anterior nucleus; 32, midline nuclei; 33, central lateral nucleus; 34, paracentral nucleus; 35, central medial nucleus; 36, ventromedial nucleus; 37, parafascicular nucleus; 38, crossed, ascending limb of brachium conjunctivum; 39, accessory brachium conjunctivum; 40, brachium conjunctivum; 41, hook bundle; 42, direct fastigiobulbar tract; 43, group X of Brodal and Pompeiano; 44, tegmental reticular nucleus. From "On Cerebellar Evolution and Organization from the Point of View of a Morphologist" by J. Jansen, 1969, in R. Llinas (Ed.), *Neurobiology of Cerebellar Evolution and Development* (pp. 881–893), Chicago: American Medical Association. Copyright 1969 by the American Medical Association. Reprinted by permission.

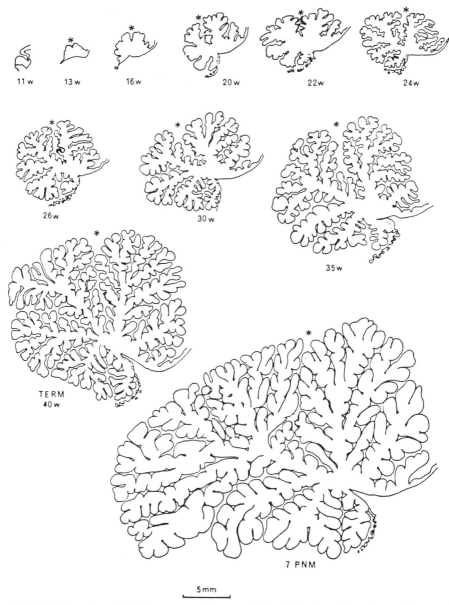

FIGURE 6-5.   Growth of the human cerebellar vermis from 11 fetal weeks (w) of age to 7 postnatal months (PNM) of age; size indicated by 5-mm scale at the bottom of the figure. The asterisks indicate the primary fissure. From "Histogenesis of Cortical Layers in Human Cerebellum, Particularly the Lamina Dissecans" by P. Rakic and R. L. Sidman, 1970, *Journal of Comparative Neurology*, 139, 473–500. Copyright 1970 by Alan R. Liss, Inc. Reprinted by permission.

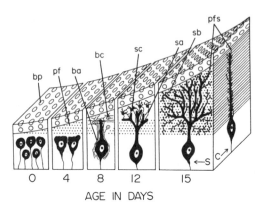

AGE IN DAYS

FIGURE 6-6. Growth of cerebellar cortex, and scheme of the major steps in the postnatal morphogenesis of rat Purkinje cells, and of the proposal for the growth of spiny branchlets in a single plane and at a right angle to the pile of parallel fibers. An "exclusion principle," which allows a single contact between a given Purkinje cell and a parallel fiber, confines outgrowth in the coronal plane (C) to the vicinity of the stem dendrite. This principle does not affect growth in the sagittal plane (S), as contacts can be established with other parallel fibers. ba, basket cell axons; bc, basket cells; pf, parallel fibers; pfs, parallel fiber synapses; sa, stellate cell axons; sb, spiny branchlets; sc, stellate cells. From "Experimental Reorganization of the Cerebellar Cortex: VII. Effects of Late X-Irradiation Schedules That Interfere with Cell Acquisition after Stellate Cells Are Formed" by J. Altman, 1976, *Journal of Comparative Neurology, 165,* 65–76. Copyright 1976 by Alan R. Liss, Inc. Reprinted by permission.

(Figure 6-9). Hypoplasia was also evident in adjacent neocerebellar hemisphere lobules VI and VII (Figure 6-9). This case was uncomplicated by mental retardation, epilepsy, or a history of drug use or neurological diseases (Courchesne *et al.*, 1987). The patient's macroscopic hypoplasia was regionally limited: Neighboring lobules of the vermis and hemispheres (I–V and VIII–X) appeared to be relatively unaffected (Figure 6-9).

Since that report, we (Courchesne *et al.*, 1988) have measured the vermis of 17 additional people with infantile autism, also uncomplicated by severe mental retardation, epilepsy, cerebral palsy, perinatal trauma, chromosomal abnormality, or a history of neurological disease or drug use during development. The Wechsler Verbal IQ of these 18 autistic subjects (17 plus our original one) ranged from 45 to 111, and the mean was 77; their Wechsler Performance IQ ranged from 70 to 112, and their mean was 88. Of the 18, 13 had Wechsler Full Scale IQs between 73 and 108; 7 either held jobs (e.g., gardeners aide, assembler of new bicycles in a bike shop, secretarial aide; most were nonpaying jobs) or attended a local college. The remaining 5 of the 18 autistic subjects had Full Scale IQs between 55 and 70 and required close custodial care.

For comparison, we also measured the vermis of 12 normal controls and of patients with (1) the Arnold–Chiari type I developmental malformation of the

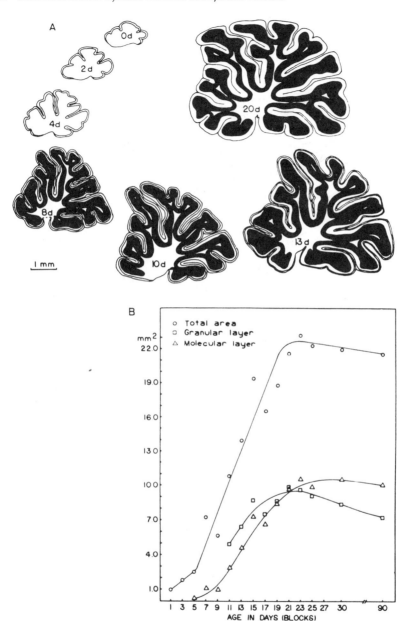

FIGURE 6-7. (A) Tracings of matched sagittal sections of the vermis from rats of different postnatal ages in days (d). Outer band, external germinal layer; black zone, granular layer; white zone between the two, molecular layers. (B) Planimetric measurement of the areal and laminar growth of the cerebellar cortex after birth. From "Autoradiographic and Histological Studies of Postnatal Neurogenesis: III. Dating the Time of Production and Onset of Differentiation of Cerebellar Microneurons in Rats" by J. Altman, 1969, *Journal of Comparative Neurology, 136,* 269–274. Copyright 1969 by Alan R. Liss, Inc. Reprinted by permission.

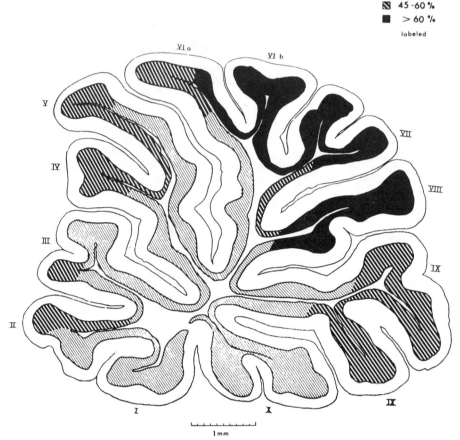

FIGURE 6-8. Schematic presentation of the percentage of granule cells labeled in the different lobules of the vermis (I–X) in rats that were injected with multiple doses of [³H]thymidine between postnatal days 11 and 16. Regions where less than 45% of the cells could be tagged are considered early-forming, while those where more than 60% of the cells were labeled are considered late-forming. From "Autoradiographic and Histological Studies of Postnatal Neurogenesis: III. Dating the Time of Production and Onset of Differentiation of Cerebellar Microneurons in Rats" by J. Altman, 1969, *Journal of Comparative Neurology, 136,* 269–274. Copyright 1969 by Alan R. Liss, Inc. Reprinted by permission.

cerebellum; (2) the Dandy–Walker developmental malformation of the cerebellum; (3) olivopontocerebellar degeneration; (4) agenesis of the corpus callosum (which is sometimes associated with developmental malformations of the cerebellum); (5) cerebellar atrophy associated with seizure disorders; and (6) very small focal lesions in cortical or subcortical areas, but no discernible pathology in the posterior fossa (Courchesne *et al.*, 1988). In collaboration with Dr. Richard Haas

NORMAL

AUTISTIC

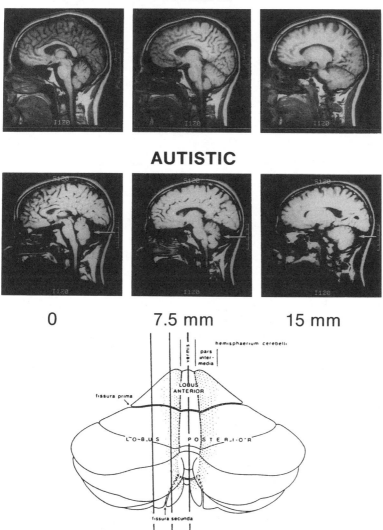

Dorsal view of the cerebellum

FIGURE 6-9. Magnetic resonance images of sagittal sections at 0.0 mm (midsagittal image), 7.5 mm (lateral to midline), and 15.0 mm (lateral to midline) from a normal subject and a nonretarded patient with infantile autism. In the latter, arrows indicate the areas of cerebellar hypoplasia which include the superior posterior vermis (i.e., vermal lobules VI and VII) and the neocerebellar hemispheres. The diagram shows the posterior view of the cerebellum with vertical lines indicating image locations. Adapted from "Abnormal Neuroanatomy in a Nonretarded Person with Autism: Unusual Findings with Magnetic Resonance Imaging" by E. Courchesne, J. R. Hesselink, T. L. Jernigan, and R. Yeung-Courchesne, 1987, *Archives of Neurology, 44,* 335–341. Copyright 1987 by the American Medical Association. Adapted by permission. Also from *Reduced Cerebellar Hemisphere Size and Its Relationship to Vermal Hypoplasia in Autism* by J. Murakami, E. Courchesne, G. A. Press, R. Yeung-Courchesne, and J. R. Hesselink, 1988, manuscript submitted for publication. Reprinted by permisison of the authors.

(Neurosciences Department, University of California at San Diego), we are currently also measuring patients with Rett syndrome; these data will be presented elsewhere and are not mentioned further herein.

We have found evidence of anatomical abnormality in the neocerebellar vermis in our autistic group (Figure 6-10). Specifically, neocerebellar vermal lobules VI and VII were statistically significantly diminished in size in the autistic group, but paleocerebellar vermal lobules I–V and VIII were normal in size. A simple index of regionally localized vermal hypoplasia was created, which further statistically confirmed that the diminished size of neocerebellar vermal lobules VI and VII was regionally localized and not the result of an overall smaller brain size in autism. This index was the ratio of the combined areas of vermal lobules VI and VII to the combined areas of vermal lobules I–V. In normals the index was 72.4% ($\pm 6.5\%$), and in autistics it was 59.1%. Of the 18 autistic subjects, 4 showed no evidence of hypoplasia, 4 fell between 1.40 and 1.59 standard deviations below normal, and 10 fell between 2.20 and 4.92 standard deviations below normal. In the latter 14, vermal lobules VI and VII were 25% smaller than those of normals. The neighboring lobules I–V and VIII were normal in size (Figure 6-10), with a single exception: Vermal lobule VIII was 2.58 standard deviations smaller than normal in one autistic person whose vermal lobules VI and VII were 4.33 standard deviations below normal and whose vermal lobules I–V were within 0.6 standard deviations of normal (see the third MRI scan from the bottom of the autistic subjects in Figure 6-10A). The 4 autistic subjects without evidence of hypoplasia, alert us to the fact that the vermis will appear macroscopically normal in some as yet to be determined portion of the autistic spectrum.

As shown in Figure 6-11, this pattern of regionally localized macroscopic hypoplasia of the vermis differs from our other comparison patient groups as well as from normals (Courchesne *et al.*, 1988). This pattern also differs from that seen in familial global cerebellar hypoplasia and other forms of cerebellar dysgenesis reported in the literature (Chaves & Frank, 1983; Gilman, Bloedel, & Lechtenberg, 1981; Jervis, 1950; Sarnat & Alcala, 1980). Thus, this form of vermal hypoplasia (i.e., macroscopic hypoplasia of vermal lobules VI and VII but not of adjacent lobules I–V and VIII) is distinctive in our autistic patients, and is not seen in patients with one of several other neurological disorders presenting in infancy, childhood, or adulthood (Figure 6-11). Comparisons to potential "neighbor" neurobehavioral disorders, such as other pervasive developmental disorders, Rett syndrome, and schizophrenia, will be important.

Hypoplasia in autism may not be restricted to only the posterior vermis. Of our 18 autistic subjects, 3 also had clinically obvious hypoplasia of portions of the neocerebellar hemispheres (e.g., Figure 6-9). We are now quantitatively mapping all regions of the cerebellum in an effort to delineate which ones (in addition to vermal lobules VI and VII) are consistently hypoplastic, which are variably so, and which are usually normal (in addition to anterior vermal lobules I–V).

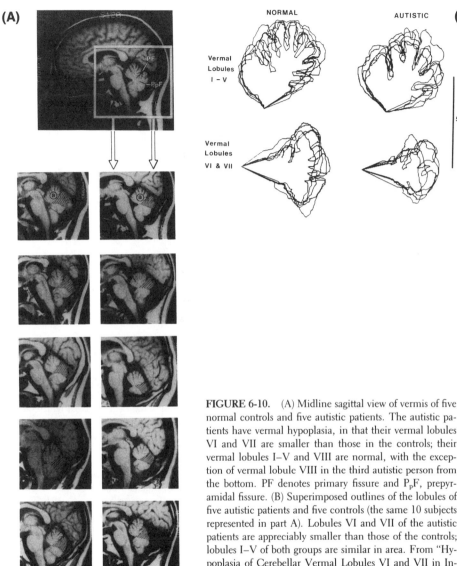

Normal   **Autistic**

(a)   *Vermal Lobules I-V*
▨   *Vermal Lobules VI-VII*

FIGURE 6-10. (A) Midline sagittal view of vermis of five normal controls and five autistic patients. The autistic patients have vermal hypoplasia, in that their vermal lobules VI and VII are smaller than those in the controls; their vermal lobules I–V and VIII are normal, with the exception of vermal lobule VIII in the third autistic person from the bottom. PF denotes primary fissure and P_pF, prepyramidal fissure. (B) Superimposed outlines of the lobules of five autistic patients and five controls (the same 10 subjects represented in part A). Lobules VI and VII of the autistic patients are appreciably smaller than those of the controls; lobules I–V of both groups are similar in area. From "Hypoplasia of Cerebellar Vermal Lobules VI and VII in Infantile Autism" by E. Courchesne, R. Yeung-Courchesne, G. A. Press, J. R. Hesselink, and T. L. Jernigan, 1988, *New England Journal of Medicine*, 318, 1349–1354. Copyright 1988 by the *New England Journal of Medicine*. Reprinted by permission.

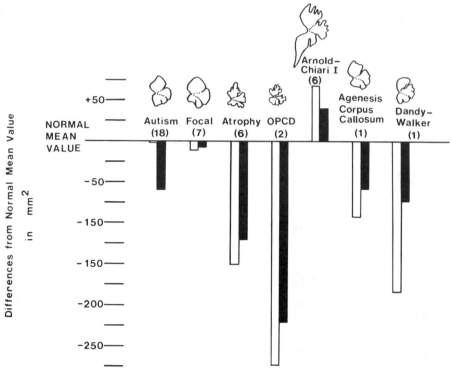

FIGURE 6-11. Differences from normal vermal area values in lobules I–V and VI and VII for autism and six other neurological disorders. The zero line represents normal mean value obtained in this study for the midsagittal area of vermal lobules I–V (i.e., 423 mm^2), and each white bar represents a difference from this value. The zero line also represents the mean normal value obtained in this study for the midsagittal area of vermal lobules VI and VII (i.e., 305 mm^2), and each filled bar represents a difference from this value for the same several neurological disorders. Also shown are examples of the midline midsagittal view of the vermis of individuals with each of the neurological disorders studied. OPCD denotes olivopontocerebellar degeneration and Focal denotes focal lesion in cerebral white matter. Values in parentheses represent the number of patients with the disorder. From "Hypoplasia of Cerebellar Vermal Lobules VI and VII in Infantile Autism" by E. Courchesne, R. Yeung-Courchesne, G. A. Press, J. R. Hesselink, and T. L. Jernigan, 1988, *New England Journal of Medicine, 318,* 1349–1354. Copyright 1988 by the *New England Journal of Medicine.* Reprinted by permission.

IMPLICATIONS

This diminished size or hypoplasia of vermal lobules VI and VII is evidence of a neuroanatomical pathology in people with classic infantile autism uncomplicated by other medical and mental disorders. Since this macroscopic abnormality was demonstrated in a large group of high-functioning as well as somewhat lower-functioning autistic people, it may be a common denominator in a large portion of people with infantile autism. It is also anatomical evidence that appears to have resulted from damage early in brain development.

These cerebellar findings may present us with a key to unraveling the biology of autism. Specifically, a precise knowledge of the cause and time at which the cerebellum was damaged could alert us to the presence of concurrent damage that might have been inflicted upon other neural structures that were also at a vulnerable point in their development. Also, if the damaging event is a genetically mediated one, study of cerebellar damage in autism could lead to the uncovering of the genetic mechanisms responsible and could point to other neural structures whose development may be disrupted by the same genetic abnormality.

Disruption of Cerebellar Development and Hypoplasia

Many factors, such as malnourishment, viruses, toxic agents, drugs, and genetic mutations, can cause abnormal cerebellar development. If these act during early development to destroy Purkinje or granule cells or to reduce the full growth of these cells, then the cerebellum will not become fully grown. It will be hypoplastic. In our autistic subjects, we have yet to detect in the maternal and postnatal histories any consistent pattern of drug exposure, illness, and the like that could potentially explain the selective macroscopic hypoplasia of vermal lobules VI and VII. Of the commonly known teratogenic agents of environmental origin (e.g., drugs, toxic chemicals, viruses, malnourishment, oxygen insufficiency), none are known to produce in humans the *specific* type of hypoplasia seen in the MRI scans of our autistic subjects. In our group of 18 autistic subjects, the tissue loss in vermal lobules VI and VII averaged 19% and was as much as 44% in several subjects. What might account for such a large amount of tissue loss in these lobules, but not in the neighboring ones?

The amount, form, and specific regions of hypoplasia depend on the type of and time of exposure to the damaging event during cerebellar development (Altman, 1982). For example, if the cerebellum of the rat is X-irradiated several times during very early postnatal development, there will be global cerebellar hypoplasia throughout much of cerebellar cortex, and Purkinje cells will be grossly shrunken, malformed, and improperly oriented (Altman, 1982; Figures 6-12 and 6-13, second row in each). On the other hand, if the cerebellum is X-irradiated briefly late during postnatal development, hypoplasia would be regionally limited, and Purkinje cells would be more nearly normally formed (e.g., Figure 6-13, last row).

Two important cell types in cerebellar cortex are Purkinje and granule cells. If Purkinje cells were destroyed during neurogenesis or halted in their migration (i.e., between 8 and 14 weeks of intrauterine development in humans), then the cerebellum might be expected to be massively reduced in size, and the formation of primary and secondary sulci and folia might be distorted. Such massive reductions and distortions were not seen in our autistic subjects. However, it is a pos-

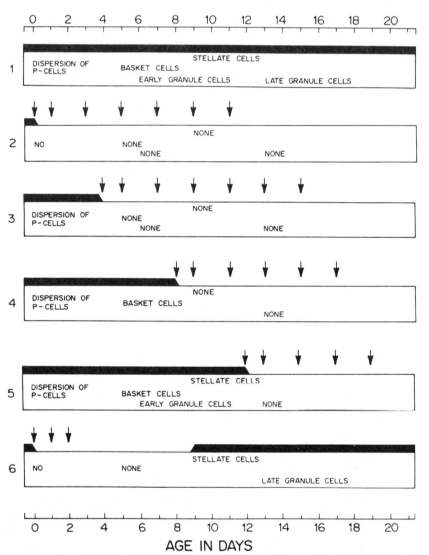

FIGURE 6-12. The expected consequences of irradiation of the cerebellum after birth with different exposure schedules on cell acquisition in the cerebellar cortex. Row 1 shows schematically the sequential production of different cell types in normal animals and approximate postnatal ages. Row 2 shows that with repeated doses of X-rays (arrows), which destroy the cells of the external germinal layer and prevent their regeneration, the acquisition of the postnatally forming microneurons can be prevented. Row 3 shows that similar effects can be obtained by delaying irradiation until postnatal day 4. However, if the exposure to X-rays is begun on postnatal day 8 (row 4), the basket cells are spared, and if it is delayed until postnatal day 12 (row 5), the stellate cells are also spared, and only the acquisition of the late granule cells is prevented. Row 6 is an example of a schedule that permits the recovery of the external germinal layer and the production of late-produced microneurons. From "Experimental Reorganization of the Rat Cerebellum and Some of Its Mechanisms" by J. Altman and W. J. Anderson, 1972, *Journal of Comparative Neurology, 146,* 355–406. Copyright 1972 by Alan R. Liss, Inc. Reprinted by permission.

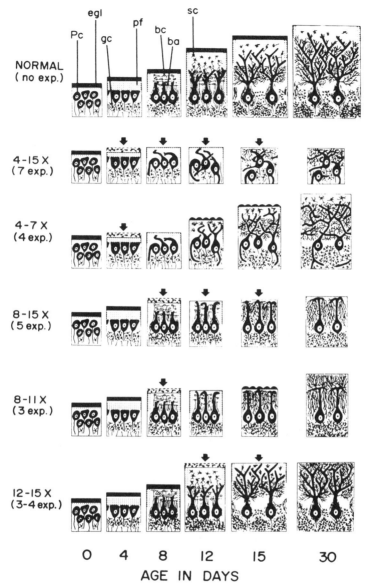

FIGURE 6-13. Schematic summary of the stages and time course of Purkinje cell dendritic development in normal rats (top row) and in rats irradiated between the postnatal days, and the number of X-ray exposures specified in the legend column on the left. Arrows indicate X-irradiation; fragmented external germinal layer (egl) symbolizes its destruction by irradiation; absence of egl indicates its failure to recover after irradiation or its natural dissolution; corrugated egl symbolizes its recovery after irradiation. ba, basket cell axons; bc, basket cell bodies; exp, exposure; gc, granule cells; Pc, Purkinje cells; pf, parallel fibers; sc, stellate cells. From "Experimental Reorganization of the Cerebellar Cortex: VII. Effects of Late X-Irradiation Schedules That Interfere with Cell Acquisition after Stellate Cells Are Formed" by J. Altman, 1976, *Journal of Comparative Neurology, 165*, 65–76. Copyright 1976 by Alan R. Liss, Inc. Reprinted by permission.

sibility that some forms of autism result from a limited loss restricted to specific regions within the cerebellum, rather than from massive and global loss of Purkinje cells. Such a specific form of maldevelopment would be expected to result from a rather discrete environmentally or genetically mediated event that acts only within a narrow window of time during fetal development.

In humans, the precise timing of genesis and migration of Purkinje cells destined for different cerebellar regions is not known. However, it is known for the rat (Altman & Bayer, 1985). Peak times and durations of Purkinje cell neurogenesis and migration differ between anterior and posterior cerebellum and between vermis and hemisphere. Nonetheless, there is considerable overlap, and it seems likely that a damaging environmental event would affect Purkinje cells destined for numerous regions of the cerebellum.

Granule cell neurogenesis and migration in human development continue through early postnatal life (Raaf & Kernohan, 1944). These cells are among the last neural building blocks to be put into place in the human cerebellum. The genesis and migration of 50 billion granule cells in the human cerebellum contributes directly and indirectly (through interactions with Purkinje cell dendritic growth) to the large increase in the size of the cerebellum during late prenatal life and the first year of postnatal life. In the rat, the final stage of cerebellar granule cell genesis and migration is in vermal lobules VI, VII, and VIII. They receive their full complement of granule cells after the anterior vermis is complete (Altman, 1969). If X-irradiation exposure is late during postnatal development, then granule cells will be lost to a much greater extent in vermal lobules VI, VII, and VIII (see Figure 6-8) than in other regions of the vermis, and hypoplasia would be regionally limited rather than global. Although other areas would be affected, the degree and form of the maldevelopment would depend on the stage of their development at the time of the late postnatal X-irradiation (Altman, 1982). For instance, cerebellar cortex in the deep fissures might be predicted to suffer less disturbance than cortex on the still-growing outer folial surfaces (e.g., Robain, Wen, Wisniewski, Shek, & Loo, 1981).

It is not known whether there are comparable regionally distinct chronologies of granule cell development in the human. If there are, then it is at least theoretically possible that exposure to teratogenic events during specific stages of granule cell genesis or migration could differentially affect the development of vermal lobules VI and VII more than that of the anterior vermis. In light of Altman's (1969) evidence, it may be worth nothing again that, besides vermal lobules VI and VII, the only other vermal region with evidence of hypoplasia in our study was vermal lobule VIII in one autistic subject (Figure 6-10A, third from the bottom).

Since there is some evidence suggestive of a genetic factor in autism (see Rimland, 1964, for a review of the early literature; see Folstein & Rutter, 1987, for a recent review; Folstein & Rutter, 1977; Ritvo, Freeman, Mason-Brothers, Mo, & Ritvo, 1985), the hypoplasia might be genetically mediated, possibly via a genetic vulnerability to particular environmental conditions or precipitators. Many genetic abnormalities that selectively create cerebellar pathology have been described in animals (Caviness & Rakic, 1978). Postnatal loss of Purkinje cells in mice is caused by two genetic mutations: the "nervous" mutation and the "Purkinje cell degeneration" mutation (Mullen, Eicher, & Sidman, 1976; Sidman & Green, 1970). Such Purkinje cell loss might be expected to result in macroscopic cerebellar hypoplasia less severe than if the loss occurred during Purkinje genesis or migration. Both mouse mutations also cause photoreceptor degeneration.

The Region of Vermal Hypoplasia in Autism: Distinctive in Three Ways

Vermal lobules VI and VII are phylogenetically, embryologically, and anatomically distinct from their vermal neighbors (i.e., anterior vermal lobules I–V and posterior vermal lobule VIII). They are the only regions of the vermis classified as neocerebellar; their neighbors, anterior vermal lobules I–V and posterior vermal lobule VIII, are classified as paleocerebellar regions (Gilman et al., 1981). Also, as just discussed, the time and the site of neurogenesis of Purkinje and granule cells in vermal lobules VI and VII differ from those in the anterior vermis (Altman, 1969; Altman & Bayer, 1985; Rakic & Sidman, 1970; Verbitskaya, 1969). These phylogenetic and embryological distinctions may hold clues to the genetically and/or environmentally mediated etiology of autism. Moreover, as will be discussed next, many of the anatomical connections of vermal lobules VI and VII *to* the brain stem and thalamus (via fastigial nucleus), and *from* the cerebral cortex and brain stem, differ from those of the anterior vermis (Beitz, 1982; Carpenter & Batton, 1982; Gilman et al., 1981; Nieuwenhuys, Voogd, & van Huijzen, 1981).

Cerebellar Hypoplasia and Symptoms of Infantile Autism

In addition to aberrant social, language, and cognitive functioning, autism may involve abnormality in attention, sensory modulation, dopamine activity, serotonergic activity, speech, memory, and complex motivated behavior such as eating. Since the cerebellum has usually been viewed as principally involved in motor control, it seems paradoxical that the anatomical pathology of some individuals with autism involves hypoplasia of neocerebellar vermal lobules VI and VII, and also hypoplasia of regions within neocerebellar hemispheres.

Normal Neocerebellar Functions and Connections

Recent publications indicate that the neocerebellum in general and vermal lobules VI and VII in particular are involved in additional functions besides motor control. Leiner, Leiner, and Dow (1986) pointed out a possible role of the neocerebellum in the acquisition and execution of skilled mental as well as motor operations. Leaton and Supple (1986a, 1986b, 1986c) have found that lesions that completely eliminate vermal lobules VI, VII, and VIII prevent both long-term habituation of the acoustic startle response and classical conditioning of heart rate responses. Comparable paradigms have never been performed with autistic people. Nonetheless, studies have shown that autistic people fail to show normal heart rate changes in response to repetitive stimulation (Kootz & Cohen, 1981) and have abnormally reduced neurophysiological responses to acoustically surprising stimuli (Courchesne, 1987; Courchesne *et al.*, 1984, 1985). The prepositus hypoglossi in the brain stem is one of only two nuclei directly controlling the noradrenergic locus ceruleus (Aston-Jones, Pieribone, Nickell, & Shipley, 1986). Degeneration studies show that a significant neural input to prepositus hypoglossi comes from the fastigial nucleus, which in turn is directly controlled by the vermal cortex; however, this neural pathway has yet to be confirmed by autoradiographic studies (Carpenter & Batton, 1982; Gilman *et al.*, 1981). Thompson and McCormick (McCormick & Thompson, 1984; Thompson, 1983, 1986) have shown that the neocerebellum is an "obligatory part" of the "discrete, adaptive response circuit" for associative learning. They suggest that the cerebellum may be the location of the memory trace for such learned responses. With regard to the relationship between the cerebellum and motivated behavior, Ito (1984) concluded, "The cerebrocerebellar relationships have so far been investigated mainly in connection with the neocortical motor functions, but it is apparent that these should also be investigated in connection with the limbic, behavioral functions. Specification of roles and mechanism of the cerebellum in animal behavior would be an important theme for future investigations" (p. 451).

The functional significance of hypoplasia of the neocerebellar vermis and hemispheres in autism may also be considered in conjunction with the normal physioanatomy of the deep cerebellar nuclei (e.g., fastigial, interpositus, and dentate nuclei). Purkinje cells in the cortex of the cerebellar vermis and hemispheres exert inhibitory control over the activity of the deep cerebellar nuclei. Neurons in the deep cerebellar nuclei are spontaneously active, and they have an excitatory output to a great variety of systems within the brain stem and thalamus (Figure 6-4). For example, the fastigial nucleus influences systems involved in arousal and attention, thalamic sensory processing, motor initiation and coordination, serotonergic activity, dopaminergic activity, and vestibular and ocular–motor activity.[1] Also, vermal lobules VI and VII and fastigial nucleus have physiological connections with the hippocampus (Newman & Reza, 1979), a structure important for

1. Vermal lobules VI and VII project to specific segments of the fastigial nucleus, which in turn project to pontine reticular formation; portions of the vestibular nuclei; superior colliculus; nucleus pontis oralis and caudalis; nucleus reticularis gigantocellularis; paramedian reticular nucleus; lateral reticular nucleus (small), the nuclei of the posterior commissure; and vental lateral thalamus, ventral posterolateral thalamus, and midline thalamic nuclei, including the intralaminar nuclei, centrum medianum, and zona incerta (Beitz, 1982; Carpenter & Batton, 1982; Gilman *et al.*, 1981; Nieuwenhuys *et al.*, 1981).

creating conscious awareness of memories of specific people, places, objects, and events that occurred in the past (Nadel & Zola-Morgan, 1984). Stimulation of fastigial nucleus affects cell activity in fields CA1 and CA3 of hippocampus, and hippocampal cell activity evoked by cutaneous stimulation is depressed when preceded by fastigial stimulation (Newman & Reza, 1979). Newman and Reza (1979) found that vermal lobules VI and VII were the only cerebellar cortical areas that responded to stimulation of hippocampus. In addition, electrical stimulation of fastigial nucleus in cats induces complex behavior such as grooming, aggression, and eating, and includes biting and chewing any object placed nearby (Reis, Doba, & Nathan, 1973).

The connections of another deep cerebellar nucleus—the dentate nucleus, which is controlled by Purkinje cells in the cerebellar hemispheres—are also to numerous systems mediating arousal and attention, intentional motor behavior, and serotonergic activity (Courchesne, 1987). Speech is influenced by the left superior paravermal region of the neocerebellar hemisphere via its connections through the dentate nucleus. Abnormalities of this region can result in dysarthria, and we have suggested that the dysarthria of one of our autistic patients is due to the presence of hypoplasia in this region of his neocerebellum (see Figure 6-9 and Courchesne *et al.*, 1987).

Speculations on Possible Consequences of Abnormal Neocerebellar Physioanatomy

The neocerebellar hypoplasia in our studies of autism (in vermal lobules VI and VII and in neocerebellar hemispheres in three of our subjects) is likely to be the result of the extensive loss of granule or Purkinje cells. Loss of granule cells creates major distortions in the development, organization and functioning of neural circuits in the damaged cerebellum (Figure 6-13) (Caviness & Rakic, 1978). Loss of Purkinje cells eliminates the only source of cortical inhibitory control over the spontaneously active, excitatory neurons in the deep cerebellar nuclei.

Such physioanatomical abnormalities in neocerebellar vermal and hemisphere cortex (i.e., either granule or Purkinje cell loss) could create abnormal functioning of neurons in deep cerebellar nuclei (fastigial, interpositus, and dentate), which in turn could interfere with the normal functioning of one or more of the systems mediating arousal and attention; thalamic sensory processing; motor initiation and coordination; serotonergic activity; dopaminergic activity; ocular–vestibular functioning; hippocampal functioning; speech; and complex motivated behavior such as eating. There is no direct evidence from developmental animal studies that speaks specifically to this possibility. However, it is interesting to consider that many of the functions mediated by these systems fall into the domains of dysfunction or abnormality characteristic of autism (e.g., attention, arousal, orienting—Cohen, Caparulo, & Shaywitz, 1976; Courchesne, 1987; Courchesne *et al.*, 1984, 1985; Kootz & Cohen, 1981; Rimland, 1964; sensory processing—

Ornitz, 1978, 1985; dopamine and serotonin—Young et al., 1982; ocular–vestibular—Ornitz, 1985; hippocampus and memory— Ameli, Courchesne, Lincoln, Kaufman, & Grillon, 1988; DeLong, 1978; speech and motor dysfunction—DeMyer, 1975; DeMyer, Hingtgen, & Jackson, 1981; peculiar eating habits—DeMyer et al., 1981).

We agree with earlier researchers that autism is a disorder affecting brain stem and thalamic systems, and that the dysfunction includes abnormal modulation of arousal, attention, thalamic sensory responses, catecholaminergic and serotonergic activity, ocular–vestibular responses, and speech and motor output (Cohen et al., 1976; Ornitz, 1985; Rimland, 1964). It would be important to determine if one or more of these dysfunctions is due to a single source of abnormal neural activity that distributes its excitatory interference to brain stem and thalamic systems mediating each of these functions, and that this single source is the deep cerebellar nuclei. If some dysfunction is due to abnormal activity in deep cerebellar nuclei, then one might hypothesize that Purkinje or granule cell loss in neocerebellar cortex is responsible.

CONCLUDING REMARKS

The macroscopic hypoplasia of vermal lobules VI and VII present in many autistic individuals appears to be the result of biological factors acting during pregnancy or early postnatal life, and is generally compatible with single-case postmortem studies of autism showing Purkinje and/or granule cell loss in the neocerebellum (Bauman & Kemper, 1985; Ritvo et al., 1986; Williams et al., 1980). The macroscopic hypoplasia in our MRI studies is unlike abnormalities found in many other congenital and childhood disorders. Vermal lobules VI and VII are phylogenetically, ontogenetically, and anatomically distinct parts of the vermis. Uncovering their functional significance may provide unexpected perspectives of normal cerebellar function as well as of autism. It must now be determined whether macroscopic hypoplasia of the neocerebellum is or is not a common denominator in the majority of people with autism and whether it is present in related developmental disorders. Similarly, it must also be determined whether or not there are other anatomic sites of abnormal development that are common denominators.

Acknowledgments

The research reported here was supported by a grant from the Children's Hospital Research Center, National Institute of Neurological and Communicative Disorders and Stroke Grant No. 5-RO1-NS19855, and National Institute of Mental Health Grant No. 1-RO1-MH36840, and awarded to Eric Courchesne. Thanks to Rachel Yeung-Courchesne, Gary Press, John R. Hesselink, and Terry L. Jernigan. This chapter is abstracted in part from Courchesne, Hesselink, Jernigan, and Yeung-Courchesne (1987) and Courchesne, Yeung-Courchesne, Press, Hesselink, and Jernigan (1988).

References

Altman, J. (1969). Autoradiographic and histological studies of postnatal neurogenesis: III. Dating the time of production and onset of differentiation of cerebellar microneurons in rats. *Journal of Comparative Neurology, 136,* 269–294.

Altman, J. (1976). Experimental reorganization of the cerebellar cortex: VII. Effects of late X-irradiation schedules that interfere with cell acquisition after stellate cells are formed. *Journal of Comparative Neurology, 165,* 65–76.

Altman, J. (1982). Morphological development of the rat cerebellum and some of its mechanisms. In S. L. Palay & V. Chan-Palay (Eds.), *The cerebellum: New vistas* (pp. 8–49). Berlin: Springer-Verlag.

Altman, J., & Anderson, W. J. (1972). Experimental reorganization of the cerebellar cortex: I. Morphological effects of elimination of all microneurons with prolonged X-irradiation started at birth. *Journal of Comparative Neurology, 146,* 355–406.

Altman, J., & Bayer, S. (1985). Embryonic development of the rat cerebellum. III. Regional differences in the time of origin, migration, and settling of Purkinje cells. *Journal of Comparative Neurology, 231,* 42–65.

Ameli, R., Courchesne, E., Lincoln, A. J., Kaufman, A. S., & Grillon, C. (1988). Visual memory processes in high-functioning individuals with autism. *Journal of Autism and Developmental Disorders, 18,* 601–615.

Aston-Jones, G., Pieribone, E. N., Nickell, W. T., Shipley, M. T. (1986). The brain nucleus locus coeruleus: Restricted afferent control of a broad efferent network. *Science, 234,* 734–737.

Bauman, M., & Kemper, T. (1985). Histoanatomic observations of the brain in early infantile autism. *Neurology, 35,* 866–874.

Beitz, A. J. (1982). Structural organization of the fastigial nucleus. In S. L. Palay & V. Chan-Palay, (Eds.), *The cerebellum: New vistas* (pp. 233–249). Berlin: Springer-Verlag.

Carpenter, M. B., & Batton, R. R., III. (1982). Connections of the fastigial nucleus in the cat and monkey. In S. L. Palay & V. Chan-Palay (Eds.), *The cerebellum: New vistas* (pp. 250–291). Berlin: Springer-Verlag.

Caviness, V. S., Jr., & Rakic, P. (1978). Mechanisms of cortical development: A view from mutations in mice. *Annual Review of Neuroscience, 1,* 297–326.

Chaves, E., & Frank, L. M. (1983). Disorders of basal ganglia, cerebellum, brain stem, and cranial nerves. In T. W. Farmer (Ed.), *Pediatric neurology* (pp. 605–648). Philadelphia: Harper & Row.

Cohen, D. J., Caparulo, B. K., & Shaywitz, B. A. (1976). Primary childhood aphasia and childhood autism. *Journal of the American Academy of Child Psychiatry, 15,* 604–646.

Courchesne, E. (1985). The missing ingredients in autism. In *Brain and behavioral development: Biosocial dimensions.* Eldridge, MD: Social Science Research Council.

Courchesne, E. (1987). A neurophysiological view of autism. In E. Schopler & G. B. Mesibov (Eds.), *Neurobiological issues in autism* (pp. 285–324). New York: Plenum.

Courchesne, E., Hesselink, J. R., Jernigan, T. L., & Yeung-Courchesne, R. (1987). Abnormal neuroanatomy in a nonretarded person with autism: Unusual findings with magnetic resonance imaging. *Archives of Neurology, 44,* 335–341.

Courchesne, E., Kilman, B., Galambos, R., & Lincoln, A. (1984). Autism: Processing of novel auditory information assessed by event-related brain potentials. *Electroencephalography and Clinical Neurophysiology, 59,* 238–248.

Courchesne, E., Lincoln, A. J., Kilman, B. A., & Galambos, R. (1985). Event-related brain potential correlates of the processing of novel visual and auditory information in autism. *Journal of Autism and Developmental Disorders, 15*(1), 55–76.

Courchesne, E., Lincoln, A. J., Yeung-Courchesne, R., Elmasian, R., & Grillon, C. (1989). Pathophysiological findings in social and language disorders: Autism and receptive developmental language disorder. *Journal of Autism and Developmental Disorders.*

Courchesne, E., Yeung-Courchesne, R., Press, G. A., Hesselink, J. R., & Jernigan, T. L. (1988). Hypoplasia of cerebellar vermal lobules VI and VII in infantile autism. *New England Journal of Medicine, 318*, 1349–1354.

Creasey, H., Rumsey, J. M., Schwartz, M., Duara, R., Rapoport, J. L., & Rapoport, S. I. (1986). Brain morphometry in autistic men as measured by volumetric computed tomography. *Archives of Neurology, 43*, 669–672.

DeLong, G. R. (1978). A neuropsychological interpretation of infantile autism. In E. Schopler & M. Rutter (Eds.), *Autism: A reappraisal of concepts and treatment* (pp. 207–218). New York: Plenum.

DeMyer, M. K. (1975). The nature of the neuropsychological disability in autistic children. *Journal of Autism and Childhood Schizophrenia, 5*, 109–128.

DeMyer, M. K., Hingtgen, J. N., & Jackson, R. K. (1981). Infantile autism reviewed: A decade of research. *Schizophrenia Bulletin, 7*(3). 390–453.

Folstein, S., & Rutter, M. (1977). Infantile autism: A genetic study of 21 twin pairs. *Journal of Child Psychology, 18*, 297–321.

Folstein, S. E., & Rutter, M. L. (1987). Autism: Familial aggregation and genetic implications. In E. Schopler & G. B. Mesibov (Eds.), *Neurobiological issues in autism* (pp. 83–105). New York: Plenum.

Gilman, S., Bloedel, J., & Lechtenberg, R. (1981). *Disorders of the cerebellum.* Philadelphia: F. A. Davis.

Ito, M. (1984). *The cerebellum and neural control.* New York: Raven Press.

Jansen, J. (1969). On cerebellar evolution and organization from the point of view of a morphologist. In R. Llinas (Ed.), *Neurobiology of cerebellar evolution and development* (pp. 881–893). Chicago: American Medical Association.

Jervis, G. A. (1950). Early familial cerebellar degeneration. *Journal of Nervous and Mental Disease, 111*, 398–407.

Kanner, L. (1943). Autistic disturbances of affective contact. *The Nervous Child, 2*, 217–250.

Kootz, J. P., & Cohen, D. J. (1981). Modulation of sensory intake in autistic children: Cardiovascular and behavioral indices. *Journal of the American Academy of Child Psychiatry, 20*, 692–701.

Leaton, R. N., & Supple, W. F. (1986a). Cerebellar vermis: Essential for long-term habituation of the acoustic startle response. *Science, 232*, 513–515.

Leaton, R. N., & Supple, W. F. (1986b). Lesions of the cerebellar vermis block classically conditioned bradycardia in rats. *Society for Neuroscience Abstracts, 12*(2), 978.

Leaton, R. N., & Supple, W. F. (1986c). Long-term habituation of acoustic startle following lesions of the cerebellar vermis or cerebellar hemisphere. *Society for Neuroscience Abstracts, 12*(2), 978.

Leiner, H. C., Leiner, A. L., & Dow, R. S. (1986). Does the cerebellum contribute to mental skills? *Behavioral Neuroscience, 100*(4), 443–454.

McCormick, D. A., & Thompson, R. F. (1984). Cerebellum: Essential involvement in the classically conditioned eyelid response. *Science, 223*, 296–299.

Mullen, R. J., Eicher, E. M., & Sidman, R. L. (1976). Purkinje cell degeneration, a new neurological mutation in the mouse. *Proceedings of the National Academy of Sciences USA, 73*, 208–212.

Nadel, L., & Zola-Morgan, S. (1984). Infantile amnesia: A neurobiological perspective. In M. Moscovitch (Ed.), *Infant memory* (pp. 145–172). New York: Plenum.

Newman, P. P., & Reza, H. (1979). Functional relationships between the hippocampus and the cerebellum: An electrophysiological study of the cat. *Journal of Physiology, 287*, 405–426.

Nieuwenhuys, R., Voogd, J., & van Huijzen, C. (1981). *The human central nervous system.* Berlin: Springer-Verlag.

Ornitz, E. M. (1978). Neurophysiological studies. In M. Rutter & E. Schopler (Eds.), *Autism: A reappraisal of concepts and treatment* (pp. 117–139). New York: Plenum.

Ornitz, E. M. (1985). Neurophysiology of infantile autism. *Journal of the American Academy of Child Psychiatry, 24,* 251–262.

Prior, M., Tress, B., Hoffman, W. L., & Boldt, D. (1984). Computed tomographic study of children with classic autism. *Journal of Autism and Developmental Disorders, 41,* 482–484.

Raaf, J., & Kernohan, J. W. (1944). A study of the external granular layer in the cerebellum. *American Journal of Anatomy, 75,* 151–172.

Rakic, P., Sidman, R. L. (1970). Histogenesis of cortical layers in human cerebellum, particularly the lamina dissecans. *Journal of Comparative Neurology, 139,* 473–500.

Reis, D. J., Doba, N., & Nathan, M. A. (1973). Predatory attack, grooming, and consummatory behaviors evoked by electrical stimulation of cat cerebellar nuclei. *Science, 182,* 845–847.

Rimland, B. (1964). *Infantile autism: The syndrome and its implications.* New York: Appleton-Century-Crofts.

Ritvo, E. R., Freeman, B. J., Mason-Brothers, A., Mo, A., & Ritvo, A. M. (1985). Concordance of the syndrome of autism in 40 pairs of afflicted twins. *American Journal of Psychiatry, 142,* 74–77.

Ritvo, E. R., Freeman, B. J., Scheibel, A. B., Duong, T., Robinson, H., Guthrie, D., & Ritvo, A. (1986). Lower Purkinje cell counts in the cerebella of four autistic subjects: Initial findings of the UCLA–NSAC autopsy research report. *American Journal of Psychiatry, 143,* 862–866.

Robain, O., Wen, G. Y., Wisniewski, H. M., Shek, J. W., & Loo, Y. H. (1981). Purkinje cell dendritic development in experimental phenylketonuria. *Acta Neuropathologica, 53,* 107–112.

Sarnat, H. B., & Alcala, H. (1980). Human cerebellar hypoplasia: A syndrome of diverse causes. *Archives of Neurology, 37,* 300–305.

Sidman, R. L., & Green, M. C. (1970). "Nervous," a new mutant mouse with cerebellar disease. In M. Sabourdy (Ed.), *Les mutants pathologiques chez l'animal: Leur intérêt pour la recherche biomedicale* (pp. 69–79). Paris: Editions du Centre National de La Recherche Scientifique.

Thompson, R. F. (1983). Neuronal substrates of simple associative learning: Classical conditioning. *Trends in Neurosciences, 6,* 270–275.

Thompson, R. F. (1986). The neurobiology of learning and memory. *Science, 233,* 941–947.

Verbitskaya, L. B. (1969). Some aspects of the ontophylogenesis of the cerebellum. In R. Llinas (Ed.), *Neurobiology of cerebellar evolution and development* (pp. 859–874). Chicago: American Medical Association.

Williams, R. S., Hauser, S. L., Purpura, D. P., DeLong, G. R., & Swisher, C. N. (1980). Autism and mental retardation: Neuropathologic studies performed in four retarded persons with autistic behavior. *Archives of Neurology, 37,* 749–753.

Young, J. G., Cohen, D. J., Shaywitz, S. E., Caparulo, B. K., Kavanaugh, M. E., Hunt, R. D., Leckman, J. F., Anderson, G. M., Detlor, J., Harcherik, D., & Shaywitz, B. A. (1982). Assessment of brain function in clinical pediatric research: Behavioral and biological strategies. *Schizophrenia Bulletin, 8,* 205–235.

CHAPTER 7

Reciprocal Subcortical–Cortical Influences in Autism

The Role of Attentional Mechanisms

GERALDINE DAWSON
ARTHUR LEWY
University of Washington

For the past three decades, the search for the locus of brain dysfunction in autism has been the focus of great attention and effort. It is now clear that the etiology of autism is varied and includes both genetic (Brown *et al.*, 1982; Folstein & Rutter, 1977; Golfine *et al.*, 1985; Ritvo, Freeman, Mason-Brothers, Mo, & Ritvo, 1985) and environmental (Chess, Fernandez, & Korn, 1978; Deykin & Mac-Mahon, 1980; Finegan & Quadrington, 1979) factors. However, the possibility that autistic individuals share certain common neuropathological features continues to motivate researchers.

The research findings to date implicate both subcortical and cortical dysfunction in autism. Evidence of subcortical dysfunction in autistic individuals consists of abnormalities in vestibular responses (Ornitz, Atwell, Kaplan, & Westlake, 1985; Ornitz, Brown, Mason, & Putnam, 1974) and autonomic abnormalities, including elevated heart rate, increased peripheral blood flow, increased heart rate variability (Cohen & Johnson, 1977; Hutt, Forrest, & Richer, 1975; Kootz & Cohen, 1981; Kootz, Marinelli, & Cohen, 1982), and a failure to exhibit normal orienting responses (James & Barry, 1980; Palkowitz & Wiesenfeld, 1980; Stevens & Gruzelier, 1984). Cortical dysfunction is suggested by studies of event-related potentials (ERPs) in autistic persons, in which a reduced P3 wave has been found (Courchesne, Kilman, Galambos, & Lincoln, 1984; Courchesne, Lincoln, Kilman, & Galambos, 1985; Dawson, Finley, Phillips, Galpert, & Lewy, in press; Novick, Vaughn, Kurtzberg, & Simson, 1980), and by studies of functional brain lateralization, in which an increased incidence of reversed or absent lateralization has been reported (Dawson, Finley, Phillips, & Galpert, 1986; Dawson, Warrenburg, & Fuller, 1982, 1983; Ogawa *et al.*, 1982; Prior & Bradshaw, 1979; Tanguay, 1976; Wetherby, Koegel, & Mendel, 1981). These findings suggest that autism is a disorder that encompasses both subcortical and cortical levels of brain processing.

In an attempt to begin integrating research findings of subcortical and cortical dysfunction in autism, this chapter explores the reciprocal influences of subcortical and cortical abnormalities and their contributions to the kinds of cognitive and affective impairments found in autism. Thus, rather than focusing on the possible effects of a specific area of brain dysfunction, we argue that autism may be better explained within a brain systems framework. Specifically, we argue that autism involves dysfunction of the cortical–limbic–reticular system that mediates attention. Before reaching this conclusion, however, it is helpful to review the research on cortical and subcortical dysfunction in autistic persons.

CORTICAL FUNCTIONING IN AUTISM: RESEARCH FINDINGS

Behavioral Profile

One of the most puzzling characteristics of autistic persons is the great variability in their abilities across functional domains. In the preschool years, autistic children exhibit severely impaired language and social skills, and a lack of imaginative play. These deficits often coexist with adequate object permanence and spatial relations skills (Dawson & Adams, 1984; Sigman & Ungerer, 1984). In later years, autistic persons show a highly variable pattern of abilities on standardized intelligence tests, which is typified by severely impaired language and abstract reasoning skills and adequate to superior visual–spatial abilities (Dawson, 1983; Lockyer & Rutter, 1970). This variability is illustrated in Figure 7-1, which displays the mean scaled scores for two language subtests (Vocabulary and Comprehension) and two

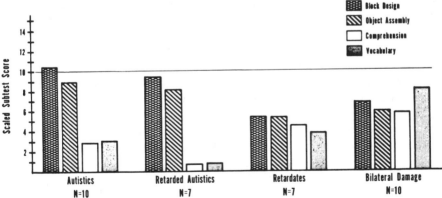

FIGURE 7-1. Mean subtest scores for selected spatial (Block Design and Object Assembly) and verbal (Comprehension and Vocabulary) subtests from the age-appropriate Wechsler intelligence scale for autistic, mentally retarded, and brain-damaged subjects. From "Lateralized Brain Dysfunction in Autism: Evidence from the Halstead–Reitan Neuropsychological Battery" by G. Dawson, 1983, *Journal of Autism and Developmental Disorders, 13,* 269–286. Copyright 1983 by Plenum Publishing Corporation. Reprinted by permission.

visual–spatial subtests (Block Design and Object Assembly) of the age-appropriate Wechsler intelligence scale for four groups of subjects: (1) autistic subjects of a wide range of intelligence ($n = 10$); (2) autistic subjects whose Full Scale IQ scores fell into the mentally retarded ($n = 7$); (3) IQ-matched mentally retarded subjects without autism ($n = 7$); and (4) age-matched nonautistic subjects with demonstrable diffuse or bilateral brain damage ($n = 10$).

This pattern of cognitive strengths and weaknesses led investigators to propose that autism primarily affects left-hemisphere functions, including language and other symbolic functions, while leaving right-hemisphere functions intact (Dawson, 1983; Dawson *et al.*, 1982, 1983; Prior & Bradshaw, 1979; Rutter, 1974; Tanguay, 1976). This position has been criticized, however, by Fein and her coworkers (Fein, Humes, Kaplan, Lucci, & Waterhouse, 1984), who pointed out that the autistic individual's difficulties with emotional comprehension and expression suggest right-hemisphere involvement as well. We return to this criticism later.

Tests of Asymmetrical Brain Activity

In this section, we review studies that have examined patterns of functional brain lateralization in autistic persons. We begin by briefly describing what is known about normal development of brain specialization.

A variety of data indicates that the two hemispheres are functionally and anatomically asymmetric at birth (Best, Hoffman, & Glanville, 1982; Crowell, Jones, Kapuniai, & Nakagawa, 1973; Entus, 1977; Glanville, Best, & Levinson, 1977; Molfese, Freeman, & Palermo, 1975; Molfese & Molfese, 1979). Current views on the development of brain lateralization hold that, although increasing specialization of the hemispheres occurs as an individual acquires functional capabilities, the propensity for certain functions to be lateralized to the right or left hemisphere is probably present at birth and does not change with age (see Witelson, 1977, for review). Thus, the failure of autistic children to exhibit normal patterns of functional brain lateralization (as reported below) cannot easily be attributed to a simple delay in the development of hemispheric specialization. Rather, autistic individuals appear to be exhibiting a deviant pattern of brain activity and development.

Two types of studies of hemispheric lateralization have been conducted with autistic individuals: dichotic listening and electrophysiological studies. Dichotic listening involves the simultaneous presentation of two different auditory stimuli (usually consonant–vowel combinations) to the right and left ears. Subjects are asked to report what they hear, and usually only report one of the stimuli. When the stimuli are of a linguistic nature, normal subjects typically show a left-hemisphere or right-ear advantage (REA) on such tests. Five studies have used dichotic listening to assess brain lateralization in autistic subjects (see Table 7-1). Of these, four studies reported that a higher than normal percentage of autistic subjects exhibited a left-ear (right-hemisphere) advantage or no ear preference. These findings are compromised by the small number of subjects used in one study (Wetherby *et al.*, 1981), and the failure of the mental-age-matched normal control group to show an REA in another study (Hoffman & Prior, 1982). Two studies (Prior & Bradshaw, 1979; Wetherby *et al.*, 1981) found that the degree or direction of lateralization was associated with level of language ability in autistic subjects. Normal patterns of lateralization were associated with improved language ability.

The two most common electrophysiological techniques used to study hemispheric lateralization are event-related potentials (ERPs) and the alpha-blocking method. ERPs (or averaged evoked potentials) require averaging of separate electrophysiological responses, which are time-locked to the onset of discrete stimuli, over many trials. When brain waves are averaged in this way, random electrical activity cancels out, and a characteristic wave form results. The amplitudes and latencies of the early components of this wave form tend to be asymmetric across the hemispheres. The second method, alpha blocking, involves the measurement of ongoing electroencephalographic (EEG) activity during the administration of various cognitive tasks. It makes use of the well-known alpha-blocking phenomenon (Butler & Glass, 1974; Doyle, Galin, & Ornstein, 1974), in which differential attenuation of EEG in the 8- to 12-Hz frequency band (alpha) is used to infer localized brain activity.

To date, five studies have used one of these EEG methods to measure right- and left-hemisphere brain activity during different information-processing tasks in autistic individuals. A sixth study (Small, 1975) only measured resting EEG, and therefore is difficult to interpret. These studies are summarized in Table 7-2.

Three of the electrophysiological studies measured ERPs to either simple, nonlinguistic (e.g., click, flash) or linguistic (e.g., "da") stimuli (Dawson *et al.*, 1986; Ogawa *et al.*, 1982; Tanguay, 1976). In each of these studies, a higher than normal percentage of autistic subjects showed either reversed (i.e., right-hemisphere-dominant) (Dawson *et al.*, 1986) or absent (Ogawa *et al.*, 1982; Tanguay, 1976) lateralization of brain activity when compared to normal control subjects. The Dawson *et al.* study differed in two important ways from those by Ogawa *et al.* and Tanguay: It utilized linguistic rather than nonlinguistic stimuli, and it required an active response from the subjects, thereby controlling for attention and motivation on the part of the subjects.

In the two studies that used the alpha-blocking method (Dawson *et al.*, 1982, 1983), a higher than normal percentage of subjects showed a reversed pattern of lateralization of brain activity during tasks involving language or other left-hemisphere-mediated functions (i.e., motor imitation). In contrast, in the one study in which right- and left-hemisphere EEG was measured during visual–spatial tasks (Dawson *et al.*, 1982), autistic subjects' pattern of hemispheric activity did not differ from that of age-matched normal controls.

Thus, the existing data suggest that autism is associated with atypical patterns of hemispheric activity—namely, right-dominant or symmetric hemispheric activity during language and other left-hemisphere-related tasks.

TABLE 7-1. Dichotic Listening Studies of Individuals with Autism

Reference	n	CA	Mean IQ	Diagnosis	Method	Results
Blackstock, 1978	11	$\overline{X} = 10.3$ yr	Not given	Autistic (Rutter's criteria)	Speakers placed to right and left of Ss. S had to put ear to speaker to hear stimuli. Stimuli: 3 musical passages, 3 verbal passages	Autistic Ss, as a group, listened to both musical and verbal passages with L ear. Normal Ss listened to musical passages with L ear, verbal passages with R ear.
	7	$\overline{X} = 5.4$ yr	Not given	Normal		
Prior & Bradshaw, 1979	19	8–13 yr	PPVT: 68 MA: 3–14 yr	Autistic (Prior's criteria)	Dichotic listening: Words	Normal: Significant group REA Autistic: 5 REA 7 LEA 7 no EA
	19	Primary-school age	PPVT MA: 8 yr	Normal		Lateralized autistic Ss more likely to have had speech before 5 years of age.
Wetherby, Koegel, & Mendel, 1981	6	8–24 yr	Not given	Autistic (NSAC criteria)	Dichotic listening: Words Two language tests (TACL and PPVT)	3 REA 2 LEA 1 no EA One S followed longitudinally; as language improved, LEA decreased.
Hoffman & Prior, 1982	10	$\overline{X} = 11$ yr (7–14 yr)	87 (76–109)	Autistic (Rutter's criteria)	Dichotic listening: Words	Both autistic and MA control group showed LEA. CA control group showed REA.
	10	Matched on CA	100 (85–112)	Normal		
	10	Matched on MA (8–10 yr)	107 (97–120)	Normal		

Arnold & Schwartz, 1983	8	6–14 yr	PPVT: 6 yr (3–12 yr)	Autistic (Rimland's Checklist)	Dichotic listening: CVs, presented dichotically with separation of 50 msec. Response: "Point to ear you heard the sound in first."	Autistic: 7 REA, 1 LEA Aphasic: 1 REA, 6 LEA Normal: 6 REA, 0 LEA
	8	7–11 yr	PPVT: 5 yr (3–7 yr)	Aphasic "varied in symptoms" MLU: $\bar{X} = 2.5$		
	8	6–13 yr	Not given	Normal		

Note. From "Cerebral Lateralization in Autism: Its Role in Language and Affective Disorders" by G. Dawson, 1988, in D. L. Molfese and S. J. Segalowitz (Eds.), *Brain Lateralization in Children: Developmental Implications* (pp. 437–461). New York: Guilford Press. Copyright 1988 by The Guilford Press. Reprinted by permission. CA, chronological age; CVs, consonant–vowel combinations; LEA, left-ear advantage; MA, mental age; MLU, mean length of utterance; NSAC, National Society for Autistic Children; PPVT, Peabody Picture Vocabulary Test; REA, right-ear advantage; TACL, Carrow Test for Auditory Comprehension of Language.

There is also evidence that the pattern of hemispheric activity is not only deviant in direction, but also in magnitude. In our study of right- and left-hemisphere speech-related brain potentials (Dawson *et al.*, 1986), we found that autistic subjects with right-hemisphere-dominant patterns showed a greater degree of asymmetry than did either normal subjects or autistic subjects with left-hemisphere dominance. Normal subjects with reversed direction showed the least degree of asymmetry, whereas the opposite was true for autistic subjects.

Relationship between Hemispheric Asymmetries and Language Ability

Studies of hemispheric lateralization in autistic individuals report substantially greater intersubject variability than is typically found in normal populations. Autistic subjects may exhibit reversed, absent, or normal asymmetries. The relationship between pattern of lateralization and language ability has been addressed in three studies. Prior and Bradshaw (1979) reported that autistic children who had developed language before the age of 5 were more likely to exhibit the normal REA during a dichotic listening task. Wetherby *et al.* (1981) found that increases in REA accompanied an improvement in language ability in one autistic subject

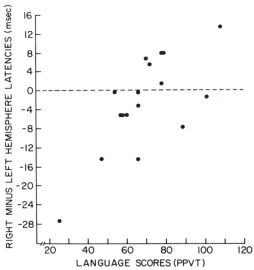

FIGURE 7-2.   Scatterplot displaying the relationship between patterns of hemispheric asymmetry, as measured by right minus left N1 latency of the speech-related brain potential, and language, as measured by the Peabody Picture Vocabulary Test, for 17 autistic subjects. From "Hemispheric Specialization and the Language Abilities of Autistic Children" by G. Dawson, C. Finley, S. Phillips, and L. Galpert, 1986, *Child Development*, 57, 1440–1453. Copyright 1986 by the Society for Research in Child Development, Inc. Reprinted by permission.

TABLE 7-2. Electrophysiological Studies of Lateralization in Individuals with Autism

Reference	n	CA	Mean IQ	Diagnosis	Method	Results
Small, 1975	7	Not given	Not given	Autistic (criteria not reported)	Resting EEG recorded from right and left occipital regions	Normal Ss showed higher mean integrated voltage values from LH than from RH. Autistic Ss showed no hemispheric asymmetry.
Tanguay, 1976	10	2–5 yr	Not given	Autistic (DSM-III criteria)	Auditory evoked potentials taken during sleep	Normal Ss showed larger RH than LH potentials during REM. Autistic Ss showed no significant hemispheric differences.
	10	4–5 yr	Not given	Normal		
Ogawa, Sugiyama, Ishiwa, Suzuki, Ishihara, & Sato, 1982	21	2–8 yr	Not given	Autistic (Kanner's criteria), R-handed	EEG activity recorded during click and flash stimulation	During click stimulation, 42% of normal Ss showed significant hemispheric asymmetry; no autistic Ss did so. During flash stimulation, 64% of normal Ss showed hemispheric asymmetry; 28% of autistic Ss did so.
	28	2–8 yr	Not given	Normal R-handed		
Dawson, Warrenburg, & Fuller, 1982	10	9–34 yr	FSIQ: 69 (40–113)	Autistic (Rutter's criteria)	RH and LH parietal alpha taken during 4 cognitive tasks: 2 verbal, 2 spatial	Autistic and normal Ss did not differ during spatial tasks; autistic Ss showed greater RH activation during verbal tasks than normal Ss. 7/10 autistic Ss showed RH dominance during verbal tasks. For autistic Ss only, greater asymmetry related to increases in IQ and age.
	10	9–34 yr	Not given	Normal matched on gender, CA, handedness		
Dawson, Warrenburg, & Fuller, 1983	10	9–34 yr	FSIQ: 69 (40–113)	Autistic (Rutter's criteria)	RH and LH parietal alpha taken during 4 motor imitation tasks: 2 manual, 2 oral	Autistic Ss showed greater RH activity than normal Ss, particularly during oral imitation. Older autistic Ss more likely to exhibit normal patterns of asymmetry.
	10	9–34 yr	Not given	Normal matched on gender, CA, handedness		
Dawson, Finley, Phillips, & Galpert, 1986	17	6–18 yr	71 (53–91)	Autistic (CARS score, DSM-III criteria)	RH and LH cortical auditory evoked potentials to linguistic stimulus; battery of language tests	11/17 autistic Ss showed RH dominance for speech. RH dominance associated with poorer language abilities and greater degree of asymmetry. Older Ss more likely to show normal direction of asymmetry.
	17	6–18 yr	PPVT: 125	Normal, matched on gender and CA		

Note. From "Cerebral Lateralization in Autism: Its Role in Language and Affective Disorders" by G. Dawson, 1988, in D. L. Molfese and S. J. Segalowitz (Eds.), *Brain Lateralization in Children: Developmental Implications* (pp. 437–461), New York: Guilford Press. Copyright 1988 by The Guilford Press. Reprinted by permission. CA, chronological age; CARS, Child Autism Rating Scale; FSIQ, Full Scale IQ, age-appropriate Wechsler intelligence scale; LH, left hemisphere; PPVT, Peabody Picture Vocabulary Test; REM, rapid eye movement; RH, right hemisphere.

who was followed longitudinally. We (Dawson, 1988; Dawson *et al.*, 1986) examined the relationship between autistic children's patterns of hemispheric asymmetries in speech-related brain potentials and language ability. Language ability
was measured by standardized tests of articulation, semantics, and vocabulary.
Levels of language ability were found to be strongly correlated with pattern of
hemispheric asymmetry. Specifically, poorer language ability was associated with
a reversed (right-hemisphere-dominant) pattern of asymmetry. This relationship is
illustrated in Figure 7-2, a scatterplot displaying individual autistic subjects' scores
on the Peabody Picture Vocabulary Test and patterns of hemispheric asymmetry,
as measured by right- minus left-hemisphere speech-related brain potentials (latency of the N1 component). Such a relationship was not found for normal subjects. Interestingly, when separate measures of right- and left-hemisphere activity
(N1 amplitudes and N1 latencies of speech-related potentials) were correlated with
language ability, significant and consistent relationships were found between *right-
hemisphere* activity and language, but not between left-hemisphere activity and
language (see Table 7-3). That is, greater right-hemisphere activity was predictive
of poorer language ability. Again, no such relationship was found for normal
subjects.

Furthermore, between-group comparisons of right- and left-hemisphere activity tended to yield *right-*, rather than left-, hemisphere differences; for the right
hemisphere only, autistic subjects tended to show shorter latencies in their re-

TABLE 7-3. Correlations between N1 Amplitude of the Averaged
Evoked Response to the Linguistic Stimulus and Language Abilities
for Each Hemisphere

	Hemisphere	
Language ability	Right	Left
Arizona Articulation Test	.43*	.01
Peabody Picture Vocabulary Test	.61†	.16
Northwestern Syntax Screening Test		
Receptive	.46**	.19
Expressive	.43*	.06
Wechsler subtests		
Vocabulary	.60†	.08
Comprehension	.61†	.21
Mean length of utterance	.52***	.00
Length complexity index	.55***	.12

Note. From "Cerebral Lateralization in Autism: Its Role in Language and
Affective Disorders" by G. Dawson, 1988, in D. L. Molfese and S. J. Segalowitz (Eds.), *Brain Lateralization in Children: Developmental Implications* (pp.
437–461), New York: Guilford Press. Copyright 1988 by The Guilford Press.
Reprinted by permission.
*$p = .08$; **$p = .05$; ***$p = .03$; †$p = .01$.

sponses to the speech stimuli than normal subjects. These data are illustrated in Figure 7-3, which displays the right- and left-hemisphere N1 latencies of the speech-related brain potentials of normal and autistic subjects. Thus, from this study, we found some evidence that *right-hemisphere overactivation* may be related to the language-processing impairments of autistic persons. We explore this idea in greater detail later in the chapter.

We were also interested in whether similar relationships between pattern of hemispheric asymmetries and language ability exist for other developmentally disabled populations, or whether they are specific to autism. To date, we have comparison data only for children with developmental language disorder (dysphasia) (Dawson, Finley, Phillips, & Lewy, in press). Ten dysphasic children, ranging from 6 to 15 years of age, were tested using the same ERP method as was used with autistic and normal subjects in our previous study (Dawson *et al.*, 1986). Their data were compared with data from 10 autistic and 10 normal children who were chosen from larger samples of subjects who had participated in the study reported above (Dawson *et al.*, 1986). Autistic and normal subject were selected to match dysphasic subjects as closely as possible on age and language ability; autistic and dysphasic subjects did not significantly differ on these two characteristics.

Similar to autistic subjects, a high percentage of dysphasic subjects (8 out of 10) showed a reversed (right-dominant) pattern of hemispheric asymmetry in their evoked responses to speech stimuli. Evoked responses from representative autistic, dysphasic, and normal subjects are shown in Figure 7-4. However, in contrast to autistic subjects, dysphasic subjects' pattern of hemispheric asymmetry, as measured by right- minus left-hemisphere differences scores for N1 amplitude and latency, was not related to language ability. These correlations are shown in Table 7-4. These results suggest that although autistic and dysphasic individuals exhibit similar patterns of hemispheric asymmetry for speech, these patterns do not bear the same relationship with language ability for the two groups. For autistic subjects, improved language ability was found to be associated with normal patterns

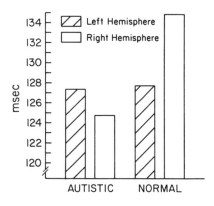

FIGURE 7-3. Mean right- and left-hemisphere N1 latency of the speech-related brain potential for autistic and normal age-matched subjects ($n = 17$ subjects, each group). From "Hemispheric Specialization and the Language Abilities of Autistic Children" by G. Dawson, C. Finley, S. Phillips, and L. Galpert, 1986, *Child Development, 57,* 1440–1453. Copyright 1986 by the Society for Research in Child Development, Inc. Reprinted by permission.

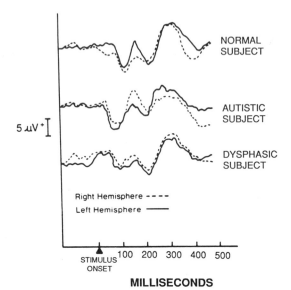

FIGURE 7-4.   Right- and left-hemisphere averaged speech-related brain potentials for representative autistic, dysphasic, and normal subjects. From "A Comparison of Patterns of Lateralization in the Speech-Related Brain Potentials of Autistic and Dysphasic Children" by G. Dawson, C. Finley, S. Phillips, and A. Lewy, in press, *Brain and Language.* Copyright by Academic Press, Inc. Reprinted by permission.

of hemispheric activity during speech processing, whereas for dysphasic subjects, the reversed (right-hemisphere) patterns of hemispheric activity persisted regardless of level of language ability. One possible interpretation of these findings is that reversed hemispheric asymmetries in dysphasia reflect inherent, and thus stable, dysfunction of the language areas of the left hemisphere, whereas in autism, reversed asymmetries may reflect a more transient abnormal functioning that changes as the child develops greater language capabilities.

Reversed Hemispheric Asymmetries: Current Hypotheses

Several hypotheses have been put forth to explain the high incidence of abnormal brain lateralization in autism. In this section, we review three of these hypotheses.

  Hypothesis 1: Abnormal Cortical Neural Organization. In earlier writings (Dawson, 1983; Dawson *et al.,* 1982), we proposed that atypical patterns of cerebral lateralization in autism may reflect inherent differences in underlying brain organization. These differences were presumed to be caused by early left-hemisphere insult, genetic influences, or other prenatal influences on cortical development. Geschwind and Galaburda (1985a, 1985b, 1985c) proposed a more elaborate version of this hypothesis. They argued that a number of developmental

TABLE 7-4. Correlations between Language Ability and Pattern of Speech Lateralization for Autistic and Dysphasic Subjects

	Language measures					
	Vocabulary	Comprehension	Articulation	NSST-R	NSST-E	PPVT
Autistic						
N1 amplitude	−.73§	−.63††	−.70†††	−.48***	−.61††	−.60††
N1 latency	.53†	.50***	.33*	.56††	.59††	.72†††
Dysphasic						
N1 amplitude	.09	.06	.36**	−.06	.04	.24
N1 latency	.20	−.04	−.03	−.47***	−.15	−.22

Note. NSST-R and -E, Northwestern Syntax Screening Test—Receptive and Expressive; PPVT, Peabody Picture Vocabulary Test. From "A Comparison of Patterns of Lateralization in the Speech-Related Brain Potentials of Autistic and Dysphasic Children" by G. Dawson, C. Finley, S. Phillips, L. Galpert, and A. Lewy, in press, *Brain and Language.* Copyright by Academic Press, Inc. Reprinted by permission.
*p = .09; **p = .08; ***p = .04; †p = .03; ††p = .02; †††p = .005; §p = .004.

disabilities, including dyslexia, dysphasia, and autism, are related to abnormal cerebral dominance for language, which is caused by intrauterine hormonal influences. These hormonal influences are believed to permanently alter the neural organization of the brain in such a way that the left hemisphere is not specialized for language processing. From evidence that the right hemisphere develops more rapidly than the left (Taylor, 1969), these authors argued that harmful hormonal influences that occur during fetal and early postnatal life are more likely to affect the development of the left hemisphere, which is at risk over a longer period of time. Furthermore, they suggest that any abnormal delay in left-hemisphere development would result in more successful competition by right-hemisphere neurons for available synapses, and thus lead to diminished rates of neuronal death in the right hemisphere. This hypothesis was given as an explanation for the enhanced right-hemisphere skills found in some language-impaired individuals.

Hypothesis 2: Abnormal Hemispheric Activation. Data from our more recent studies (Dawson *et al.*, 1986; Dawson, Finley, Phillips, Galpert, & Lewy, in press), which are inconsistent with Hypothesis 1, have led us to propose a different explanation to account for reversed asymmetries. First, the fact that not all autistic individuals exhibit abnormal patterns of lateralization suggests that this is not a universal causal mechanism in autism, as Geschwind and Galaburda proposed. Second, our finding that patterns of speech lateralization were strongly related to levels of language acquisition raises the possibility that patterns of hemispheric asymmetry for speech processing may actually shift toward normal left-hemisphere dominance as the autistic individual acquires language abilities. Such a shift in pattern of hemispheric dominance would not be expected if permanent abnormalities in underlying brain organization existed. Thus, in more recent writings (Dawson, 1987, 1988; Dawson *et al.*, 1986), we have proposed that reversed asymmetries may reflect abnormal activation of the hemispheres. Here we are making a distinction between the terms "specialization" and "activation." Kinsbourne (1987) and others (Levy, Heller, Banich, & Burton, 1983) have suggested that the term "hemispheric specialization" specifically be used to refer to the underlying structural organization of the hemispheres. On the other hand, "hemispheric activation" is used to refer to individual differences in temporary and task-related, as well as characteristic, patterns of asymmetric hemispheric arousal. These patterns of hemispheric arousal interact with the underlying cortical organization to produce lateralized responses during perceptual and cognitive tasks. In this chapter, we have adopted this distinction and terminology, and agree with Kinsbourne (1987) that autism may be related to abnormal activation of the hemispheres. Furthermore, we suggest that the autistic individual's patterns of hemispheric activation may change with development. A longitudinal study including measures of both speech lateralization and language ability would be necessary to test this developmental hypothesis.

   Hypothesis 3: Subgroups. Variations in patterns of speech lateralization may reflect distinct subgroups of autistic individuals that differ in degree of specific left-hemisphere pathology (Soper & Satz, 1984). This explanation is consistent with our finding that more severely language-impaired autistic children are more likely to exhibit reversed speech lateralization. As mentioned above, only a longitudinal study of brain activity and language development in autistic individuals will allow us to determine whether a developmental (Hypothesis 2) or subgroup (Hypothesis 3) explanation can better account for the variability in patterns of brain lateralization found in autistic persons. The subgroup hypothesis would predict greater intrasubject stability over time.

Reduced P3 Component of the Event-Related Potential

One of the most consistent findings in autism research is a reduction in the long-latency, P3 component of the ERP (Courchesne *et al.*, 1984, 1985; Dawson, Finley, Phillips, Galpert, & Lewy, in press; Novick, Kurtzberg, & Vaughn, 1979; Novick *et al.*, 1980). This ERP component is associated with the detection of novel, unpredictable stimuli (Hillyard & Picton, 1979; Pritchard, 1981; Tueting, 1978). The reduction in P3 found in autistic persons is illustrated in Figure 7-5, which displays ERPs elicited by the target stimulus "da," and recorded from central cortex (Cz) of 17 autistic and 17 normal individuals. The target stimulus was intermixed with nontargets and with background clicks. In addition to the dramatically reduced P3 component in these data, there appeared to be a general reduction of amplitude in the other long-latency components as well (N1, P2); however, only the difference in P3 reached statistical significance.

   The question of whether the reduced P3 of autistic individuals is specific to particular types of stimuli has not been fully explored. Most studies of autistic persons have been concerned with auditory processing (Courchesne *et al.*, 1984, 1985; Dawson, Finley, Phillips, Galpert, & Lewy, in press; Novick *et al.*, 1979, 1980). These studies have consistently found reductions in P3 to auditory stimuli,

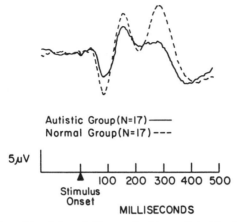

Autistic Group(N=17) ──────
Normal Group(N=17) ─ ─ ─

5μV

100 200 300 400 500
Stimulus
Onset

MILLISECONDS

FIGURE 7-5. ERPs from 17 autistic and 17 normal subjects, elicited by the target stimulus "da" and recorded from central cortex (Cz). The target stimulus was intermixed with nontargets, and background clicks. Note the dramatically reduced P3 component. Adapted from "Reduced P3 Amplitude of the Event-Related Brain Potential: Its Relationship to Language Ability in Autism" by G. Dawson, C. Finley, S. Phillips, L. Galpert, and A. Lewy, in press, *Journal of Autism and Developmental Disorders*. Copyright by Plenum Publishing Corporation. Adapted by permission.

including both simple, nonlinguistic stimuli (e.g., tones) and complex, linguistic stimuli (e.g., words). In two studies of the P3 response to visual stimuli, inconsistent results have been reported. Novick *et al.* (1979) found that both visual and auditory responses were abnormal in autistic adolescents. Courchesne *et al.* (1985), on the other hand, found that novel visual stimuli were associated with abnormalities in an earlier component of the ERP, but not with a reduced P3 component. Courchesne *et al.*, however, studied a very selective group of older autistic subjects who were not mentally retarded; it is uncertain whether their results would generalize to more impaired autistic persons.

An interesting question is whether the reduced P3 component found in autistic persons indicates that they are failing to differentiate novel from familiar stimuli. To address this question, Courchesne (1987) presented normal and autistic, nonretarded subjects with a repetitive series of background stimuli that also included an occasional, unpredictable, and novel stimulus. Auditory and visual novel stimuli were presented in separate conditions. ERPs were recorded to both background and novel stimuli from Cz (auditory) and the frontocentral cortex (visual). Courchesne found that the autistic group's P3 response to auditory novel stimuli was reduced, compared to the normal group's response. As indicated above, visual novel stimuli were associated with abnormalities in an earlier component of the ERP, but not with a reduced P3 component. Two additional important findings emerged. First, the autistic subjects' P3 responses to auditory and visual novel stimuli were significantly larger than to background stimuli, indicating that the autistic subjects were, in fact, capable of detecting and responding to novelty.

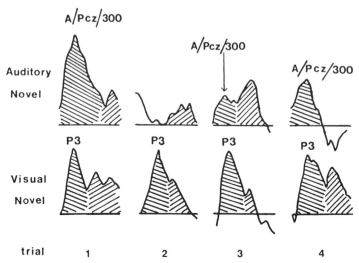

FIGURE 7-6. Single-trial evoked responses from a 15-year-old autistic male elicited by the first four auditory and visual novel stimuli, showing A/Pcz/300 and frontocentral P3 components (A, auditory modality; P, positive in polarity; cz, central cortex; 300, mean latency of 300 msec). Note large initial response to auditory novel stimulus, but extreme variability to subsequent auditory novel stimuli. In contrast, large and consistent responses to visual novel stimuli are shown. From "A Neurophysiological View of Autism" by E. Courchesne, 1987, in E. Schopler and G. Mesibov (Eds.), *Neurobiological Issues in Autism* (pp. 285–324), New York: Plenum. Copyright 1987 by Plenum Publishing Corporation. Reprinted by permission.

Second, when Courchesne examined ERP trials to auditory novel stimuli, he found that the autistic subjects usually had a normal, or even large, P3 response amplitude to the very first novel stimulus (see Figure 7-6). However, after this first trial, each of the following responses to novel stimuli was usually very much smaller. Courchesne (1987) suggests that these data indicate that the neural generators involved in detecting novelty have the capacity for normal functioning, and occasionally do respond normally. Moreover, the author suggests that *"this evidence raises the possibility that the operation of this apparently otherwise normal neural system is usually abnormally interfered with or hindered by some other system"* (p. 302, italics in original). This possibility is explored in some detail below.

SUBCORTICAL FUNCTIONING IN AUTISM: RESEARCH FINDINGS

Brain Stem Auditory Evoked Responses

Several studies of brain stem evoked responses have been conducted with autistic individuals of a wide range of functioning (Gillberg, Rosenhall, & Johansson,

1983; Novick *et al.*, 1980; Rumsey, Grimes, Pikus, Duara, & Ismond, 1984; Skoff, Mirsky, & Turner, 1980; Tanguay, Edwards, Buchwald, Schwafel, & Allen, 1982; Taylor, Rosenblatt, & Linschoten, 1982; Courchesne, Yeung-Courchesne, Hicks, & Lincoln, 1985). These studies have not consistently demonstrated brain stem dysfunction; rather, prolonged brain stem transmission times are found only in a subgroup of autistic children. Ornitz (1985) has pointed out that the brain stem auditory evoked responses reflect the integrity of a very select subset of neurons within the brain stem. He has further argued that although brain stem dysfunction is a basic feature of autism (see Ornitz, Chapter 8, this volume), it need not involve this specific group of neurons.

Vestibular and Autonomic Studies

Ornitz and his coworkers have carried out several studies demonstrating vestibular abnormalities in autistic children (see Ornitz, 1985, for review). These abnormalities include various abnormal visual–vestibular responses (Ornitz *et al.*, 1974), such as reduced secondary nystagmus (Ornitz *et al.*, 1985).

Subcortical dysfunction is also suggested by studies of autonomic responsivity in autistic individuals. Before we describe these studies, however, we provide some background on how autonomic responsivity is measured.

Brain stem mechanisms are involved in both phasic (short-latency responses to novel stimuli) and tonic (sustained) autonomic regulation. Autonomic responses are known to be sensitive correlates of attention (Graham & Clifton, 1966; Porges, 1980, 1984). An orienting response, which typically is elicited by novel, unpredictable stimuli, is accompanied by several physiological changes. These include an initial slowing of heart rate, suppression of respiratory frequency, decreased peripheral blood flow, increased electrodermal activity, and EEG desynchronization. The orienting response is associated with enhanced stimulus intake (Lacey, 1967) and facilitates stimulus recognition and recall (Clarkson & Berg, 1983). If the stimulus is presented repeatedly, these physiological indices will return to prestimulus baseline (i.e., habituation occurs). In contrast, aversion to stimuli, such as occurs if the stimulus is intense or noxious, is accompanied by an initial heart rate *increase* that fails to habituate or habituates slowly when the stimulus is repeated. The aversive (or defensive) response is associated with stimulus rejection and limits the influences of the external stimulation on the organism (Lacey, 1967).

Several studies of cardiovascular responses to the presentation of novel stimuli suggest that autistic individuals have an abnormal orienting response. Findings include accelerations in heart rate, reductions in rate of habituation (Palkowitz & Wiesenfeld, 1980), a failure to habituate (James & Barry, 1980), and a failure to reinstate to novelty when habituation occurs (Bernal & Miller, 1971). James and Barry (1980) also report a failure to habituate for respiratory responses to novel stimuli. Studies of electrodermal responses to novel, repetitive stimuli have

yielded less consistent findings with regard to specific type of abnormality. However, most authors have reported some abnormality, including reduced response
to the first trials (Bernal and Miller, 1971; van Engeland, 1984); reduced or absent habituation (Stevens & Gruzelier, 1984); and higher mean levels of skin
conductance, which were accompanied by greater intraindividual variability
(Palkowitz & Wiesenfeld, 1980). Based on the available research, it is quite
likely that autistic children often fail to show the adaptive orienting response
to novel stimuli that is associated with sensory intake and processing. The
evidence thus far suggests that novel stimuli may elicit an aversive response
(characterized by slow or absent habituation), which is associated with sensory
rejection.

Several investigators (e.g., Charlop, 1986; Ferrara & Hill, 1980; Lord & Magill, Chapter 14, this volume; Runco, Charlop, & Schreibman, 1986; Schopler,
Brehm, Kinsbourne, & Reichler, 1971) have examined autistic children's behavioral responses to novelty and unpredictability in their environments. These studies have examined the effects of familiarity of therapist, peers, and room, and
predictability of task stimuli. The studies found that novelty and unpredictability
are associated with an increase in autistic behaviors, including social withdrawal,
decreased eye contact, echolalic speech, and stereotypies.

Studies of tonic autonomic indices have revealed elevated heart rates, increased peripheral blood flow, and greater heart rate variability in autistic as
compared to normal children (Cohen & Johnson, 1977; Hutt *et al.*, 1975;
Kootz & Cohen, 1981; Kootz *et al.*, 1982). Kootz *et al.* (1982) found that
lower-functioning autistic children were more likely than higher-functioning
autistic children to exhibit increased heart rates in response to changes in their
environment. Although some studies report negative findings, lower than
normal values on measures of tonic autonomic arousal have not been reported.
Although the research is by no means conclusive, the data thus far, taken
together, suggest that many autistic individuals have chronically high levels of
arousal.

Some authors have argued that, in normal populations, high levels of arousal
may be associated with specific information-processing impairments. Easterbrook
(1959) argued that overarousal leads to a restriction of cue utilization—an idea
that is consistent with studies of overselectivity in autism (Lovaas, Schreibman,
Koegel, & Rehm, 1971). Recent experimental studies with normal infants, children, and adults have demonstrated that stimulus recognition and recall are correlated with physiological indices (such as heart rate) that reflect optimal states of
arousal (e.g., Clarkson & Berg, 1983; Coles, 1974; Linnemeyer & Porges, 1986).
Thus, if autistic children are, in fact, in a chronic state of high arousal, this may
be associated with specific information-processing deficits. This possibility needs
to be explored more fully in future research.

SUMMARY OF EVIDENCE ON BRAIN FUNCTIONING
IN AUTISM

To review, the available evidence supports several important characteristics of brain functioning in autism:

1. Impairments in social, emotional, and language functioning are, by definition, universally found in autism; however, visual–spatial functions are not necessarily deficient.

2. Autistic individuals often exhibit right-hemisphere-dominant patterns of brain activation, suggestive of hemispheric imbalance (relative right-hemisphere overactivation).

3. Autistic individuals' cortical event-related responses to unpredictable, novel stimuli suggest that novelty is detected but that further processing of novel information is deficient, as reflected in a reduced P3 component of the ERP.

4. The orienting response that usually occurs upon detection of novelty appears to be abnormal in autistic individuals; physiological responses to novel stimuli are more consistent with an aversive response. Since aversive responses in normal individuals occur when stimuli are perceived as intense, noxious, or painful; the occurrence of these responses to novel stimuli of moderate intensity in autistic persons suggests that these stimuli may be overstimulating for them (i.e., they are experienced as intense or noxious). The behavioral responses of autistic individuals to novel situations (increased withdrawal, anxiety, and perseverative behavior) also suggest that these situations may be aversive to them.

5. There is some evidence of chronic levels of overarousal in autism (e.g., chronically elevated heart rates).

RECIPROCAL SUBCORTICAL–CORTICAL INFLUENCES
IN AUTISM

In this section, we propose a framework for integrating cortical and subcortical findings in autism. This framework posits that autism involves those brain systems that mediate attention to novel and unpredictable stimuli. We begin by providing a brief description of the neural systems that mediate attention in normal individuals. This is followed by a discussion of how abnormalities of these neural systems may account for both cortical and subcortical findings in autistic individuals.

Neural Model of Attention

The act of attending to novel, unpredictable stimuli is based on a complex interaction of cortical and subcortical systems (Thatcher & John, 1977). According to

Sokolov's (1963, 1975) model, analysis of the stimulus properties is mediated by the primary sensory cortex and hippocampus. Furthermore, the novelty detectors of the hippocampus, excited by the novel stimulus, influence the activity of the reticular system, which in turn enhances the activity of the cortex. This enhancement includes EEG desynchronization and is part of several physiological changes (including autonomic changes) that comprise the orienting response.

It has been suggested (Sokolov, 1975) that, during relaxed states, the neurons of the hippocampus maintain the activity of a tonic synchronizing system of the thalamus. When a novel stimulus is presented, there is a decrease in the spontaneous activity of these neurons. This decrease disrupts the thalamic synchronizing system and its influence on the cortical EEG. The novel stimulus enhances the functional state of the cerebral cortex by both increasing the activity of the reticular activating systems and disrupting the synchronizing mechanisms of the thalamus so that desynchronization of neural generators occurs. Enhanced attention is associated with desynchronization of the EEG, since, presumably, desynchronization allows for more generators to be available to respond to the stimulus. When neural activity is highly synchronized (such as during deep sleep), minimal information processing occurs, since a large number of neurons are doing the same thing (Spinelli & Pribram, 1966). In contrast, an aroused neural state is characterized by relatively independent but cooperative neural groupings, which are available to process different aspects of information.

Thus, attention to a novel stimulus involves changes in neural coherence. There is a tonic desynchronization of neural generators, as evidenced by EEG desynchronization, as well as increased phasic coherence, as evidenced by increased amplitude of the evoked response during attending states. Thatcher and John (1977) have pointed out that the increased amplitude of the evoked response during attention may be related to two factors. First, there is the tendency for more generators to be available to respond to the stimulus, due to desynchronization. Second, during attention, there is a reduction in the variance of the latency of the evoked response, which results in higher-amplitude averaged responses. This is believed to be due to an increased tendency of aroused (and thus desynchronized) neural generators to become synchronized in response to external stimuli.

With development, social and language representational systems exert increasing influence on attentional control. These representational systems allow the young child to go beyond a basic reflex-type attentional response to novelty, described above, to acquire voluntary attentional control. Stored representations interact with stimulus properties to influence stimulus value for the child. These higher-order cortical processes influence the direction of voluntary attention (Thatcher, 1976).

Dysfunction of the Cortical–Limbic–Reticular System in Autism

Reduced P3 Response and Habituation

To turn now to what is known about autistic individuals, it seems quite possible that autism involves dysfunction of the cortical–limbic–reticular system or loop (Heilman & Van Den Abell, 1980), which is the basis for attention. As reviewed above, the behavioral and physiological evidence suggests that autism is associated with aversive responses to novelty and with chronic high levels of autonomic arousal (e.g., high heart rates). Aversive responses to novelty could be related to overresponsivity to novel stimuli at the cortical level and/or subsequent overactivation of the subcortical mechanisms responsible for regulating cortical activation (Kinsbourne, 1987). If novelty detectors of the cortex are oversensitive to changes in the environment, this may result in an aversive response and a failure to attend to that stimulus. In this regard, Courchesne's (1987) study of autistic adolescents provides an important clue. He found normal or large-amplitude P3 responses to first presentation of a novel stimulus and subsequent attenuation of the P3 response. This finding suggests that the cortical detectors of stimulus properties and novelty are functional on the first presentation of a novel stimulus. If so, subsequent distortion of cortical processing may be caused by overactivation of the reticular and thalamic arousal-regulating mechanisms. Such overactivation would preclude the two facilitatory actions of the reticular formation and the thalamus. Recall that the reticular formation and thalamus influence cortical arousal, resulting in desynchronization of cortical neurons. Theoretically, desynchronization facilitates phasic neural synchronization, which is reflected in enhanced averaged evoked responses. Thus, without the facilitatory actions of the reticular and thalamic regulating mechanisms, succeeding ERPs would be diminished. This would be consistent with findings from several studies (cited above) in which a reduced P3 component of the *averaged* ERP has been found in autistic subjects.

Similarly, the slow or absent habituation of autonomic responses to repetitive stimuli may be explained by dysfunction at different levels in the cortical–limbic–reticular loop. Habituation depends on the activity of inhibitory neurons of the hippocampus, which increases with repeated presentations of a stimulus. These inhibitory neurons activate the synchronizing thalamic system and suppress reticular system activity (Sokolov, 1975). Overactivation of the excitatory neurons of the hippocampus, or the failure of the reticular formation and/or thalamic synchronizing system to be adequately responsive to the inhibitory influences of the hippocampus, would result in absent or diminished habituation. As has been described earlier in this chapter, several studies of the orienting response in autistic individuals have found absent or reduced habituation of autonomic responses, to novel stimuli.

Right-Hemisphere Overactivation

Admittedly, the evidence for right-hemisphere overactivation in autism rests on only three studies (Dawson *et al.*, 1982, 1983, 1986), and must be considered tentative. However, with this caution in mind, in this section we consider how dysfunction of the cortical–limbic–reticular attentional mechanisms may be related to abnormal patterns of hemspheric activation—in particular, right-hemiophere overactivation.

As described above, Sokolov's (1963, 1975) attention–arousal model involves both cortical analysis of the stimulus for specific properties, novelty, and significance, and reticular–thalamic mediation of cortical arousal. Based on research findings from both brain-damaged and normal persons, Heilman and Van Den Abell (1979, 1980) and others (Kinsbourne & Bemporad, 1984) have proposed that each hemisphere has its own cortical–limbic–reticular loop, with the right hemisphere exhibiting dominance for novelty detection, involuntary and voluntary attention, and arousal. Specifically, there is evidence that the temporoparietal area has a large number of "fixation" cells that activate mechanisms to direct attention (Bushnell, Goldberg, & Robinson, 1981; Goldberg & Robinson, 1977). The temporoparietal area receives polymodal sensory, limbic, and frontal input related to stimulus properties and significance. Temporoparietal damage results in the failure to report, respond to, or orient toward novel or meaningful stimuli (Heilman, Bowers, Valenstein, and Watson, 1986). However, this neglect is more frequent and more severe after right- than after left-hemisphere lesions (Brain, 1941; Critchley, 1966).

Hcilman and his coworkers have carried out several studies of both normal and brain-damaged individuals that provide supportive evidence for differential hemispheric involvement in attention. In studies of normal adults, Heilman and Van Den Abell (1979, 1980) presented lateralized visual stimuli and recorded right- and left-hemisphere EEG, as well as reaction times. Although the left parietal lobe desynchronized most after right-sided stimuli, the right parietal lobe desynchronized equally after right- or left-sided stimuli. Furthermore, visual stimuli projected to the right hemisphere resulted in faster reaction times than did visual stimuli projected to the left hemisphere. The fact that the subjects were using their right (left-hemisphere-mediated) hands to respond to the stimuli makes this finding even more striking.

Right-hemisphere mechanisms may also mediate general level of arousal. Heilman, Schwartz, and Watson (1978) demonstrated that patients with right-hemisphere disease had dramatically smaller arousal responses, as measured by galvanic skin response, than aphasic (left-hemisphere) patients or control patients without disease. Heilman *et al.* suggest that this may account, in part, for the typical affective indifference exhibited by right-hemisphere-damaged patients.

In autism, findings of enhanced right-hemisphere activity may reflect overactivation of the right-hemisphere-mediated cortical–limbic–reticular system, which is involved in novelty detection, involuntary and voluntary attention, and arousal.

Theoretically, such right-hemisphere overactivation may lead to increased sensitivity to novelty and arousal; this increased sensitivity would account for the autistic child's tendency to respond to novel stimuli of normal intensity with aversive reactions (Kinsbourne, 1987). Since aversive responses are associated with reduced stimulus intake and processing (Lacey, 1967), higher levels of right-hemisphere activation would be expected to be correlated with more severe functional impairments, as was found in our study of the relationship between hemispheric activity and language abilities (Dawson *et al.*, 1986).

Right-hemisphere overactivation may be caused by dysfunctional subcortical mechanisms that influence cortical arousal. Because the cortical, limbic, and reticular subsystems that regulate arousal and attention are interdependent, dysfunction of any part of the larger system would be manifested at all levels of brain function.

Selective Functional Deficits

How would oversensitivity to novelty and chronic high levels of arousal differentially affect the acquisition of social knowledge (language and socioemotional development) versus nonsocial knowledge (i.e., concepts about objects and space)? We speculate that the functional consequences of overarousal are related to basic differences in the nature of information provided by animate versus inanimate objects. Social, emotional, and linguistic stimuli are, by nature, unpredictable and indeterminate. Thus, these types of stimuli are more likely to be novel and arousal-producing. In contrast, object-related stimuli, such as pattern, space, and the mechanical aspects of an object, tend to be more predictable (by the characteristics of the object and/or actions on the object), repeatable, and determinate. Such types of information, over which the autistic child may have control and which may be repeated, are less likely to elicit overarousal and aversion. It is possible that, for autistic children, subtle changes in degree of novelty and predictability may have significant consequence for information processing. As mentioned above, a number of autistic behaviors, including eye contact, motor stereotypies, and general social responsiveness, have been shown to vary as a function of the degree of structure, familiarity, and predictability in the environment (Charlop, 1986; Ferrara & Hill, 1980; Lord and Magill, Chapter 14, this volume; Runco *et al.*, 1986; Schopler *et al.*, 1971; Tiegerman & Primavera, 1981). Thus, without a therapeutic environment that entails a high level of routine and structure, it is not uncommon to find an autistic child who is highly focused on an activity involving repetitive, predictable stimulation (e.g., spinning an object), and who responds to social bids for attention with apparent indifference or distress and withdrawal.

The ability of autistic children to carry out certain right-hemisphere tasks, such as complex visual–spatial tasks, may reflect the degree to which the children have control of the stimulus input. Any task that requires ongoing processing of novel, unpredictable information, such as would be involved in comprehension of spontaneous language and facial expressions, would be difficult. Here we agree with Fein *et al.* (1984) that the information-processing capabilities of autistic persons may reflect attentional deficits, rather than falling into a strict pattern of right- versus left-hemisphere skills. We are speculating that the selective linguistic and social deficits found in autism are related to the arousal-producing qualities of language and social stimulation and to the negative consequences of over-arousal on attention and information processing.

Differential Hemispheric Involvement in Emotion: Implications for Autism

In this last section, we consider how differential patterns of hemispheric activation may be involved in the characteristic affective responses of autistic individuals. We begin by providing an overview of the research on hemispheric specialization for emotion in normal persons.

A substantial experimental and clinical literature indicates the two cerebral hemispheres mediate different emotional responses (see Fox & Davidson, 1984; Kinsbourne & Bemporad, 1984; and Weber & Sackeim, 1984, for recent reviews). Clinical observations of brain-damaged patients suggest that right-hemisphere damage is associated with indifference, carefree attitudes, and euphoria, whereas left-hemisphere damage is associated with feelings of anxiety, depression, and despair (Gainotti, 1972; Hecaen, 1962; Sackeim *et al.*, 1982). Sackeim *et al.* (1982) have argued that emotional changes resulting from unilateral brain damage are a result of disinhibition of the contralateral and intact hemisphere.

Experimental studies of normal adults and infants have also supported differential involvement of the hemispheres in emotion. EEG studies of both adults and young infants have found that positive emotional states are associated with relative activation of the left frontal lobe, whereas negative emotional states are associated with relative activation of the right frontal lobe (Davidson & Fox, 1982; Davidson, Schwartz, Saron, Bennett, & Goleman, 1979; Fox & Davidson, 1987; Tucker, Stenslie, Roth, & Shearer, 1981). In an EEG study of 10-month-old infants, Fox and Davidson (1987) recently demonstrated relative left-hemisphere activation during approach sequences with the mother, and relative right-hemisphere activation during avoidance responses to a stranger.

Kinsbourne and Bemporad (1984) and Fox and Davidson (1984) have theorized that behavioral responses of approach and withdrawal may be related to left- and right-hemisphere activity, respectively. The positive emotions such as interest and joy, for which the left hemisphere appears to be specialized, are involved in stimulus approach; negative emotions such as distress and anxiety, for which the right hemisphere appears to be specialized, are involved in stimulus withdrawal. Furthermore, the individual's emotional and motoric responses to the environment may reflect interhemispheric balance and interactions (Kinsbourne & Bemporad, 1984). For example, there is some evidence that left-hemisphere development, as reflected in increasing language ability, may allow for inhibition of right-hemisphere distress reactions via verbal mediation (Fox & Davidson, 1984). Kinsbourne and Bemporad (1984) have argued that adaptive responses to external stimuli require an integration of right- and left-hemisphere mechanisms: The right hemisphere is specialized for detection of novelty, which causes temporary disequilibration as reflected in the orienting response, whereas the left hemisphere is specialized for various vocal- and motor-skilled action plans and sequences that allow restoration of equilibrium. These authors further suggest that stimulation of moderate intensity or complexity, which is assimilable to the individual's behavioral and representational repertoire, is more likely to lead to the motivation to exert "action control" (left-hemisphere-mediated). In contrast, overly intense or complex stimulation, which disequilibrates the system, leads to emotional responses of anxiety and withdrawal (right-hemisphere-mediated) unless actions (left-hemisphere-mediated) are carried out that can restore equilibrium.

Autistic individuals tend to become anxious, to withdraw, and often to show uncontrollable distress reactions in situations (social or otherwise) that are unfamiliar and/or unpredictable. We offer the hypothesis that these emotional responses to the environment are related to an imbalance of hemispheric activity in the direction of right-hemisphere overactivation. This hypothesis has also been offered by Kinsbourne (1979, 1987). Although we suspect that right-hemisphere overactivation is an inherent part of a cortical–limbic–reticular system dysfunction, it is also likely that this original dysfunction is further reinforced by three factors: (1) the failure to develop language and other representational systems, which normally allow for greater potential for assimilation of novel events to existing schemes and for verbal mediation of emotional responses; (2) the overreliance on certain right-hemisphere-mediated information-processing strategies, related to a preference for right-hemisphere activities, such as puzzles, maps, and music; and (3) the tendency for certain stimuli or situations (e.g., social situations) to be associated with feelings of anxiety, which may lead to conditioned right-hemisphere-mediated avoidance reactions.

GENERAL SUMMARY AND CONCLUSION

Until recently, investigators have tended to focus exclusively on cortical or subcortical areas in their explanations of the nature of brain dysfunction in autism. However, the research evidence strongly supports involvement of all levels of brain processing. The ideas presented in this chapter represent an attempt to begin integrating research findings of subcortical and cortical dysfunction in autism. We have explored the possibility of reciprocal influences of subcortical and cortical abnormalities and their contributions to autistic persons' impairments in information processing.

To summarize, we propose that autism involves dysfunction of the cortical–

limbic–reticular system, which is the basis for attention to novelty. Dysfunction of the cortical–limbic–reticular system would account for the findings of a reduced P3 response, and absent or reduced habituation of autonomic responses, to novel stimuli. Furthermore, findings of enhanced right-hemisphere activity may reflect overactivation of the right-hemisphere-mediated cortical–limbic–reticular system, which may be dominant for novelty detection, attention, and arousal. Right-hemisphere overactivation, in theory, may lead to increased sensitivity to novelty and arousal; this increased sensitivity would account for the autistic child's tendency to respond to novel stimuli of normal intensity with aversive reactions. Moreover, we speculate that increased sensitivity to novelty will selectively impair processing of social (including linguistic) information, as compared to visual–spatial information, because such information is, by nature, novel and unpredictable. We predict that autistic individuals will tend to excel on tasks that allow them to have control over stimulus input and that may be repeated (e.g., puzzles), since, theoretically, these tasks would be less likely to elicit overarousal and aversive responses. In general, we are suggesting that subtle changes in degree of novelty and predictability may have significant consequences for information processing for individuals with autism.

We acknowledge that some of these ideas rest on sparse evidence, and fully expect that they will require substantial revision as additional data are acquired. However, it is our hope that these ideas will serve to inspire research that attempts to integrate measures of cortical and subcortical functioning in autistic persons. The data gathered so far raise several important questions that are amenable to study: Are autistic persons' attentional deficits related to specific stimulus characteristics? If so, which stimulus characteristics are most relevant: modality, social versus nonsocial nature, complexity, novelty, or predictability? Are measures of autonomic responsivity to novelty, such as the orienting response, correlated with measures of cortical processing of novelty, such as the ERP? Are both of these measures predictive of level of language and socioemotional impairment in autism? Finally, are measures of right-hemisphere activity correlated with measures of attention and emotional responses to novelty in autistic individuals? It is our hope that answers to questions such as these may help us to better understand the unusual attentional, cognitive, and affective characteristics of persons with autism.

Acknowledgments

We want to express our appreciation to several people who provided helpful feedback on earlier versions of this chapter: Larry Galpert, Laura Grofer, Deborah Hill, Earl Hunt, John Palmer, and Sid Segalowitz. Preparation of this chapter was supported in part by a grant from the John D. and Catherine T. MacArthur Foundation awarded to Geraldine Dawson.

References

Arnold, G., & Schwartz, G. E. (1983). Hemispheric lateralization of language in autistic and aphasic children. *Journal of Autism and Developmental Disorders, 13,* 129–139.

Bernal, M. E., & Miller, W. H. (1971). Electrodermal and cardiac responses of schizophrenic children to sensory stimuli. *Psychophysiology, 7,* 155–168.

Best, C. T., Hoffman, H., & Glanville, B. B. (1982). Development of right ear asymmetries for speech and music. *Perception and Psychophysics, 31,* 75–85.

Blackstock, E. (1978). Cerebral asymmetry and the development of early infantile autism. *Journal of Autism and Developmental Disorders, 8,* 339–353.

Brain, W. R. (1941). Visual disorientation with special reference to lesions of the right cerebral hemisphere. *Brain, 64,* 244–271.

Brown, W. T., Jenkins, E. C., Friedman, E., Brooks, J., Wisniewski, K., Raguthu, S., & French, J. (1982). Autism is associated with the fragile X syndrome. *Journal of Autism and Developmental Disorders, 12,* 303–308.

Bushnell, M. C., Goldberg, M. E., & Robinson, D. L. (1981). Behavioral enhancement of visual responses in monkey cerebral cortex: I. Modulation in posterior parietal cortex related to selected visual attention. *Journal of Neurophysiology, 46,* 755–772.

Butler, S. R., & Glass, A. (1974). Asymmetries in the electroencephalogram associated with cerebral dominance. *Electroencephalography and Clinical Neurophysiology, 36,* 481–491.

Charlop, M. H. (1986). Setting effects on the occurrence of autistic children's immediate echolalia. *Journal of Autism and Developmental Disorders, 16,* 473–483.

Chess, S., Fernandez, P. B., & Korn, S. J. (1978). Behavioral consequences of congenital rubella. *Journal of Pediatrics, 93,* 699–703.

Clarkson, M. G., & Berg, W. K. (1983). Cardiac orienting and vowel discrimination in newborns: Crucial stimulus parameters. *Child Development, 54,* 162–171.

Cohen, D. J., & Johnson, W. T. (1977). Cardiovascular correlates of attention in normal and psychiatrically disturbed children. *Archives of General Psychiatry, 34,* 561–567.

Coles, M. G. H. (1974). Physiological activity and detection: The effects of attentional requirements and the prediction of performance. *Biological Psychology, 2,* 113–125.

Courchesne, E. (1987). A neurophysiological view of autism. In E. Schopler & G. Mesibov (Eds.), *Neurobiological issues in autism.* New York: Plenum.

Courchesne, E., Kilman, B. A., Galambos, R., & Lincoln, A. J. (1984). Autism: Processing of novel auditory information assessed by event-related brain potentials. *Electroencephalography and Clinical Neurophysiology, 59,* 238–248.

Courchesne, E., Lincoln, A. J., Kilman, B. A., & Galambos, R. (1985). Event-related brain potential correlates of the processing of novel visual and auditory information in autism. *Journal of Autism and Developmental Disorders, 15,* 55–75.

Courchesne, E., Yeung-Courchesne, R., Hicks, G., & Lincoln, A. J. (1985). Functioning of brainstem auditory pathway in non-retarded autistic individuals. *Electroencephalography and Clinical Neurophysiology: Evoked Potentials, 61,* 491–501.

Critchley, M. (1966). *The parietal lobes.* New York: Hafner.

Crowell, P., Jones, R., Kapuniai, L., & Nakagawa, J. (1973). Unilateral cortical activity in newborn humans: An early index of cerebral dominance. *Science, 180,* 205–208.

Davidson, R. J., & Fox, N. A. (1982). Asymmetrical brain activity discriminates between positive versus negative affective stimuli in human infants. *Science, 218,* 1235–1237.

Davidson, R. J., Schwartz, G. E., Saron, C., Bennett, J., & Goleman, D. J. (1979). Frontal versus parietal EEG asymmetry during positive and negative affect. *Psychophysiology, 16,* 202–203.

Dawson, G. (1983). Lateralized brain dysfunction in autism: Evidence from the Halstead–Reitan Neuropsychological Battery. *Journal of Autism and Developmental Disorders, 13,* 269–286.

Dawson, G. (1987). The role of abnormal hemispheric specialization in autism. In E. Schopler & G. Mesibov (Eds.), *Neurobiological issues in autism.* New York: Plenum.

Dawson, G. (1988). Cerebral lateralization in autism: Its role in language and affective disorders. In D. L. Molfese & S. J. Segalowitz (Eds.), *Brain lateralization in children: Developmental implications.* New York: Guilford Press.

Dawson, G., & Adams, A. (1984). Imitation and social responsiveness in autistic children. *Journal of Abnormal Child Psychology, 12,* 209–225.

Dawson, G., Finley, C., Phillips, S., & Galpert, L. (1986). Hemispheric specialization and the language abilities of autistic children. *Child Development, 57,* 1440–1453.

Dawson, G., Finley, C., Phillips, S., Galpert, L., & Lewy, A. (in press). Reduced P3 amplitude of the event-related brain potential: Its relationship to language ability in autism. *Journal of Autism and Developmental Disorders.*

Dawson, G., Finley, C., Phillips, S., & Lewy, A. (in press). A comparison of patterns of lateralization in the speech-related brain potentials of autistic and dysphasic children. *Brain and Language.*

Dawson, G., Warrenburg, S., & Fuller, P. (1982). Cerebral lateralization in individuals diagnosed as autistic in early childhood. *Brain and Language, 15,* 353–368.

Dawson, G., Warrenburg, S., & Fuller, P. (1983). Hemisphere functioning and motor imitation in autistic persons. *Brain and Cognition, 2,* 346–354.

Deykin, E. Y., & MacMahon, B. (1980). Pregnancy, delivery and neonatal complications among autistic children. *American Journal of Diseases of Children, 134,* 860–864.

Doyle, J., Galin, D., & Ornstein, R. E. (1974). Lateral specialization of cognitive mode: EEG frequency analysis. *Psychophysiology, 11,* 567–578.

Easterbrook, J. A. (1959). The effect of emotion on cue utilization and the organization of behavior. *Psychological Review, 66,* 183–201.

Entus, A. K. (1977). Hemispheric asymmetry in processing of dichotically presented speech and non-speech sounds by infants. In S. Segalowitz & F. A. Gruber (Eds.), *Language development and neurological theory.* New York: Academic Press.

Fein, D., Humes, M., Kaplan, E., Lucci, D., & Waterhouse, L. (1984). The question of left hemisphere dysfunction in autistic children. *Psychological Bulletin, 95,* 258–281.

Ferrara, C., & Hill, S. (1980). The responsiveness of autistic children to the predictability of social and nonsocial toys. *Journal of Autism and Development Disorders, 10,* 51–57.

Finegan, J., & Quadrington, B. (1979). Pre-, peri-, and neonatal factors and infantile autism. *Journal of Child Psychology and Psychiatry, 20,* 119–128.

Folstein, S., & Rutter, M. (1977). Infantile autism: A genetic study of 21 twin pairs. *Journal of Child Psychology and Psychiatry, 18,* 297–231.

Fox, N. A., & Davidson, R. J. (1984). Hemispheric substrates of affect: A developmental model. In N. A. Fox & R. J. Davidson (Eds.), *The psychobiology of affective development.* Hillsdale, NJ: Erlbaum.

Fox, N. A., & Davidson, R. J. (1987). Electroencephalogram asymmetry in response to the approach of a stranger and maternal separation in 10-month-old infants. *Developmental Psychology, 23,* 233–240.

Gainotti, G. (1972). Emotional behavior and hemispheric side of the lesion. *Cortex, 8,* 41–55.

Geschwind, N., & Galaburda, A. M. (1985a). Cerebral lateralization: Biological mechanisms, association, and pathology. I. A hypothesis and a program for research. *Archives of Neurology, 42,* 428–459.

Geschwind, N., & Galaburda, A. M. (1985b). Cerebral lateralization: Biological mechanisms, association, and pathology. II. A hypothesis and a program for research. *Archives of Neurology, 42,* 521–552.

Geschwind, N., & Galaburda, A. M. (1985c). Cerebral lateralization: Biological mechanisms, associations, and pathology. III. A hypothesis and a program for research. *Archives of Neurology, 42,* 634–654.

Gillberg, C., Rosenhall, U., & Johansson, E. (1983). Auditory brainstem responses in childhood psychosis. *Journal of Autism and Developmental Disorders, 13,* 181–195.

Glanville, B. B., Best, C. T., & Levinson, R. (1977). A cardiac measure of cerebral asymmetries in infant auditory perception. *Developmental Psychology, 13,* 54–59.

Goldberg, M. E., & Robinson, D. L. (1977). Visual responses of neurons in monkey inferior parietal lobule: The physiologic substrate of attention and neglect. *Neurology*, 27, 350.

Golfine, P. E., McPherson, P. M., Heath, G. A., Hardesty, V. A., Beauregard, L. J., & Gordon, S. (1985). Association of fragile X syndrome with autism. *American Journal of Psychiatry*, 142, 108–110.

Graham, F. K., & Clifton, R. K. (1966). Heart rate changes as a component of the orienting response. *Psychological Bulletin*, 65, 305–320.

Hecaen, H. (1962). Clinical symptomatology in right and left hemispheric lesions. In V. B. Mountcastle (Ed.), *Interhemispheric relations and cerebral dominance*. Baltimore: Johns Hopkins University Press.

Heilman, K. M., Bowers, D., Valenstein, E., & Watson, R. T. (1986). The right hemisphere: Neuropsychological functions. *Journal of Neurosurgery*, 64, 693–704.

Heilman, K. M., & Van Den Abell, T. (1979). Right hemispheric dominance for mediating cerebral activation. *Neuropsychologia*, 17, 315–321.

Heilman, K. M., & Van Den Abell, T. (1980). Right hemisphere dominance for attention: The mechanism underlying hemispheric asymmetries of inattention (neglect). *Neurology*, 30, 327–330.

Heilman, K. M., Schwartz, H. D., & Watson, R. T. (1978). Hypoarousal in patients with the neglect syndrome and emotional indifference. *Neurology*, 28, 229–232.

Hillyard, S. A., & Picton, R. W. (1979). Event-related brain potentials and selective information processing in man. In J. E. Desmedt (Ed.), *Progress in clinical neurophysiology* (Vol. 6). Basel: S. Karger.

Hoffman, W., & Prior, M. (1982). Neuropsychological dimensions of autism in children: A test of the hemispheric hypothesis. *Journal of Clinical Psychology*, 4, 27–41.

Hutt, S. J., Forrest, S. J., & Richer, J. (1975). Cardiac arhythmia and behavior in autistic children. *Acta Psychiatrica Scandinavica*, 51, 361–372.

James, A., & Barry, R. J. (1980). Respiratory and vascular responses to simple visual stimuli in autistics, retardates and normals. *Psychophysiology*, 17, 541–547.

Kinsbourne, M. (1979). The neuropsychology of autism. In L. A. Lockman, K. F. Swaiman, J. S. Drage, K. B. Nelson, & K. M. Marsden (Eds.), *Workshop on the neurological basis of autism* (NINCDS Monograph No. 23). Bethesda, MD: U.S. Department of Health, Education and Welfare.

Kinsbourne, M. (1987). Cerebral–brainstem relations in infantile autism. In E. Schopler & G. Mesibov (Eds.), *Neurobiological issues in autism*. New York: Plenum.

Kinsbourne, M., & Bemporad, B. (1984). Lateralization of emotion: A model and the evidence. In N. A. Fox & R. J. Davidson (Eds.), *The psychobiology of affective development*. Hillsdale, NJ: Erlbaum.

Kootz, J. P., & Cohen, D. J. (1981). Modulation of sensory intake in autistic children: Cardiovascular and behavioral indices. *Journal of the American Academy of Child Psychiatry*, 20, 692–701.

Kootz, J. P., Marinelli, B., & Cohen, D. J. (1982). Modulation of response to environmental stimulation in autistic children. *Journal of Autism and Developmental Disorders*, 12, 185–193.

Lacey, J. I. (1967). Somatic response in patterning and stress: Some revisions of activation theory. In M. H. Appley & R. Trumbull (Eds.), *Psychological stress: Issues in research*. New York: Appleton-Century-Crofts.

Levy, J., Heller, W., Banich, M. T., & Burton, L. A. (1983). Are variations among right-handed individuals in perceptual asymmetries caused by characteristic arousal differences between hemispheres? *Journal of Experimental Psychology: Human Perception and Performance*, 9, 329–359.

Linnemeyer, S. A., & Porges, S. W. (1986). Recognition memory and cardiac vagal tone in 6-month-old infants. *Infant Behavior and Development*, 9, 43–56.

Lockyer, L., & Rutter, M. (1970). A five to fifteen year follow up study of infantile psychosis: IV. Patterns of cognitive ability. *British Journal of Social and Clinical Psychology*, 31, 152–163.

Lovaas, O. I., Schreibman, L., Koegel, R. L., & Rehm, R. (1971). Selective responding by autistic children to multiple sensory input. *Journal of Abnormal Psychology*, 77, 211–222.

Molfese, D. L., Freeman, R. B., & Palermo, D. S. (1975). The ontogeny of brain lateralization for speech and non-speech stimuli. *Brain and Language, 2,* 356–368.

Molfese, D. L., & Molfese, V. J. (1979). Hemisphere and stimulus differences as reflected in the cortical responses of newborn infants to speech stimulus. *Developmental Psychology, 15,* 505–511.

Novick, B., Kurtzberg, D., & Vaughn, H. G. (1979). An electrophysiologic indication of defective information storage in childhood autism. *Psychiatry Research, 1,* 101–108.

Novick, B., Vaughn, Jr., H. G., Kurtzberg, D., & Simson, R. (1980). An electrophysiological indication of auditory processing defects in autism. *Psychiatry Research, 3,* 107–114.

Ogawa, T., Sugiyama, A., Ishiwa, S., Suzuki, M., Ishihara, T., & Sato, K. (1982). Ontogenic development of EEG-asymmetry in early infantile autism. *Brain and Development, 4,* 439–449.

Ornitz, E. M. (1985). Neurophysiology of infantile autism. *Journal of the American Academy of Child Psychiatry, 24,* 251–262.

Ornitz, E. M., Atwell, C. W., Kaplan, A. R., & Westlake, J. R. (1985). Brainstem dysfunction in autism. *Archives of General Psychiatry, 42,* 1018–1025.

Ornitz, E. M., Brown, M. B., Mason, A., & Putman, N. H. (1974). Effect of visual input on vestibular nystagmus in autistic children. *Archives of General Psychiatry, 31,* 369–375.

Palkowitz, R. W., & Wiesenfeld, A. R. (1980). Differential autonomic responses of autistic and normal children. *Journal of Autism and Developmental Disorders, 10,* 347–360.

Porges, S. W. (1980). Individual differences in attention: A possible physiological substrate. *Advances in Special Education, 2,* 111–134.

Porges, S. W. (1984). Physiological correlates of attention: A core process underlying learning disorders. *Pediatric Clinics of North America, 31,* 371–385.

Prior, M. R., & Bradshaw, J. L. (1979). Hemisphere functions in autistic children, *Cortex, 15,* 73–81.

Pritchard, W. S. (1981). Psychophysiology of P300. *Psychological Bulletin, 89,* 506–540.

Ritvo, E. R., Freeman, B. J., Mason-Brothers, B., Mo, A., & Ritvo, A. M. (1985). Concordance for the syndrome of autism in 40 pairs of afflicted twins. *American Journal of Psychiatry, 142,* 74–77.

Rumsey, J. M., Grimes, A. M., Pikus, A. M., Duara, R., & Ismond, D. R. (1984). Auditory brainstem responses in pervasive developmental disorders. *Biological Psychiatry, 19,* 1403–1418.

Runco, M. A., Charlop, M. H., & Schreibman, L. (1986). The occurrence of autistic children's self-stimulation as a function of familiar versus unfamiliar stimulus conditions. *Journal of Autism and Developmental Disorders, 16*(1), 31–44.

Rutter, M. (1974). The development of infantile autism. *Psychological Medicine, 4,* 147–163.

Sackeim, H. A., Greensberg, M. S., Weiman, A. L., Gur, R. C., Hungerbuhler, J. P., & Geschwind, N. (1982). Hemispheric asymmetry in the expression of positive and negative emotions: Neurological evidence. *Archives of Neurology, 39,* 210–218.

Schopler, E., Brehm, S., Kinsbourne, M., & Reichler, R. J. (1971). Effect of treatment structure on development in autistic children. *Archives and General Psychiatry, 24,* 415–421.

Sigman, M., & Ungerer, J. (1984). Cognitive and language skills in autistic, mentally retarded, and normal children. *Developmental Psychology, 20,* 293–302.

Skoff, B. F., Mirsky, A. F., & Turner, D. (1980). Prolonged brainstem transmission time in autism. *Psychiatry Research, 2,* 157–166.

Small, J. (1975). EEG and neurophysiological studies of early infantile autism. *Biological Psychiatry, 10,* 385–389.

Soper, H. V., & Satz, P. (1984) Pathological left-handedness and ambiguous handedness: A new explanatory model. *Neuropsychologia, 22,* 511–515.

Sokolov, E. N. (1963). *Perception and the conditioned reflex.* New York: Macmillan.

Sokolov, E. N. (1975). The neuronal mechanisms of the orienting reflex. In E. N. Sokolov & O. S. Vinogradova (Eds.), *Neuronal mechanisms of the orienting reflex.* Hillsdale, NJ: Erlbaum.

Spinelli, D. N., & Pribram, K. H. (1966). Changes in visual recovery functions produced by temporal lobe stimulation in monkeys. *Electroencephalography and Clinical Neurophysiology, 20,* 44–49.

Stevens, S., & Gruzelier, J. (1984). Electrodermal activity to auditory stimuli in autistic, retarded, and normal children. *Journal of Autism and Developmental Disorders, 14,* 245–260.

Tanguay, P. E. (1976). Clinical and electrophysiological research. In E. R. Ritvo (Ed.), *Autism: Diagnosis, current research and management.* New York: Spectrum.

Tanguay, P., Edwards, R. M., Buchwald, J., Schwafel, J., & Allen, V. (1982). Auditory brainstem evoked responses in autistic children. *Archives of General Psychiatry, 39,* 174–180.

Taylor, D. C. (1969). Differential rates of cerebral maturation between sexes and between hemispheres: Evidence from epilepsy. *Lancet, ii,* 140–142.

Taylor, M. J., Rosenblatt, B., & Linschoten, L. (1982). Electrophysiological study of the auditory system in autistic children. In A. Rothenberger (Ed.), *Event-related potentials in children.* New York: Elsevier.

Thatcher, R. W. (1976). Electrophysiological correlates of animal and human memory. In R. Terry & S. Gershon (Eds.), *The neurobiology of aging.* New York: Raven Press.

Thatcher, R. W., & John, E. R. (1977). *Foundations of cognitive processes: Functional neuroscience* (Vol. 1). New York: Wiley.

Tiegerman, E., & Primavera, L. (1981). Object manipulation: An interactional strategy with autistic children. *Journal of Autism and Developmental Disorders, 11,* 427–438.

Tucker, D. J., Stenslie, C. E., Roth, R. S., & Shearer, S. L. (1981). Right frontal lobe activation and right hemisphere performance decrement during a depressed mood. *Archives of General Psychiatry, 38,* 169–174.

Tueting, P. (1978). Event-related potentials, cognitive events, and information processing. In D. A. Otto (Ed.), *Multidisciplinary perspectives in event-related brain potential research.* Washington, DC: U.S. Government Printing Office.

van Engeland, H. (1984). The electrodermal orienting response to auditive stimuli in autistic children, normal children, mentally retarded children, and child psychiatric patients. *Journal of Autism and Developmental Disorders, 14,* 261–279.

Weber, S. L., & Sackeim, H. A. (1984). The development of functional brain asymmetry in the regulation of emotion. In N. A. Fox & R. J. Davidson (Eds.), *The psychobiology of affective development.* New Jersey: Erlbaum.

Wetherby, A. M., Koegel, R. L., & Mendel, M. (1981). Central auditory nervous system dysfunction in echolalic autistic individuals. *Journal of Speech and Hearing Research, 24,* 420–429.

Witelson, S. F. (1977). Early hemisphere specialization and inter-hemispheric plasticity: An empirical and theoretical review. In S. J. Segalowitz & F. A. Gruber (Eds.), *Language development and neurological theory.* New York: Academic Press.

CHAPTER 8

Autism at the Interface between Sensory and Information Processing

EDWARD M. ORNITZ

UCLA School of Medicine

Autism is a behavioral syndrome consisting of specific disturbances of social relating and communication, language, response to objects, and sensory modulation and motility (Ornitz, 1973, 1983, 1985). I have recently proposed a neurophysiological model of infantile autism that stresses the autistic disturbances of sensory modulation and motility (Ornitz, 1983, 1985). This model assumes that the disturbances of sensory modulation are the primary symptoms and that disturbances of social relating, communication, language, and the bizarre responses to the environment are consequences of a dysmodulation of sensory input. This neurophysiological model suggests a dysfunction of the neuronal networks in the brain stem and diencephalon that are involved in the initial processing of sensory input before such input has informational value. Thus, this is a model for a subcortical dysfunction of sensory processing. It assumes that distorted sensory input, when transmitted to higher centers, becomes distorted information, and that this in turn becomes the basis of the deviant language and social communication.

Other lines of investigation have focused on the language disorder, attempting to identify specific areas of cortical dysfunction, notably involving the left hemisphere (Hoffman & Prior, 1982). Although there is some evidence suggesting failure of hemispheric lateralization (Fein, Humes, Kaplan, Lucci, & Waterhouse, 1984; see reviews in Ornitz, 1983, 1985), autism is clearly more than a language-processing disorder, and the view that it can be explained as the result of a specific cognitive defect (Rutter, 1978) fails to account for its incredibly complex symptomatology, which involves reactivity both to simple raw sensation and to the intricacies of human relationships. The "cognitive" and language disorder hypothesis cannot explain the disturbances of social relating, sensory modulation, and motility of autistic children (A. R. Damasio, 1984; Ornitz, 1983).

Nevertheless, the failure of even very high-functioning autistic individuals to respond appropriately to social cues and nuances does suggest some subtle cognitive dysfunction that can be considered in the context of information processing. For the considerations in this chapter, the notion of a disorder of information processing provides a more operational context for behavioral and neurophysiological studies than does the notion of a disorder of cognition. Information processing can be considered in terms of more discrete functions, such as attention, learning, and memory (Donchin *et al.*, 1984). It is the function of attention, and particularly directed attention, which is the focus of this chapter, since both the autistic disturbances of sensory modulation and the autistic disturbances of response to objects ("bizarre responses to various aspects of the environment"; American Psychiatric Association, 1980, p. 90) are indicative of deviant direction of attention to stimuli in the environment. There is also evidence that even language (and therefore language disorders) may originate in early selective orienting to environmental stimuli (Lempert & Kinsbourne, 1985). Directed attention can be considered as an element of both sensory processing at lower levels of the neuraxis and information processing at higher levels.

The relationship between the dysfunction of sensory modulation and a dysfunction of information processing requires elaboration. The earlier suggestion that distorted sensory input becomes distorted information (Ornitz, 1983, 1985) seems intuitively correct but is clearly imprecise. The purpose of this presentation is to extend the sensory-processing dysfunction hypothesis to an information-processing dysfunction hypothesis by utilizing the Jacksonian principle that higher levels of the nervous system represent and re-represent, but do not replace, lower levels. Through an analysis of recent experimental neurophysiological findings, I attempt to demonstrate (1) the influence of the brain stem and diencephalic regions involved in the modulation of sensory input on those cortical centers involved with information processing; (2) the relevance of the functions of those higher centers to autistic behavior; and (3) the way in which these higher centers might elaborate an autistic dysfunction of sensory processing to a disorder of information processing.

To facilitate the development of these hypotheses, I review neurophysiological investigations of autism in the context of the behavioral disturbances observed in autistic children. I then propose that autistic behavior can be understood as a disorder of directed attention involving neurophysiological mechanisms primarily, though not necessarily exclusively, in the right hemisphere. I attempt to show that this disorder of directed attention can be conceptualized as occurring at the interface between sensory processing and information processing. Sensory processing involves brain stem and other subcortical mechanisms that modulate the rostral flow of sensory input along the neuraxis. It is subject to caudally directed influences from cortical and other more rostral structures that regulate the direction of attention. Distortions of sensory input during sensory processing can compromise the conversion of sensation into information. Thus distorted sensory processing can induce distorted information processing. Further distortions of information processing can occur at cortical levels when cortical structures elaborate the distorted sensory input.

Autistic behavioral disturbances of sensory modulation—that is, underreactivity and overreactivity to sensory stimuli—suggest subcortical dysfunction resulting in disordered sensory processing. Autistic behavioral disturbances of language and cognition suggest cortical dysfunction resulting in disordered information processing. There is neurophysiological evidence for and against both the hypothesis of subcortical dysfunction and that of cortical dysfunction.

THE AUTISTIC BEHAVIORAL SYNDROME

First, it is necessary to consider the nature of the autistic behavioral syndrome. The behavioral syndrome of autism is unique; as noted earlier, it consists of specific disturbances of social relating and communication, language, response to objects, and sensory modulation and motility (Ornitz, 1973, 1983, 1985). When first described, the autistic disturbances of social relating and communication, manifested by disturbances of affective contact, were considered to be the primary components of the autistic syndrome (Kanner, 1943). Subsequently, the primacy of the social and emotional dysfunction was usurped by an emphasis on the language disturbance and the assumption that it could be explained by a special cognitive deficit (Rutter, 1968, 1978). More recently, Rutter (1983) has allowed that the cognitive deficit may be specific for emotional and social meaning. Currently, the primacy of the disturbance of social relating, including a basic dysfunction of emotional response, is back in fashion (Cohen, Paul, & Volkmar, 1986; Denckla, 1986; Fein, Pennington, Markowitz, Braverman, & Waterhouse, 1986) and is incorporated in the *Diagnostic and Statistical Manual of Mental Disorders*, third edition (DSM-III), along with the autistic disturbance of language and the disturbance of response to objects.

Curiously, the disturbance of sensory modulation has not been recognized by most authorities in the field of autism and has not been incorporated into DSM-III, even though very specific and easy-to-describe deviant responses to raw sensory stimuli occur in most autistic children when they are observed prior to 6 years of age or when their parents are questioned about specific behaviors that occurred during the preschool period (Ornitz, 1969, 1973, 1974, 1983, 1985; Ornitz, Guthrie, & Farley, 1977, 1978). Part of the problem may have been insufficient observation of the preschool autistic child, and part of the problem has been the manner of thinking about and classifying the observed behavior. For example, underreactivity and overreactivity to sound were considered symptoms of the language disturbance (Rutter & Lockyer, 1967); more recently, behaviors such as preoccupation with noises, textures, or spinning objects, ignoring noises, and failure to notice painful stimuli have been grouped with "responses to the environment" or "affective responses" (Volkmar, Cohen, & Paul, 1986), obscuring the recognition of such behaviors as deviant responses to sensory input (i.e., collectively, as a disturbance of sensory modulation). Additional obfuscation occurred when DSM-III (American Psychiatric Association, 1980) mandated a differential diagnosis between infantile autism and childhood-onset pervasive developmental disorder (COPDD) on the dubious basis of age of onset. DSM-III includes disturbances of sensory modulation ("hyper- or hyposensitivity to sensory stimuli") along with other symptoms of infantile autism ("oddities of motor movement," "monotonous voice," "resistance to change") among the diagnostic criteria for COPDD (age of onset over 30 months), while relegating the hyper- and hyposensitivities to associated symptoms in infantile autism (age of onset under 30 months). In fact, hyper- and hyposensitivities to sensory stimuli occur in children diagnosed as autistic with onset prior to 30 months of age with the same frequencies as the disturbances of relating to people and to objects (Ornitz et al., 1977, 1978).

The disturbance of sensory modulation involves all sensory modalities, and is manifested as both under- and overreactivity to sensory stimuli and as self-stimulation (e.g., visual scrutiny of spinning objects). Some of the motility disturbances (e.g., hand flapping) may provide such input through proprioceptive and kinesthetic channels. Before the age of 6 years, parental reports on a developmental inventory indicated that the disturbances of sensory modulation and motility were observed with almost the same frequencies as the disturbance of relating to people and objects (Ornitz et al., 1977, 1978). Using the identical developmental inventory, and considering behaviors that exemplify under- or overreactivity to sensory stimuli, Volkmar et al. (1986) have replicated these findings on an independent sample of autistic subjects. The manner in which individual autistic children express the disturbance of sensory modulation has not been systematically studied. My own observations of preschool autistic children suggest that most manifest both the under- and overreactivity to sensory stimuli, while some may show a preponderance of one or the other type of behavior.

The uniqueness of the autistic syndrome suggests a single underlying pathophysiological mechanism (Ornitz, 1983). However, multiple etiologies, which could activate or replicate such a mechanism, are suggested by the association with some cases of autism of many pre-, peri-, and neonatal conditions that putatively are likely to insult fetal or neonatal brain function (Ornitz, 1983). In other cases, autism has been associated with various congenital structural and metabolic disorders (Ornitz, 1983) and also with certain chromsomal disorders (Brown et al., 1986; Fisch et al., 1986). In most cases, potential etiological factors have not been identified, although there is some evidence from family studies suggesting a subgroup with a genetic component (Folstein, 1985; see reviews in Ornitz, 1983). There is a paucity of pathological studies, and the very few autistic brains that have been examined have failed to reveal consistent neuropathology (Coleman, Romano, Lapham, & Simon, 1985; Williams, Hauser, Purpura, DeLong, & Swisher, 1980), although the single brain recently examined by Bauman and Kemper (1985) merits particular attention and is discussed later in this chapter. Biochemical investigations have not revealed any consistent neuromodulator or neurotransmitter abnormalities (Cohen, Caparulo, Shaywitz, & Bowers, 1977), although elevated blood serotonin in about 30% of the cases remains an unexplained finding (Hanley, Stahl, & Freedman, 1977; Yuwiler, Geller, & Ritvo, 1985).

NEUROPHYSIOLOGICAL INVESTIGATION

Neurophysiological studies tend to examine mechanism rather than etiology. They have taken two general directions, one stressing the disturbances of language and cognition and the other stressing the disturbances of sensory modulation and motility. The disturbances of language and cognition suggest cortical dysfunction, and the disturbances of sensory modulation and motility suggest subcortical dysfunction. Neurophysiological studies of autism are reviewed here in the context of cortical and subcortical, particularly brain stem, activity.

Neurophysiological Studies of Cortical Activity

Neurophysiological studies of cortical events are relevant to the autistic disturbances of language and communication. The neurophysiological research that has focused on cortical mechanisms has included electroencephalographic (EEG) studies, radiological studies (including several computerized tomography [CT] investigations), and event-related potential studies.

Quantitative EEG studies, both during wakefulness without (Small, 1975) and with (Dawson, Warrenburg, & Fuller, 1982, 1983) tasks, and during sleep (Ogawa *et al.*, 1982), suggest abnormal patterns of hemispheric lateralization. Compared to age-matched controls, autistic subjects showed reduced left-hemisphere (relative to right-hemisphere) alpha attenuation specifically during tasks requiring language (Dawson *et al.*, 1982) and motor imitation (Dawson *et al.*, 1983). These findings are relevant to the autistic language and motor imitation impairments.

Evoked potential studies also suggest alteration of normal hemispheric asymmetry, both during sleep (Tanguay, 1976) and in the waking state (Dawson, Finley, Phillips, & Galpert, 1986). The amplitude of wave N1 of the auditory evoked response to the syllable "da" was larger over the right than the left temporoparietal scalp in 12 out of 17 normal subjects, whereas only 7 out of 17 autistics showed this pattern. The 10 autistics who showed the reversed pattern showed a greater relative right-sided decrement than did the 5 normals who showed the reversed pattern (Dawson, *et al.*, 1986).

These findings are not consistently supported by dichotic listening studies (Arnold & Schwartz, 1983) or CT scans (Tsai, Jacoby, & Stewart, 1983; Tsai, Jacoby, Stewart, & Beisler, 1982). Autistic children preferred nonverbal (music) to verbal auditory stimuli (Blackstock, 1978), and listened to both music and speech with the left ear, rather than listening to speech with the right ear, as did normals—observations that might reflect only their lack of interest in speech. In a dichotic listening task, autistics did not show the normal right-ear advantage in one investigation (Prior & Bradshaw, 1979). This finding appeared to be limited to autistics who were echolalic (Wetherby, Koegel, & Mendel, 1981) and could not be confirmed at all in a more recent study, which was designed to avoid confounding laterality with the more general linguistic disadvantage of autistics (Arnold & Schwartz, 1983). Hoffman and Prior (1982) used a control group matched for mental age (MA) in a dichotic listening task and concluded that "since the left-ear advantage was exhibited by both the autistic and MA control groups, it is not possible to attribute differences specifically to the autistic syndrome" (p. 36). Using reaction times to monaural presentation of tones in a study controlled for age, James and Barry (1983) have demonstrated a significant developmental delay in ear advantage, and (by inference) the establishment of cerebral lateralization, in autistic children.

Hier, LeMay, and Rosenberger (1979) used CT to measure the parieto-occipital width in 16 autistics. In 57% (9 cases) of these autistics, the right parieto-occipital width was wider than the left—a pattern which occurred only in 23% and 25%, respectively, of larger groups of mentally retarded and neurological patients. This finding was not replicated in another CT study of autistics (H. Damasio, Maurer, Damasio, & Chui, 1980). These investigations also could not confirm the left temporal lateral cleft enlargement observed by Hauser, DeLong, and Rosman (1975). They found reversal of the normal lateral ventricular asymmetry in only 6 of 17 cases. More recently, comparisons between autistic and neurological patients (Tsai *et al.*, 1982, 1983) failed to reveal any significant increase in unfavorable brain asymmetries in autism. CT scans have shown abnormal structural configurations in only about one-quarter of autistic subjects (Campbell *et al.*, 1982; Gillberg & Svendsen, 1983), and abnormal findings in CT scans may have little if any relation to infantile autism (Prior, Tress, Hoffman, & Boldt, 1984).

In summary, there is evidence from quantitative EEG and evoked potential studies, and from one study of the maturation of ear advantage, for unfavorable hemispheric lateralization in autism. This concept does not receive support from either dichotic listening studies or CT scan studies. Although the electrophysiological studies do suggest deficient hemispheric lateralization, particularly the normal left-hemisphere dominance in the processing of auditory stimuli, the lack of normal asymmetry in autism is not necessarily of cerebral origin. Normal right–left asymmetries, with larger amplitudes for right-ear stimulation, have been demonstrated in human brain stem auditory evoked responses (BAERs; Levine & McGaffigan, 1983). It has been suggested that cerebral asymmetries for language could be related to asymmetries in the brain stem auditory pathways. Therefore, lack of normal hemispheric asymmetry in autism could be related to deviant brain stem function.

Although the evidence for an abnormal pattern of hemispheric lateralization is inconsistent, and the source of any possible deviant or deficient asymmetry may or may not be cortical, deviant left or right cortical function in autism remains a possible explanation of many aspects of autistic behavior. Deviant left or right cortical function may occur independently of deviant asymmetry (i.e., independently of the issue of cerebral lateralization). I return to the issue of possible cortical dysfunction, particularly right-hemisphere dysfunction, later in this chapter in the discussion of deviant and deficient directed attention in autism. Autistic patients show a deficient capacity to direct attention toward emotionally relevant stimuli in their environment. It is this capacity that is most strongly represented in the right hemisphere (Bear, 1983; Mesulam, 1983).

The amplitude of the P300 wave in response to a stimulus increases with increasing confidence in stimulus detection and increasing use of information about the stimulus. Therefore, impaired information processing has been suggested by reports of small or absent P300 waves in the evoked EEG response to different types of stimuli (Courchesne, Kilman, Galambos, & Lincoln, 1984; Courchesne, Lincoln, Kilman, & Galambos, 1985; Niwa, Ohta, & Yamazaki, 1983; Novick, Kurtzberg, & Vaughan, 1979; Novick, Vaughn, Kurtzberg, & Simon, 1980). Conclusions from some of these studies are based on rather small sample sizes. Three autistic adolescents in one study and five in another detected and made behavioral responses to rare missing stimuli in series of tones or flashes, and showed small or absent P300 waves recorded from parietal scalp derivations (Novick *et al.*, 1979, 1980). In similar experiments, Novick *et al.* (1980) (five autistic adolescents) and Courchesne *et al.* (1984) (seven autistic adolescents) found smaller P300 waves in autistic adolescents (than in normals) who were required to detect rare target auditory stimuli interspersed among background stimuli. Courchesne *et al.* (1985) replicated these findings in a somewhat larger population (10 nonretarded autistic adolescents or adults) with auditory stimuli. However, there were no significant differences when the study was extended to visual stimuli. When a response to the rare sounds was not required, there were no differences in P300 between autistics and normals for either auditory or visual stimuli (Courchesne *et al.*, 1984, 1985). Niwa *et al.* (1983) also found nonsignificant differences between four autistic adolescents and both normal and Down syndrome controls in amplitudes of P300 responses to rare auditory stimuli in a nontask experiment. In another type of experiment, subjects were presented with rare novel stimuli (such that each auditory or visual stimulus was different from every other one) to which responses were not required (Courchesne *et al.*, 1984, 1985). Autistic adolescents had significantly smaller responses to these nontask but novel stimuli than did normals.

Three of the studies described above (Courchesne *et al.*, 1984, 1985; Novick *et al.*, 1980) also reported P300 and P2 response amplitudes to the background stimuli among which the target or novel stimuli were embedded. Although there were usually no statistically significant group differences, these responses to background stimuli were in almost all cases smaller in the autistics than in the normal controls. For example, in the data of Courchesne *et al.* (1985), the P300 amplitudes of the autistics to target and novel stimuli were 43% and 34%, respectively, of the normal amplitudes, whereas the P300 amplitudes of the autistics to *background* stimuli in the auditory task and the auditory no-response-required experimental conditions were 52% and 31%, respectively, of the normal amplitudes. Thus, the reduced amplitude of the P300 response in autistics reflects a generally smaller evoked response, irrespective of the stimulus characteristics. In this regard,

Courchesne *et al.* (1985) also found significantly smaller N1 responses in autistics than in normals to target, novel, and also background auditory stimuli, suggesting nonspecific attentional differences, and Novick *et al.* (1980) found smaller P2 responses in autistics to background auditory stimuli presented alone. In view of these findings, smaller P300 responses in autistics cannot be interpreted as reflecting limited information processing unless it can be shown that the reduction in response to signal stimuli is proportionally smaller than the reduction in response to background stimuli. Courchesne *et al.* (1985) have demonstrated this for novel and target auditory stimuli but not for visual stimuli.

Since the amplitude of the P300 increases as a function of the confidence with which a stimulus is detected and the degree to which information about the stimulus is used (Hillyard, 1985), the interest of the subject in the novel or target stimuli relative to the stimulus context in which such stimuli are embedded will affect the amplitude of the P300 response. The general reduction of most evoked response components to background stimuli in autistics suggests that the reduced P300 response to specific stimuli must be interpreted in the context of the general response of the autistic subject to the total experimental environment. Therefore, it may be premature to interpret the P300 findings as unequivocally indicative of a dysfunction in information processing per se. The significantly smaller N1 responses to target, novel, and also background auditory stimuli found in autistics (Courchesne *et al.*, 1985) deserve consideration in regard to the issue of directed attention, since the "processing negativity" (Naatanen, 1982) or wave N_d (Hillyard, 1985) associated with selective attention can contribute to the amplitude of N1. This negativity in the event-related potential has an onset contiguous with that of wave N1, about 60 milliseconds poststimulus, and it increases with increased selective attention toward the stimulus. The generally smaller N1 amplitudes in autistics suggest that, relative to normal controls, the autistics were not directing their attention toward auditory features in the laboratory environment, whether the sounds were novel, targeted or not targeted, or background. The autistics may simply have had less interest in any auditory feature of the environment than the normals, suggesting a deficiency of the *intensive* and *sustaining* components of directed attention. These components, along with the *selective* component of directed attention, are described later in this chapter in the context of a neurophysiology of directed attention.

Neurophysiological Studies of Subcortical Activity

Neurophysiological studies of subcortical events are relevant to the autistic disturbances of sensory modulation and motility. These investigations have included autonomic, vestibular, and BAER studies. It has been proposed that the increased heart rate variability of autistic children may reflect reticular formation responses to insignificant stimuli (MacCulloch & Williams, 1971). Also, increased heart rate variability is greatest during autistic stereotypic behavior (Hutt, Forrest, &

Richer, 1975), linking dysmodulation of autonomic responsivity to the motility disturbances. Failure to habituate respiratory responses and enhancement of vascular responses to visual stimuli, indicating incapacity to reduce stimulus novelty and therefore sensory overload (James & Barry, 1980), link the abnormal autonomic responses to the disturbances of sensory modulation. The increased reactivity of autonomic responses may reflect the inability to "gate" or "filter" trivial sensory stimuli, thereby compromising appropriate selective attention. The vestibular response studies have demonstrated abnormal visual–vestibular interactions (Ornitz, Brown, Mason, & Putnam, 1974), prolonged time constants, and reduced secondary nystagmus (Ornitz, Atwell, Kaplan, & Westlake, 1985). Abnormalities of vestibular adaptation and the influence of excessive reverberation in multisynaptic brain stem pathways have been proposed to account for these findings (Ornitz, 1985).

Both the vestibular and autonomic responses distinguish autistic from normal populations rather than suggesting subgroups within the autistic population which show the abnormality. BAER studies, on the other hand, have not consistently demonstrated brain stem dysfunction; prolonged brain stem transmission times are found only in a minority of autistic children (Gillberg, Rosenhall, & Johansson, 1983; see reviews in Ornitz, 1983, 1985). The vestibular and autonomic responses probably involve widespread interconnecting neuronal fields within the brain stem. BAERs are responses of a subset of neurons within the brain stem. The mechanism underlying the autistic behavioral syndrome is likely to involve a system dysfunction rather than a pathological change in a specific group of neurons.

Some studies of the phasic activity of rapid eye movement (REM) sleep have also suggested a system dysfunction involving subcortical mechanisms. The quality of REM sleep was degraded in autistic children who showed a significant increase in sleep spindles (EEG components of non-REM sleep) during REM sleep and a significant reduction in the number of single REMs and in the precentage of REM sleep time taken up by REM bursts (Ornitz *et al.*, 1969). The significance of the EEG finding requires further evaluation, since sleep spindles have been reported during REM sleep in both normal adults (Gaillard & Blois, 1981) and mentally retarded children (Shibagaki, Kiyono, Watanabe, & Hakamada, 1982). The REM findings were only partially supported in subsequent studies. When sinusoidal vestibular stimulation was applied to the bed throughout the night, autistic children failed to show the progressive increase in the organization of the REMs into bursts that was characteristic of normal children (Ornitz, Forsythe, & de la Pena, 1973). Using a different definition of REM burst from that in the Ornitz *et al.* (1969) study—that is, the interval between any two successive eye movements should not exceed 1 second, rather than 3 seconds—and adjusting REM parameters for time of night, we (Tanguay, Ornitz, Forsythe, & Ritvo, 1976) found that the percentage of REM sleep time with bursts was not different in autistics and normal controls, but that the mean duration of the bursts was significantly longer in the autistics. In this respect the autistics were more like younger normal children, limiting the finding to a maturational delay.

Deficiencies in the organization of REMs into REM bursts in autistic children were not found in a recent study that evaluated the intervals between individual eye movements (Hashimoto & Tayama, 1984). These investigators did find a significant increase in the twitch movements recorded from the submental muscle in autistics (compared to normal controls) during stages 2, 3, and 4 and REM sleep when the muscular activity was expressed as a percentage of the activity occurring during stage 1 sleep. This finding, together with abnormalities in the circadian sleep–wake rhythm found in a study of 62 autistic children compared with their normal siblings (Segawa, 1985), suggests a possible disturbance in brain stem regulating mechanisms. The inconsistent findings from the several sleep studies indicate the need for greater attention to such factors as adaptation to the sleep laboratory environment, control for time from sleep onset, definition of REM bursts, and age of subjects.

Abnormal patterns of locomotion involving alterations in flexor–extensor dominance were found in 14 out of 17 autistics aged 3–13, suggesting a possible disturbance in descending brain stem influence over spinal mechanisms (Yamashita, Nagata, Nomura, & Segawa, 1986).

BRAIN STEM DYSFUNCTION MODEL OF AUTISM

In an attempt to integrate the evidence for both cortical and subcortical neurophysiological dysfunction, it has been proposed that the disturbances of sensory modulation and motility reflect the pathophysiological mechanism and that the other abnormal behavior can be understood as consequences of distorted sensory input (Ornitz, 1983, 1985). This suggests a neurophysiological dysfunction involving a cascading series of interacting neuronal loops in the brain stem and diencephalon that subserve modulation of sensory input. These include the brain stem reticular formation, the substantia nigra, specific and nonspecific thalamic nuclei, and the rostral projections from these structures to neostriatal and cortical structures (see review in Ornitz, 1983). Some of these same systems modulate motor output in response to sensory input, and their dysfunction may release the abnormal perseverative motility of infantile autism. In one animal model, lesions of the substantia nigra disrupt neostriatal inhibition of neuronal response to sensory input recorded at the centromedian–parafascicularis complex, while inducing repetitive stereotyped flexion–extension movements of the forepaw and arrests of ongoing purposeful activity (Dalsass & Krauthamer, 1981). Thus, dysmodulation of both sensory input and motor output (analogous to the abnormal reactions to sensation, the hand flapping, and the postural arrests of young autistic children) can be attributed to disruption of a complex interaction of mesencephalic, diencephalic, and neostriatal structures.

In addition to the role of brain stem mechanisms in sensory processing (and the modulation of motor expression), there is a broad base of data that also argues strongly for the role of the brain stem in the generation of adaptive behavior

(Berntson & Micco, 1976). In addition, neurophysiological studies of vocalization (Kirzinger & Jurgens, 1985; Larson & Kistler, 1984), and analyses of behavior and neuropathology in encephalitis lethargica, suggest that normal and abnormal language (such as the vocalizations in Tourette syndrome) can also be produced in brain stem centers (Devinksy, 1983). Stimulation and lesion studies suggest that brain stem mechanisms can not only integrate complex behavior, but also influence the function of more rostral levels. Berntson and Micco (1976) concluded that prosencephalic systems are "involved more in the further elaboration and control rather than the fundamental organization of adaptive behaviors" generated in the brain stem (p. 478). The development of generalized learning deficits following median raphe and pontine reticular formation lesions (Thompson, Gibbs, Ristic, Cotman, & Yu, 1986; Thompson, Ramsay, & Yu, 1984), and reduced exploratory and orienting behavior following mesencephalic reticular formation lesions (Mager, Mager, & Klingberg, 1983), provide further illustrations of this principle. Simon and Le Moal (1984) have suggested that a relatively small group of dopaminergic cells in the ventral mesencephalon influence cognition, emotion, and the initiation of motor responses through innervation of prefrontal cortex, septum, and nucleus accumbens. This group of neurons is described as a phylogenetically older regulatory system that, through dopaminergic activity, tunes, arouses, and organizes phylogenetically more recent cortical, limbic, and striatal integrating systems. After experimental destruction of the brain stem regulatory neurons, the integrating systems are characterized by "rigidity and automation."

NEUROPHYSIOLOGY OF NEGLECT

As we move rostrally from brain stem structures, we can observe replication, with elaboration and differentiation, of behavior generated in the brain stem. This is well demonstrated by the neurophysiology of attention and its disruption in neglect syndromes. In neglect syndromes, patients with unilateral brain injury may show neglect for events that occur within the contralateral half of space. Left-sided neglect after right-hemisphere lesions is more frequent and severe, and persists longer, than right-sided neglect following left-hemisphere lesions. This has suggested right-hemisphere specialization for directed attention (Mesulam, 1981, 1983). The right hemisphere attends to both contra- and ipsilateral stimuli, whereas the left hemisphere is more limited to contralateral attention. These clinically based observations have received experimental support from studies of alpha desynchronization after lateralized visual stimulation, lending support to the hypothesis that the right hemisphere is dominant for directed attention (Heilman & Van Den Abell, 1980). Consideration of the neglect syndromes facilitates expansion of the brain stem dysfunction model of autism to a model involving the interaction of neuronal activity generated in the brain stem with neuronal activity generated at higher levels of the neuraxis. This expanded model emphasizes the right hemisphere, where specialization for directed attention, the use of prosodic (nonverbal) aspects of communication, and the recognition of emotion all occur. It is in these same functions that autistics show severe and persisting deficits.

Neglect of contralateral hemispace can be induced by lesions—particularly in the right hemisphere (Heilman & Van Den Abell, 1980); in pontine, mesencephalic, and thalamic reticular structures; in basal ganglia; and in cingulate, frontal, and parietal cortex (Mesulam, 1981, 1983). In reticular neglect, attentional deficits reflect tonic disturbances of vigilance. Following mesencephalic reticular formation lesions, "neglect is secondary to an inability of sensory stimuli to alert an organism, resulting from a corticolimbic reticular activating disconnection" (Watson, Heilman, Miller, & King, 1974, p. 296). Thalamic neglect may be characterized by hypokinesia associated with disruption of nonspecific thalamic reticular pathways to cortical, particularly cingulate, structures. There is a reduction of arousal and motor response to novel or painful stimuli (Schott, Laurent, Mauguiere, & Chazot, 1981; Watson, Valenstein & Heilman, 1981). Cingulectomy induces neglect (Watson, Heilman, Cauthern, & King, 1973), which may reflect the added dimension of "loss in the perception of biological importance associated with events in the contralateral hemispace" (Mesulam, 1981, p. 318). Frontal (Heilman & Valenstein, 1972) and perhaps striatal neglect (A. R. Damasio, Damasio, & Chui, 1980) add an additional motor component, a "hypokinesia for exploration and manipulation within the contralateral hemispace" (Mesulam, 1981, p. 317). Parietal neglect is particularly a defect of spatial awareness and perception, involving a deficit of directed attention to events in contralateral hemispace (Mesulam, 1981, 1983). The deficit has been attributed to an inability to disengage attention from its current focus before attention can be diverted to a new event (Posner, Walker, Friedrich, & Rafal, 1984). Thus the neglect syndrome is manifested at every level of the neuraxis, from mesencephalic reticular formation to high-order association cortex, with dysfunction at higher levels elaborating the attentional deficit associated with pathology at lower levels.

Based on studies of patients with right- or left-hemisphere lesions at various levels of the neuraxis, Heilman, Bowers, Valenstein, and Watson (1986) have characterized unilateral neglect as "an attention–arousal–activation defect caused by dysfunction in a corticolimbic–reticular loop" (p. 702). They note that since "neglect occurs more often after right hemisphere lesions . . . the right hemisphere may be dominant for mediating an attention–arousal response" (p. 702). Heilman *et al.* (1986) have reviewed a large body of evidence from neurophysiological and neuropsychological studies of patients with right-hemisphere disease, which suggests that such patients show emotional indifference and have "dramatically smaller arousal responses (galvanic skin response) than aphasic patients with left hemisphere disease or control patients without hemispheric lesions" (p. 701). Thus the neglect syndromes suggest an association between deficits of arousal and activation and deficits of emotion, secondary to right-hemisphere dysfunction—as association that prepares the way for the following discussions of the neurophysiology of directed attention and its dysfunction in autism. It will be seen that directed attention requires both a state of activation–arousal and a state of heightened emotion in relation to attended features of the environment. It will also be seen that these functions reside in interconnected loops involving cortical, limbic, and reticular structures that, in the right hemisphere, are involved in the neglect syndromes.

NEUROPHYSIOLOGY OF DIRECTED ATTENTION

Now we can consider the neurophysiology of information processing and speculate on its relationship to the autistic syndrome. As we move rostrally from midbrain and diencephalic structures, modulated sensation assumes increasingly complex informational value, and this requires directed attention. Directed attention involves a *selective process* for distinguishing the relevant from the trivial; an *intensive process* that determines the distribution of attention across a set of stimuli, by attaching value to certain stimuli; and an *alerting and sustaining process* that involves vigilance (i.e., the energy sustaining the attentional state) (Davies, 1983; Posner, 1975). In addition, there is a motor component to these perceptual processes, enabling and modulating perceptual activity (e.g., visual scanning).

In the posterior parietal cortex, the inferior parietal lobule mediates functions involving directed attention to stimuli of emotional significance (Lynch, 1980; Mesulam, 1981, 1983; Mesulam, Van Hoesen, Pandya, & Geschwind, 1977). Within the inferior parietal lobule, the area designated PG appears to integrate sensory input transmitted from polymodal association cortex and thalamic centers, limbic input, and reticular input (Mesulam, 1981, 1983). Output is to regions involved with motor responses (such as visual scanning and reaching) to emotionally significant stimuli (Mesulam, 1983). Mountcastle and his colleagues (Motter & Mountcastle, 1981; Mountcastle, Andersen, & Motter, 1981) have described light-sensitive cells within PG that receive ambient (nonfoveal) visual input from the retinal periphery through retinocollicular pathways (Benevento & Fallon, 1975), providing for the redirection of attention from one foveated object to the next. They have proposed that these neurons generate an internal neural construction of surrounding space, and objects in it, in relation to the position and movement of one's own body within that space. Two types of ambient (nonfoveal) vision may provide the necessary input. Egocentric ambient vision locates objects in the environment in respect to the observer; exteroceptive ambient vision orients the observer in respect to his or her position in space (Dichgans, 1977). Both functions depend on input from the peripheral retina as it sweeps the environment and interpretation by the light-sensitive (optokinetic) cells of area PG (Motter & Mountcastle, 1981). Mesulam (1983) has reviewed the experimental data documenting the motivational aspects of these scanning behaviors. Neurons in the inferior parietal lobule "increase firing when the animal detects, looks at, or reaches toward a motivationally relevant" (Mesulam, 1983, p. 384) object. Thus the activity of certain neurons in the inferior parietal lobule is contingent upon novel sensory input, motivational relevance, motor responses toward novel input of interest (e.g., looking and reaching), and also the level of vigilance.

Such neuronal activity is the neurophysiological basis of directed attention. The area PG in fact receives inputs from polymodal sensory association cortex, limbic structures, and reticular structures, and sends efferents to frontal eye fields, striatum, and superior colliculus—areas involved with looking, reaching, and other perceptual activities (Mesulam, 1983). Its neurons obey a "sensory contingency," responding to sensory events; a "motor contingency," providing the motility necessary for directed attention; and a "limbic contingency," or a sensitivity to emotional relevance (Mesulam, 1983). Thus, the inputs and outputs to this area provide the essential circuitry for directed attention. The selective process depends on the sensory input from polymodal association cortex and polymodal thalamic structures (e.g., the pulvinar) involved in selective attention (Mesulam, 1983; Mesulam et al., 1977; Petersen, Robinson, & Keys, 1985). The intensive process depends on the limbic input, particularly from the cingulate cortex (Mesulam, 1983; Mesulam et al., 1977). The alerting and sustaining process depends on reticular input from nonspecific thalamic and brain stem regions (Mesulam, 1983; Mesulam et al., 1977). The efferents provide the necessary motor components of directed attention, for directed attention, as Mesulam (1981) points out, is not merely seeing, hearing, and feeling, but looking, listening, and touching.

As already indicated, disruption of directed attention is manifested as neglect. Neglect, which is recognized as lack of an appropriate motor response to a sensory event, may have a sensory or motor component or both. Neglect can be due to a loss of *attention* to stimuli, so that a motor response is not made to the unattended stimuli; or it can be due to loss of *intention* to perform a motor response to perceived stimuli. Watson, Miller, and Heilman (1978) have demonstrated experimentally that neglect induced by either frontal or reticular formation lesions is characterized by a defect of (motor) intention rather than (sensory) attention. They found no difference in the intentional deficits produced by the cortical or subcortical lesions. Simon and Le Moal (1984, 1985) have described a dopaminergic mechanism by which neurons in the ventral mesencephalon regulate the function and interaction of prefrontal cortical, limbic, and striatal centers. This reticular modulation of higher centers regulates the process of attention in prefrontal and associated medial striatal centers and the process of intention in limbic and associated lateral striatal centers (Simon & Le Moal, 1985). Thus, brain stem reticular structures that provide the energy for the alerting and sustaining process underlying directed attention (Davies, 1983) influence both the sensory (attention) and motor (intention) contingencies obeyed by inferior parietal lobule neurons as they mediate the process of directed attention (Mesulam, 1983). Simon and Le Moal (1985) attribute the intentional component to the intensive process underlying directed attention.

Among the various structures considered here as participating in the neurophysiology of directed attention, Margulies (1985) has attributed the attentional component of directed attention almost exclusively to the hippocampus and the intentional component to the nucleus accumbens. A pathway from hippocampus via the subiculum to nucleus accumbens projects to substantia innominata and provides limbic input to the area PG in the inferior parietal lobule (Mesulam & Geschwind, 1978), paralleling the limbic input to this same area from cingulate cortex. Such a pathway is likely to contribute substantially to the process of directed attention, particularly to the intensive process. However, directed attention is a complex neuropsychological construct that is more likely to be distributed throughout the neural structures discussed in this section than to be localized to one specific pathway.

DEVIANT AND DEFICIENT DIRECTED ATTENTION IN AUTISM

Autistic children suffer from severe distortions of directed attention and fail to sustain appropriate motor responses, such as eye contact to socially relevant stimuli. Deficient and deviant eye contact is a cardinal symptom of autism. The failure to maintain an interested fixation of gaze can readily be attributed to a failure of neuronal linkage in the inferior parietal lobule; that is, the limbic contribution to motivated selective attention or the reticular energy to maintain a vigilant state of interest in the environment, or both, are deficient. However, the abnormalities of autistic eye contact are characterized not only by deficient gaze, but also by abnormally protracted fixation. This is most apparent in response to spinning and whirling objects. It is particularly interesting that neurons in area PG of the inferior parietal lobule respond uniquely to rotation of visual stimuli (Sakata, Shibutani, Ito, & Turugai, 1986). Could the perseverative interest of young autistic children in spinning and whirling objects be attributed to dysfunctional input to cells in the inferior parietal lobule?

On the output side, the efferents from the inferior parietal lobule to the frontal eye fields (Mesulam, 1983) and from there to pontine reticular gaze control centers (Schnyder, Reisine, Hepp, & Henn, 1985) would not convey sufficient information. This could compromise presaccadic activity and voluntary control over eye movements, which reside in the cortex of the frontal eye fields (Bruce & Goldberg, 1984).[1] Alternatively, autistic behavior such as the deficient and deviant eye contact could result from inadequate reticular regulation of prefrontal (perhaps also including frontal eye fields), limbic, and striatal mechanisms involved in the attentional (seeing, hearing, feeling) and intentional (looking, listening, touching, and reaching) aspects of directed attention. Whether attributed to dysfunction of very high-level integration of sensory, limbic, and reticular inputs

1. Similar suggestions regarding dysfunction in the frontal eye fields and the modulation of visual attention have been made for schizophrenia (Levin, 1984), and the development course of some autistic children leads to a schizophrenic outcome (Petty, Ornitz, Michelman, & Zimmerman, 1984).

to parietal cortex, or to reticular dysmodulation of prefrontal–limbic–striatal circuitry, the deviant and distorted directed attention in autism involves both attentional and intentional components.

The deviant directed attention in autism may underlie the autistic emotional,
cognitive, and language deficits. Bear (1983) has described patients with right-
hemisphere lesions who fail to detect and sustain attention to emotionally significant stimuli, and therefore fail to develop appropriate emotional responses. This
failure of emotional surveillance has been attributed by Bear (1983) to dysfunction
of the same neuronal system under consideration here, with extension through
efferents from the inferior parietal lobule via the cingulate cortex to dorsolateral
prefrontal cortex.

The complexity, extensiveness, and vagueness of prefrontal cortical function
(Stuss & Benson, 1984) precludes attribution of prefrontal dysfunction to specific
aspects of the autistic behavioral syndrome. However, the hypokinesia, lack of
initiative and spontaneity, and compulsive repetition of initiated behavior (perseveration) seen in frontal lobe syndromes (Stuss & Benson, 1984) is similar to the
behavior of some autistic patients, particularly those who are more severely retarded. It is also noteworthy that just as the inferior parietal lobule receives con-
verging sensory, limbic, and reticular input, the prefrontal cortex receives sensory
input from thalamic afferents, limbic input from amygdala, and reticular input
from brain stem neurons (Sarter & Markowitsch, 1984).

Both Bear (1983) and Mesulam (1983) have reviewed the evidence suggesting
that the function under consideration, the ability to direct attention toward emotionally relevant stimuli in the environment, is more strongly represented in the
right hemisphere. Heilman *et al.* (1986) have demonstrated the association between the states of activation–arousal (the alerting and sustaining process of directed attention) and emotional responsiveness (the intensive process of directed
attention), which reside in right-hemisphere mechanisms. Also represented in the
right hemisphere are the capacities to recognize the nonverbal components of
certain types of emotional expression, particularly those emanating from facial
expression (Benowitz *et al.*, 1983; Natale, Gur, & Gur, 1983; Ross, 1984; Rueter-
Lorentz, Givis, & Moscovitch, 1983), and to produce and modulate the affective
components of prosody and gesture (i.e., nonverbal communication) (Ross, 1981,
1984; Ross & Mesulam, 1979).[2] The severe autistic deficiencies in directed attention, in the use and recognition of nonverbal communication (particularly the
prosodic aspects of speech, gesture, and expression), and in the recognition of

2. See also Rinn (1984) for alternative hypotheses in respect to the production of facial expression. The representation of emotional recognition and expression in the two hemispheres is complex.
There is evidence that the right hemisphere is specialized for the perception of emotional valence and
negative emotion, whereas the left hemisphere is biased toward positive (e.g., happiness-producing)
emotional stimuli (Natale *et al.*, 1983; Rueter-Lorenz *et al.*, 1983). Nevertheless, right-hemisphere
damage seriously impairs the evaluation of nonverbal emotional stimuli, whereas major left-hemisphere damage leads to significantly milder deficits (Benowitz *et al.*, 1983).

emotional valence all suggest right-hemisphere dysfunction.[3] Weintraub and Mesulam (1983) have described a group of patients with neurological and neuropsychological evidence of right-hemisphere dysfunction, emotional and interpersonal difficulties, and pathological shyness, who, while not considered autistic, shared many features with high-functioning communicative autistics: namely, poor eye contact, deficient use of prosody and gesture, inability to display emotion, poor social perception, and social isolation. Voeller (1986) has described a group of children with neurological or CT scan evidence of right-hemisphere lesions or dysfunction who failed to understand social nuances, had atypical prosody (e.g., "monotonous, robot-like intonations"), rocked, and failed to make adequate eye contact.

NEUROPHYSIOLOGICAL MODEL FOR DYSFUNCTION AT THE INTERFACE BETWEEN SENSORY AND INFORMATION PROCESSING IN AUTISM

As indicated in Figure 8-1, brain stem and diencephalic centers project rostrally to telencephalic structures. In particular, the inferior parietal lobule and the neostriatum receive inputs from the brain stem reticular formation, raphe nuclei, and nucleus locus ceruleus, either directly or via thalamic intralaminar nuclei or limbic pathways through the hippocampal formation and cingulate cortex. Together with efferents to the frontal eye fields, striatum, and superior colliculus, the neuronal connectivity in the area PG (particularly in the right hemisphere) provides the neurophysiological basis for directed attention as proposed by Mesulam (1981, 1983).

I have previously suggested that dysmodulation of sensory input in brain stem and reticular diencephalic structures could explain the autistic behavioral responses to both simple and complex sensory stimuli and provide the basis for an autistic disorder of sensory processing (Ornitz, 1983, 1985). Figure 8-1 indicates the widespread reticular input to telencephalic structures where information processing takes place. The suggested interface between sensory processing and information processing is to be found in the same functional neuroanatomy that Mesulam (1983) has described for directed attention. The basic behavioral disorder

3. An older hypothesis of left-hemisphere dysfunction in autism (Hoffman & Prior, 1982; Prior & Bradshaw, 1979; Tanguay, 1976) was based on a too narrowly drawn clinical picture of autism as a language and cognitive disorder (Rutter, 1974, 1978). The inadequacies of this position have been discussed (Fein *et al.*, 1984; Ornitz, 1983). Others (e.g., Dawson, 1988) have argued for the role of left-hemisphere dysfunction in autism, and the more recent emphasis on right-hemisphere dysfunction need not exclude consideration of the left hemisphere. The intellectual deficiencies, particularly the symbolic deficiencies, associated with autism suggest left-hemisphere dysfunction. Dawson (1988) has postulated dysfunction of a complex developmentally determined interaction between the two hemispheres in autism. Much work will be needed to determine whether such a pathological process is intrinsic to cortical disturbance or is initiated by brain stem dysfunction, which could affect both right and left cortical regions.

AUTISM: AT THE INTERFACE BETWEEN SENSORY
AND INFORMATION PROCESSING

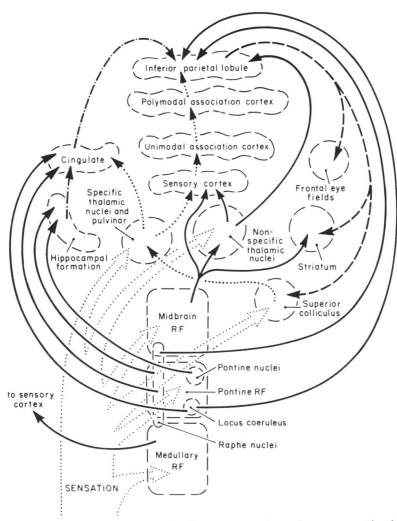

FIGURE 8-1. Schematic representation of the three major ascending pathways—sensory (dotted lines), limbic (dot-and-dash lines), and reticular (solid lines)—that uniquely converge on cells in area PG in the inferior parietal lobule (Mesulam, 1981, 1983; Mesulam *et al.*, 1977). Efferents (dashed lines) project to frontal eye fields, superior colliculus, and striatum. For simplicity, limbic–striatal pathways; important interconnections between frontal eye fields, striatum, and superior colliculus; prefrontal cortical connections; and all the reciprocal pathways are not shown.

in autistic children can be described equally well as "deviant and distorted directed attention"[4] or as "dysfunction at the interface between sensory processing and information processing."

The following review of the neurophysiological connections represented in Figure 8-1 encompasses those structures and connections that subserve the several processes and components of directed attention discussed in this chapter. The possible contributions of dysfunction at some of these levels to the suggested disorder of directed attention in autism are indicated. The alerting and sustaining process utilizes reticular and reticular–limbic connections. The intensive process involves limbic afferent and efferent pathways and is centered around limbic, particularly hippocampal, function. The selective process takes place at all levels, but is particularly centered in polymodal thalamocortical connections to parietal structures. Hippocampal function, modulated by brain stem influence, reflects the intertwined sensory (attentional) and motor (intentional) components of directed attention. The parietal efferents to frontal eye fields, superior colliculus, and basal ganglia provide the circuitry by which the intentional component is effected.

Reticular Influence

The widespread brain stem influence on directed attention is carried to higher structures through numerous pathways, some of which are indicated in Figure 8-1. Reticular structures, the locus ceruleus, raphe nuclei, and pretectal region of the brain stem, along with intralaminar (IL) thalamic nuclei, project directly to the inferior parietal lobule (area PG) (Mesulam *et al.*, 1977). Raphe nuclei also project to IL and other thalamic nuclei (Peschanski & Besson, 1984). Serotonin derived from the dorsal raphe nucleus inhibits transmission in the reticular and lateral geniculate nuclei of the thalamus (Yoshida, Sasa, & Takaori, 1984). Midbrain reticular formation (MRF) neurons may project to cortex via IL synapses (Eberhart, Morrell, Krieger, & Pfaff, 1985; Steriade & Glenn, 1982). MRF stimulation produces metabolic activation in IL and other thalamic structures while inducing metabolic suppression of cortical and limbic structures (Gonzalez-Lima & Scheich, 1985). Thalamic structures, through the reticular nucleus of the thalamus, feed back upon the MRF (Parent & Steriade, 1984).

Dysfunction of reticular brain stem mechanisms and their projection to higher centers could be responsible for the autistic inability to modulate sensory input, resulting in the under- and overreactivity to sensory stimuli.

Reticular–Limbic Connections

Reticular influence is also conveyed rostrally to limbic structures via thalamic relays (Baleydier & Mauguiere, 1985; Finch, Derian, & Babb, 1984a, 1984b),

4. Such *deviant and distorted* directed attention is not to be confused with merely *deficient* directed attention (i.e., distractibility), as seen, for example, in children with attention deficit disorders.

which may be regulated by cholinergic mechanisms (Sofroniew, Priestley, Consolazione, Eckenstein, & Cuello, 1985; Vogt, 1984). There are also direct connections to limbic structures from brain stem regions that both receive sensory input and modulate sensory processing in higher structures by the reticular control of vigilance during directed attention (Mesulam, 1983). Other brain stem–limbic pathways modulate complex behaviors. These include projections from midbrain central gray (Eberhart *et al.*, 1985) and pontine noradrenergic and medullary neurotensin-producing regions (Kawakami *et al.*, 1984) to amygdala. The amygdaloid complex projects to the hippocampal formation (Finch *et al.*, 1986; Krettek & Price, 1977) through a disynaptic relay in entorhinal cortex, where it modulates corticohippocampal neurotransmission (Thomas, Assaf, & Iverson, 1984). Pathways involved in directed attention include serotonergic (Crunelli & Segal, 1985; Moore & Halaris, 1975; Winson, 1984; Zhou & Azmitia, 1983) and also nonserotonergic projections (Crunelli & Segal, 1985) from the median raphe nuclei to hippocampus; noradrenergic projections from locus ceruleus (Jones & Moore, 1977, Winson, 1984) to hippocampus; and ventral mesencephalic dopaminergic projections to hippocampus (Simon & Le Moal, 1984). These and other projections from the brain stem to the hippocampus may modulate the excitability of hippocampal neurons through a process of neuronal gating, which alters information flow through the hippocampus according to the behavioral state, which in turn is determined by the brain stem activity (Winson, 1984).

These reticular–limbic reciprocal interconnections integrate the alerting and sustaining process and the intensive process of directed attention. Dysfunction at the level of these interconnections could be the neurophysiological substrate of the autistic failure to invest attended aspects of the environment with the appropriate emotional cathexis. In the next several sections, the mechanisms by which the limbic-mediated intensive process of directed attention subserves information processing are described. Dysfunction of these reticular–limbic connections could result in distortions of information processing at limbic levels of the neuraxis; such dysfunction could be manifested in the cognitive and language disturbances of autism as the distorted information is transmitted to higher cortical levels of the neuraxis.

Modulation of Hippocampal Theta Rhythm, Information Processing, and Directed Attention

Lasting changes in synaptic function in the dentate gyrus can be induced by MRF stimulation (Bloch & Laroche, 1985), and brain stem stimulation modulates the frequency and spectral characteristics of the hippocampal theta rhythm according to the density of impulses arriving at the hippocampus (Arnolds, Lopes de Silva, Boeijinga, Kamp, & Aitink, 1984). Information processing (e.g., spatial memory) in the hippocampus is dependent on the integrity of the hippocampal theta rhythm (Winson, 1984), which is frequency-modulated by pontine reticular formation (synchronization) and median raphe (desynchronization) neurons (Vertes, 1982).

There are at least two components to the hippocampal theta rhythm, and these are related to behavior (Buzsaki, Rappelsberger, & Kellenyi, 1985). The behavioral immobility in response to novel and frightening stimuli and the accompanying changes in hippocampal theta rhythm are mediated by a septohippocampal cholinergic mechanism (B. H. Bland, Seto, Sinclair & Fraser, 1984; S. K. Bland & Bland, 1986), with further modulation by inhibitory noradrenergic and serotonergic influences arising in the brain stem (Fontani & Farabollini, 1984). The septal pathway conveys modulating striatal influence over the hippocampal theta rhythm (Sabatino, Ferraro, Liberti, Vella, & La Grutta, 1985; Sabatino, Savatteri, Liberti, Vella, & La Grutta, 1986); this striatal influence is in turn modulated by limbic input via the nucleus accumbens (Taghzouti, Simon, Louilot, Herman, & Le Moal, 1985). Behavior that involves locomotion and head movement is accompanied by hippocampal theta, which is mediated by a perforant pathway noncholinergic influence (Vanderwolf, Leung, & Cooley, 1985). This complex modulation is subject to saturation effects (desynchronization) from excessive input, the type of sensory input, and species differences (Arnolds et al., 1984). Arnolds et al. (1984) have also drawn attention to the fact that the hippocampal theta reflects both the sensory input *and* the motor output associated with orienting behavior. Thus the brain stem–hippocampal linkage reflects the intertwined sensory *and* motor components of directed attention, as discussed by Mesulam (1983) in respect to the connectivity of area PG in the inferior parietal lobule.

Limbic Afferents and Efferents

The hippocampal formation sends subicular projections to the cingulate cortex (Finch et al., 1984a), where there is excitatory synaptic integration with thalamic afferents (Finch et al., 1984b). Brain stem influence is transmitted rostrally to cingulate cortex via hippocampal synaptic networks, where increasingly complex sensory and information processing takes place. Other brain stem pathways, including raphe nuclei, locus ceruleus, substantia nigra, and tegmentum, transmit input directly to cingulate cortex (see reviews in Calvo & Fernandez-Guardiola, 1984; Finch et al., 1984a). From cingulate cortex, information that has received extensive limbic and reticular processing is transmitted to the inferior parietal lobule (Mesulam et al., 1977; Pandya, Van Hoesen, & Mesulam, 1981) for integration with highly processed sensory input from polymodal association cortex and direct input from brain stem reticular structures (Mesulam, 1983). A parallel limbic pathway to area PG in the inferior parietal lobule goes from hippocampus to nucleus accumbens to substantia innominata to area PG (Mesulam & Geschwind, 1978). At several levels, there are reciprocal pathways through which the higher cortical centers may modify the input received from lower centers. These include cingulate cortex projections to periaqueductal gray, ventral pontine nuclei, the lateral tegmental region, and the superior colliculus (Wyss & Sripanidkulchai,

1984), and inferior parietal lobule projections to cingulate cortex (Pandya & Kuypers, 1969).

The "Limbic Contingency" and the Intensive Process of Directed Attention

The "limbic" structures, including the hippocampal formation and its connections with amygdala, entorhinal cortex, cingulate cortex, and septum, are of considerable theoretical importance to the central hypothesis of this chapter: that autism can be understood as a disorder of directed attention or a dysfunction at the interface between sensory and information processing. These structures provide the "limbic contingency" (i.e., the "motivational relevance") to the process of directed attention (Mesulam, 1983) by attaching relative value to stimuli. They can be understood to comprise the neuronal circuitry underlying the intensive process (Davies, 1983) of directed attention. As just described, the limbic structures convey sensory input modulated by brain stem to the highest levels of association cortex, particularly area PG within the inferior parietal lobule; and limbic function, particularly in the hippocampal formation, is subject to extremely complex modulation by brain stem structures. In addition to the hypothesis put forward in this chapter—that in autism the distorted direction of attention to environmental stimuli (i.e., the deficient and deviant emotional cathexis toward both people and things) can be attributed to dysfunction in the brain stem–limbic–neocortical processing of sensory input—there is also histoanatomical evidence from one autistic brain of limbic neuropathology (Bauman & Kemper, 1985). The principal findings were increased neuronal cell-packing density throughout the hippocampal formation and mammillary bodies; also involved were parts of the entorhinal cortex, amygdala, and septum, but not the cingulate or parietal cortices or brain stem. The pathological findings were attributed by the investigators to early prenatal changes rather than to other factors, such as the history of seizure disorder and both anticonvulsive and neuroleptic medication in this single autistic adult. If replicated, this finding would provide anatomical evidence of a disruption in the processing of sensory input at one of the levels of the neuraxis where sensory processing takes on the attributes of information processing.

Parietal Efferents and the Intentional (Motor) Component of Directed Attention

The efferents from the inferior parietal lobule, in addition to feeding back on the sensory, limbic, and reticular structures from which it receives highly processed sensory input, project to the frontal eye fields, superior colliculus, and striatum—areas involved in the motor aspects of directed attention, particularly looking and reaching toward objects of interest (Mesulam, 1981, 1983). Autistic children utilize looking and reaching, but these behaviors are often deviant and distorted (e.g., the autistic child's absence of eye-to-eye contact, coupled with intense staring at his or her own hand movements or spinning objects).

Frontal Eye Fields, Superior Colliculus, and Their Connections: Deviant Eye Contact in Autism

The frontal eye fields contain visual cells that fire whether or not a saccade occurs in response to a visual stimulus, movement cells that discharge just before responsive saccades, and visual–movement cells that fire tonically from the onset of the visual stimulus until the responsive saccade is made (Bruce & Goldberg, 1984). The presaccadic responses of these cells are enhanced during attention, as are the cells of posterior parietal cortex that project to them. The parietal cells also show enhancement during attention that is independent of saccadic activity (Goldberg & Bruce, 1985). Thus the parietal cells appear to be involved in the preparation for focused attention, whereas the frontal eye fields are involved in the act of focusing attention. The ability of the frontal eye fields to elicit eye movements, and the size of the eye movements, are modulated by the degree to which active fixation on environment stimuli occurs (Goldberg, Bushnell, & Bruce, 1986). Limbic input, processed by parietal structures as described earlier or transmitted directly to frontal eye fields (Barbas & Mesulam, 1981), may provide the motivational relevance for these attentional processes. Could the deviant eye contact of autistic children reflect a disturbed component of one or more of these processes?

In addition to their projections to striatum and thalamus (Kunzle & Akert, 1977) and pontine gaze control centers (Schnyder et al., 1985), the frontal eye fields project to the superior colliculus (Bruce & Goldberg, 1984; Kunzle & Akert, 1977), which also receives direct projections from cells in area PG of the interior parietal lobule (Mesulam, 1983). Along with the pontine centers, the superior colliculus mediates eye movement activity generated in the frontal eye fields. This brain stem structure receives visual input, projects that input rostrally for cortical processing via thalamic nuclei (Benevento & Fallon, 1975), and appears to be instrumental in mediating the utilization of ambient (nonfoveal) vision during directed attention (Lines & Milner, 1985)—a process that is elaborated by the light-sensitive cells of area PG in parietal cortex (Motter & Mountcastle, 1981). Here we have an example of the elaboration but not the replacement of a brain stem function by a cortical mechanism. The autistic failure to make eye contact seems to be both a failure to redirect attention from one foveated target to another and to maintain gaze toward targets (i.e., faces) that should be motivationally relevant. Such disturbed behavior suggests a system disturbance of the mechanisms by which ambient (nonfoveal, peripheral retinal) visual input stimulates refoveation. Such a system disturbance is not likely to be localized, since it involves sensory, motor, and motivational components (the sensory, motor, and limbic contingencies of inferior parietal lobule neurons as suggested by Mesulam [1983]), and a distribution across both brain stem and cortical structures.

Basal Ganglia and Their Collicular, Limbic, and Reticular Connections

The superior colliculus, in addition to mediating visual attention, is also involved with the integration of visual and auditory information (King & Palmer, 1985), and is intimately involved with nonvisual motor behavior through nigral connections with the striatum. A pathway from neostriatum to substantia nigra pars reticulata to superior colliculus (Beckstead, 1983) mediates circling behavior (Vaccarino, Franklin, & Prupas, 1985) and tonic electromyographic (EMG) activity (Ellenbroek, Schwarz, Sontag, Jaspers, & Cools, 1985) initiated in substantia nigra pars compacta. While the striatum functions in the preparation for the execution and guidance of voluntary movement (Groves, 1983), caudate cells also respond to simple sensory stimuli (Schneider & Lidsky, 1981; Strecker, Steinfels, Abercrombie, & Jacobs, 1985), and there are some caudate cells that only respond when sensory stimuli are behaviorally significant (Rolls, Thorpe, & Maddison, 1983). Evarts, Kimura, Wurtz, and Hikosaka (1984) and Schneider (1984) have stressed that the responses of many basal ganglia neurons are contingent on the behavioral relevance of the sensory input or the movement to be initiated. This motivation could be provided directly to the striatum by limbic input via amygdalostriatal projections (Kelley, Domesick, & Nauta, 1982) and hippocampal connections to the nucleus accumbens (Nauta, 1982), or indirectly via descending limbic modulation of brain stem dopaminergic and serotonergic innervations of the striatum (Louilot, Simon, Taghzouti, & Le Moal, 1985; Nauta, 1982). The amygdalostriatal projections could mediate the outward (i.e., motor) expression of emotion (Russchen, Bakst, Amaral, & Price, 1985), and disruption of limbic–striatal connections by lesions of nucleus accumbens results in a syndrome of perseveration, decreased behavioral flexibility, and reduced behavioral initiation (Taghzouti *et al.*, 1985). Dysfunction in these limbic–striatal pathways could contribute to the autistic deficits in conveying emotion, as through facial expression, and to the autistic intolerance of change and novelty.

Schneider (1984) has further emphasized the role of the basal ganglia in sensory modulation, particularly the control of the access of sensory input to regions concerned with motor expression. This "sensory gating" concerns both the shifting of attention among sensory inputs and the consequent effect on motor activity. Such attentional effects on motor response may have a motivational aspect mediated by the limbic–striatal influences just described. Feedback could occur via striatal–limbic projections—for example, septal and pallidal cholinergic pathways to cingulate cortex (Stewart, MacCabe, & Leung, 1985), interacting with thalamic–cingulate projections (Finch *et al.*, 1984b). Conceptualized in this way, the basal ganglia would subserve the same function of directed attention that

Mesulam (1983) has attributed to parietal cortical structures and that Berntson and Micco (1976) have attributed to brain stem structures. Again we see the replication but not the replacement of the function of more caudal and phylogenetically older systems of behavioral expression and control by more rostral and recent systems (Jackson, 1884/1958). Although Schneider (1984) stresses the influence of basal ganglia on brain stem as well as other structures, the direction of influence appears to be reciprocal. For example, a brain stem structure (the locus coeruleus) inhibits basal ganglia responses to nigral or limbic input through noradrenergic mechanisms (Fujimoto, Sasa, & Takaori, 1981; Unemoto, Sasa, & Takaori, 1985).

CONCLUSIONS

It is not possible at the present time, and may not be necessary, to attribute autistic behavior exclusively to dysfunction of one or another neurobehavioral level—brain stem, limbic, striatal, or cortical.[5] Instead, we can conceptualize a general principle of central nervous system organization of the mechanisms mediating directed attention. This organization involves sensory modulation, behavioral relevance (motivation), reticular activation, and motility directed toward the source of the sensory input. It is stratified in a hierarchical fashion, with phylogenetically newer structures elaborating the activity of older structures by providing increasing levels of behavioral differentiation and diversity. As a corollary of this increasing complexity, sensory processing at more primitive, caudal levels takes on the characteristics of information processing at newer, more rostral levels. Autism may be the disease that is a manifestation of dysfunction of this sensory-processing–information-processing system—a system that is distributed throughout the central ner-

5. It may be relevant to consider the cerebellum in this context, since in the same autistic brain in which Kemper described hippocampal histopathology, he also observed atrophy of the neocerebellar cortex, with marked loss of Purkinje cells, and reduced numbers of neurons in the cerebellar roof nuclei (Bauman & Kemper, 1985). Professor Arnold Scheibel (Ritvo et al., 1986) has replicated the Purkinje cell finding in four additional autistic brains. The cerebellum, like brain stem, limbic, striatal, and cerebral cortical structures, also appears to be involved in the modulation of attentional mechanisms and complex behavior, since stimulation of cerebellar cortex modulates midbrain and forebrain sensory responses (Crispino & Bullock, 1984), and stimulation of a cerebellar efferent structure (the fastigial nucleus) modulates brain stem behavioral mechanisms (i.e., eating and grooming behavior) (Berntson & Paulucci, 1979). The loss of Purkinje cells in autistic brains, if replicated, could be related to dysfunction of a distributed sensory-processing–information-processing system or could be a functionally unrelated marker of some early embryological insult to the autistic fetal brain. Recent reports of enlargement of the fourth ventricle (Gaffney, Kuperman, Tsai, Minchin, & Hassanein, 1987) and reduced area of cerebellar vermal lobules VI and VII (Courchesne, Yeung-Courchesne, Press, Hesselink, & Jernigan, 1988) seen on magnetic resonance imaging (MRI) scans are also suggestive of cerebellar pathology. However, the latter investigation suffers from the use of "normal" controls that were defined as subjects with "normal" MRI scans (selected from a pool of scans that were done for clinical reasons); that is, the controls may not be representative of the true range of normality of MRI scans. Ritvo and Garber (in press) have recently failed to find cerebellar vermal differences between autistic patients and normal controls on MRI scans.

vous system but is arranged in a hierarchical manner, stratified by overlapping layers such that phylogenetically more recent and more rostral structures elaborate and also depend on the persisting activity of older and more caudal structures. In this model, hypotheses of rostrally and caudally directed sequences of pathoneurophysiological dysfunction in autism merge, so that autism can be explained in terms of dysfunction of brain stem and related diencephalic behavioral systems and the cascading impact of such dysfunction on selected higher neural structures that elaborate, refine, and modulate the activities of the lower centers. The autistic neurobehavioral dysfunction can be located at the interface between sensory processing and information processing.

Acknowledgments

My research described in this chapter was supported in part by National Institute of Mental Health Grant No. MH-29798, National Eye Institute Grant No. EY-02612, and the Alice and Julius Kantor Charitable Trust. Ellen Patton provided invaluable help in preparation of the manuscript and the References section.

References

Author. American Psychiatric Association. (1980). *Diagnostic and statistical manual of mental disorders* (3rd ed.). Washington, DC.

Arnold, G., & Schwartz, S. (1983). Hemispheric lateralization of language in autistic and aphasic children. *Journal of Autism and Developmental Disorders, 13*, 129–139.

Arnolds, D.E.A.T., Lopes de Silva, F. H., Boeijinga, P., Kamp, A., & Aitink, W. (1984). Hippocampal EEG and motor activity in the cat: The role of eye movements and body acceleration. *Behavioural Brain Research, 12*, 121–135.

Baleydier, C., & Mauguiere, F. (1985). Anatomical evidence for medial pulvinar connections with the posterior cingulate cortex, the retrosplenial area, and the posterior parahippocampal gyrus in monkeys. *Journal of Comparative Neurology, 232*, 219–228.

Barbas, H., & Mesulam, M.-M. (1981). Organization of afferent input to subdivisions of area 8 in the rhesus monkey. *Journal of Comparative Neurology, 200*, 407–431.

Bauman, M., & Kemper, T. L. (1985). Histoanatomic observations of the brain in early infantile autism. *Neurology, 35*, 866–874.

Bear, D. M. (1983). Hemispheric specialization and the neurology of emotion. *Archives of Neurology, 40*, 195–202.

Beckstead, R. M. (1983). Long collateral branches of substantia nigra pars reticulata axons to thalamus, superior colliculus and reticular formation in monkey and cat. *Neuroscience, 10*, 767–779.

Benevento, L. A., & Fallon, J. H. (1975). The ascending projections of the superior colliculus in the rhesus monkey (*Macaca mulatta*). *Journal of Comparative Neurology, 160*, 339–362.

Benowitz, L. I., Bear, D. M., Rosenthal, R., Mesulam, M.-M., Zaidel, E., & Sperry, R. W. (1983). Hemispheric specialization in nonverbal communication. *Cortex, 19*, 5–11.

Berntson, G. G., & Micco, D. J. (1976). Organization of brainstem behavioral systems. *Brain Research Bulletin, 1*, 471–483.

Berntson, G. G., & Paulucci, T. S. (1979). Fastigial modulation of brainstem behavioral mechanisms. *Brain Research Bulletin, 4*, 549–552.

Blackstock, E.G. (1978). Cerebral asymmetry and the development of early infantile autism. *Journal of Autism and Developmental Disorders, 8,* 339–353.

Bland, B. H., Seto, M. G., Sinclair, B. R., & Fraser, S. M. (1984). The pharmacology of hippocampal theta cells: Evidence that the sensory processing correlate is cholinergic. *Brain Research, 299,* 121–131.

Bland, S. K., & Bland, B. H. (1986). Medial septal modulation of hippocampal theta cell discharges. *Brain Research, 375,* 102–116.

Bloch, V., & Laroche, S. (1985). Enhancement of long-term potentiation in the rat dentate gyrus by post-trial stimulation of the reticular formation. *Journal of Physiology, 360,* 215–231.

Brown, W. T., Jenkins, E. C., Cohen, I. L., Fisch, G. S., Wolf-Schein, E. G., Gross, A., Waterhouse, L., Fein, D., Mason-Brothers, A., Ritvo, E., Ruttenberg, B. A., Bently, W., & Castells, S. (1986). Fragile X and autism: A multicenter survey. *American Journal of Medical Genetics, 23,* 341–352.

Bruce, C. J., & Goldberg, M. E. (1984). Physiology of the frontal eye fields. *Trends in Neuroscience, 7,* 436–441.

Buzsaki, G., Rappelsberger, P., & Kellenyi, L. (1985). Depth profiles of hippocampal rhythmic slow activity ("theta rhythm") depend on behaviour. *Electroencephalography and Clinical Neurophysiology, 61,* 77–88.

Calvo, J. M., & Fernandez-Guardiola, A. (1984). Phasic activity of the basolateral amygdala, cingulate gyrus, and hippocampus during REM sleep in the cat. *Sleep, 7,* 202–210.

Campbell, M., Rosenbloom, S., Perry, R., George, A. E., Dricheff, I. I., Anderson, L., Small, A. M., & Jennings, S. J. (1982). Computerized axial tomography in young autistic children. *American Journal of Psychiatry, 139,* 510–512.

Cohen, D. J., Caparulo, B. J., Shaywitz, B. A., & Bowers, M. B., Jr. (1977). Dopamine and serotonin metabolism in neuropsychiatrically disturbed children. *Archives of General Psychiatry, 34,* 545–550.

Cohen, D. J., Paul, R., & Volkmar, F. R. (1986). Issues in the classification of pervasive and other developmental disorders: Toward DSM-IV. *Journal of the American Academy of Child Psychiatry, 25,* 213–220.

Coleman, P. D., Romano, J., Lapham, I., & Simon, W. (1985). Cell counts in cerebral cortex of an autistic patient. *Journal of Autism and Developmental Disorders, 15,* 245–256.

Courchesne, E., Kilman, B. A., Galambos, R., & Lincoln, A. J. (1984). Autism: Processing of novel auditory information assessed by event-related brain potentials. *Electroencephalography and Clinical Neurophysiology, 59,* 238–248.

Courchesne, E., Lincoln, A. J., Kilman, B. A., & Galambos, R. (1985). Event-related brain potential correlates of the processing of novel visual and auditory information in autism. *Journal of Autism and Developmental Disorders, 15,* 55–76.

Courchesne, E., Yeung-Courchesne, R., Press, G. A., Hesselink, J. R., & Jernigan, T. L. (1988). Hypoplasia of cerebellar vermal lobules VI and VII in autism. *New England Journal of Medicine, 318,* 1349–1354.

Crispino, L., & Bullock, T. H. (1984). Cerebellum mediates modality-specific modulation of sensory responses of midbrain and forebrain in rat. *Proceedings of the National Academy of Sciences USA, 81,* 2917–2920.

Crunelli, V., & Segal, M. (1985). An electrophysiological study of neurones in the rat median raphe and their projections to septum and hippocampus. *Neuroscience, 15,* 47–60.

Dalsass, M., & Krauthamer, G. M. (1981). Behavioral alterations and loss of caudate modulation in the centrum medianum–parafascicular complex of the cat following electrolytic lesions of the substantia nigra. *Brain Research, 208,* 67–79.

Damasio, A. R. (1984). Editorial: Autism. *Archives of Neurology, 41,* 481.

Damasio, A. R., Damasio, H., & Chui, H. C. (1980). Neglect following damage to frontal lobe or basal ganglia. *Neuropsychologia, 18,* 123–132.

Damasio, H., Maurer, R. G., Damasio, A. R., & Chui, H. C. (1980). Computerized tomographic scan findings in patients with autistic behavior. *Archives of Neurology, 37,* 504–510.

Davies, D. R. (1983). Attention, arousal and effort. In A. Gale & J. A. Edwards (Eds.), *Physiological correlates of human behaviour* (pp. 9–34). London: Academic Press.

Dawson, G. (1988). Cerebral lateralization in autism: Clues to its role in language and affective development. In D. L. Molfese & S. J. Segalowitz (Eds.), *Brain lateralization in children: Developmental implications* (pp. 437–461). New York: Guilford Press.

Dawson, G., Finley, C., Phillips, S., & Galpert, L. (1986). Hemispheric specialization and the language abilities of autistic children. *Child Development, 57,* 1440–1453.

Dawson, G., Warrenburg, S., & Fuller, P. (1982). Cerebral lateralization in individuals diagnosed as autistic in early childhood. *Brain and Language, 15,* 353–368.

Dawson, G., Warrenburg, S., & Fuller, P. (1983). Hemisphere functioning and motor imitation in autistic persons. *Brain and Cognition, 2,* 346–354.

Denckla, M. B. (1986). Editorial: New diagnosis criteria for autism and related behavioral disorders— guidelines for research protocols. *Journal of the American Academy of Child Psychiatry, 25,* 221–224.

Devinsky, O. (1983). Neuroanatomy of Gilles de la Tourette's syndrome. *Archives of Neurology, 40,* 508–514.

Dichgans, J. (1977). Neuronal mechanisms in visual perception: IV. Visual–vestibular interaction. *Neurosciences Research Progress Bulletin, 15,* 376–385.

Donchin, E., Heffley, E., Hillyard, S. A., Loveless, N., Maltzman, I., Ohman, A., Öhman, A., Rösler, F., Ruchkin, D., & Siddle, D. (1984). Cognition and event-related potentials: II. The orienting reflex and P300. *Annals of the New York Academy of Sciences, 425,* 39–57.

Eberhart, J. A., Morrell, J. I., Krieger, M. S., & Pfaff, D. W. (1985). An autoradiographic study of projections ascending from the midbrain central gray, and from the region lateral to it, in the rat. *Journal of Comparative Neurology, 241,* 285–310.

Ellenbroek, B., Schwarz, M., Sontag, K.-H., Jaspers, R., & Cools, A. (1985). Muscular rigidity and delineation of a dopamine specific neostriatal subregion: Tonic EMG activity in rats. *Brain Research, 345,* 132–140.

Evarts, E. V., Kimura, M., Wurtz, R. H., & Hikosaka, O. (1984). Behavioral correlates of activity in basal ganglia neurons. *Trends in Neuroscience, 7,* 447–453.

Fein, D., Humes, M., Kaplan, E., Lucci, D., & Waterhouse, L. (1984). The question of left hemisphere dysfunction in infantile autism. *Psychological Bulletin, 95,* 258–281.

Fein, D., Pennington, B., Markowitz, P., Braverman, M., & Waterhouse, L. (1986). Toward a neuropsychological model of infantile autism: Are the social deficits primary? *Journal of the American Academy of Child Psychiatry, 25,* 198–212.

Finch, D. M., Derian, E. L., & Babb, T. L. (1984a). Afferent fibers to rat cingulate cortex. *Experimental Neurology, 83,* 468–485.

Finch, D. M., Derian, E. L., & Babb, T. L. (1984b). Excitatory projection of the rat subicular complex to the cingulate cortex and synaptic integration with thalamic afferents. *Brain Research, 301,* 25–37.

Finch, D. M., Wong, E. E., Derian, E. L., Chen, X. H., Nowlin-Finch, N. L., & Brothers, L. A. (1986). Neurophysiology of limbic system pathways in the rat: Projections from the amygdala to the entorhinal cortex. *Brain Research, 370,* 273–284.

Fisch, G. S., Cohen, I. L., Wolf, E. G., Brown, W. T., Jenkins, E. C., & Gross, A. (1986). Autism and the fragile X syndrome. *American Journal of Psychiatry, 143,* 71–73.

Folstein, S. E. (1985). Genetic aspects of infantile autism. *Annual Review of Medicine, 36,* 415–419.

Fontani, G., & Farabollini, F. (1984). Effect of DSP-4, pCPA, and haloperidol on hippocampal electrical activity and behavior in rabbits. *Behavioral and Neural Biology, 40,* 213–226.

Fujimoto, S., Sasa, M., & Takaori, S. (1981). Inhibition from locus coeruleus of caudate neurons activated by nigral stimulation. *Brain Research Bulletin, 6,* 267–274.

Gaffney, G. R., Kuperman, S., Tsai, L. Y., Minchin, S., & Hassanein, K. M. (1987). Midsagittal magnetic resonance imaging of autism. *British Journal of Psychiatry, 151,* 831–833.

Gaillard, J.-M., & Blois, R. (1981). Spindle density in sleep of normal subjects. *Sleep, 4,* 385–391.

Gillberg, C., & Svendsen, P. (1983). Childhood psychosis and computed tomographic brain scan findings. *Journal of Autism and Developmental Disorders, 13,* 19–32.

Gillberg, C., Rosenhall, U., & Johansson, E. (1983). Auditory brainstem responses in childhood psychosis. *Journal of Autism and Developmental Disorders, 13,* 181–195.

Goldberg, M. E., & Bruce, C. J. (1985). Cerebral cortical activity associated with the orientation of visual attention in the rhesus monkey. *Vision Research, 25,* 471–481.

Goldberg, M. E., Bushnell, M. C., & Bruce, C. J. (1986). The effect of attentive fixation on eye movements evoked by electrical stimulation of the frontal eye fields. *Experimental Brain Research, 61,* 579–584.

Gonzalez-Lima, F., & Scheich, H. (1985). Ascending reticular activating system in the rat: A 2-deoxyglucose study. *Brain Research, 344,* 70–88.

Groves, P. M. (1983). A theory of the functional organization of the neostriatum and the neostriatal control of voluntary movement. *Brain Research Reviews, 5,* 109–132.

Hanley, H. G., Stahl, S. M., & Freedman, D. X. (1977). Hyperserotonemia and amine metabolites in autistic and retarded children. *Archives of General Psychiatry, 34,* 521–531.

Hashimoto, T., & Tayama, M. (1984). Polysomnographic study on autism: Phasic events during sleep. In *Proceedings of the 1984 annual meeting of the Research Committee of the Ministry of Health and Welfare of Japan: The study of prevention and treatment of early infantile autism from the standpoint of developmental neurobiology* (pp. 11–18). Tokyo: Ministry of Health and Welfare of Japan.

Hauser, S. L., DeLong, G. R., & Rosman, N. P. (1975). Pneumographic findings in the infantile autism syndrome: A correlation with temporal lobe disease. *Brain, 98,* 667–688.

Heilman, K. M., Bowers, D., Valenstein, E., & Watson, F. T. (1986). The right hemisphere: Neuropsychological functions. *Journal of Neurosurgery, 64,* 693–704.

Heilman, K. M., & Valenstein, E. (1972). Frontal lobe neglect in man. *Neurology, 22,* 660–664.

Heilman, K. M., & Van Den Abell, T. (1980). Right hemisphere dominance for attention: The mechanism underlying hemispheric asymmetries of inattention (neglect). *Neurology, 30,* 327–330.

Hier, D. B., LeMay, M., & Rosenberger, P. B. (1979). Autism and unfavorable left–right asymmetries of the brain. *Journal of Autism and Developmental Disorders, 9,* 153–159.

Hillyard, S. A. (1985). Electrophysiology of human selective attention. *Trends and Neuroscience, 8,* 400–405.

Hoffman, W. L., & Prior, M. R. (1982). Neuropsychological dimensions of autism in children: A test of the hemispheric dysfunction hypothesis. *Journal of Clinical Neuropsychology, 4,* 27–41.

Hutt, C., Forrest, S. J., & Richer, J. (1975). Cardiac arrhythmia and behavior in autistic children. *Acta Psychiatrica Scandinavica, 51,* 361–372.

Jackson, J. H. (1958). Evolution and dissolution of the nervous system. In J. Taylor (Ed.), *Selected writings of John Hughlings Jackson* (Croonian Lectures, 1884). New York: Basic Books. (Original work published 1884)

James, A. L., & Barry, R. J. (1980). Respiratory and vascular responses to simple visual stimuli in autistics, retardates, and normals. *Psychophysiology, 17,* 541–547.

James, A. L., & Barry, R. J. (1983). Developmental effects in the cerebral lateralization of autistic, retarded and normal children. *Journal of Autism and Developmental Disorders, 13,* 43–54.

Jones, B. E,. & Moore, R. Y. (1977). Ascending projections of the locus coeruleus in the rat: II. Autoradiographic study. *Brain Research, 127,* 23–53.

Kanner, L. (1943). Autistic disturbances of affective contact. *The Nervous Child, 2,* 217–250.

Kawakami, F., Fukui, K., Okamura, H., Morimoto, N., Yanaihara, N., Nakajima, T., & Ibata, Y. (1984). Influence of ascending nonadrenergic fibers on the neurotensin-like immunoreactive perikarya and evidence of direct projection of ascending neurotensin-like immunoreactive fibers in the rat central nucleus of the amygdala. *Neuroscience Letters, 51,* 225–230.

Kelley, A. E., Domesick, V. B., & Nauta, W. J. H. (1982). The amygdalostriatal projection in the rat: An anatomical study by anterograde and retrograde tracing methods. *Neuroscience, 7,* 615–630.

King, A. J., & Palmer, A. R. (1985). Integration of visual and auditory information in bimodal neurones in the guinea-pig superior colliculus. *Experimental Brain Research, 60,* 492–500.

Kirzinger, A., & Jurgens, U. (1985). The effects of brainstem lesions on vocalization in the squirrel monkey. *Brain Research, 358,* 150–162.

Krettek, J. E., & Price, J. L. (1977). Projections from the amygdaloid complex and adjacent olfactory structures to the entorhinal cortex and subiculum in the rat and the cat. *Journal of Comparative Neurology, 172,* 723–752.

Kunzle, H., & Akert, K. (1977). Efferent connections of cortical, area 8 (frontal eye field) in *Macaca fascicularis:* A reinvestigation using the autoradiographic technique. *Journal of Comparative Neurology, 173,* 147–164.

Larson, C. R., & Kistler, M. K. (1984). Periaqueductal gray neuronal activity associated with laryngeal and vocalization in the awake monkey. *Neuroscience Letters, 46,* 261–266.

Lempert, H., & Kinsbourne, M. (1985). Possible origin of speech in selective orienting. *Psychological Bulletin, 97,* 62–73.

Levin, S. (1984). Frontal lobe dysfunctions in schizophrenia: I. Eye movement impairments. *Journal of Psychiatric Research, 18,* 27–55.

Levine, R. A., & McGaffigan, P. M. (1983). Right–left asymmetries in the human brain stem: Auditory evoked potentials. *Electroencephalography and Clinical Neurophysiology, 55,* 532–537.

Lines, C. R., & Milner, A. D. (1985). A deficit in ambient visual guidance following superior colliculus lesions in rats. *Behavioral Neuroscience, 99,* 707–716.

Louilot, A., Simon, H., Taghzouti, K., & Le Moal, M. (1985). Modulation of dopaminergic activity in the nucleus accumbens following facilitation or blockade of the dopaminergic transmission in the amygdala: A study by *in vivo* differential pulse voltammetry. *Brain Research, 346,* 141–145.

Lynch, J. C. (1980). The functional organization of posterior parietal association cortex. *Behavioral and Brain Sciences, 3,* 485–534.

MacCulloch, M. J., & Williams, C. (1971). On the nature of infantile autism. *Acta Psychiatrica Scandinavica, 47,* 295–314.

Mager, P., Mager, R., & Klingberg, F. (1983). Open field behaviour of rats after various mesencephalic lesions. *Biomedica Biochimica Acta, 42,* 1257–1267.

Margulies, D. M. (1985). Selective attention and the brain: A hypothesis concerning the hippocampal–ventral striatal axis, the mediation of selective attention, and the pathogenesis of attentional disorders. *Medical Hypotheses, 18,* 221–264.

Mesulam, M.-M. (1981). A cortical network for directed attention and unilateral neglect. *Annals of Neurology, 10,* 309–325.

Mesulam, M.-M. (1983). The functional anatomy and hemispheric specialization for directed attention. The role of the parietal lobe and its connectivity. *Trends in Neuroscience, 6,* 384–387.

Mesulam, M.-M., & Geschwind, N. (1978). On the possible role of neocortex and its limbic connections in the process of attention and schizophrenia: Clinical cases of inattention in man and experimental anatomy in monkey. *Journal of Psychiatric Research, 14,* 249–259.

Mesulam, M.-M., Van Hoesen, G. W., Pandya, D. N., & Geschwind, N. (1977). Limbic and sensory connections of the inferior parietal lobule (area PG) in the rhesus monkey: A study with a new method for horseradish peroxidase histochemistry. *Brain Research, 136,* 393–414.

Moore, R. Y., & Halaris, A. E. (1975). Hippocampal innervation by serotonin neurons of the midbrain raphe in the rat. *Journal of Comparative Neurology, 164,* 171–184.

Motter, B. C., & Mountcastle, V. B. (1981). The functional properties of the light-sensitive neurons of the posterior parietal cortex studied in waking monkeys: Foveal sparing and opponent vector organization. *Journal of Neuroscience, 1,* 3–26.

Mountcastle, V. B., Andersen, R. A., & Motter, B. C. (1981). The influence of attentive fixation upon the excitability of the light sensitive neurons of the posterior parietal cortex. *Journal of Neuroscience, 1,* 1218–1235.

Naatanen, R. (1982). Processing negativity: An evoked-potential reflection of selective attention. *Psychological Bulletin, 92,* 605–640.

Natale, M., Gur, R. E., & Gur, R. C. (1983). Hemispheric asymmetries in processing emotional expressions. *Neuropsychologia, 21,* 555–565.

Nauta, W. J. H. (1982). Limbic innervation of the striatum. In A. J. Friedhoff & T. N. Chase (Eds.), *Gilles de la Tourette syndrome* (pp. 41–47). New York, Raven Press.

Niwa, S., Ohta, M., & Yamazaki, K. (1983). P300 and stimulus evaluation process in autistic subjects. *Journal of Autism and Developmental Disorders, 13,* 33–42.

Novick, B., Kurtzberg, D., & Vaughan, H. G. (1979). An electrophysiologic indication of defective information storage in childhood autism. *Psychiatry Research, 1,* 101–108.

Novick, B., Vaughan, H. G., Kurtzberg, D., & Simon, R. (1980). An electrophysiologic indication of auditory processing defects in autism. *Psychiatry Research, 3,* 107–114.

Ogawa, T., Sugiyama, A., Ishiwa, S., Suzuki, M., Ishihara, T., & Sato, K. (1982). Ontogenic development of EEG-asymmetry in early infantile autism. *Brain Development, 4,* 439–449.

Ornitz, E. M. (1969). Disorders of perception common to early infantile autism and schizophrenia. *Comprehensive Psychiatry, 10,* 259–274.

Ornitz, E. M. (1973). Childhood autism: A review of the clinical and experimental literature. *California Medicine, 118,* 21–47.

Ornitz, E. M. (1974). The modulation of sensory input and motor output in autistic children. *Journal of Autism and Childhood Schizophrenia, 4,* 197–215.

Ornitz, E. M. (1983). The functional neuroanatomy of infantile autism. *International Journal of Neuroscience, 19,* 85–124.

Ornitz, E. M. (1985). Neurophysiology of infantile autism. *Journal of the American Academy of Child Psychiatry, 24,* 251–262.

Ornitz, E. M., Atwell, C. W., Kaplan, A. R., & Westlake, J. R. (1985). Brain-stem dysfunction in autism. *Archives of General Psychiatry, 42,* 1018–1025.

Ornitz, E. M., Brown, M. B., Mason, A., & Putnam, N. H. (1974). Effect of visual input on vestibular nystagmus in autistic children. *Archives of General Psychiatry, 31,* 369–375.

Ornitz, E. M., Forsythe, A. B., & de la Pena, A. (1973). Effect of vestibular and auditory stimulation on the REMs of REM sleep in autistic children. *Archives of General Psychiatry, 29,* 786–791.

Ornitz, E. M., Guthrie, D., & Farley, A. J. (1977). The early development of autistic children. *Journal of Autism and Childhood Schizophrenia, 7,* 207–229.

Ornitz, E. M., Guthrie, D., & Farley, A. J. (1978). The early symptoms of childhood autism. In G. Serban (Ed.), *Cognitive defects in the development of mental illness* (pp. 24–42). New York: Brunner/Mazel.

Ornitz, E. M., Ritvo, E. R., Brown, M. B., La Franchi, S., Parmelee, T., & Walter, R. D. (1969). The EEG and rapid eye movements during REM sleep in normal and autistic children. *Electroencephalography and Clinical Neurophysiology, 26,* 167–175.

Pandya, D. N., & Kuypers, K. G. J. M. (1969). Cortico-cortical connections in the rhesus monkey. *Brain Research, 12,* 13–36.

Pandya, D. N., Van Hoesen, G. W., & Mesulam, M.-M. (1981). Efferent connections of the cingulate gyrus in the rhesus monkey. *Experimental Brain Research, 42,* 319–330.

Parent, A., & Steriade, M. (1984). Midbrain tegmental projections of nucleus reticularis thalami of cat and monkey: A retrograde transport and antidromic invasion study. *Journal of Comparative Neurology, 229,* 548–558.

Peschanski, M., & Besson, J. M. (1984). Diencephalic connections of the raphe nuclei of the rat brainstem: An anatomical study with reference to the somatosensory system. *Journal of Comparative Neurology, 224,* 509–534.

Petersen, S. E., Robinson, D. L., & Keys, W. (1985). Pulvinar nuclei of the behaving rhesus monkey: Visual responses and their modulation. *Journal of Neurophysiology, 54,* 867–886.

Petty, L. K., Ornitz, E. M., Michelman, J. D., & Zimmerman, E. G. (1984). Autistic children who become schizophrenic. *Archives of General Psychiatry, 41,* 129–135.

Posner, M. (1975). Psychobiology of attention. In M. S. Gazzaniga & C. Blakemore (Eds.), *Handbook of psychobiology* (pp. 441–480). New York: Academic Press.

Posner, M. I., Walker, J. A., Friedrich, F. J., & Rafal, R. D. (1984). Effects of parietal injury on covert orienting of attention. *Journal of Neuroscience, 4,* 1863–1874.

Prior, M. R., & Bradshaw, J. L. (1979). Hemispheric functioning in autistic children. *Cortex, 15,* 73–81.

Prior, M. R., Tress, B., Hoffman, W. L., & Boldt, D. (1984). Computed tomographic study of children with classic autism. *Archives of Neurology, 41*, 482–484.

Rinn, W. E. (1984). The neuropsychology of facial expression: A review of the neurological and psychological mechanisms for producing facial expressions. *Psychological Bulletin, 95*, 52–77.

Ritvo, E. R., Freeman, B. J., Scheibel, A. B., Duong, T., Robinson, H., Guthrie, D., & Ritvo, A. (1986). Lower Purkinje cell counts in the cerebella of four autistic subjects: Initial findings of the UCLA–NSAC autopsy research report. *American Journal of Psychiatry, 143*, 862–866.

Ritvo, E. R., & Garber, H. J. (in press). Normal size cerebellar vermal lobules VI and VII in autism. *New England Journal of Medicine* (Correspondence).

Rolls, E. T., Thorpe, S. J., & Maddison, S. P. (1983). Responses of striatal neurons in the behaving monkey: 1. Head of the caudate nucleus. *Behavioural Brain Research, 7*, 179–210.

Ross, E. D. (1981). The aprosodias: Functional–anatomic organization of the affective components of language in the right hemisphere. *Archives of Neurology, 38*, 561–569.

Ross, E. D. (1984). Right hemisphere's role in language, affective behavior and emotion. *Trends in Neuroscience, 7*, 342–346.

Ross, E. D., & Mesulam, M.-M. (1979). Dominant language functions of the right hemisphere. *Archives of Neurology, 36*, 144–148.

Rueter-Lorenz, P. A., Givis, R. P., & Moscovitch, M. (1983). Hemispheric specialization and the perception of emotion: Evidence from right-handers and from inverted and non-inverted left-handers. *Neuropsychologia, 21*, 687–692.

Russchen, F. T., Bakst, I., Amaral, D. G., & Price, J. L. (1985). The amygdalostriatal projections in the monkey: An anterograde tracing study. *Brain Research, 329*, 241–257.

Rutter, M. (1968). Concepts of autism: A review of research. *Journal of Child Psychiatry, 9*, 1–5.

Rutter, M. (1974). The development of infantile autism. *Psychological Medicine, 4*, 147–163.

Rutter, M. (1978). Language disorder and infantile autism. In M. Rutter & E. Schopler (Eds.), *Autism: A reappraisal of concepts and treatment* (pp. 85–104). New York: Plenum.

Rutter, M. (1983). Cognitive deficits in the pathogenesis of autism. *Journal of Child Psychology and Psychiatry, 24*, 513–531.

Rutter, M., & Lockyer, L. (1967). A five-to-fifteen year follow-up study of infantile psychosis: I. Description of sample. *British Journal of Psychiatry, 113*, 1169–1182.

Sabatino, M., Ferraro, G., Liberti, G., Vella, N., & La Grutta, V. (1985). Striatal and septal influence on hippocampal theta and spikes in the cat. *Neuroscience Letters, 61*, 55–59.

Sabatino, M., Savatteri, V., Liberti, G., Vella, N., & La Grutta, V. (1986). Effects of substantia nigra and pallidum stimulation on hippocampal interictal activity in the cat. *Neuroscience Letters, 64*, 293–298.

Sakata, H., Shibutani, H., Ito, Y., & Tsurugai, K. (1986). Parietal cortical neurons responding to rotary movement of visual stimulus in space. *Experimental Brain Research, 61*, 658–663.

Sarter, M., & Markowitsch, H. J. (1984). Collateral innervation of the medial and lateral prefrontal cortex by amygdaloid, thalamic, and brain-stem neurons. *Journal of Comparative Neurology, 224*, 445–460.

Schneider, J. S. (1984). Basal ganglia role in behavior: Importance of sensory gating and its relevance to psychiatry. *Biological Psychiatry, 19*, 1693–1710.

Schneider, J. S., & Lidsky, T. I. (1981). Processing of somatosensory information in striatum of behaving cats. *Journal of Neurophysiology, 45*, 841–851.

Schnyder, H., Reisine, H., Hepp, K., & Henn, V. (1985). Frontal eye field projection to the paramedian pontine reticular formation traced with wheat germ agglutinin in the monkey. *Brain Research, 329*, 151–160.

Schott, B., Laurent, B., Mauguiere, F., & Chazot, G. (1981). Négligence motrice par hematome thalamique droit. *Revue de Neurologie (Paris), 137*, 447–455.

Segawa, M. (1985). Circadian rhythm in early infantile autism (English abstract). *Advances in Neurological Sciences (Tokyo), 29*, 140–153.

Shibagaki, M., Kiyono, S., Watanabe, K., & Hakamada, S. (1982). Concurrent occurrence of rapid eye movement with spindle burst during nocturnal sleep in mentally retarded children. *Electroencephalography and Clinical Neurophysiology, 53*, 27–35.

Simon, H., & Le Moal, M. (1984). Mesencephalic dopaminergic neurons: Functional role. In E. Usdin, A. Carlsson, A. Dahlstrom, & J. Engel (Eds.), *Catecholamines: Neuropharmacology and central nervous system—theoretical aspects* (pp. 293–307). New York: Alan R. Liss.

Simon, H., & Le Moal, M. (1985). Influence des neurones dopaminergiques du mesencephale sur les processus d'attention et d'intention. *Psychologie Medicale, 17*, 939–945.

Small, J. G. (1975). EEG and neurophysiological studies of early infantile autism. *Biological Psychiatry, 10*, 385–397.

Sofroniew, M. V., Priestley, J. V., Consolazione, A., Eckenstein, F., & Cuello, A. C. (1985). Cholinergic projections from the midbrain and pons to the thalamus in the rat, identified by combined retrograde tracing and choline acetyltransferase immunohistochemistry. *Brain Research, 329*, 213–223.

Steriade, M., & Glenn, L. L. (1982). Neocortical and caudate projections of intralaminar thalamic neurons and their synaptic excitation from midbrain recticular core. *Journal of Neurophysiology, 48*, 352–371.

Stewart, D. J., MacCabe, D. F., & Leung, W. S. (1985). Topographical projection of cholinergic neurons in the basal forebrain to the cingulate cortex in the rat. *Brain Research, 358*, 404–407.

Strecker, R. E., Steinfels, G. F., Abercrombie, E. D., & Jacobs, B. L. (1985). Caudate unit activity in freely moving cats: Effects of phasic auditory and visual stimuli. *Brain Research, 329*, 350–353.

Stuss, D. T., & Benson, D. F. (1984). Neuropsychological studies of the frontal lobes. *Psychological Bulletin, 95*, 3–28.

Taghzouti, K., Simon, H., Louilot, A., Herman, J. P., & Le Moal, M. (1985). Behavioral study after local injection of 6-hydroxydopamine into the nucleus accumbens in the rat. *Brain Research, 344*, 9–20.

Tanguay, P. E. (1976). Clinical and electrophysiological research. In E. R. Ritvo (Ed.), *Autism: Diagnosis, current research and management* (pp. 75–84). New York: Spectrum.

Tanguay, P. E., Ornitz, E. M., Forsythe, A. B., & Ritvo, E. R. (1976). Rapid eye movement (REM) activity in normal and autistic children during REM sleep. *Journal of Childhood Schizophrenia, 6*, 275–288.

Thomas, S. R., Assaf, S. Y., & Iverson, S. D. (1984). Amygdaloid complex modulates neurotransmission from the entorhinal cortex to the dentate gyrus of the rat. *Brain Research, 207*, 363–365.

Thompson, R., Gibbs, R. B., Ristic, G. A., Cotman, C. W., & Yu, J. (1986). Learning deficits in albino rats with early median raphe or pontine reticular formation lesions. *Physiology and Behavior, 32*, 107–114.

Tsai, L., Jacoby, C. G., & Stewart, M. A. (1983). Morphologic cerebral asymmetries in autistic children. *Biological Psychiatry, 18*, 317–327.

Tsai, L., Jacoby, C. G., Stewart, M. A., & Beisler, J. M. (1982). Unfavorable left–right asymmetries of the brain and autism. *British Journal of Psychiatry, 140*, 312–319.

Unemoto, H., Sasa, M., & Takaori, S. (1985). Inhibition from locus coeruleus of nucleus accumbens neurons activated by hippocampal stimulation. *Brain Research, 338*, 376–379.

Vaccarino, F. J., Franklin, K. B. J., & Prupas, D. (1985). Opposite locomotor asymmetries elicited from the medial and lateral substantia nigra: Role of the superior colliculus. *Physiology and Behavior, 35*, 741–747.

Vanderwolf, C. H., Leung, L.-W.S., & Cooley, R. K. (1985). Pathways through cingulate, neo- and entorhinal cortices mediate atropine-resistant hippocampal rhythmical slow activity. *Brain Research, 347*, 58–73.

Vertes, R. P. (1982). Brain stem generation of the hippocampal EEG. *Progress in Neurobiology, 19*, 159–186.

Voeller, K. K. S. (1986). Right-hemisphere deficit syndrome in children. *American Journal of Psychiatry, 143*, 1004–1009.

Vogt, B. A. (1984). Afferent specific localization of muscarinic acetylcholine receptors in cingulate cortex. *Journal of Neuroscience, 4,* 2191–2199.

Volkmar, F. R., Cohen, D. J., & Paul, R. (1986). An evaluation of DSM-III criteria for infantile autism. *Journal of the American Academy of Child Psychiatry, 25,* 190–197.

Watson, R. T., Heilman, K. M., Cauthen, J. C., & King, F. A. (1973). Neglect after cingulectomy. *Neurology, 23,* 1003–1007.

Watson, R. T., Heilman, K. M., Miller, B. D., & King, F. A. (1974). Neglect after mesencephalic reticular formation lesions. *Neurology, 24,* 294–298.

Watson, R. T., Miller, B. D., & Heilman, K. M. (1978). Nonsensory neglect. *Annals of Neurology, 3,* 505–508.

Watson, R. T., Valenstein, E., & Heilman, K. M. (1981). Thalamic neglect: Possible role of the medial thalamus and nucleus reticularis in behavior. *Archives of Neurology, 38,* 501–506.

Weintraub, S., & Mesulam, M.-M. (1983). Developmental learning disabilities of the right hemisphere: Emotional, interpersonal, and cognitive components. *Archives of Neurology, 40,* 463–468.

Wetherby, A. M., Koegel, R. L., & Mendel, M. (1981). Central auditory nervous system dysfunction in echolalic autistic individuals. *Journal of Speech and Hearing, 24,* 420–429.

Williams, R. S., Hauser, S. L., Purpura, D. P., DeLong, G. R., & Swisher, C. N. (1980). Autism and mental retardation: Neuropathologic studies performed in four retarded persons with autistic behavior. *Archives of Neurology, 37,* 749–753.

Winson, J. (1984). Neuronal transmission through the hippocampus: Dependence on behavioral state. In F. Reinoso-Suarez & C. Ajmone-Marsan (Eds.), *Cortical integration* (pp. 131–146). New York: Raven Press.

Wyss, J. M., & Sripanidkulchai, K. (1984). The topography of the mesencephalic and pontine projections from the cingulate cortex of the rat. *Brain Research, 293,* 1–15.

Yamashita, K., Nagata, E., Nomura, Y., & Segawa, M. (1986). Locomotion in early infantile autism. *Brain and Development, 8,* 90–96.

Yoshida, M., Sasa, M., & Takaori, S. (1984). Serotonin-mediated inhibition from dorsal raphe nucleus of neurons in dorsal lateral geniculate and thalamic reticular nuclei. *Brain Research, 290,* 95–105.

Yuwiler, A., Geller, E., & Ritvo, E. (1985). Biochemical studies in autism. In A. Lejtha (Ed.), *Handbook of neurochemistry* (Vol. 10, pp. 671–691). New York: Plenum.

Zhou, F. C., & Azmitia, E. C. (1983). Effects of 5,7-dihydroxytryptamine on HRP retrograde transport from hippocampus to midbrain raphe nuclei in the rat. *Brain Research Bulletin, 10,* 445–451.

CHAPTER 9

Neurochemical Perspectives
on Infantile Autism

FRED R. VOLKMAR
GEORGE M. ANDERSON
Yale University School of Medicine

Most investigators would now agree with the proposition that a disorder (or disorders) of central nervous system (CNS) functioning underlies the expression of the behavioral syndrome we recognize as autism. Although the exact nature of any etiological mechanism or mechanisms remains to be elucidated, the evidence in favor of neurobiological factors is impressive in its breadth and frustrating in that no single biological marker for the disorder has yet been identified. The mechanism or mechanisms underlying the disorder may be of various forms—for example, in patterns of connection of neuronal systems or in disturbed patterns of neuronal transmission (Ciaranello, VandenBerg, & Anders, 1982). Particular interest has focused on neurochemical factors; this interest derives from the success of pharmacological treatments for certain limited aspects of the disorder and from recent advances in basic neuroscience. In this chapter, research findings from the past 20 years of research in the neurochemistry of autism are critically reviewed. Other aspects of neurobiological research (e.g., neuroendocrine, neuroanatomical, etc.) are noted only as they relate to neurochemical studies, and the interested reader is advised to consult other sources for fuller treatment of these studies (Anderson & Hoshino, 1987; Maurer, 1986; Yuwiler, Geller, & Ritvo, 1985). The chapter is organized around major neurotransmitter systems of interest; this format is convenient for purposes of presentation, but should not be taken to suggest that such systems function in isolation from one another.

In evaluating research in this area, both historical and methodological factors must be considered. Historically, several controversies posed obstacles to neurobiological studies of autism. In important ways, these controversies stem from Kanner's (1943) original description of the autistic syndrome. Kanner proposed that his first 11 cases suffered from an inborn disorder of affective contact, or early infantile autism, which was unrelated to other psychiatric disorders, unrelated to known medical conditions, and not associated with mental retardation. Disagreements about the validity of Kanner's diagnostic concept continued for many years; many investigators assumed, largely on the basis of severity, that infantile autism was the earliest manifestation of schizophrenia. Particularly in the 1950s, many clinicians assumed that Kanner's initial speculation regarding the inborn nature of the condition was incorrect and that the disorder developed as a result of deviant early parent–child interaction. Kanner's suggestion that the disorder was unrelated to medical conditions proved incorrect, as it became apparent that the disorder was often observed in association with a variety of medical conditions, such as congenital rubella (Chess, Fernandez, & Korn, 1974). Similarly, as autistic children were followed over time, it became apparent that many suffered from seizures in adolescence (Rutter, 1972) and that most autistic people were, and remained, retarded. These disagreements were significant obstacles to early research efforts, particularly in relation to syndrome definition. The lack of overarching diagnostic schemes made patterns of subject selection idiosyncratic and generalizations across studies difficult, if not impossible. As longitudinal, family history, psychological, and other data became available, many of these disagreements were resolved. In the 1960s, evidence regarding the validity of the syndrome and its biological basis became more coherent, and investigators began to turn to a study of neurobiological factors (Rimland, 1964). Although autism was not accorded official diagnostic status until 1980 (American Psychiatric Association, 1980), the previous two decades witnessed an impressive increase in biological studies, as it became apparent that autism was associated with CNS dysfunction.

However, even after the early controversies were largely resolved, other issues proved problematic for neurobiological studies of the autistic syndrome. These issues continue to complicate the interpretation of research studies. Some of these issues are intrinsic to the disorder itself. Autism is a relatively uncommon disorder, and subject recruitment can prove difficult. Although the validity of the diagnostic concept is now generally recognized, issues in the elaboration of readily applicable, explicit criteria for the disorder remain (Cohen, Volkmar, & Paul, 1986). Furthermore, it has become apparent that autism is a rather heterogeneous disorder associated with various degrees of gross organic involvement, differing intellectual levels, and so on. The variability of the syndrome poses substantial problems for research studies. Similarly, issues of subject selection complicate interpretation of research studies. The frequency of autistic-like behaviors increases with the degree of mental retardation (Freeman, Schroth, Ritvo, Guthrie, & Wake, 1980; Wing & Gould, 1979). Some aspects of the syndrome (e.g., social relatedness) change with age (Rutter, 1970); sex differences have also been observed (Lord, Schopler, & Revick, 1982). Effects of treatment, either educational or pharmacological, may confound results. All these factors make subject selection difficult.

Additional problems are posed for neurochemical research (Young, Kavanagh, Anderson, Shaywitz, & Cohen, 1982). Assay methods may differ between laboratories. Only a few subjects are typically studied. Generally, indirect methods are required, given the inaccessibility of brain tissue. The indirect methods required are understandable, but fundamental questions of relationships to central processes and potential confounding effects of other variables complicate interpretation of research studies. The lack of information about more fundamental mechanisms (e.g., the neurobiology of social relatedness or the interrelationships of neuronal systems), and the lack of animal models of the disorder, are also serious obstacles to research. Similarly, changes in neurotransmitter systems with age complicate the interpretation of research studies. Despite these problems, a considerable number of studies have been conducted, and the information generated has been substantial.

SEROTONIN

Background

Serotonin (5-hydroxytryptamine, or 5-HT) is an important central neurotransmitter that is synthesized from the amino acid tryptophan (TRP) and metabolized to 5-hydroxyindoleacetic acid (5-HIAA). The synthesis of serotonin is illustrated in Figure 9-1. The cell bodies of serotonergic neurons are located in the hindbrain and project widely; these neuronal systems have modulatory effects on a variety of important behavioral–physiological processes (e.g., sleep, pain and sensory perception, motor function, appetite, learning, and memory) (Young *et al.*, 1982). 5-HT has been implicated in various psychiatric disorders, particularly depression (Coppen & Wood, 1982). It is also found peripherally, most notably in the intestinal wall and bound to blood platelets.

Research Studies

The most widely replicated biological finding in autism has been that of an elevated group mean blood 5-HT level in autistic subjects as compared to control subjects (Anderson & Hoshino, 1987; Yuwiler *et al.*, 1985). This observation, made first in 1961 by Schain and Freedman, is even more impressive, given the variety of assay methods and procedures used (Anderson *et al.*, 1987). Mean levels in autistic groups have been observed to be from 17% to 128% higher than in control subjects (Anderson & Hoshino, 1987). The term "hyperserotonemic" has been used to describe individuals in the upper 5% of the normal population; by this criterion, typically 30%–50% of autistic subjects examined can be considered hyperserotonemic. However, it should be noted that 5-HT levels in the autistic population appear to be normally distributed, and the subgroup termed "hyperserotonemic" is arbitrarily defined. A number of research groups have attempted to elucidate the mechanism(s) responsible for this increase. Research has focused on three major areas: the synthesis of 5-HT by the gut, the degradation of 5-HT by the enzyme monoamine oxidase (MAO), and the uptake and storage of 5-HT by the platelet.

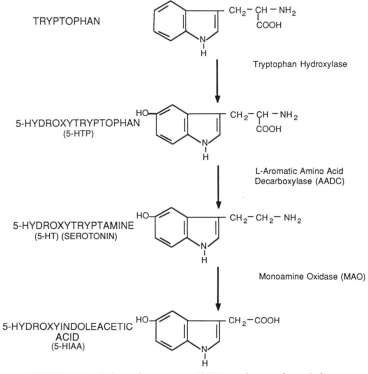

FIGURE 9-1. Pathway for serotonin (5-HT) synthesis and metabolism.

Gut synthesis of 5-HT has been examined by measuring urinary excretion rates of the endpoint metabolite, 5-HIAA. In some studies TRP, the amino acid precursor to 5-HT (see Figure 9-1), was given (orally) in large amounts in order to test the metabolic pathway. Most studies of baseline urinary excretion of 5-HIAA have not found differences between autistic and normal subjects (Minderaa, *et al.*, 1987; Partington, Tu, & Wong, 1973; Schain & Freeman, 1961). A report of higher 5-HIAA excretion in autistic subjects (Hanley, Stahl, & Freedman, 1977) also indicated that autistic subjects excreted higher levels of 5-HIAA after a TRP load than did control subjects. Other studies of urinary 5-HIAA excretion following a TRP load have found lower (Sutton, Read, & Arbor, 1958) or similar (Schain & Freeman, 1961; Shaw, Lucas, & Rabinovitch, 1959) excretion rates in autistic subjects compared to normals. Overall, the research would appear to indicate that the elevation of blood 5-HT is not a result of increased gut synthesis, for this increase would presumably result in increased excretion rates of 5-HIAA.

The activity of the degradative enzyme MAO has been examined by measuring platelet levels of MAO and by measuring urinary levels of monoamines and their oxidized metabolites. Studies of platelet MAO are unanimous in finding no differences between autistic and normal subjects (Boullin *et al.*, 1982; Cohen, Young, & Roth, 1977; Lake, Ziegler, & Murphy, 1977). These studies are somewhat compromised by the fact that most 5-HT is thought to be catabolized by the A form of MAO (MAO-A), whereas platelet MAO is of the B form (MAO-B). Recent studies (Minderaa *et al.*, 1988a, 1988b) have found normal or slightly decreased ratios of urinary amines to their respective oxidized metabolites. This has been found to be the case for 5-HT and 5-HIAA, dopamine and homovanillic acid (HVA), and norephinephrine and 3-methoxy-4-hydroxyphenylglycol (MHPG) or vanillylmandelic acid (VMA) (see Figures 9-1 and 9-2). These findings strongly indicate that the *in vivo* functioning of both MAO-A and MAO-B is normal in autism.

Finally, a number of studies have examined the uptake and efflux of 5-HT by the platelet. Direct measurements of platelet uptake and efflux have generally suggested that these processes are unaltered in autism (Boullin *et al.*, 1982). Autistic subjects have also been reported to have normal numbers (and affinities) of platelet imipramine-binding sites, further suggesting that their regulation of 5-HT uptake is normal (Anderson *et al.*, 1984). However, two recent studies of platelet

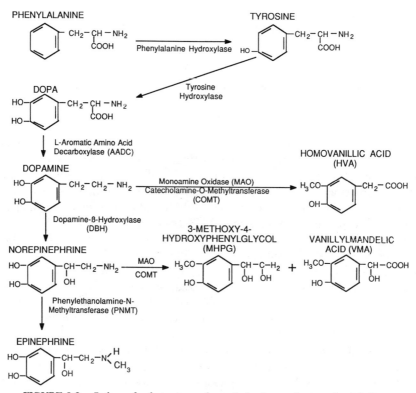

FIGURE 9-2. Pathway for dopamine and catecholamine synthesis and metabolism.

5-HT uptake have found higher rates of uptake in autistic subjects (Katsui, Okuda, Usuda, & Koizumi, 1986; Rotman, Caplan, & Szekely, 1980). In addition, the recent finding of slightly decreased urinary 5-HT in autistic subjects in our laboratory strongly indicates that plasma-free 5-HT levels are normal or slightly reduced in autism. This, in turn, suggests that the increased platelet levels seen in autism are a result of increased uptake or facilitated storage of 5-HT by the platelet. This issue would appear to warrant further careful study.

Despite the significant number of publications relating to elevations in peripheral serotonin levels in autism, few studies have addressed the critical question of relationships to central or cerebrospinal fluid (CSF) levels of 5-HT metabolites. CSF 5-HIAA is particularly interesting, since most CNS 5-HT is metabolized to 5-HIAA and the CSF appears to be a major route of elimination. Some studies have used probenecid to block 5-HIAA transport from the CSF; Cohen, Shaywitz, Johnson, and Bowers (1974) and Cohen, Young, and Roth (1977) found CSF levels to be similar in autistic and control subjects.

Although precise relationships of 5-HT levels to specific behaviors or symptoms remain to be established, it appears that the strongest association with 5-HT have been with intellectual level or IQ rather than with diagnostic group per se (Campbell, Friedman, DeVito, Greenspan, & Collins, 1974; Partington, *et al.*, 1973). The initial report (Schain & Freedman, 1961) of hyperserotonemia in autism indicated that subjects exhibited mixed features of autism and retardation. A relationship between peripheral 5-HT levels and activity has been variably reported (Campbell *et al.*, 1974; Partington *et al.*, 1973; Takahashi, Kanai, & Miyamoto, 1976). A study at our center (Volkmar, Minderaa, Anderson, Hoder, & Cohen, 1983) found essentially no relationship between a variety of behavioral parameters and peripheral 5-HT level.

The recent report of behavioral improvement in autistic children following administration of fenfluramine (Geller, Ritvo, Freeman, & Yuwiler, 1982), a potent 5-HT-depleting agent structurally related to amphetamine, has increased interest in serotonergic mechanisms in autism. Studies of this agent have been complicated by the observation of side effects (Volkmar, Paul, Cohen, & Shaywitz, 1983); in adults, the emergence of such side effects impairs the "blindness" of study design (Brownell & Stunkard, 1982). Although some children appear to respond the usefulness of this agent can not yet be regarded as clearly established (Gualtieri, 1986).

Issues and Prospects for Future Research

Although the finding of elevated peripheral 5-HT levels in autism is well replicated, its significance remains unclear. Studies explicating the basic mechanism responsible for hyperserotemia will be particularly important, for it appears that only when the mechanism of the observed increase is elucidated will it be possible to understand its relevance to CNS functioning. At this time, careful study of the platelet would appear to be the most promising direction to take in this regard.

DOPAMINE

Background

Dopamine is a catecholamine synthesized from the amino acids phenylalanine and tyrosine; it is metabolized to homovanillic acid (HVA) and dihydroxyphenylacetic acid (DOPAC) (see Figure 9-2). Several dopaminergic neuronal pathways have been described; most have cell bodies in the midbrain and are particularly important in the regulation of motor and other activities (Roberts, Woodruff, & Iversen, 1978). Dysfunction in these pathways has been implicated in the pathogenesis of Parkinson disease and in schizophrenia (Bowers, 1980). The major tranquilizers or neuroleptics act to block dopamine receptors; stimulant medications, such as amphetamines, act to facilitate dopaminergic activity. The observation that major tranquilizers may reduce levels of stereotypy and other maladaptive behaviors in autism, whereas stimulants generally increase these behaviors in autistic individuals, suggests some role of dopaminergic mechanisms in autism (Mikkelsen, 1982).

Research Studies

In animals, administration of stimulants produces increased levels of stereotyped behaviors, activity, and rotational behaviors, particularly in relation to specific neuroanatomical lesions (Young et al., 1982). This effect is dose-related, with higher stimulant doses producing more restricted and intense behaviors (Iversen, 1977); particular behavior patterns have been related to specific dopaminergic pathways (Pijnenburg, Honig, van der Heyden, & van Rossum, 1973). The analogy to some aspects of the autistic syndrome is apparent. The implications of dopamine in amphetamine-produced stereotypies in animals, the role of dopaminergic systems in other psychiatric disorders, and the effects of stimulant and neuroleptic administration in autistic children lend interest to the study of dopamine in autism.

Various methods have been used to assess dopaminergic activity, including studies of CSH metabolites, urinary and blood studies, and postmortem analyses of dopaminergic systems. Measures of peripheral (plasma or urinary) dopamine or HVA offer the most convenient methods for study. However, the relation of peripheral measures to central activity is not straightforward. Only a fraction of peripheral HVA is derived from central turnover of dopamine (Maas, Hattox, Greene, & Landis, 1980), and most peripheral dopamine appears to be of peripheral origin. Findings in autism have been contradictory. Boullin and O'Brien (1972) and Minderaa et al. (1987) found no significant differences between autistic and comparison groups. Garreau *et al.* (1980) reported elevated urinary HVA levels in autism, with higher levels associated with greater severity of autistic symptoms. Some alteration in urinary HVA after the administration of vitamin B_6 has been observed (Lelord *et al.*, 1978; Martineau, Garreau, Barthelmy, Callaway, & Lelord, 1981), but the significance of this observation remains unclear. Studies of CSF provide more direct methods of assessing dopaminergic functions.

Studies of CSF levels of HVA, the major dopamine metabolite, have not found significant differences between autistic and other neuropsychiatrically disturbed control groups when probenecid is administered to block transport of metabolites out of CSF (Cohen *et al.*, 1974; Cohen, Caparulo, Shaywitz, & Bowers, 1977). In one study (Cohen *et al.*, 1974), lower HVA values were suggested to be associated with greater degrees of disturbance. The use of probenecid, although theoretically attractive, has practical disadvantages that probably make CSF measurements made after its administration no better indices of monoamine turnover than baseline measures. Gillberg, Svennerholm, & Hamilton-Hellberg (1983) did not employ probenecid to block HVA and observed an elevation of HVA in an autistic group as compared to an age- and sex-matched control group. The observation that HVA levels are higher in younger subjects (Leckman *et al.*, 1980; Riddle *et al.*, 1986; Shaywitz, Anderson, & Cohen, 1985) might be taken to suggest that a relative immaturity in the development of dopaminergic systems exists in autistic subjects. However, theorizing in this area is probably premature, especially considering that one group has failed to replicate the finding of increased CSF HVA in autism (Ross, Klykylo, & Anderson, 1985).

Issues and Prospects for Future Research

Various lines of evidence suggest some role of dopaminergic systems in the pathogenesis of autism, and it is somewhat surprising that studies of dopaminergic functioning have been relatively uncommon. The limitations inherent in existing measures of peripheral activity have clearly impeded research in this area. The use of pharmacological agents that block the peripheral production of dopamine metabolites (e.g., debrisoquin; Riddle *et al.*, 1986) may help to provide more feasible measures of central dopaminergic activity. Despite the circumstantial evidence implicating these systems in at least some aspects of the autistic syndrome, the clear presence of central dopaminergic dysfunction in autism remains to be demonstrated.

NOREPINEPHRINE

Background

The catecholamines norepinephrine (NE) and epinephrine serve both as neurotransmitters and hormones; these compounds are found both in the central and peripheral nervous systems and in the general circulation. The adrenal medulla synthesizes most of the peripheral epinephrine, which has an important role in the regulation of a wide variety of physiological processes. NE serves as a central and peripheral neurotransmitter and is synthesized from dopamine by the action of the enzyme dopamine-β-hydroxylase (DBH) (see Figure 9-2). Most NE neurons in the brain are located in the locus ceruleus in the hindbrain, and central NE pathways have a broad range of effects on respiratory and cardiac function, attention, arousal, movement, memory, and anxiety (Amaral & Sinnamon, 1977; Moore & Bloom, 1979). Central NE is metabolized to 3-methoxy-4-hydroxy-phenylglycol (MHPG), whereas peripheral NE is metabolized to both MHPG and vanillylmandelic acid (VMA). As with dopamine, both animal studies and the activity of certain pharmacological agents in nonautistic populations have suggested a role of NE in the expression of various disorders (Young *et al.*, 1982).

Research Studies

Some pharmacological agents (e.g., clonidine) act to reduce the activity of central NE and can be used to reduce the severity of opiate withdrawal (Redmond & Huang, 1979) and the severity of tics in Tourette syndrome (Cohen, Young, Nathanson, & Shaywitz, 1979). Agents that act to increase NE activity (e.g., desipramine) are effective antidepressants and act to increase arousal. The apparent involvement of such systems in regulating attention and arousal lends interest to these mechanisms in autism.

Measures of NE activity have included both CSF levels of NE and its metabolite MHPG, as well as blood and urinary levels of these compounds. CSF measures offer the most direct techniques for assessing central NE functioning, although the presence of spinal cord and peripheral NE activity complicate interpretation of these measures (Kopin, Gordon, Jimerson, & Polinsky, 1983). Two studies have examined CSF MHPG in autistic and control subjects. Young, Cohen, Kavanagh, *et al.*, (1981) reported that CSF levels of MHPG were in the normal range in the autistic group; Gillberg *et al.* (1983) studied a larger group of autistic individuals and age- and sex-matched controls and observed only a slight, nonsignificant mean elevation of MHPG in the autistic group.

Blood and urinary levels of MHPG reflect both central and peripheral activity. Lake *et al.* (1977) noted elevations in plasma NE in autistic subjects, but lower levels of plasma DBH, an enzyme released along with NE, were also observed. Other studies of DBH activity have not observed differences between autistic and normal subjects (Coleman *et al.*, 1974; Young, Kyprie, Ross, & Cohen, 1980). Young, Cohen, Brown, and Caparulo (1978) and Young, Cohen, Caparulo, Brown, and Maas (1979) observed significantly lower levels of urinary MHPG in autism; this result is not consistent with the hypothesis that increased levels of NE might be responsible for increased arousal or activity levels in autism. Subsequent studies (Young, Cohen, Kavanagh, *et al.*, 1981; Minderaa *et al.*, 1988a) found that autistic and normal subjects were very similar in plasma MHPG levels.

Minderaa *et al.* (1988a) also observed that urinary levels of MHPG and NE were only slightly lower in autistic subjects.

Studies of the enzyme catechol-O-methyltransferase, which is involved in the extraneuronal degradation of NE, have not revealed significant differences in autism (Anderson & Hoshino, 1987).

Issues and Prospects for Future Research

Although noradrenergic mechanisms might reasonably be expected to be implicated in the pathogenesis of autism, research studies have failed to demonstrate consistent differences among diagnostic groups. The limited number of studies and the relatively small number of patients studied suggest the need for additional research with larger samples. Studies that relate noradrenergic mechanisms to clinical features (e.g., attention, arousal) are needed to facilitate our understanding of basic mechanisms of action.

PEPTIDES

Background

Certain peptides have recently been demonstrated to act as neurotransmitters (Snyder & Childers, 1979). These compounds have been implicated in various processes, including pain perception, emotion, appetite, and sexual behaviors. Particular interest has centered on compounds such as the enkephalins and the endorphins, which appear to act as endogenous opioids. Animals treated with exogenous opiate compounds display a number of characteristics, including decreased response to painful stimuli and self-injurious behavior, which suggest some similarity to behaviors seen in autism (Panskepp, 1979).

Research Studies

The observation that some opiate-induced behaviors in animals resemble autistic behaviors has led to the clinical use of opiate antagonists for treatment of severe self-injurious behaviors. Initial reports (Sandman *et al.*, 1983) suggest some potential usefulness of these agents; these results await future replication in double-blind studies with larger samples. Coid, Allolio, and Rees (1983) reported significantly increased plasma levels of the endogenous opioid metenkephalin in self-abusive adults. Weizman *et al.* (1984) reported significantly lower plasma levels of endorphins in autistic subjects. Although differences in methodology may account for the apparent discrepancy between these two reports, the limited available evidence is contradictory. Several studies (Gillberg, 1980; Gillberg, Trygstad, & Foss, 1982) have reported unusual patterns of urinary peptide excretion in autism. Unfortunately, the implications of this observation are unclear, given the nature of the studies and methods employed, as the specific peptides that might have been altered were not identified.

Issues and Prospects for Future Research

Investigations of the various neuropeptides, particularly those with opiate-like activity, are of interest in the light of possible clinical usefulness of opiate blockers in autism. As with other aspects of the neurochemistry of autism, the use of these pharmacological agents suggests a role for them as probes of the endogenous opioid system. Although results of initial studies have not been consistent, further research may help to clarify fundamental mechanisms underlying patterns of self-injury and isolation in autism. The observation of unusual peptide excretion patterns awaits replication; the analysis and identification of the specific compounds found to be altered in autism would strengthen research in this area.

OTHER COMPOUNDS

A variety of other compounds have been examined. The observation that some chronic schizophrenic patients excreted unusual psychoactive compounds led to a series of studies with autistic individuals; these unusual methylated metabolites of neurotransmitters produced hallucinations, and initial reports suggested that such compounds were observed in some autistic individuals (Himwich, Jenkins, Fujimori, & Narashimhachari, 1972; Widelitz & Feldman, 1969). The etiological significance of such compounds remains to be established. Studies of other neurotransmitter systems (e.g., acetylcholine) have not revealed systematic differences in autism.

Various neuroendocrine compounds have also been examined, particularly thyroid hormone and cortisol. Thyroid functioning has been evaluated in autistic individuals in a series of studies (Campbell, Hollander, Ferris, & Greene, 1978; Campbell, Small, et al., 1978; Cohen, Young, Lowe, & Harcherik, 1980), and studies of the efficacy of thyroid hormone administration in autism have also been conducted (Campbell, Hollander, et al., 1978). Only minimal improvement has been observed in carefully designed studies (e.g., Campbell, Small, et al., 1978).

Failure to suppress cortisol production after the administration of dexamethasone has been reported in depressed patients and has been thought to result from altered hypothalamic–pituitary functioning in depression. Levels of cortisol and its metabolites and the response to dexamethasone have also been examined in autism. Baseline differences were not apparent, but the results suggested that lower-functioning subjects fail to suppress cortisol production after dexamethasone. The failure to suppress cortisol secretion has been suggested to be due to alterations in central NE functioning (Hoshino et al., 1984).

Autism has been observed in association with some inborn disorders of the metabolism of amino acids, particularly phenylketonuria, histidinemia, and homocystinuria (Kotsopoulos & Kutty, 1979; Lowe, Tanaka, Seashore, Young, & Cohen, 1980). Although the increased frequency of autistic-like behaviors with severe and profound mental retardation complicates this observation (i.e., the differentiation of "autistic" and "autistic-like" individuals becomes more complicated in the profoundly and severely retarded), the study of autism in association with specific metabolic deficits is intriguing. Studies of excretion of other amino acids have not generally revealed specific syndromes.

SUMMARY

Of all the various biochemical findings, the most widely replicated has been that of the increased peripheral levels of 5-HT in autism. The meaning of this finding remains unclear and is an important priority for future research. Studies of dopaminergic systems also suggest an important area for future research. The availability of specific pharmacological probes (e.g., fenfluramine, neuroleptics) may help to clarify these issues. Studies of endogenous peptides are also of interest; careful clinical investigations of the opiate antagonists using double-blind procedures remain to be done.

Given the clear evidence of CNS dysfunction in autism, it is surprising how relatively little research has been conducted and how few findings have been replicated. No specific biochemical markers for autism have yet been identified. Various problems have contributed to this situation. Assay methods have often not been comparable across studies. Sample descriptions are often all too brief, and the selection of autistic subjects for research studies has often been idiosyncratic. Typically, only small numbers of subjects are studied. Important and potentially confounding effects of developmental level, age, sex, medication status, and so on have not received sufficient attention. Additional problems have been posed by the nature of the indirect methods employed to assess CNS neuronal systems. The lack of suitable animal models that closely mimic the autistic syndrome has also been an obstacle to research in this area. A review of the available research makes it clear that theoretical models or mechanisms and pharmacological probes have often been borrowed from studies of psychiatric disorders that are, at best, only tenuously related to autism. The use of larger, better-characterized samples and the use of comparable assay methods across laboratories would be helpful. To this end, multicenter and collaborative studies should be encouraged.

Several factors may act to facilitate research in the coming decade. Advances in analytical methods and in the basic neurosciences should facilitate research studies. Despite the problems (Volkmar, Cohen, & Paul, 1986) with current diagnostic criteria (e.g., American Psychiatric Association, 1980), the use of such criteria to define study populations more rigorously will aid in the interpretation of research. The relation of behavioral to biochemical markers is an area of great interest. Most fundamentally, a greater appreciation of the biological basis for the social-communicative dysfunction of autism may help to suggest specific neuronal systems that might most profitably be studies. For example, although much interest has focused on problems in arousal and attention in the pathogenesis of autism, comparatively few studies have related such deficits to neural systems that regulate these processes. Given the range of problems confronting investigators and the relative novelty of many methods currently employed in the study of the neurochemistry of autism, it is not surprising that much work remains to be done.

Acknowledgments

The support of the W. T. Grant Foundation, the John Merck Fund, the Stallone Fund for Autism Research, National Institute of Mental Health Grant No. MH00418, National Institute of Child Health and Human Development Grant No. HD-03008, Mental Health Clinical Research Center Grant No. 30929, Children's Clinical Research Center Grant No. RR00125, and Mr. Leonard Berger is gratefully acknowledged.

References

Amaral, D. G., & Sinnamon, H. M. (1977). The locus coeruleus: Neurobiology of a central noradrenergic nucleus. *Progress in Neurobiology, 9,* 147–196.

American Psychiatric Association. (1980). *Diagnostic and statistical manual of mental disorders* (3rd ed.). Washington, DC: Author.

Anderson, G. M., & Hoshino, Y. (1987). Neurochemical studies of autism. In D. J. Cohen & A. Donnellan (Eds.), *Handbook of autism and pervasive developmental disorders* (pp. 166–191). New York: Wiley.

Anderson, G. M., Minderaa, R. B., van Bentem, P. P. G., Volkmar, F. R., & Cohen, D. J. (1984). Platelet imipramine binding in autistic subjects. *Psychiatry Research, 11,* 133–141.

Anderson, G. M., Volkmar, F. R., Hoder, E. L., McPhedran, P., Minderaa, R. B., Young, J. G., Hansen, C. R., & Cohen, D. J. (1987). Whole blood serotonin in autistic and normal subjects. *Journal of Child Psychiatry and Psychology, 28,* 885–900.

Boullin, D. J., Freeman, B. J., Geller, E., Ritvo, E., Rutter, M., & Yuwiler, A. (1982). Toward the resolution of conflicting findings. *Journal of Autism and Developmental Disorders, 12,* 97–98.

Boullin, D. J., & O'Brien, R. A. (1972). Uptake and loss of ^{14}C-dopamine by platelets from children with infantile autism. *Journal of Autism and Childhood Schizophrenia, 2,* 67–74.

Bowers, M. B., Jr. (1980). Biochemical process in schizophrenia: an update. *Schizophrenia Bulletin, 6,* 393–412.

Brownell, K. D., & Stunkard, A. J. (1982). The double blind in danger: Untoward consequences of informed consent. *American Journal of Psychiatry, 139,* 1487–1489.

Campbell, M., Friedman, E., DeVito, E., Greenspan, L., & Collins, P. J. (1974). Blood serotonin in psychotic and brain-damaged children. *Journal of Autism and Childhood Schizophrenia, 4,* 33–41.

Campbell, M., Hollander, C. S., Ferris, S., & Greene, L. W. (1978a). Response to thyrotropin-releasing hormone stimulation in young psychotic children: A pilot study. *Psychoneuroendocrinology, 3,* 195–201.

Campbell, M., Small, A. M., Hollander, C. S., Korein, J., Cohen, I. L., Kalmijn, M., & Ferris, S. (1978). A controlled crossover study of triiodothyronine in autistic children. *Journal of Autism and Childhood Schizophrenia, 8,* 371–381.

Chess, S., Fernandez, P., & Korn, S. (1974). Behavioral consequences of congenital rubella. *Journal of Pediatrics, 93,* 699–712.

Ciaranello, R. D., VandenBerg, S. R., & Anders, T. G. (1982). Intrinsic and extrinsic determinants of neuronal development: Relation to infantile autism. *Journal of Autism and Developmental Disorders, 12,* 115–145.

Cohen, D. J., Caparulo, B. K., Shaywitz, B. A., & Bowers, M. B., Jr. (1977). Dopamine and serotonin metabolism in neuropsychiatrically disturbed children: CSF homovanillic acid and 5-hydroxyindoleacetic acid. *Archives of General Psychiatry, 34,* 545–550.

Cohen, D. J., Shaywitz, B. A., Johnson, W. T., & Bowers, M. B. (1974). Biogenic amines in autistic and atypical children: Cerebrospinal fluid measures of homovanillic acid and 5-hydroxyindole-acetic acid. *Archives of General Psychiatry, 31,* 845–853.

Cohen, D. J., Volkmar, F. R., & Paul, R. (1986). Issues in the classification of pervasive developmental disorders and associated conditions: History and current status of nosology, *Journal of the American Academy of Child Psychiatry, 25,* 158–161.

Cohen, D. J., Young, J. G., Lowe, T. L., & Harcherik, D. (1980). Thyroid hormone in autistic children. *Journal of Autism and Developmental Disorders, 10,* 445–450.

Cohen, D. J., Young, J. G., Nathanson, J. A., & Shaywitz, B. A. (1979). Clonidine in Tourette's syndrome. *Lancet, ii,* 551–553.

Cohen, D. J., Young, J. G., & Roth, J. A. (1977). Platelet monoamine oxidase in early childhood autism. *Archives of General Psychiatry, 34,* 534–537.

Coid, J., Allolio, B., & Rees, L. H. (1983). Raised plasma metenkephalin in patients who habitually mutilate themselves. *Lancet, ii,* 545.

Coleman, M., Campbell, M., Freedman, L. S., Roffman, M., Ebstein, R. P., & Goldstein, M. (1974). Serum dopamine-β-hydroxylase levels in Down's syndrome. *Clinical Genetics, 5,* 312–315.

Coppen, A., & Wood, K. (1982). 5-Hydroxytryptamine in the pathogenesis of affective disorders. *Advances in Biochemical Pharmacology, 34,* 249–258.

Freeman, B. J., Schroth, P., Ritvo, E., Guthric, D., & Wake, L. (1980). The Behavior Observation Scale for Autism (BOS): Initial results of factor analyses. *Journal of Autism and Developmental Disorders, 10,* 343–346.

Garreau, B., Barthelemy, C., Domenech, J., Sauvage, D., Num, J. P., Lelord, G., & Callaway, E. (1980). Disturbances in dopamine metabolism in autistic children: Results of clinical tests and urinary dosages of homovanilic acid (HVA). *Acta Psychiatrica Belgica, 80,* 249–265.

Geller, E., Ritvo, E. R., Freeman, B. J., & Yuwiler, A. (1982). Preliminary observations on the effect of fenfluramine on blood serotonin and symptoms in three autistic boys. *New England Journal of Medicine, 307,* 165–169.

Gillberg, C. (1980). Identical triplets with infantile autism and fragile X syndrome. *British Journal of Psychiatry, 143,* 256–260.

Gillberg, C., Svennerholm, L., & Hamilton-Hellberg, C. (1983). Childhood psychosis and monoamine metabolites in spinal fluid. *Journal of Autism and Developmental Disorders, 13,* 383–396.

Gillberg, C., Trygstad, O., & Foss, J. (1982). Childhood psychosis and urinary excretion of peptides and protein-associated peptide complexes. *Journal of Autism and Developmental Disorders, 12,* 229–241.

Gualtieri, C. T. (1986). Fenfluramine and autism: A careful reappraisal is in order. *Journal of Pediatrics, 108,* 417–419.

Hanley, H. G., Stahl, S. M., & Freedman, D. X. (1977). Hyperserotonemia and amine metabolites in autistic and retarded children. *Archives of General Psychiatry, 34,* 521–531.

Himwich, H. E., Jenkins, R. L., Fujimori, M., & Narashimhachari, N. (1972). A biochemical study of early infantile autism. *Journal of Autism and Childhood Schizophrenia, 2,* 114–126.

Hoshino, Y., Ohno, Y., Yamamoto, T., Tachibana, R., Murata, S., Yokoyama, F., Kaneko, M., & Kamashiro, H. (1984). Dexamethasone suppression test in autistic children. *Japanese Journal of Clinical Psychiatry, 26,* 100–102.

Inverson, S. D. (1977). Brain dopamine systems and behavior. In L. L. Iversen, S. D. Iversen, & S. H. Snyder (Eds.), *Handbook of psychopharmacology* (Vol. 8, pp. 333–384). New York: Plenum.

Kanner, L. (1943). Autistic disturbances of affective contact. *The Nervous Child, 2,* 227–250.

Katsui, T., Okuda, M., Usuda, S., & Koizumi, T. (1986). Kinetics of ^{3}H-serotonin uptake by platelets in infantile autism and developmental language disorder (including five pairs of twins). *Journal of Autism and Developmental Disorders, 16,* 69–76.

Kopin, I. J., Gordon, E. K., Jimerson, D. C., & Polinsky, R. J. (1983). Relationship between plasma and cerebrospinal fluid levels of 3-methoxy-4-hydroxyphenylglycol. *Science, 219,* 73–75.

Kotsopoulos, S., & Kutty, K. M. (1979). Histidinemia and infantile autism. *Journal of Autism and Developmental Disorders, 9,* 55–60.

Lake, R., Ziegler, M. G., & Murphy, D. L. (1977). Increased norepinephrine levels and decreased DBH activity in primary autism. *Archives of General Psychiatry, 35,* 553–556.

Leckman, J. F., Cohen, D. J., Shaywitz, B. A., Caparulo, B. K., Heninger, G. R., & Bowers, M. B., Jr. (1980). CSF monoamine metabolites in child and adult psychiatric patients. *Archives of General Psychiatry, 37,* 677–681.

Lelord, G., Callaway, E., Muh, J. P., Arlot, J. C., Sauvage, D., Garreau, B., & Domenech, J., (1978). Modifications in urinary homovanillic acid after ingestion of vitamin B6: Functional study in autistic children. *Revue Neurologique, 134,* 797–801.

Lord, C., Schopler, D., & Revick, E. (1982). Sex differences in autism. *Journal of Autism and Developmental Disorders, 12,* 317–330.

Lowe, T. L., Tanaka, K., Seashore, M. R., Young, J. G., & Cohen, D. J. (1980). Detection of phenylketonuria in autistic and psychotic children. *Journal of the American Medical Association, 243,* 126–128.

Maas, J. W., Hattox, S. E., Greene, N. M., & Landis, B. H. (1980). Estimates of dopamine and serotonin synthesis by the awake human brain. *Journal of Neurochemistry, 34,* 1547–1551.

Martineau, J., Garreau, B., Barthelemy, C., Callaway, E., & Lelord, G. (1981). Effects of vitamin B6 on averaged evoked potentials in infantile autism. *Biological Psychiatry, 16,* 627–641.

Maurer, R. G. (1986). Neuropsychology of autism. *Psychiatric Clinics of North America, 9,* 367–380.

Mikkelsen, E. (1982). Efficacy of neuroleptic medication in pervasive developmental disorders of childhood. *Schizophrenia Bulletin, 8,* 320–328.

Minderaa, R. B., Anderson, G. M., Volkmar, F. R., Harcherik, D., Akkerhuis, G. W., & Cohen, D. J. (1987). Urine 5-hydroxy-indoleacetic acid, whole blood serotonin and tryptophan in autistic and normal subjects, *Biological Psychiatry, 22,* 933–940.

Minderaa, R. B., Anderson, G. M., Volkmar, F. R., Harcherik, D., Akkerhuis, G. W., & Cohen, D. J. (1988a). *Plasma levels of 3-methoxy-4-hydroxyphenylglycol (MHPG) and urinary excretion of norepinephrine, epinephrine, and MHPG in autistic and normal subjects.* Manuscript submitted for publication.

Minderaa, R. B., Anderson, G. M., Volkmar, F. R., Harcherik, D., Akkerhuis, G. W., & Cohen, D. J. (1988b). *Plasma levels of homovanillic acid and prolactin and urinary excretion of homovanillic acid and dopamine in autism.* Manuscript submitted for publication.

Moore, R. Y., & Bloom, F. E. (1979). Central catecholamine neuron systems: Anatomy and physiology of the dopamine systems. *Annual Review of Neuroscience, 1,* 129–169.

Panskepp, J. (1979). A neurochemical theory of autism. *Trends in Neuroscience, 2,* 174–177.

Partington, M. W., Tu, J. B., & Wong, C. Y. (1973). Blood serotonin levels in severe mental retardation. *Developmental Medicine and Child Neurology, 15,* 616–627.

Pijnenburg, A. J. J., Honig, W. M. M., van der Heyden, J. A., M., & van Rossum, J. M. (1973). Effects of chemical stimulation of the mesolimbic dopamine system upon locomotor activity. *European Journal of Pharmacology, 35,* 45–58.

Redmond, D. E., & Huang, Y. H. (1979). New evidence for a locus coeruleus–norepinephrine connection with anxiety. *Life Sciences, 25,* 2149–2162.

Riddle, M. A., Shaywitz, B. A., Leckman, J. F., Anderson, G. M., Hardin, M. T., Ort, S., & Cohen, D. J. (1986). Brief debrisoquin loading to assess central dopaminergic function in children. *Life Sciences, 38,* 1041–1048.

Rimland, B. (1964). *Infantile autism.* New York: Appleton-Century-Crofts.

Roberts, P. J., Woodruff, G. N., & Iversen, L. L. (1978). *Advances in biochemical psychopharmacology: Vol. 19. Dopamine.* New York: Raven Press.

Ross, D. L., Klykylo, W. M., & Anderson, G. M. (1985). Cerebrospinal fluid indoleamine and monoamine effects of fenfluramine treatment of infantile autism. *Annals of Neurology, 18,* 394.

Rotman, A., Caplan, R., & Szekely, G. A. (1980). Platelet uptake of serotonin in psychotic children. *Psychopharmacology, 67,* 245–248.

Rutter, M. (1970). Autistic children: Infancy to adulthood. *Seminars in Psychiatry, 2,* 435–450.

Rutter, M. (1972). Childhood schizophrenia reconsidered. *Journal of Autism and Childhood Schizophrenia, 2,* 435–450.

Sandman, C. A., Patta, P. C., Banon, J., Hoehler, F. K., Williams, C., Williams, C., & Swanson, J. M. (1983). Naloxone attenuates self-abusive behavior in developmentally disabled clients. *Applied Research in Mental Retardation, 4,* 5–11.

Schain, R. J., & Freedman, D. X. (1961). Studies on 5-hydroxyindole metabolism in autistic and other mentally retarded children. *Journal of Pediatrics, 58,* 315–320.

Shaw, C. R., Lucas, J., & Rabinovitch, R. D. (1959). Metabolic studies in childhood schizophrenia. *Archives of General Psychiatry, 1,* 366–371.

Shaywitz, B. A., Anderson, G. M., & Cohen, D. J. (1985). Cerebrospinal fluid (CSF) and brain monoamine metabolites in the developing rat pup. *Developmental Brain Research, 17,* 225–232.

Snyder, S. H., & Childers, S. (1979). Opiate receptors and endorphins. *Annual Review of Neuroscience, 2,* 35–64.

Sutton, H. E., Read, J. H., & Arbor, A. (1958). Abnormal amino acid metabolism in a case suggesting autism. *American Journal of Diseases of Children, 96,* 23–28.

Takahashi, S., Kanai, H., & Miyamoto, Y. (1976). Reassessment of elevated serotonin levels in blood platelets in early infantile autism. *Journal of Autism and Childhood Schizophrenia, 6,* 317–326.

Volkmar, F., Cohen, D. J., & Paul, R. (1986). An evaluation of DSM III criteria for infantile autism. *Journal of the American Academy of Child Psychiatry, 25,* 190–197.

Volkmar, F. R., Minderaa, R. B., Anderson, G. M., Hoder, E. L., & Cohen, D. J. (1983, October). *The relation of serotonin level to behavioral characteristics in autistic children.* Paper presented at the annual meeting of the American Academy of Child Psychiatry, San Francisco.

Volkmar, F. R., Paul, R., Cohen, D. J., & Shaywitz, B. (1983). Irritability in autistic children treated with fenfluramine [Letter to the editor]. *New England Journal of Medicine, 309,* 187.

Weizman, R., Weizman, A., Tyano, S., Szekely, B., Weissman, B. A., & Sarne, Y. (1984). Humoral–endorphin blood levels in autistic, schizophrenic and healthy subjects. *Psychopharmacology (Berlin), 82,* 368–370.

Widelitz, M. M., & Feldman, W. (1969). Pink spot in childhood schizophrenia. *Behavioral Neuropsychiatry, 1,* 29–30.

Wing, L., & Gould, J. (1979). Severe impairments of social interaction and associated abnormalities in children: Epidemiology and classification. *Journal of Autism and Development Disorders, 9,* 11–30.

Young, J. G., Cohen, D. J., Brown, S.-L., & Caparulo, B. K. (1978). Decreased urinary free catecholamines in childhood autism. *Journal of the American Academy of Child Psychiatry, 17,* 671–678.

Young, J. G., Cohen, D. J., Caparulo, B. K., Brown, S.-L., & Maas, J. W. (1979). Decreased 24-hour urinary MHPG in childhood autism. *American Journal of Psychiatry, 136,* 1055–1057.

Young, J. G., Cohen, D. J., Kavanagh, M. E., Landis, H. D., Shaywitz, B. A., & Maas, J. W. (1981). Cerebrospinal fluid, plasma, and urinary MHPG in children. *Life Sciences, 28,* 2837–2845.

Young, J. G., Kavanagh, M. E., Anderson, G. M., Shaywitz, B. A., & Cohen, D. J. (1982). Clinical neurochemistry of autism and associated disorders. *Journal of Autism and Developmental Disorders, 12,* 147–165.

Young, J. G., Kyprie, R. M., Ross, N. Y., & Cohen, D. J. (1980). Serum dopamine-beta-hydroxylase activity: Clinical applications in child psychiatry. *Journal of Autism and Developmental Disorders, 10,* 1–14.

Yuwiler, A., Geller, E., & Ritvo, E. (1985). Biochemical studies of autism. In E. Lajtha (Ed.), *Handbook of neurochemistry* (pp. 671–691). New York: Plenum.

CHAPTER 10

Genetic Influences in Autism and Assessment of Metalinguistic Performance in Siblings of Autistic Children

ELAINE R. SILLIMAN
University of South Florida
MAGDA CAMPBELL
New York University Medical Center
ROBIN S. MITCHELL
Private practice, St. Ives, New South Wales, Australia

Recent research indicates that genetic factors may play a role in infantile autism, and that a broad range of cognitive and language disorders is implicated in the description of autism as the most severe form of disrupted development. Evidence supportive of genetic influences also derives from findings with siblings of autistic children. These siblings tend to show a higher incidence of delays in cognitive and language development in comparison to control groups. The major evidence on the language development lags of siblings of autistic children derives from two patterns of performance on the Wechsler Intelligence Scale for Children—Revised (WISC-R; Wechsler, 1974) and the Wechsler Preschool and Primary Scale of Intelligence (WPPSI; Wechsler, 1967). One consistent pattern is that the Verbal IQs of siblings are significantly lower than the Verbal IQs of matched controls; the other pattern is that, within siblings, Verbal IQs are lower than Performance IQs by 15 points or more (Campbell, Minton, Green, Jennings, & Samit, 1981; Minton, Campbell, Green, Jennings, & Samit, 1982). The specific meaning of this discrepancy remains unknown, as does its contribution to illuminating possible genetic influences in autism.

In addressing the discrepancy issue, one conceptualization is that standardized measures of verbal intelligence may be actually assessing different aspects of metalinguistic ability. By "metalinguistic ability" is generally meant skill in reflecting consciously on, or analyzing in a controlled way, various components of the linguistic-communicative system as an internalized means for the self-regulation of thinking. Currently, no single methodology is available that systematically assesses a range of metalinguistic skills (Nesdale & Tunmer, 1984)—for example,

225

in the age range from 6 years to 9 years. During this period of development, many different metalinguistic skills begin to flower.

The intent of this chapter is to provide a foundation for developing more refined descriptions of possible connections among kinship, metalinguistic modes of language processing, and genetic influences in autism. In building this foundation, a working hypothesis is that the discrepancy commonly found between Verbal and Performance IQs in siblings of autistic children may have a metalinguistic component, given the metalinguistic bias of the WISC-R Verbal Scale, as an example.

INTRODUCTION: GENETIC ISSUES IN AUTISM

Infantile autism is a syndrome defined by history, age of onset of illness, and behavioral criteria; therefore, it is doubtful that it is an etiologically homogeneous disorder (Campbell & Green, 1985; Coleman & Gillberg, 1985; DeMyer, Hingtgen, & Jackson, 1981, Rimland, 1964). Although in most cases the factors leading to the clinical picture of autism are unknown, in rare instances it is found to be the result of identifiable causes, such as phenylketonuria (Lowe, Tanaka, Seashore, Young, & Cohen, 1980), congenital rubella (Chess, Corn, & Fernandez, 1971), or the fragile X syndrome (for review, see Coleman & Gillberg, 1985; Rutter, 1985). Pre- and perinatal complications are also among factors that may contribute to this condition (Campbell *et al.*, 1978; Coleman & Gillberg, 1985; Folstein & Rutter, 1977, 1978; Green *et al.*, 1984; Kolvin, 1971; Torrey, Hersh, & McCabe, 1975). Brain dysfunction of various degrees that is due to complications of pregnancy and birth has been found in many autistic children, resulting in seizure disorder in later life (Deykin & MacMahon, 1979; Kolvin, 1971; Rutter, 1985). The clinical picture of autism may be modified by the child's intellectual functioning or degree of mental subnormality (Campbell & Green, 1985; Freeman *et al.*, 1981; Rutter, 1978).

The results of a carefully designed study based on 21 pairs of monozygotic (MZ) and dizygotic (DZ) twins suggest that genetic factors too may play a role in some cases (Folstein & Rutter, 1977, 1978; for review, see Campbell & Green, 1985; Campbell *et al.*, 1988). The biological influences in infantile autism have been recently reviewed (Campbell & Green, 1985; Coleman & Gillberg, 1985; Young, Kavanagh, Anderson, Shaywitz, & Cohen, 1982; Young, Leven, Togasaki, & Knott, 1986; Young, Ludman, & Knott, 1986). In 1976, in a careful review and analysis of the pertinent literature, Hanson and Gottesman came to the conclusion that there is no clear evidence indicating that genetic factors play a role in infantile autism. These same authors found no adequately documented cases of infantile autism in almost 400 siblings of autistics in the literature. However, the 7 (or 1.8%) undocumented cases of autism among siblings did suggest a familial clustering of autism compatible with multifactorial models. Only 18 pairs of twins were reported in the literature before 1976; Hanson and Gottesman found the data inadequate for genetic analysis. There was no report on offspring of autistic individuals.

In the same year, Spence (1976) addressed the following questions: "What are the possible genetic factors" (p. 169) in this condition, and how would one test for the presence of such factors? She forwarded several genetic hypotheses and considered them very thoughtfully. No hard data were available at that time. Since then, in the past decade, suggestive evidence has accumulated indicating that genetic influences, though weak, may play a contributory role in the development of autism in a subgroup of such children. Thus, various factors, including genetic, neurobiological, and developmental, may be operating and leading to this final clinical pathway called infantile autism.

Shifting from contributing factors to the mode of inheritance of autism, Ritvo, Ritvo, and Mason-Brothers (1982) suggest on the basis of their twin studies, that autosomal recessive inheritance is operative. Spence (1976), in contrast, in a thoughtful discussion, argues for a polygenic or multifactorial mode of transmission—a hypothesis supported by others, based on their research findings (Campbell et al., 1988; Tsai, Stewart, & August, 1981). Moreover, unraveling the mode of inheritance is complicated further because of the low incidence of either marriage or parenthood in individuals with the autistic syndrome (Ludlow & Cooper, 1983; Vandenberg & Streng, 1984). Siblings of autistic children therefore offer an opportunity to examine the role of familial transmission. Evidence supportive of genetic factors shows that siblings of autistic children tend to have a higher incidence of cognitive and language development delays than do children without autistic siblings (August, Stewart, & Tsai, 1981; Campbell et al., 1981; Folstein & Rutter, 1978; Minton et al., 1982).

A complex genetic model, a polygenic or multifactorial mode of inheritance, suggests that many genes affect the expression of the trait. This theoretical concept was applied in the 1960s to such human conditions as a cleft lip, cleft palate, and clubfoot. The trait measured can be height, weight, or a theoretical liability for a disease or condition like autism. For height and weight, we see a bell-shaped curve. For a condition like autism, we see only two categories, affected or normal. The breakpoint between the two is called the "threshold" on the liability scale. If the individual has enough contributions from genes and environment, his or her own liability value will fall above the threshold point, and he or she will be classified as affected. With this model, it is possible to account for the small recurrence risk in families and the slightly different rate in the two sexes.

Multifactorial models have been utilized in the analysis of family data of psychiatric syndromes, such as antisocial personality, criminality, alcoholism, and schizophrenia (Cloninger, Christiansen, Reich, & Gottesman, 1978; Cloninger, Lewis, Rice, & Reich, 1981; Gottesman & Shields, 1972; Reich, Rice, Cloninger, Wette, & James, 1979). With the multifactorial models, it is possible to interpret the different rate of a condition in sexes and the very small occurrence of the same condition in families. Actually, these findings—that is, the differences related to sex and severity of the condition—may be used, first, to get a better understanding of the roles played by genetic and environmental contributions in a condition, and, second, to test the mode of transmission of various psychiatric syndromes (Cloninger et al., 1978; Spence, 1976).

The sex effect has been explored also with family data in psychiatric disorders such as alcoholism, criminality, and psychopathy (Cloninger et al., 1978). Phenotypic heterogeneities of multifactorial traits were interpreted by using multiple thresholds and segregation analysis of family data (Cloninger et al., 1981; Reich et al., 1979). For example, antisocial personality or criminality is less common in women than in men. Females may have a higher threshold than men for manifesting this condition. When females do show manifestations of criminal behavior, they are more deviant and more of their relatives are affected (Cloninger et al., 1978).

Thus, it is interesting to hypothesize that infantile autism lies at an extreme pole of a spectrum of cognitive–language disorders, with some learning and/or language disorders being milder variants of the same continuum or diathesis (Folstein, 1985). This continuum may include cases where there are large discrepancies between Verbal and Performance IQs. It is also recognized that developmental deviations in language and cognition can be multiply determined. It seems reasonable to speculate that there are probably polygenically determined reaction ranges that find expression and modification through multiple interactions with many environmental factors, including intrauterine insult, complications of birth, subsequent physical health or illness, cultural–familial experiences, and others.

OVERVIEW OF THE PERTINENT LITERATURE:
TWIN AND SIBLING STUDIES

Twins Concordant and Discordant for Autism

One type of genetic study is the twin study. Twin studies suggest that there is a greater concordance rate for autism in MZ twins than in DZ twins.

Autism, however, is a very rare condition. Most reports agree that 2–4 children in 10,000 are autistic (Gillberg, 1984; Gillberg & Schaumann, 1982; Lotter, 1966, 1967; Steinhausen, Gobel, Breinlinger, & Wohlleben, 1986). Furthermore, only about 1 of 86 live births are twins. As a result, there are only two major twin studies, 26 reports on one or two cases, and additional passing references to autistic twins in the literature (for review, see Campbell et al., 1988).

In a 1964 review, Rimland found reports on a total of 11 pairs of MZ twins, all of whom were concordant for autism. Subsequent to 1964, there were six additional case reports on MZ twins, until the publication of the important work of Folstein and Rutter (1977, 1978). Their carefully designed study consisted of 11 pairs of MZ twins and 10 pairs of same-sex DZ twins. Of the 11 MZ pairs, 4 were concordant for autism, while none of the DZ pairs were concordant.

Following a few case reports, Ritvo, Freeman, Mason-Brothers, Mo, and Ritvo (1985) published their findings on 23 pairs of MZ and 17 pairs of DZ twins, based on the UCLA Registry for Genetic Studies in Autism. Of the 61 pairs enrolled in this registry, the 40 pairs studied by Ritvo *et al.* met the Research Diagnostic Criteria for autism. Of the 23 MZ pairs, 22 were concordant for autism, whereas only 4 of the 17 DZ twins were so. However, only 12 pairs of MZ twins and 5 pairs of the 12 pairs of same-sex DZ twins had blood grouping studies; furthermore, this is not a representative sample of twinships in the population of autistic patients.

A more representative, although smaller, sample consisted of seven pairs of twins who were part of a total of 278 preschool-age autistic children, admitted from 1961 to the present time to the Therapeutic Nursery of Bellevue Hospital, Psychiatric Division (Campbell *et al.*, 1988). All 278 patients were carefully studied and diagnosed as having infantile autism. Of the seven twin pairs, five were same-sex pairs; three of these had studies for blood grouping. Two pairs were found to be MZ (males), and one was a DZ pair (females). The two MZ pairs had additional studies, for fingerprints and hair whorl. The two MZ twin pairs were concordant for autism, but all three DZ pairs were discordant. The other two pairs of same-sex male twins did not have studies for blood grouping; one pair was concordant for autism, and the other was not. Table 10-1 presents a survey of the pertinent literature on twins. Tables 10-2 and 10-3 list the well-documented MZ and DZ twins, respectively.

Finally, since 1982, several reports in the literature suggest that, in a subgroup of autistic children, there is a specific association of autism and the fragile X syndrome. No agreement is apparent, however, on the frequency of this syndrome in populations of autistics (W. T. Brown *et al.*, 1982; Coleman & Gillberg, 1985, p. 65, Figure 6-1; Fisch *et al.*, 1986; Gillberg & Walhstrom, 1985; Goldfine *et al.*, 1985; Levitas *et al.*, 1983). For details, a chapter by Rutter (1985) is recommended.

Rate of Autism in Siblings of Autistic Children

As previously mentioned, autism is a rare occurrence. In siblings of autistic children, however, the incidence of autism is approximately 50 times greater than in the general child population (August *et al.*, 1981; Campbell *et al.*, 1981; Coleman & Rimland, 1976; Eisenberg & Kanner, 1956; Gillberg & Wahlstrom, 1985; Minton *et al.*, 1982; Rimland, 1971; Rutter, 1967). Specifically, 1.3% to 2.8% of siblings are themselves autistic.

A few studies report on three siblings in the same family, all having autism (Rivto *et al.*, 1982; Ritvo, Spence, *et al.*, 1985; Shell, Campion, Minton, Caplan, & Campbell, 1984). Coleman and Rimland (1976) found an 8% incidence of autism in extended families of autistic subjects.

TABLE 10-1.   Twins: Survey of the Literature

Author(s)	Zygosity (MZ–DZ)	Evidence	Concordant or discordant for autism	Sex
Sherwin (1953)	MZ	NA	Concordant	Males
Bakwin (1954)	MZ	B, 1P, S	Concordant	Males
Eisenberg & Kanner (1956)	MZ	NA	One twin died at 5 months	Males
Chapman (1957)	MZ	S	Concordant	Females
Keeler, cited in Kanner & Eisenberg (1957)	MZ DZ	NA NA	Concordant Discordant	? ?
Lehman, Haber, & Lesser (1957)	MZ	NA	Concordant	Males
Keeler (1958)	MZ	NA	Concordant	Males
Bruch (1959)	MZ	NA	Concordant	Males
Polan & Spencer (1959)	MZ	NA	Concordant	Males
Chapman (1960)	MZ	NA	Concordant	? (two pairs)
Creak & Ini (1960)	DZ	NA	Discordant	?
Ward & Hoddinott (1962)	DZ	NA, 2P	Concordant	Females
Vaillant (1963)	DZ ?	B, 1P, S 1P, S	Discordant Discordant	Males Females
Book, Nichtern, & Gruenberg (1963)	DZ	NA	Discordant	Male autistic, female normal
Kamp (1964)	MZ	B, FP	Discordant	Females
Ornitz, Ritvo, & Walter (1965)	MZ	NA	Concordant	Males
Lovaas, Schaeffer, & Simmons (1965)	MZ	NA	Concordant	Males
Havelkova (1967)	MZ DZ	NA	Concordant Discordant	Females Female autistic, male normal
Kean (1975)	MZ	NA	Concordant	Males
McQuaid (1975)	MZ	B	Concordant	Males
Kotsopoulos (1976)	DZ		Concordant	Male Female
Folstein & Rutter (1977, 1978)	11 MZ 10 DZ	B, S, FP	4 concordant, 7 discordant All discordant	Same-sexed Same-sexed
Campbell, Dominijanni, & Schneider (1977)	MZ	B, S, FP	Concordant	Males
Sloan (1978)	DZ		Discordant	Male female autistic
Wessels & Van Meerdervoort (1979)	MZ	B	Concordant	Males

(continued)

TABLE 10-1.   (Continued)

Author(s)	Zygosity (MZ–DZ)	Evidence	Concordant or discordant for autism	Sex
Salimi-Eshkevari (1979)	MZ	B	Concordant	Males
Gillberg (1983)	MZ (triplets)	S	Concordant	Males
Salimi-Eshkevari (1985)	MZ	B	Concordant	Males
Ritvo, Freeman, Mason-Brothers, Mo, & Ritvo (1985)	23 MZ 17 DZ	B (for 12 pairs) B (for 5 pairs of 10 same-sexed pairs)	22 concordant 4 concordant, 13 discordant	Males, females Same- and opposite-sexed
Campbell *et al.* (1988)	2 MZ 3 DZ	B, S, FP B	Concordant Discordant	Males 1 female, same-sexed; 2 opposite-sexed (males, autistic)

Note. MZ, monozygotic; DZ, dizygotic; concordant, concordant for autism; discordant, discordant for autism; NA, not available; B, blood grouping; P, placenta (1P or 2P); S, similarity; FP, fingerprints.

Cognitive and Language Impairments in Twins, Siblings, and Parents of Autistic Children

Folstein and Rutter (1977, 1978) forwarded a hypothesis that a genetic vulnerability to develop language and/or cognitive dysfunction, "of which autism constitutes but one part" (Rutter, 1985, p. 553), exists in certain families. For infantile autism to emerge, however, additional factors are necessary in many but not in all cases (e.g., pre- or perinatal insult to the central nervous system; Folstein & Rutter, 1977, 1978). In effect, a genetic influence may be inherited and contribute to a wide range of cognitive impairments. Autism is only one of the expressions of genetic influence, but does represent the severest form of disruption in the development of cognition and communication.

The Folstein and Rutter hypothesis, as noted earlier, was based on a genetic study of 21 pairs of same-sex twins and their siblings and parents. The nonautistic cotwins in the MZ twin pairs discordant for autism frequently showed some kind of cognitive–language deficit. This finding was true in only one or two cases for DZ twins, all of whom were discordant for autism. The deficit included wide discrepancy between Verbal and Performance IQs on age-appropriate Wechsler intelligence tests. In three cases, the Verbal IQ was lower by 14 to 23 points than the Performance IQ in cotwins who were of normal intelligence. Furthermore, in 3 of the 21 families, a severe delay in the use of speech was reported for the siblings or for the parents.

August *et al.*, (1981), in a genetic study designed to assess the spectrum of possible expressions of infantile autism, also report "a significant familial clustering of cognitive disabilities in the siblings of autistic probands" (p. 416). Their study was a comparison of 71 siblings of (41) autistic children, and 38 controls, all of whom were siblings of (15) Down syndrome children. Age-appropriate Wechsler intelligence tests were administered to all siblings, as was the Wide Range Achievement Test (WRAT) where appropriate. Cognitive disabilities were found to be significantly greater in the siblings of autistics ($n = 11$, or 15.5%) than in the controls (3%). Of the 11 siblings of probands, 4 evidenced problems in the comprehension or production of language; 9 had IQs below 80; and 2 had reading disability. Other investigators have also made similar observations in siblings of autistic children (Cohen, Caparulo, & Shaywitz, 1976; Steffenburg *et al.*, 1988; Ritvo, Freeman, *et al.*, 1985; see also Coleman & Gillberg, 1985, pp. 61–62). In a controlled study, nonautistic siblings of autistic children ($n = 50$) had significantly lower verbal scores than performance scores on Wechsler intelligence scales, and 10% were mentally retarded (Minton *et al.*, 1982).

It is of interest that, though developmental language impairment and infantile autism are considered different diagnostic entities (Cohen *et al.*, 1976; Rutter, 1978), a family history of speech delay exists in about 25% of cases in both conditions (Bartak, Rutter, & Cox, 1975; Cohen *et al.*, 1976; Rutter, 1978). There is the increasing awareness across disciplinary boundaries that learning disabilities in nonautistic and nonretarded children are often associated with language disabilities (Denckla, 1983; Duane, 1985; Mann, 1986). In all autistic children, how-

TABLE 10-2. Well-Documented Monozygotic Twins: Survey of the Literature

Investigator(s)	No. pairs	Concordant or discordant	Sex
Bakwin (1954)	1	Concordant	M M
Kamp (1964)	1	Discordant	F F
McQuaid (1975)	1	Concordant	M M
Campbell *et al.* (1977)	1	Concordant	M M
Folstein & Rutter (1977, 1978)	11	4 concordant, 7 discordant	M & F
Wessels & Van Meerdervoort (1979)	1	Concordant	M
Salimi-Eshkevari (1979)	1	Concordant	M
Salimi-Eshkevari (1985)	1	Concordant	M
Ritvo *et al.* (1985)	12	11 concordant, 1 discordant	M & F
Campbell *et al.* (1988)	1[a]	Concordant	M

Note. Total = 31 pairs; concordant = 22, discordant = 9.
[a] In addition to the Campbell *et al.* (1977) report.

TABLE 10-3. Well-Documented Dizygotic Twins: Survey of the Literature

Investigator(s)	No. pairs	Concordant or discordant	Sex
Ward & Hoddinott (1962)	1	Concordant	F[a] F[a]
Vaillant (1963)	1	Discordant	M[a] M
Book et al. (1963)	1	Discordant	A? M[a] B? F
Kotsopoulos (1976)	1	Concordant	M[a] F[a]
Folstein & Rutter (1977, 1978)	10	Discordant	Same-sexed
Sloan (1978)	1	Discordant	M F[a]
Ritvo et al. (1985)	10	3 concordant, 7 discordant	3 same-sexed, 7 opposite-sexed
Campbell et al. (1988)	3	Discordant	F/F[a], F/M[a], F/M[a]

Note. Total = 28 pairs; concordant = 5, discordant = 23. A, first-born twin; B, second-born twin.
[a] Autistic.

ever, developmental disruptions of cognition and communication result in learning disabilities of various degrees, which constitute the pathogenic features of this clinical syndrome (Rutter, 1978, 1985).

Thus, the expression of the diathesis for developing cognitive and language disabilities can be viewed on a continuum: Infantile autism is the most severe expression of this diathesis, while language-learning disabilities, including significant discrepancies between Verbal and Performance IQs, are milder forms of the same diathesis. Table 10-4 summarizes the pertinent literature on the language and cognitive deficits in twins and siblings of autistic children.

Some Limitations of the Sibling Studies

The interpretations of language ability in the sibling research have several limitations. Among these limitations are (1) inconsistency across studies in conceptually distinguishing between speech as the vocalized form by which meaning and intent are expressed and language as "a code whereby ideas about the world are represented through a conventional system of arbitrary signals for communication" (Bloom & Lahey, 1978, p. 4); (2) the use of discrepancies between Verbal and Performance IQs obtained from the WISC-R as diagnostic indicators of impairment in either language or learning ability (Algozzine & Ysseldyke, 1986; Tindal & Marston, 1986); and (3) the general focus on language behaviors as a set of discrete skills that can be isolated for assessment purposes.

TABLE 10-4. Representative Literature for the Influence of Genetic and Environmental Factors in Infantile Autism: Language or Cognitive Deficits

Authors	Numbers	Subjects	Controls	Findings
Vaillant (1963)	2 pairs of DZ twins discordant for autism	The 2 DZ twins with autism	The 2 nonautistic twins	Deviant speech and intellectual development in both nonautistic twins
Whittam, Simon, & Mittler (1966)	43	Psychotic	66 siblings (43 males)	8 (12%) of siblings had delay in language
Havelkova (1967)	18	Schizophrenic (autistic) children with one or more abnormal siblings	42 siblings	13 (27.1%) of siblings were retarded; 8 (16.7%) of siblings had delayed speech
Bartak, Rutter, & Cox (1975)	19	Autistic	23 uncomplicated developmental language disorder ("dysphasia"); 5 mixed with autistic features	In both groups, over 25% of the patients had parents or siblings with a history of language or speech disorder
Folstein & Rutter (1978)	21 pairs of same-sexed twins	Autistic twins: 7 MZ and 10 DZ twins discordant for autism and 4 MZ twins corcordant for autism	The 17 nonautistic twins	Language or cognitive delay or deficit in 5 MZ twins and in 2 DZ twins discordant for autism
August, Stewart, & Tsai (1981)	71	Siblings of autistic children	38 siblings of Down syndrome children	15.5% of the siblings of autistics had cognitive disabilities (language, learning, and 9.8% mental retardation), and 2.8% had infantile autism; 3% of controls had cognitive disability
Minton, Campbell, Green, Jennings, & Samit (1982)	50	Siblings of autistic children	Wechsler standardization sample	Siblings had significantly lower Verbal than Performance scores on Wechsler IQ tests; 10% were mentally retarded; 2% had infantile autism

Note. From "Pervasive Developmental Disorders of Childhood" by M. Campbell and W. H. Green, 1985, in H. I. Kaplan and B. J. Sadock (Eds.), *Comprehensive Textbook of Psychiatry/IV* (4th ed., Vol. 2, pp. 1672–1683), Baltimore: Williams & Wilkins. Copyright 1985 by the Williams & Wilkins Co. Reprinted by permission.

A fourth variable affecting the interpretation of sibling studies stems from the discrete skills orientation. This variable involves the inherent metalinguistic bias of the tasks used to assess facets of language ability. In effect, normative measures of language knowledge, including measures of verbal intelligence, may actually be assessing proficiency in the metalinguistic mode of use (Flood & Salus, 1982; Silliman, 1984; van Kleeck, 1984a). Although these normative measures are not specifically designed to elicit metalinguistic awareness, the practical outcome is a metalinguistic bias (Flood & Salus, 1982). In the analysis of van Kleeck (1984a), standardized tests assess language skills by requiring that the child reflect on aspects of the linguistic code apart from real-world interactional contexts of use—for example, in comparing whether two words have a similar or different sound structure or considering what a word means. Often, adequate performance is also dependent on the child's ability to suspend everyday rules for how to participate in conversational interaction, as when he or she is required to engage in sentence imitation. The adequacy of a child's performance, then, may depend on how well that child can infer expectations for how to perform (Silliman, 1987).

METALINGUISTIC DEVELOPMENT AND ITS ASSESSMENT

Metalinguistic Awareness and Metacognition

Metalinguistic knowledge appears to be a specialized application of metacognitive knowledge (Hirsh-Pasek, Gleitman, & Gleitman, 1980; Pratt & Grieve, 1984a, 1984b; Valtin, 1984b; van Kleeck, 1984b). Metacognition, although not operationally well defined, generally entails thinking about thinking or cognizing about one's cognitive products, including strategies for their use (Borkowski & Kurtz, 1984; Yussen, 1985). Much of mental activity appears to be conducted through automatic modes of processing (Gazzaniga, 1985) or the effortless performance that results from extensive familiarity (Hutchins, 1986; Sternberg, 1987a). Both metacognitive and metalinguistic activity are viewed as directed or controlled processes, however, and are engaged when information must be actively organized and utilized for a specific goal (A. L. Brown, 1977; A. L. Brown & DeLoache, 1983; Tunmer & Herriman, 1984).

A number of unresolved issues pertain to more precise description of metacognition and its relationship to metalinguistic awareness. These issues include (1) variability in definition (Cavanaugh & Perlmutter, 1982); (2) sequences and rates of development (Pratt & Grieve, 1984b; Yussen, 1985); (3) the significance of differences in either the structure or functioning of automatic versus controlled processing modes (Gazzaniga, 1985); (4) the exact boundary between cognition and metacognition, and how to measure the point of awareness (Yussen, 1985); and (5) whether conscious awareness is an invariant precondition for metacognitive activity (Day, French, & Hall, 1985; Pressley, Forrest-Pressley, Elliot-Faust, & Miller, 1985; Tunmer & Herriman, 1984; Yussen, 1985). Although there is minimal research on the metacognitive abilities of autistic individuals, metacognitive limitations have been identified as characteristic of performance by learning-disabled children (for reviews, see Silliman, 1987; Sternberg, 1987a; Wong, 1985).

Metalinguistic Development

In common with the definitional ambiguity of metacognition, metalinguistic awareness also lacks a unifying theoretical framework, including a specification of its components, sequences, and rates of development (Pratt & Grieve, 1984a; Tunmer & Herriman, 1984; Valtin, 1984b). What have been elaborated are descriptions of metalinguistic awareness, including its general relationship to a metacognitive processing mode, and the content that may comprise its knowledge base.

Descriptions of Metalinguistic Awareness

Cazden (1983) offers the "glass theory" of metalinguistic awareness. In this analysis, language forms used for everyday, or routine, communicative purposes are transparent: "We hear through them to the meaning intended" (Cazden, 1983, p. 303). Thus, children learn to use language in this transparent way in their dual roles as speakers and listeners. But children also develop the ability to make language forms opaque. That is, children also develop the ability to consider linguistic elements as independent objects of analysis separate from the intention, or purposes, of communicative acts and their meaning. The ability to attend selectively to linguistic elements as units disembedded from practical, everyday uses of communication (van Kleeck, 1984b) appears to be a special kind of language performance. This mode of use makes different demands on cognitive processes, is a less easily and universally acquired ability, and is an essential aspect of proficiency with literacy activities (Cazden, 1983; Denckla, 1983; Flood & Menyuk, 1983; Flood & Salus, 1982; Menyuk, 1983; Valtin, 1984a, 1984b; Vellutino & Shub, 1982).

   The ability to shift the focus of attention from the practical, or implicit, system of use to the metalinguistic mode implies, then, that a controlled mode of processing is activated at some level (Hakes, 1980; Pratt & Grieve, 1984a; Tunmer & Herriman, 1984). It is the nature of this shift as a function of the contextual variables occasioning its occurrence, as well as the level and degree of occurrence, that is of theoretical and empirical interest for a more precise understanding of childhood language impairment. Many of the academic and developmental problems in language learning displayed by these children appear to have a metalinguistic base, at least partially (Kamhi & Koenig, 1985; Kamhi, Lee, & Nelson,

1985; Liles, Schulman, & Bartlett, 1977; Nippold & Fey, 1983; Seidenberg & Bernstein, 1986; van Kleeck, 1984b).

Although a variety of metalinguistic acquisitions have been identified, a number of issues remain controversial: (1) how metalinguistic development occurs—that is, whether it is intertwined with the basic language acquisition process (Clark, 1980), whether it is related to and the result of a more general transformation in cognitive capacities during middle childhood (Tunmer & Herriman, 1984), or whether it is facilitated by literacy instruction (Ehri, 1984); (2) the nature of emergence—specifically, whether different metalinguistic abilities emerge synchronously or asynchronously (Nesdale & Tunmer, 1984); and (3) the levels of awareness required by different kinds of metalinguistic performances (Pratt & Grieve, 1984a). In regard to this last controversy, Valtin (1984b) distinguishes three stages of explicit awareness. Only the third stage, controlled processing, meets rigorous requirements for a metalinguistic mode of use in a formal sense. These stages and the characteristic behaviors defining each are outlined in Table 10-5.

Metalinguistic Content

Menyuk (1983) cites the dependence of skillful reading comprehension on the degree of accessibility, or the availability, of the linguistic categories and relations comprising one's knowledge of the oral means of communication. Aspects of metalinguistic content that become accessible include the conscious awareness (1) that phonological segments have categorical standing separate from word meaning (e.g., as reflected in tasks requiring the production of words having identical sound sequences or the segmenting of words into their phonemic constituents); (2) that morphophonological rules can be applied in flexible ways, either to derive new syntactic categories (e.g., altering stressing rules from *per-mit'* to *per'-mit*) or to derive new lexical items through compounding or by change in affix (e.g., *mis + chief*); (3) that the individual meaning of words varies with the context of use and that words also come to represent categories of meaning (e.g., as manifested in tasks requiring definition of words); and (4) that the understanding of utterances is mutually dependent on both semantic and syntactic knowledge, which is knowledge about the relations holding among "word meanings in the context of varying structures" (Menyuk, 1983, p. 153).

The progressive understanding of the mutuality described by Menyuk (1983) has been demonstrated primarily through three kinds of tasks. Typical tasks include grammaticality (acceptability) judgments of individual sentence types (Flood & Menyuk, 1983; Flood & Salus, 1982; Menyuk, 1983; Tunmer & Grieve, 1984); synonomy judgments, which focus on the equivalence of meaning between different sentences (Hakes, 1980; Hirsh-Pasek *et al.*, 1980); and the resolution of ambiguous meaning as reflected through figurative or nonliteral forms of language

TABLE 10-5. Development of Language Awareness

Type of awareness	Behaviors	Examples[a]
I. *Unconscious awareness* (automatic uses of language)—preconscious, or implicit, monitoring of own speech production	Detects failure to be understood by others	Repairs own speech spontaneously; can evaluate whether or not the listener has understood and repair accordingly; corrects the utterances of others
II. *Actual awareness*—the momentary shifting of attention from communicative intention to the linguistic means by which intentions are realized	In role playing, can talk about aspects of language in a given context, but cannot disembed these aspects from the specific context of use	Able to adjust communicative style of the age and status of the listener, including "doing the voices" for different roles; can comment on own utterances and those of others
	Increasing ability to separate linguistic units (sounds, words, phrases, and sentences) from their communicative functions; that is, can better separate function and meaning from the forms that express them	Able to *judge* which utterances might be more polite or appropriate for a specific speaker; can *correct* violations of word order in sentences earlier judged as "silly"; can *practice* (play) with new sound, word, and sentence combinations as a deliberate strategy to learn new information
III. *Conscious awareness*—explicit knowledge of linguistic units and their possible combinations	Able to deliberately focus on and manipulate linguistic elements disembedded from their actual communicative functions and meanings or specific contexts of use	Can now *explain* in linguistic terms why a word is a word, the meaning of words, alternate interpretations, ambiguous meaning, including metaphors, idioms, riddles, jokes, and puns, and why certain sentences are permissible

Note. Summarized from Valtin (1984b).
[a]Examples are modifications of Clark (1980, p. 34).

use, such as verbal riddles and jokes (Fowles & Glantz, 1977; Hirsh-Pasek *et al.*, 1980; Pepicello & Weisberg, 1983; Shultz & Horibe, 1974).

As a general developmental trend, it appears that the practical, or social-communicative, awareness of linguistic representations precedes the ability to recognize that an incongruity exists in either the form or the meaning of representation (Hakes, 1980; Hirsh-Pasek *et al.*, 1980; Menyuk, 1983; Tunmer & Grieve, 1984). Recognition of violation, in turn, precedes the ability to correct the block element (Pepicello & Weisberg, 1983), through which awareness of a rule violation occurs (Menyuk, 1983), whereas the ability to explain one's interpretation of linguistic events emerges last (Hakes, 1980; Hirsh-Pasek *et al.*, 1980; Ryan & Ledger, 1984).

Additional corroboration for this developmental trend in the process of metalinguistic awareness is found in the Valtin (1984b) model outlined in Table 10-5. Across studies, which vary considerably in methodology, there appears to be a general consensus that the most stringent test of metalinguistic behaviors is the ability to interpret, or explicitly evaluate, plausible possibilities about what one can do with linguistic elements—a pattern of performance most consistent with Valtin's third stage of conscious awareness.

The nature of this development is not an all-or-none phenomenon, however. Successful performance on either recognition (judgment), correction, or explanation tasks will vary. Reasons for individual variation in performance include (1) the type of structural-relational awareness being assessed (e.g., linguistic synonymy versus linguistic ambiguity); (2) whether the domain of assessment is literal or figurative; (3) the cognitive complexity of the material to be acted on, including the extent of short-term memory demands; (4) the clarity of instructions, the design of practice trials and feedback, and the appropriateness of task procedures; and (5) response style preferences related to cultural differences (Flood & Salus, 1982; Fowles & Glantz, 1977; Hirsh-Pasek *et al.*, 1980; Menyuk, 1983; Nesdale & Tunmer, 1984; Pepicello & Weisberg, 1983; Valtin, 1984b).

Finally, in a substantively different approach to the description of metalinguistic content, van Kleeck (1984b) recasts the Bloom and Lahey (1978) definition of language into three focuses of metalinguistic awareness. Table 10-6 summarizes this reformulation and recognizes the kinds of tasks from which developmental inferences have been drawn. Van Kleeck (1984b) acknowledges the difficulty of agreeing on the exact behaviors constituting metalinguistic activity, given the range of behaviors that could be classified. She argues that a taxonomy of metalinguistic knowledge initially "should be based on a clear and consistent definition of language" (van Kleeck, 1984b, p. 132). A major contribution of this framework, therefore, is its definitional refinement in connecting aspects of metalinguistic knowledge to the three interactive components of language: language content or meaning, language form, and language use. The framework also permits a more parsimonious explanation of standardized measures of "language knowledge" as measures soliciting a metalinguistic mode of performance (van Kleeck, 1984a).

TABLE 10-6. Focuses of Language Awareness and Examples of Experimental Tasks Related to Each Focus of Awareness

Focus of awareness	Examples of experimental tasks
1. *Language is an arbitrary conventional code that represents* (content component)—refers to the awareness that words are separate from that which they represent in the real world and that words have different underlying meanings as agreed upon by the members of a linguistic community	• Understanding words as distinct linguistic units • Providing conventional definitions of words • Judging whether varying word orders are synonymous in meaning • Recognizing and resolving linguistic ambiguity (similar sentence forms can have different meanings)
2. *Language is a rule-governed system* (form component)—refers to the awareness that linguistic elements, from phonemic to syntactic rules for combining elements, function in a systematic and predictable manner	• Segmentation of words into syllabic and phonemic components • Judging the grammatical acceptability of sentences
3. *Language is used for different communicative purposes* (use component)—refers to the awareness that how content and form is conveyed or interpreted is inseparable from intention and the social features comprising the communicative context	• Judging utterance appropriateness as a function of context • Explaining appropriateness choices

Note. Summarized from van Kleeck (1984b), based on Bloom and Lahey (1978).

An existing weakness of this reformulation is lack of differentiation within each component for levels of awareness.

METALINGUISTIC AWARENESS IN SIBLINGS OF AUTISTIC CHILDREN: SOME PRELIMINARY EVIDENCE

The study to be described here was designed with two specific objectives. One aim was to determine types of metalinguistic tasks potentially most sensitive to possible performance differences between siblings and a set of matched controls (children without autistic siblings). A second objective was to ascertain the nature of performance differences, if any, in the comprehension and use of certain forms of metalinguistic knowledge.

Sample Selection

To maximize sample homogeneity, siblings of autistic children were selected from a pool of siblings aged 6 to 9 years, made available from Bellevue Hospital, Psychiatric Division. Five children (mean chronological age [CA] = 7 years, 6 months; range = 6 years, 2 months to 8 years, 9 months), four males and one female, met the sample selection criteria to be discussed shortly. The diagnosis of infantile autism in their siblings was made using American Psychiatric Association (1980) criteria. In addition, all five children's autistic siblings had been hospitalized at one time in the Therapeutic Nursery of the Psychiatric Division at Bellevue Hospital. Excluded from the final sample were siblings for whom causes for the autistic syndrome in their brothers or sisters were known, as well as those having seizure disorders, gross neurological deficits, or hearing impairments. All of the five children were younger than their autistic siblings; one had a normal older sibling and another had a younger normal sibling, as well. Of the five siblings, three had a parental report of some developmental or academic difficulties, such as problems in language comprehension or performing on grade level.

A pool of control children, selected from a parochial school in New York City, were matched to the siblings on five criteria: (1) age; (2) sex; (3) WISC-R performance (the measure was individually administered and interpreted by a clinical psychologist for both groups); (4) comparable native language, as documented through parental report and school officials; and (5) comparable socioeconomic status (middle-class) (Hollingshead, 1965). Using this set of selection criteria, four males and one female (mean CA = 7 years, 7 months; range = 6 years, 2 months to 8 years, 2 months) were included in the final sample. Selection characteristics for pairs of siblings and control children, shown in Table 10-7, were not possible to fit for every independent variable, given the small number of siblings who met the criteria. All control children had one or more siblings; three were the oldest, one was the youngest, and one had both younger and older siblings. Parental information indicated normal patterns of language development for the five control children; one of the five was reported as inconsistent in his school work.

Table 10-8 displays means and standard deviations for both groups on the Verbal, Performance, and Full Scales of the WISC-R. Significant mean differences, using t-test comparisons, were not found for CA ($t = 0.111$, $df = 8$) or for performance on the Performance Scale ($t = 1.16$; $df = 8$) and on the Full Scale ($t = 2.02$, $df = 8$). Consistent with previous findings (Minton *et al.*, 1982), however, significant mean differences between the two groups were obtained for performance on the Verbal Scale ($t = 2.71$, $df = 8$, $p > .05$).

Task Selection and Procedures

The van Kleeck (1984b) framework was employed as the theoretical basis for task construction because of its relatedness to an interactive definition of language (Bloom & Lahey, 1978) (see Table 10-6). Aspects of language awareness considered here are knowledge of language as a conventional code and as a rule-governed system.

Criteria for task selection included (1) how adequately a task assessed either

TABLE 10-7. Sample Characteristics for Pairs of Siblings of Autistic Children (S) (n = 5) and Normal Controls (C) (n = 5)

Pairs	CA[a]	Sex	WISC-R IQ Full Scale	Verbal	Perf.	Ethnic background[b]	Native language[c]	Second language
S₁	6, 2	M	89	87	92	White	English	—
C₁	6, 2	M	121	123	112	White	English	—
S₂	7, 2	M	101	101	101	Hispanic	English	Spanish
C₂	7, 8	M	108	109	105	Hispanic	Spanish	English
S₃	7, 2	M	89	86	95	Hispanic	English	—
C₃	7, 11	M	97	108	86	White	English	—
S₄	8, 4	F	96	84	112	Hispanic	Spanish	English
C₄	8, 2	F	87	87	102	Hispanic	Spanish	English
S₅	8, 9	M	78	78	81	White	English	—
C₅	8, 1	M	114	106	121	Hispanic	Spanish	English

[a]Chronological age, in years and months.
[b]The designation of "Hispanic" ethnicity refers to children who were of nonwhite Hispanic origin.
[c]Children having Spanish as their native language (S₄, C₂, C₄, and C₅) also spoke English fluently, according to parental report.

comprehension of metalinguistic concepts or the appropriate production of language within a metalinguistic context; (2) the extent to which each task was in accord with current conceptions of metalinguistic content, as discussed in the previous section; and (3) the frequency of use in research for the age span from 6 years to 9 years.

Awareness of Language as an Arbitrary Conventional Code

Three types of tasks were selected as exemplars of the awareness of language as a conventional code: word consciousness, word definition, and verbal riddle recall and explanation.

A word consciousness task purports to examine the comprehension of words as lexical concepts and involves judgments and explanations about word properties. The Papandropoulou and Sinclair (1974) tasks and developmental scoring criteria were used to assess performance (see also Berthoud-Papandropoulou, 1980; Sinclair & Berthoud-Papandropoulou, 1984).

The WISC-R Vocabulary items were selected to evaluate the ability to define words, essentially an explanation task involving a production component. The standard binary scoring system of the WISC-R was compared with the Litowitz (1977) scoring system, which consists of five developmental levels.

The third task, verbal riddle recall and explanation, a production task, involves the resolution of figurative linguistic ambiguity through focusing on the arbitrary relation between sound and meaning. For example, in the riddle "How do you keep fish from smelling?/You cut off their nose," the literal (conventional) meaning of "smelling" is violated. The eight riddles and scoring criteria developed by Fowles and Glantz (1977) were used for both the riddle repetition and explanation conditions.

Awareness of Language as a Rule-Governed System

The awareness of language as a rule-governed system, the form of awareness most often assessed by norm-referenced measures of language knowledge (Romaine,

TABLE 10-8.   IQs of Siblings of Autistic Children and Controls

WISC-R scale	Siblings		Controls		
	M	SD	M	SD	t
Verbal	87.2	8.4	106.6	12.8	2.71*
Performance	96.2	11.43	105.2	13.0	1.16
Full Scale	90.6	8.68	105.5	13.5	2.06

*p<.05 (df=8).

1984; van Kleeck, 1984a), was gauged here by two comprehension tasks (phoneme segmentation and judgments of grammatical acceptability) and one production task (phoneme synthesis). The phoneme segmentation task, originated by Liberman, Shankweiler, Fisher, and Carter (1974), entails the presentation of 20 items consisting of one, two, or three phonemes (e.g., "/i/," "my," "mine"). For each, the child repeats it first and then gives the number of phonemes by either clapping or saying the number. Responses are scored as correct or incorrect (Liberman *et al.*, 1974). Explaining the basis of segmentation is not required. A task of this kind appears to evoke, therefore, recognition of phonemes as linguistic units separate from meaning (Menyuk, 1983; Valtin, 1984b; van Kleeck, 1984b).

The grammaticality judgment task consisted of 12 sentences (6 negation and 6 interrogative structures) (Scholl & Ryan, 1980). Of the 12 sentences, 6 were anomalous and involved word order violations. Detection of word order violations in anomalous structures appears to be least complex for children in the early primary grades (Flood & Menyuk, 1983; Flood & Salus, 1982). Children are instructed to judge (i.e., recognize) each sentence as either a "good" or "silly" sentence. If a sentence is judged as "silly," the subsequent instruction is "Make the sentence good." This request thus solicits correction of the unacceptable element. Justification is not required (Scholl & Ryan, 1980).

In contrast to the analytical properties of phoneme segmentation, phoneme synthesis as a production task requires uniting single phonemes into a single, cohesive whole, that of the word. Tasks of this kind, often referred to as "sound blending," are typical of early reading instruction, but their value as predictors of decoding skill remains debatable (Lewkowicz, 1980; Valtin, 1984a). Research (Helfgott, 1976) suggests that, for example, segmenting "fish" into its three phonemic components is easier than presenting the components separately and then having the child derive the unit. Recognition of the word as an independent unit appears to be prerequisite for successful performance, therefore. The Sound Blending subtest from the Illinois Test of Psycholinguistic Ability (ITPA; Kirk, McCarthy, & Kirk, 1968) was used as the basis of assessment. Instructions and scoring followed manual procedures.

Finally, tasks were audiotaped and administered in random order, with matched pairs receiving the same order. Interjudge agreement was also assessed for those tasks requiring assignment of a developmental level, such as definitions and riddles. Agreement ranged from a low of 74% for the developmental levels for definitions (Litowitz, 1977) to above 90% for verbal riddles. Interjudge agreement was not assessed for the concept-of-the-word task, because of the difficulty found in reliably training a second rater according to the existing criteria for assignment of responses (Papandropoulou & Sinclair, 1974). Variability in agreement for both the definition and word consciousness tasks may indicate, therefore, that classification criteria for levels are insufficiently defined or that the levels are not distinctly different from one another.

Results and Discussion

Tasks *not* differentiating the sibling group from the control group generally appeared to have in common the requirement to make judgments about aspects of linguistic form, as opposed to the requirement to correct a rule violation or to explain the basis for a response. This pattern cut across the classification of tasks as either comprehension or production. Differences were not found for the judgment or recognition of (1) sound structure as a constituent element of the larger word unit (phonemic segmentation); (2) the reciprocal of sound structure as a larger unit built up from smaller elements (phonemic synthesis) (Lewkowicz, 1980; Sinclair & Berthoud-Papandropoulou, 1984); and (3) minor violations in the well-formedness of syntactic structure (Scholl & Ryan, 1980), an instance in which meaning was less necessary for the analysis of form (Ryan & Ledger, 1984).

Performance differences were obtained, however, when the task focus required an explanation of analyzed knowledge or when the requirement entailed the encoding of linguistic elements into longer stretches of language use for an explicit purpose. Included in this category were justifying the word as a discrete linguistic unit, defining the meaning of words, and recalling and explaining verbal riddles. Patterns of results and some preliminary implications are presented next. Where appropriate, parallel findings from language-impaired populations are included in the discussion.

Awareness of Language as an Arbitrary Conventional Code

Concept of the Word as a Linguistic Unit. Differences in performance were not found between the two groups in their ability to judge lexical items as words representing different parts of speech (e.g., "Is 'happy' a word?" or "Is 'the' a word?"). Significant differences were obtained when the frequency distributions of responses were analyzed according to four developmental levels for the explanation of why a word is a word ($X^2 = 11.68$, $df = 4$, $p < .05$). Sibling explanations were distributed over the less mature level 1 (48%) or level 2 (9%). A level 1 explanation is one in which an explicit distinction is not made between words and their referents; a level 2 explanation is characterized by defining why a word is a word on the basis of personal experience. At the more advanced levels, 16% of explanations were classified as level 3 (i.e., justification refers to the word as a constituent of a linguistic unit). For example, "A long word has many letters or syllables" is a level 3 response, as opposed to a level 2 response that "A long word is 'train.' " Only 7% of responses met the criterion for level 4 classifications (i.e., words are defined as autonomous linguistic units). Unclassifiable responses totaled 20%.

The explanations produced by the control children, in comparison, were more equally distributed over levels 1, 2, and 3 (42%, 21%, and 25%, respectively), while 3% of responses met level 4 criteria. Only 8% of their justifications were unclassifiable.

Defining Conventional Word Meaning. A significant difference was also found in the frequency distributions of word definitions, which were analyzed according to the five developmental levels offered by Litowitz (1977) ($X^2 = 27.35$, $df = 5$, $p < .05$). However, differences in the distribution of responses were not found when the same responses were examined using the 3-point scale of the WISC-R. Moreover, when the WISC-R raw scores were converted to scaled scores, the mean scaled score of siblings ($M = 6.2$) was more than one standard deviation below the mean ($M = 10$, $SD = 3$), whereas the mean scaled score of the control group was within one standard deviation of the mean ($M = 8.2$). A *t* test for independent measures applied to scaled score values did not yield significant differences. One inference, therefore, is that the WISC-R scoring criteria were not as sensitive a measure of potential differences as were the Litowitz (1977) criteria. For example, using developmental levels, patterns indicated that proportionately more of the siblings' responses were unclassifiable (level 0). Of those that were classifiable, most were distributed over level 2 (in which words are defined associatively to the stimulus word in terms of personal experience; e.g., the response to "What does 'hat' mean?" is "Head"), and level 3 (typified by a functional definition also linked to personal experience; e.g., "A hat is something you wear on your head"). Responses of the control group, however, were more often distributed across levels 3 and 4. A level 4 response indicates some awareness of the formal definitional form—for instance, when personal experience is modified into a hypothetical social situation (e.g., "A knife is when you cut with it" (Litowitz, 1977, p. 296).

Verbal Riddle Recall and Explanation (Nonconventional Meaning). Because over 97% of responses for the recall condition for both groups occurred at levels 1 and 2, level 3 was omitted from analysis to eliminate the effect of zero cells. Level 1, the most advanced, is characterized by near-verbatim maintenance of the question–answer format in recall; level 2 involves a disruption of the format either in content or structure; and a level 3 response indicates lack of familiarity with the riddle format. Distributions for recall indicated a significant difference between the two groups ($X^2 = 6.64$, $df = 1$, $p < .05$).

For the explanation condition, level 1 was excluded from analysis because of the presence of zero cells across both groups. As the most advanced form of explanation, a level 1 justification focuses solely on linguistic attributes. A level 2 explanation may entail a recognition of incongruity, but a resolution that literally refers to sources external to linguistic aspects (e.g., "How do you keep a fish from smelling? You cut off its nose" is explained as "If you cut off a fish's nose, he wouldn't be able to smell anything"). The least advanced, level 3 responses, include lack of awareness of the intended humor and "I don't know" responses. Again, a significant difference was obtained in the frequency distributions between groups in the level of explanation ($X^2 = 6.64$, $df = 1$, $p < 0.05$).

Although the patterns of distributions were similar for the two groups, control children more often were able to recall the riddle format verbatim and to attempt explanations for the source of ambiguity. These kinds of performances are consistent with expectations for this age range (Fowles & Glantz, 1977; Hirsh-Pasek *et al.*, 1980; Pepicello & Weisberg, 1983; Schultz & Horibe, 1974). In addition, control children less often evidenced lack of sensitivity to ambiguity. Only one-fifth of their explanations were classified as level 3, compared to nearly half of the siblings' explanations.

Some Implications. Performance differences between the siblings and their peer counterparts were not consistently obtained when the task requirement involved explaining aspects of word knowledge. It remains speculative whether this kind of pattern may represent discrete differences in how word knowledge is organized and used in certain groups of children with autistic siblings, or whether differences index a continuum of variation in the rate of fully developed word awareness. In refining the clinical sensitivity of word awareness tasks for addressing the scope and nature of differences, two issues deserve consideration.

One issue is lack of precision in classification criteria for the various developmental levels proposed for the emergence of word consciousness (Papandropoulou & Sinclair, 1974) and word definitions (Litowitz, 1977). Lack of precision affects the accuracy with which explanations can be reliably categorized. For example, Kahmi *et al.* (1985) investigated the level of word awareness in a sample of language-impaired children and matched controls. The language-impaired children performed similarly to the siblings in this study on the explanatory component, according to the Papandropoulou and Sinclair (1974) criteria; however, Kamhi *et al.* (1985) also found interjudge agreement to be problematic for classifying explanation levels.

A broader issue pertains to how the acquisition of different kinds and levels of word awareness should be assessed and interpreted when the intent is to explore possible linkages between language-processing patterns and genetic influences in autism. Bowey and Tunmer (1984, p. 73) surmise that mature understanding of the word as a linguistic concept consists of three components: (1) awareness of the word as a linguistic unit; (2) awareness of the word as an arbitrary phonological label, which refers to the word–referent distinction; and (3) comprehension of the metalinguistic term "word," a prerequisite for being able to define the meaning of a word—for example, as assessed by "What is a word? How do you know if something's a word?" (Papandropoulou & Sinclair, 1974). Each of these components may develop independently, rather than simultaneously, and at different rates (Bowey & Tunmer, 1984) as a function of individual differences or even the effects of schooling; hence, a child may provide evidence of understanding word–referent relations without necessarily having the adult understanding of what the term "word" means (Peters, 1983). In support of this point, Valtin (1984b) delineates nonmetalinguistic strategies that children aged 5 to 7 years may utilize for making sense of what the term "word" means on experimental tasks of the kind administered in the sibling study. One strategy is visually based, in which the number of letters in a word serves as the child's interpretative criterion; another is a pragmatic strategy, by which the child's own experience with what a word means functions as the basis for comprehension. More fine-grained attunement to the components of word awareness and attention to differences in strategy use, or task approach procedures, would enhance the potential sensitivity of tasks in future sibling research.

To turn to the tasks in which awareness of linguistic ambiguity was the focus, a reasonable statement is that how the knowledge base of word meaning is organized influences, in ways not clearly understood, the availability of processing strategies for recognizing and resolving ambiguous information. The converse of this statement is that the structure of the information to be understood influences the selection of specific strategies for executing the processing activity (Menyuk, 1983; Pressley *et al.*, 1985; Yussen, 1985). Furthermore, it appears that all linguistic ambiguity, whether literal or nonliteral in intent, involves semantic judgments (Pepicello & Weisberg, 1983)—a point not always clear in definitions of linguistic ambiguity—and requires, in addition, more metacognitive control than other types of linguistic judgments, such as synonymy (Bialystok & Ryan, 1985) or awareness of the word as a linguistic notion (Bowey & Tunmer, 1984).

The sibling pattern of performance on verbal riddle recall and explanation was similar to patterns found for language-impaired children and adolescents on tasks requiring the disambiguation of nonliteral language, such as metaphors and similes (Nippold & Fey, 1983; Seidenberg & Bernstein, 1986). In these studies, language-impaired youngsters manifested less difficulty with literal comprehension tasks, more often failed to transcend literal interpretations in their explanations of which semantic elements had alternate meanings, and were less able to recognize that a metaphoric interpretation was implicated in the task. Generalization to the verbal riddle recall and explanations of the siblings must be carefully drawn; however, similar to these findings for language-impaired samples, siblings were also less accurate in recall of the verbal riddles and more often gave explanations indicating less awareness of the linguistic origin of the humor.

Some speculations can be offered about the siblings' less proficient performance. Siblings may have had a network of multiple meanings less available to retrieve from their lexical–semantic storehouse. Less availability could have resulted in their not recognizing that an incongruity was present in a particular riddle; hence, familiarity with the underlying catagories and relations would have been a factor in recognition (Menyuk, 1983). Alternately, recognition may have occurred, but what was recognized may have been identified as nonsense rather than as a resolvable incongruity (Suls, 1983). Another possibility is that semantic representations of possible meanings were formed (i.e., representations were accessible) but could not be retained in an active state (Hakes, 1980), suggesting an inefficiency either in the appropriate selection or monitoring of a metamemory strategy (Pressley *et al.*, 1985). Other possible factors, identified by Fowles and Glantz (1977) and more closely aligned with riddle design, are riddle length, social familiarity with particular riddles, and complexity of syntactic structure. Clarifying possible sources of differences, whether based in content knowledge, strategy selection, or strategy application, is related, then, to the choice of a riddle classification schema, to the social and linguistic properties of riddle construction, and to how the incongruity–resolution structure is operationally defined for assigning justifications to various levels of awareness (Fowles & Glantz, 1977; Pepicello & Weisberg, 1983; Suls, 1983).

Awareness of Language as a Rule-Governed System

The lack of significant findings for phoneme segmentation and synthesis may have been the product of ceiling effects, since skill in phonemic analysis, as well as word recognition, is known to be facilitated by formal instruction in decoding grapheme–phoneme relations (Ehri, 1984; Lewkowicz, 1980; Valtin, 1984a). In the case of grammatical, or structural-relational, awareness, the level at which awareness was assessed seemed to be a factor contributing to task insensitivity.

Procedural Issues Affecting Task Sensitivity. A major methodological issue in the assessment of structural-relational awareness, similar to that raised for judgments of the word as a linguistic concept and linguistic ambiguity, concerns how tasks are initially defined and operationally implemented. For example, across studies with normally developing children, marked variation is apparent for the types of sentences meeting rigorous criteria for deviance or unacceptability (Flood & Salus, 1982; Hakes, 1980; Hirsh-Pasek *et al.*, 1980) and for the effects of different kinds of practice trials and instructions on children's ability to make acceptability judgments that are based on analysis of the internal structure of sentences (Hakes, 1980; Ryan & Ledger, 1984; Tunmer & Grieve, 1984). For both children and adults, therefore, the recognition–correction–explanation sequence appears to vary as a function of these factors, making difficult the separation of procedural variables from performance patterns indicative of various levels of metalinguistic awareness.

Some Implications. In establishing criteria for task selection, the distinction is seldom made between the semantic–syntactic knowledge base, aspects of which become the object of analysis in grammaticality judgments, and the metacognitive or strategic processes regulating how internal analysis is approached and self-evaluated. Bialystok and Ryan (1985) and Ryan and Ledger (1984) reinforce the need for this distinction by pointing out that typical procedures for selecting grammatical awareness tasks confound a controlled mode of processing linguistic elements with the elements being analyzed. To illustrate the distinction between what is known and how it is used, these authors suggest that sentence evaluation and explanation require the same amount of controlled processing in the basic attention to structure rather than to meaning, but differ in the *level* of metalinguistic analysis demanded. In applying this framework, tasks emphasizing analyzed knowledge are ranked from moderate to high metalinguistic demand according to whether they solicit recognition of acceptability, error location of the unacceptable

part, correction, explanation, rule statement, or statement of a system of interrelated rules. Other forms of tasks tap grammatical awareness differently. For example, sentence repetition of slightly deviant sentences requires inhibiting the
tendency to normalize; therefore, more controlled processing seems necessary in
the context of the same level of analyzed knowledge (Bialystok & Ryan, 1985;
Ryan & Ledger, 1984).

At least four potential benefits accrue from incorporating this framework into
future cross-sectional research with siblings of autistic children on their awareness
of language as a rule-governed system. First, the formulation potentially offers a
means to differentiate experimentally between metacognitive strategies directing
analysis and the kind of analysis required by different sentence acceptability tasks.
Second, it also provides for a more direct test of the Menyuk (1983) assumption
that a shift from an automatic to a controlled mode of processing requires familiarity with the sentential relations to be analyzed. In other words, these categories
and relations must exist at an automatic level in the knowledge base of oral language in order to be brought to conscious awareness. Third, the framework might
permit refinement of Valtin's (1984b) developmental model of language awareness, through examining the fluctuating nature of awareness across the three stages
as an outcome of variations in processing demands. Fourth, use of the framework
might illuminate the kinds of structural–relational awareness that should be expected of all children, since this is far from clear—particularly in relation to the
demands of literacy instruction across grade levels, as opposed to expectations that
derive from individual variation in verbal talent (Hakes, 1980; Hirsh-Pasek *et al.*,
1980). An approach of this kind may ultimately explain, as well, certain aspects
of the Verbal–Performance IQ discrepancy consistently observed in siblings of
autistic children.

CONCLUDING REMARKS

At this point, the question posed by Spence (1976) is again relevant. That question, in part, addresses how the presence of possible genetic factors in autism
might be assessed. To limit the scope of this question to future kinship studies
with siblings of autistic children, an answer is in part dependent on the resolution
of certain procedural problems. On one level, these procedural issues involve the
selection and interpretation of tasks presumed to solicit, in both theoretical and
operational senses, metamodes of cognitive processing and linguistic analysis. On
another, more complex level, resolution is also linked to the viability of the continuum hypothesis of cognitive–communicative disorders. This hypothesis specu-
lates that autism is the most extreme expression of a genetic propensity for developmental disruption. An extension of this hypothesis is the Prizant (1983) thesis
that a holistic processing mode is characteristic of how many autistic youngsters
operate on linguistic information. In effect, language processing is approached
through the chunking of linguistic elements into wholes that remain totally or

partially unanalyzed. Dependence on this inflexible mode of processing could account for the serious breakdown of the communicative system in autistic children and would explain the stereotypical quality of their language use.

The siblings reported on in this review could not be said to demonstrate the kind of holistic processing that might be particular to their autistic kin. However, as a group, the siblings' history of developmental and educational lags, combined with their performance patterns on tasks requiring deeper levels of controlled processing, suggested a profile consistent with the features of a language impairment as these symptoms are manifested during the early school-age years. The point pertinent here for the continuity hypothesis is that holistic or formulaic processing is also a property of normal language use (Peters, 1983), and, in addition, may be a strategy inappropriately activated in some language-impaired children when confronted with problem-solving activities for which their knowledge base is insufficient (Pressley *et al.*, 1985; Wallach & Liebergott, 1984; Wong, 1985).

In normal language use, formulaic processing can occur as a means for coping with the constraints imposed by short-term memory on the speed of information processing, especially when communicative pressure is present (Peters, 1983). This type of processing strategy functions to conserve available processing resources through the storage of prefabricated or preassembled chunks of grammar, which then allow communication to be maximized with a minimum of attention to the linguistic aspects of constructing utterances. Among the tactics identified by Peters (1983) as short-cutting devices are the rote memorization of long chunks to be called up for use in the appropriate situation; the fusion of frequently used sequences, such as greetings, small talk, social control regulators, and idioms; and the automatization of often-used processes. Each of these devices offers the opportunity for fast retrieval when necessary.

This form of holistic processing is distinguishable from the holistic mode to which Prizant (1983) refers in two ways. First, prefabricated chunks are potentially analyzable by the language user "either as a single unit or as a complex construction with internal structure (e.g., words can be inserted into or deleted from the phrase, or the grammatical structure can be changed as needed)" (Peters, 1983, p. 3). Next, unlike the holistic processing of autism, the prefabricated wholes of normal language use are always applied in socially and linguistically appropriate manners. Hence, holistic processing may not be uniquely peculiar to autism; rather, its expression in autism may be a primitive form of what Peters describes as a continuum of grammatical knowledge, which in the mature language user eventually operates as a flexible schema for retrieving linguistic behaviors appropriate for the shifting processing demands of ongoing interaction. Whether differences in processing modes among autistic, language-impaired, and normally developing children are best explained as discrete or continuous differences remains conjectural at this time; however, in agreement with others (Menyuk, 1983; Prizant, 1983; Sternberg, 1987b), a tenable hypothesis is that how oral language is processed affects what is learned about the content, form, and use of oral language.

In summary, twin and sibling studies present a potentially effective means by which to address the nature of genetic influences in autism and, more broadly, the question of whether superficially heterogeneous clusters of atypical language learning represent a continuum of developmental disruption or are qualitatively different disorders. Genetic factors could conceivably be expressed in phenotypically different ways if, as Galaburda (1983) and Geschwind (1985) infer, the genotype possesses a defect in cellular programming for neuronal migration. Galaburda's (1983) model of the developing neural substrate for language predicts that programming mechanisms differentially affect the *in utero* rate of neuronal growth for certain regions within the left and right hemispheres. The severe cognitive, social, linguistic, and communicative abnormalities associated with autism may be one expression of genetic influences or other forms of pathological alterations to the uterine environment (Galaburda, 1983), as these influences interact with other factors, both internal and external. Developmental language impairment may reflect a less extreme variation of a cellular programming defect. An inadequate neural substrate would then differentially disrupt the interdependence among how information is processed, what is learned, and how it is used as a consequence.

Acknowledgments

This work was supported in part by National Institute of Mental Health Grant Nos. MH-32212 and MH-40177; by a grant from the Stallone Fund for Autism Research; and by Social and Behavioral Sciences Research Grant No. 12-108 from the March of Dimes Birth Defects Foundation to Magda Campbell.

References

Algozzine, B., & Ysseldyke, J. E. (1986). The future of the LD field: Screening and diagnosis. *Journal of Learning Disabilities, 19*, 394–398.

American Psychiatric Association. (1980). *Diagnostic and statistical manual of mental disorders* (3rd ed.). Washington, DC: Author.

August, G. J., Stewart, M. A., & Tsai, L. (1981). The incidence of cognitive disabilities in the siblings of autistic children. *British Journal of Psychiatry, 138*, 416–422.

Bakwin, H. (1954). Early infantile autism. *Journal of Pediatrics, 45*, 492–497.

Bartak, L., Rutter, M., & Cox, A. (1975). A comparative study of infantile autism and specific developmental receptive language disorder: I. The children. *British Journal of Psychiatry, 126*, 127–145.

Berthoud-Papandropoulou, I. (1980). An experimental study of children's ideas about language. In A. Sinclair, R. J. Jarvella, & W. J. M. Levelt (Eds.), *The child's concept of language* (pp. 55–64). New York: Springer-Verlag.

Bialystok, E., & Ryan, E. B. (1985). A metacognitive framework for the development of first and second language skills. In D. L. Forrest-Pressley, G. E. MacKinnon & T. G. Waller (Eds.), *Metacognition, cognition, and human performance* (Vol. 1, pp. 207–252). New York: Academic Press.

Bloom, L., & Lahey, M. (1978). *Language development and language disorders.* New York: Wiley.

Book, J. A., Nichtern, S., & Gruenberg, E. (1963). Cytogenetical investigations in childhood schizophrenia. *Acta Psychiatrica Scandinavica, 39*, 309–323.

Borkowski, J. G., & Kurtz, B. E. (1984). Metacognition and special children. In B. Gholson & T. L. Rosenthal (Eds.), *Application of cognitive-developmental theory* (pp. 193–213). New York: Academic Press.

Bowey, J. A., & Tunmer, W. E. (1984). Word awareness in children. In W. E. Tunmer, C. Pratt, & M. L. Herriman (Eds.), *Metalinguistic awareness in children* (pp. 73–91). New York: Springer-Verlag.

Brown, A. L. (1977). Development, schooling, and the acquisition of knowledge about knowledge: Comments on Chapter 7 by Nelson. In R. C. Anderson, R. J. Spiro, & W. E. Montague (Eds.), *Schooling and the acquisition of knowledge* (pp. 241–253). Hillsdale, NJ: Erlbaum.

Brown, A. L., & DeLoache, J. S. (1983). Metacognitive skills. In M. Donaldson, R. Grieve, & C. Pratt (Eds.), *Early childhood development and education* (pp. 280–289). New York: Guilford Press.

Brown, W. T., Jenkins, E. C., Friedman, E., Brooks, J., Wisniewski, K., Raguthu, S., & French J. (1982). Autism is associated with the fragile X syndrome. *Journal of Autism and Developmental Disorders, 12,* 303–308.

Bruch, H. (1959). Studies in schizophrenia. *Acta Psychiatrica et Neurologica Scandinavica, 130* (Suppl.), 15.

Campbell, M., Dominijanni, C., & Schneider, B. (1977). Monozygotic twins concordant for autism: Follow-up. *British Journal of Psychiatry, 131,* 616–622.

Campbell, M., & Green, W. H. (1985). Pervasive developmental disorders of childhood. In H. I. Kaplan & B. J. Sadock (Eds.), *Comprehensive textbook of psychiatry* (4th ed., Vol. 2, IV pp. 1672–1683). Baltimore: Williams & Wilkins.

Campbell, M., Hardesty, A. S., Burdock, E., Cleary, P. A., Polevoy, N., & Geller, B. (1978). Demographic and paranatal profile of 105 autistic children: A preliminary report. *Psychopharmacology Bulletin, 14*(2), 36–39.

Campbell, M., Minton, J., Green, W. H., Jennings, S. J., & Samit, C. (1981). Siblings and twins of autistic children. In C. Perris, G. Struwe, & B. Jansson (Eds.), *Biological psychiatry 1981* (pp. 993–996). Amsterdam: Elsevier/North-Holland.

Campbell, M., Polevoy, N. T., Peselow, E., Fish, B., Shapiro, T., Rainer, J. D., Nobler, M., & Addrizzo, D. (1988). *A twin study of preschoolage autistic children.* Manuscript submitted for publication.

Cavanaugh, J. C., & Perlmutter, M. (1982). Metamemory: A critical examination. *Child Development, 53,* 11–28.

Cazden, C. B. (1983). Play with language and metalinguistic awareness: One dimension of language experience. In M. Donaldson, R. Grieve, & C. Pratt (Eds.), *Early childhood development and education* (pp. 302–307). New York: Guilford Press.

Chapman, A. H. (1957). Early infantile autism in identical twins. *Archives of Neurology and Psychiatry, 78,* 621–623.

Chapman, A. H. (1960). Early infantile autism: A review. *American Journal of Diseases of Children, 99,* 783–786.

Chess, S., Korn, S., & Fernandez, P. B. (1971). *Psychiatric disorders of children with congenital rubella.* New York: Brunner/Mazel.

Clark, E. V. (1980). Awareness of language: Some evidence from what children say and do. In A. Sinclair, R. J. Jarvella, & W. L. M. Levelt (Eds.), *The child's conception of language* (pp. 17–43). New York: Springer-Verlag.

Cloninger, C. R., Christiansen, K. O., Reich, T., & Gottesman, I. I. (1978). Implications of sex differences in the prevalence of antisocial personality, alcoholism, and criminality for familial transmission. *Archives of General Psychiatry, 35,* 941–951.

Cloninger, C. R., Lewis, C., Rice, J., & Reich, T. (1981). Strategies for resolution of biological and cultural inheritance. In E. S. Gershon, S. Matthysse, X. D. Breakefield, & R. D. Ciaranello (Eds.), *Psychobiology and psychopathology: Vol. 1. Genetic research strategies in psychobiology and psychiatry* (pp. 319–332). Pacific Grove, CA: Boxwood Press.

Cohen, D. J., Caparulo, B., & Shaywitz, B. (1976). Primary childhood aphasia and childhood autism. *Journal of the American Academy of Child Psychiatry, 15,* 604–645.

Coleman, M., & Gillberg, C. (1985). *The biology of the autistic syndromes.* New York: Praeger.

Coleman, M., & Rimland, B. (1976). Familial autism. In M. Coleman (Ed.), *The autistic syndromes* (pp. 175–182). Amsterdam: North-Holland.

Creak, M., & Ini, S. (1960). Families of psychotic children. *Journal of Child Psychology and Psychiatry, 1,* 156–175.

Day, J. D., French, L. A., & Hall, L. K. (1985). Social influences on cognitive development. In D. L. Forrest-Pressley, G. E. MacKinnon, & T. G. Waller (Eds.), *Metacognition, cognition, and human performance* (Vol. 1, pp. 33–56). New York: Academic Press.

DeMyer, M. K., Hingtgen, J. N., & Jackson, R. K. (1981). Infantile autism reviewed: A decade of research. *Schizophrenia Bulletin, 7,* 388–451.

Denckla, M. B. (1983). Learning for language and language for learning. In U. Kirk (Ed.), *Neuropsychology of language, reading, and spelling* (pp. 33–43). New York: Academic Press.

Deykin, E. Y., & MacMahon, B. (1979). The incidence of seizures among children and autistic symptoms. *American Journal of Psychiatry, 136,* 1310–1312.

Duane, D. (1985). Written language underachievement: An overview of theoretical and practical issues. In F. H. Duffy & N. Geschwind (Eds.), *Dyslexia: A neuroscientific approach to clinical evaluation* (pp. 3–32). Boston: Little, Brown.

Ehri, L. C. (1984). How orthography alters spoken language competencies in children learning to read and spell. In J. Downing & R. Valtin (Eds.), *Language awareness and learning to read* (pp. 119–147). New York: Springer-Verlag.

Eisenberg, L., & Kanner, L. (1956). Early infantile autism 1943–1953. *American Journal of Orthopsychiatry, 26,* 556–566.

Falconer, D. S. (1965). The inheritance of liability to certain diseases, estimated from the incidence among relatives. *Annals of Human Genetics, 29,* 51–76.

Fisch, G. S., Cohen, I. L., Wolf, E. G., Brown, W. T., Jenkins, E. C., & Gross, A. (1986). Autism and the fragile X syndrome. *American Journal of Psychiatry, 143*(1), 71–73.

Flood, J., & Menyuk, P. (1983). The development of metalinguistic awareness and its relation to reading achievement. *Journal of Applied Developmental Psychology, 4,* 65–80.

Flood, J., & Salus, M. W. (1982). Metalinguistic awareness: Its role in language development and its assessment. *Topics in Language Disorders, 2*(4), 56–64.

Folstein, S. E. (1985). Genetic aspects of infantile autism. *Annual Review of Medicine, 36,* 415–419.

Folstein, S. E., & Rutter, M. (1977). Infantile autism: A genetic study of 21 twin pairs. *Journal of Child Psychology and Psychiatry, 18,* 297–321.

Folstein, S. E., & Rutter, M. (1978). A twin study of individuals with infantile autism. In M. Rutter & E. Schopler (Eds.), *Autism: A reappraisal of concepts and treatment* (pp. 219–241). New York: Plenum.

Fowles, B., & Glantz, M. E. (1977). Competence and talent in verbal riddle comprehension. *Journal of Child Language, 4,* 433–452.

Freeman, B. J., Ritvo, E. R., Schroth, P. C., Tonick, I., Guthrie, D., & Wake, L. (1981). Behavioral characteristics of high- and low-IQ autistic children. *American Journal of Psychiatry, 138,* 25–29.

Galaburda, A. M. (1983). Definition of the anatomical phenotype. In C. L. Ludlow & J. A. Cooper (Eds.), *Genetic aspects of speech and language disorders* (pp. 71–84). New York: Academic Press.

Gazzaniga, M. S. (1985). *The social brain: Discovering the networks of the mind.* New York: Basic Books.

Geschwind, N. (1985). Biological foundations of reading. In F. H. Duffy & N. Geschwind (Eds.), *Dyslexia: A neuroscientific approach to clinical evaluation* (pp. 197–211). Boston: Little, Brown.

Gillberg, C. (1983). Identical triplets with infantile autism and the fragile-X syndrome. *British Journal of Psychiatry, 143,* 256–260.

Gillberg, C. (1984). Infantile autism and other childhood psychoses in a Swedish urban region: Epidemiological aspects. *Journal of Child Psychology and Psychiatry, 25,* 35–43.

Gillberg, C., & Schaumann, H. (1982). Social class and infantile autism. *Journal of Autism and Developmental Disorders, 12,* 223–228.

Gillberg, C. & Wahlstrom, J. (1985). Chromosome abnormalities in infantile autism and other childhood psychoses: A population study of 66 cases. *Developmental Medicine and Child Neurology*, 27, 293–304.

Goldfine, P. E., McPherson, P. M., Heath, G. A., Hardesty, V. A., Beauregard, L. J., & Gordon, B. (1985). Association of fragile X syndrome with autism. *American Journal of Psychiatry*, 142(1), 108–110.

Gottesman, I. I., & Shields, J. (1972). *Schizophrenia and genetics: A twin study vantage point*. New York: Academic Press.

Green, W. H., Campbell, M., Hardesty, A. S., Grega, D. M., Padron-Gayol, M., Shell, J., & Erlenmeyer-Kimling, L. (1984). A comparison of schizophrenic and autistic children. *Journal of the American Academy of Child Psychiatry*, 23, 399–409.

Hakes, D. T. (1980). *The development of metalinguistic abilities in children*. New York: Springer-Verlag.

Hanson, D. R., & Gottesman, I. I. (1976). The genetics, if any, of infantile autism and childhood schizophrenia. *Journal of Autism and Childhood Schizophrenia*, 6, 209–234.

Havelkova, M. (1967). Abnormalities of siblings of schizophrenic children. *Canadian Psychiatric Association Journal*, 12, 363–367.

Helfgott, J. A. (1976). Phonemic segmentation and blending skills of kindergarten children: Implications for beginning reading acquisition. *Contemporary Educational Psychology*, 1, 157–169.

Hirsh-Pasek, K., Gleitman, L. R., & Gleitman, H. (1980). What did the brain say to the mind? A study of the detection and report of ambiguity by young children. In A. Sinclair, R. J. Jarvella, & W. J. M. Levelt (Eds.), *The child's conception of language* (pp. 97–132). New York: Springer-Verlag.

Hollingshead, A. B. (1965). *Two factor index of social position*. New Haven, CT: Privately printed.

Hutchins, E. (1986). Mediation and automatization. *Quarterly Newsletter of the Laboratory of Comparative Human Cognition*, 8, 47–58.

Kamhi, A. G., & Koenig, L. A. (1985). Metalinguistic awareness in normal and language disordered children. *Language, Speech, and Hearing Services in Schools*, 16, 199–210.

Kamhi, A. G., Lee, R., & Nelson, L. K. (1985). Word, syllable, and sound awareness in language disordered children. *Journal of Speech and Hearing Disorders*, 50, 207–212.

Kamp, L. N. J. (1964). Autistic syndrome in one of a pair of monozygotic twins. *Psychiatria, Neurologia, Neurochirurgia*, 67, 143–147.

Kanner, L., & Eisenberg, L. (1957). Early infantile autism 1943–55. *Psychiatric Research Report*, No. 7, 67–76.

Kean, J. M. (1975). The development of social skills in autistic twins. *New Zealand Medical Journal*, 81, 204–207.

Keeler, W. R. (1958). Autistic patterns and defective communication in blind children with retrolental fibroplasia. In P. H. Hoch & S. Zubin (Eds.), *Psychopathology of communications* (pp. 64–83). New York: Grune & Stratton.

Kirk, S., McCarthy, J., & Kirk, W. (1968). *The Illinois Test of Psycholinguistic Ability* (rev. ed.). Urbana: University of Illinois Press.

Kolvin, I. (1971). Psychoses in childhood—a comparative study. In M. Rutter (Ed.), *Infantile autism: Concepts, characteristics and treatment* (pp. 7–26). London: Churchill Livingstone.

Kotsopoulos, S. (1976). Infantile autism in dizygotic twins: A case report. *Journal of Autism and Childhood Schizophrenia*, 6, 133–138.

Lehman, E., Haber, J., & Lesser, S. R. (1957). The use of reserpine in autistic children. *Journal of Nervous and Mental Disease*, 125, 351–356.

Levitas, A., Hagerman, R. J., Braden, M., Rimland, B., McBogg, P., & Matus, I. (1983). Autism and the fragile X syndrome. *Journal of Developmental Pediatrics*, 4, 151–158.

Lewkowicz, N. K. (1980). Phonemic awareness training: What to teach and how to teach it. *Contemporary Educational Psychology*, 72, 686–700.

Liberman, I. Y., Shankweiler, D., Fisher, F., & Carter, B. (1974). Explicit syllable and phoneme segmentation in the young child. *Journal of Experimental Psychology*, 18, 201–212.

Liles, B., Schulman, M., & Bartlett, S. (1977). Judgments of grammaticality in normal and language-disordered children. *Journal of Speech and Hearing Disorders, 42,* 199–209.

Litowitz, B. (1977). Learning to make definitions. *Journal of Child Language, 4,* 289–304.

Lotter, V. (1966). Epidemiology of autistic conditions in young children: I. Prevalence. *Social Psychiatry, 1,* 124–137.

Lotter, V. (1967). Epidemiology of autistic conditions in young children: Some characteristics of the parents and children. *Social Psychiatry, 1,* 163–173.

Lovaas, O. I., Schaeffer, B., & Simmons, J. Q. (1965). Building social behavior in autistic children by use of electric shock. *Journal of Experimental Research in Personality, 1,* 99–109.

Lowe, T. L., Tanaka, K., Seashore, M. R., Young, J. G., & Cohen, D. J. (1980). Detection of phenylketonuria in autistic and psychotic children. *Journal of the American Medical Association, 243,* 126–128.

Ludlow, C. L., & Cooper, J. A. (1983). Genetic aspects of speech and language disorders: Current status and future directions. In C. L. Ludlow & J. A. Cooper (Eds.), *Genetic aspects of speech and language disorders* (pp. 1–20). New York: Academic Press.

Mann, V. A. (1986). Why some children encounter reading problems: The contributions of difficulties with language processing and phonological sophistication to early reading disability. In J. K. Torgesen & B. Y. L. Wong (Eds.), *Psychological and educational perspectives on learning disabilities* (pp. 133–159). New York: Academic Press.

McQuaid, P. E. (1975). Infantile autism in twins. *British Journal of Psychiatry, 127,* 530–534.

Menyuk, P. (1983). Language development and reading. In T. M. Gallagher & C. A. Prutting (Eds.), *Pragmatic assessment and intervention issues in language* (pp. 151–170). San Diego: College-Hill Press.

Minton, J., Campbell, M., Green, W. H., Jennings, S., & Samit, C. (1982). Cognitive assessment of siblings of autistic children. *Journal of the American Academy of Child Psychiatry, 21,* 256–261.

Nesdale, A. R., & Tunmer, W. E. (1984). The development of metalinguistic awareness: A methodological overview. In W. E. Tunmer, C. Pratt, & M. L. Herriman (Eds.), *Metalinguistic awareness in children* (pp. 36–54). New York: Springer-Verlag.

Nippold, M. A., & Fey, S. H. (1983). Metaphoric understanding in preadolescents having a history of language acquisition difficulties. *Language, Speech, and Hearing Services in Schools, 14,* 171–180.

Ornitz, E. M., Ritvo, E. R., & Walter, R. D. (1965). Dreaming sleep in autistic twins. *Archives of General Psychiatry, 12,* 77–79.

Papandropoulou, I., & Sinclair, H. (1974). What is a word? *Human Development, 17,* 241–258.

Pepicello, W. J., & Weisberg, R. W. (1983). Linguistics and humor. In P. E. McGhee & J. H. Goldstein (Eds.), *Handbook of humor research* (Vol. 1, pp. 59–83). New York: Springer-Verlag.

Peters, A. M. (1983). *The units of language acquisition.* New York: Cambridge University Press.

Polan, C. G., & Spencer, B. L. (1959). A check list of symptoms of autism in early life. *West Virginia Medical Journal, 55,* 198–204.

Pratt, C., & Grieve, R. (1984a). The development of metalinguistic awareness: An introduction. In W. E. Tunmer, C. Pratt, & M. L. Herriman (Eds.), *Metalinguistic awareness in children* (pp. 2–11). New York: Springer-Verlag.

Pratt, C., & Grieve, R. (1984b). Metalinguistic awareness and cognitive development. In W. E. Tunmer, C. Pratt, & M. L. Herriman (Eds.), *Metalinguistic awareness in children* (pp. 128–143). New York: Springer-Verlag.

Pressley, M., Forrest-Pressley, D. L., Elliot-Faust, D., & Miller, G. (1985). Children's use of cognitive strategies, how to teach strategies, and what to do if they can't be taught. In M. Pressley & C. J. Brainerd (Eds.), *Cognitive learning and memory in children: Psychological foundations* (pp. 1–47). New York: Springer-Verlag.

Prizant, B. M. (1983). Language acquisition and communicative behavior in autism: Toward an understanding of the "whole" of it. *Journal of Speech and Hearing Disorders, 48,* 296–307.

Reich, T., Rice, J., Cloninger, C. R., Wette, R., & James, J. (1979). The use of multiple thresholds and segregation analysis in analyzing the phenotypic heterogeneity of multifactorial traits. *Annals of Human Genetics, 42*, 371–390.

Rimland, B. (1964). *Infantile autism.* Englewood Cliffs, NJ: Prentice-Hall.

Rimland, B. (1971). The differentiation of childhood psychoses: An analysis of checklists for 2,218 psychotic children. *Journal of Autism and Childhood Schizophrenia, 1*(2), 161–174.

Ritvo, E. R., Freeman, B. J., Mason-Brothers, A., Mo, A., & Ritvo, A. M. (1985). Concordance for the syndrome of autism in 40 pairs of afflicted twins. *American Journal of Psychiatry, 142*, 74–77.

Ritvo, E. R., Ritvo, E. C., & Mason-Brothers, M. A. (1982). Genetic and immunohematologic factors in autism. *Journal of Autism and Developmental Disorders, 12*, 109–114.

Ritvo, E. R., Spence, A., Freeman, B. J., Mason-Brothers, A., Mo, A., & Marazita, M. L. (1985). Evidence of autosomal recessive inheritance in 46 families with multiple incidences of autism. *American Journal of Psychiatry, 142*, 187–192.

Romaine, S. (1984). *The language of children and adolescents.* Oxford: Blackwell.

Rutter, M. (1967). Psychotic disorders in early childhood. In A. Coppen & A. Walk (Eds.), *Recent developments in schizophrenia: A symposium (British Journal of Psychiatry*, Special Publication No. 1, pp. 133–158). Ashford, England: Headley Brothers.

Rutter, M. (1978). Diagnosis and definition. In M. Rutter & E. Schopler (Eds.), *Autism: A reappraisal of concepts and treatment* (pp. 1–25). New York: Plenum.

Rutter, M. (1985). Infantile autism and other pervasive developmental disorders. In M. Rutter & L. Hersov (Eds.), *Child and adolescent psychiatry* (pp. 545–566). Oxford: Blackwell.

Ryan, E. B., & Ledger, G. W. (1984). Learning to attend to sentence structure: Links between metalinguistic development and reading. In J. Downing & R. Valtin (Eds.), *Language awareness and learning to read* (pp. 149–171). New York: Springer-Verlag.

Salimi-Eshkevari, H. (1979). Early infantile autism in monozygotic twins. *Journal of Autism and Developmental Disorders, 9*, 105–109.

Salimi-Eshkevari, H. (1985). Infantile autism in monozygotic twins. *Journal of the American Academy of Child Psychiatry, 24*(5), 643–646.

Scholl, D. M., & Ryan, E. B. (1980). Development of metalinguistic performance in the early school years. *Language and Speech, 23*, 199–211.

Seidenberg, P. L., & Bernstein, D. K. (1986). The comprehension of similes and metaphors by learning-disabled and nonlearning-disabled children. *Language, Speech, and Hearing Services in Schools, 17*, 219–229.

Shell, J., Campion, J. F., Minton, J., Caplan, R., & Campbell, M. (1984). A study of three brothers with infantile autism: A case report with follow-up. *Journal of the American Academy of Child Psychiatry, 23*, 498–502.

Sherwin, A. C. (1953). Reactions to music of autistic (schizophrenic) children. *American Journal of Psychiatry, 109*, 823–831.

Shultz, J. R,. & Horibe, F. (1974). Development of the appreciation of verbal jokes. *Developmental Psychology, 10*, 13–20.

Silliman, E. R. (1984). Interactional competencies in the instructional context: The role of teaching discourse in learning. In G. P. Wallach & K. G. Butler (Eds.), *Language learning disabilities in school-age children* (pp. 288–317). Baltimore: Williams & Wilkins.

Silliman, E. R. (1987). Individual differences in the classroom performance of language impaired children. *Seminars in Speech and Language, 8*, 357–375.

Sinclair, A., & Berthoud-Papandropoulou, I. (1984). Children's thinking about language and their acquisition of literacy. In J. Downing & R. Valtin (Eds.), *Language awareness and learning to read* (pp. 79–91). New York: Springer-Verlag.

Sloan, J. L. (1978). Differential development of autistic symptoms in a pair of fraternal twins. *Journal of Autism and Childhood Schizophrenia, 8*, 191–202.

Spence, M. A. (1976). Genetic studies. In E. R. Ritvo (Ed.), *Autism: Diagnosis, current research and management* (pp. 169–174). New York: Spectrum.

Steffenburg, S., Gillberg, C., Hellgren, L., Anderson, L., Gillberg, I. C., Jacobson, G., & Bohman, M. (1988). A twin study of autism in Denmark, Finland, Iceland, Norway and Sweden. *Journal of Child Psychology and Psychiatry.*

Steinhausen, H.-C., Gobel, D., Breinlinger, M., & Wohlleben, B. (1986). A community survey of infantile autism. *Journal of the American Academy of Child Psychiatry*, 25(2), 186–189.

Sternberg, R. J. (1987a). A unified theory of intellectual exceptionality. In J. D. Day & J. G. Borkowski (Eds.), *Intelligence and exceptionality* (pp. 135–172). Norwood, NJ: Ablex.

Sternberg, R. J. (1987b). A united theoretical perspective on autism. In D. J. Cohen & A. M. Donnellan (Eds.), *Handbook of autism and pervasive developmental disorders* (pp. 690–702). New York: Wiley.

Suls, J. M. (1983). Cognitive processes in humor appreciation. In P. E. McGhee & J. H. Goldstein (Eds.), *Handbook of humor research* (Vol. 1, pp. 39–57). New York: Springer-Verlag.

Tindal, G., & Marston, D. (1986). Approaches to assessment. In J. K. Torgesen & B. Y. L. Wong (Eds.), *Psychological and educational perspectives on learning disabilities* (pp. 55–84). New York: Academic Press.

Torrey, E. F., Hersh, S. P., & McCabe, K. D. (1975). Early childhood psychosis and bleeding during pregnancy. *Journal of Autism and Childhood Schizophrenia*, 5, 287–297.

Tsai, L., Stewart, M. A., & August, G. (1981). Implications of sex differences in the familial transmission of infantile autism. *Journal of Autism and Developmental Disorders*, 11, 165–173.

Tunmer, W. E., & Grieve, R. (1984). Syntactic awareness in children. In W. E. Tunmer, C. Pratt, & M. L. Herriman (Eds.), *Metalinguistic awareness in children* (pp. 92–104). New York: Springer-Verlag.

Tunmer, W. E., & Herriman, M. L. (1984). The development of metalinguistic awareness: A conceptual overview. In W. E. Tunmer, C. Pratt, & M. L. Herriman (Eds.), *Metalinguistic awareness in children* (pp. 12–35). New York: Springer-Verlag.

Vaillant, G. E. (1963). Twins discordant for early infantile autism. *Archives of General Psychiatry*, 9, 163–167.

Valtin, R. (1984a). Awareness of features and functions of language. In J. Downing & R. Valtin (Eds.), *Language awareness and learning to read* (pp. 227–260). New York: Springer-Verlag.

Valtin, R. (1984b). The development of metalinguistic abilities in children learning to read and write. In J. Downing & R. Valtin (Eds.), *Language awareness and learning to read* (pp. 207–226). New York: Springer-Verlag.

van Kleeck, A. (1984a). Assessment and intervention: Does "meta" matter? In G. P. Wallach & K. G. Butler (Eds.), *Language learning disabilities in school-age children* (pp. 179–198). Baltimore: Williams & Wilkins.

van Kleeck, A. (1984b). Metalinguistic skills: Cutting across spoken and written language and problem-solving abilities. In G. P. Wallach & K. G. Butler (Eds.), *Language learning disabilities in school-age children* (pp. 128–153). Baltimore: Williams & Wilkins.

Vandenberg, S. G., & Streng, J. (1984). The genetics of abnormal behavioral development. In E. S. Gollin (Ed.), *Malformations of development* (pp. 315–356). New York: Academic Press.

Vellutino, F. R., & Shub, M. J. (1982). Assessment of disorders in formal school language: Disorders in reading. *Topics in Language Disorders*, 2, 20–33.

Wallach, G. P., & Liebergott, J. W. (1984). Who shall be called "learning disabled": Some new directions. In G. P. Wallach & K. G. Butler (Eds.), *Language learning disabilities in school-age children* (pp. 1–14). Baltimore: Williams & Wilkins.

Ward, T. F., & Hoddinott, B. A. (1962). Early infantile autism in fraternal twins. *Canadian Psychiatric Association Journal*, 7, 191–194.

Wechsler, D. (1967). *Manual for the Wechsler Preschool and Primary Scale of Intelligence.* New York: Psychological Corporation.

Wechsler, D. (1974). *Manual for the Wechsler Intelligence Scale for Children—Revised.* New York: Psychological Corporation.

Wessels, W. H., & Van Meerdervoort, M. P. (1979). Monozygotic twins with early infantile autism. A case report. *South African Medical Journal*, 55(2), 955–957.

Whittam, H., Simon, G. B., & Mittler, P. J. (1966). The early development of psychotic children and their sibs. *Developmental Medicine and Child Neurology, 8,* 552–560.

Wong, B. Y. L. (1985). Metacognition and learning disabilities. In D. L. Forrest-Pressley, G. E. MacKinnon, & T. G. Waller (Eds.), *Metacognition, cognition, and human performance: Vol. 2. Instructional practices* (pp. 137–180). New York: Academic Press.

Young, J. G., Kavanagh, M. E., Anderson, G. M., Shaywitz, B. A., & Cohen, D. J. (1982). Clinical neurochemistry of autism and associated disorders. *Journal of Autism and Developmental Disorders, 12,* 147–165.

Young, J. G., Leven, L. I., Togasaki, D. M., & Knott, P. J. (1986, July). *Neurobiological research on infantile autism.* Paper presented at the International Association for Child and Adolescent Psychiatry and Allied Professions, 11th International Congress, Paris.

Young, J. G., Ludman, W. L., & Knott, P. J. (1986). Advances in biological studies of the pervasive developmental disorders. In C. Shagass, R. C. Josiassen, W. H. Bridger, K. J. Weiss, D. Stoff, & G. M. Simpson (Eds.), *Biological psychiatry 1985* (pp. 1495–1497). New York: Elsevier.

Yussen, S. R. (1985). The role of metacognition in contemporary theories of cognitive development. In D. L. Forrest-Pressley, G. E. MacKinnon, & T. Waller (Eds.), *Metacognition, cognition, and human performance* (Vol. 1, pp. 253–283). New York: Academic Press.

SECTION II

New Directions in the Diagnosis and Treatment of Individuals with Autism

CHAPTER 11

Re-Evaluating the Syndrome of Autism in the Light of Empirical Research

LYNN WATERHOUSE
Trenton State College
LORNA WING
Institute of Psychiatry, London
DEBORAH FEIN
Boston University School of Medicine

INTRODUCTION

Ever since Leo Kanner (1943) posited the existence of a "syndrome" he called "early infantile autism," there has been a nonstop but fragmented effort to discover the basis for the cluster of features he described.

There is an unresolved paradox at the heart of these attempts. On the one hand, a large number of medical and other professional workers have found the concept of autism useful in clinical practice. Many of those who have lived or worked with autistic children are sure that they could instantly identify any other child with the same type of handicap. Autistic children in mainstream schools tend to stand out as markedly different from the other students, and there is no doubt that they present special educational problems, regardless of their overall level of intellectual ability. Furthermore, until they contact others in the same position, parents of such children characteristically feel isolated because their children's problems have little or nothing in common with most other forms of handicap. They experience great relief when they eventually read descriptions of autism and meet parents with similar children. Thus, there is something in common among these children that needs to be identified and explained.

On the other hand, investigation of the nature of this common factor is made difficult by the existence of a number of sets of diagnostic criteria, which overlap but are not identical, although they each purport to identify typical autism. Kanner himself originally laid down five criteria in his 1943 paper, but later, Kanner and Eisenberg (1956) reduced this list to two. Other definitions of autism include those by Rutter (1972), Ritvo and Freeman (1977), and Rimland (1964), and those found in the *Diagnostic and Statistical Manual of Mental Disorders*, third edition (DSM-III; American Psychiatric Association, 1980), the new revision of DSM-III (DSM-IIIR; American Psychiatric Association, 1987), and the 9th and 10th editions of the *International Classification of Diseases* (ICD-9 and ICD-10; World Health Organization, 1978, in press). The prevalence rate found in epidemiological studies is affected by the criteria chosen for diagnosis and by the ages of the subjects at the time the criteria are applied (Wing, 1988). In the present chapter, "autism," "autistic," or "autistic syndrome" should be taken to refer to the hypothetical concept of typical autism, as opposed to the wider range of conditions that share some clinical features with autism, such as the "triad of social impairments" (Wing, 1988; Wing & Gould, 1979) and the closely similar concept of "pervasive developmental disorder" (PDD; American Psychiatric Association, 1980, 1987).

Despite clinical impressions of a unity among typically autistic children, investigations of the group, regardless of which set of diagnostic criteria has been used, have found no shared etiology, no shared uniquely pathognomonic neural deficit, no shared cognitive functional deficit, no distinct shared behavioral pattern, no shared specific life course, and no shared response to drug treatment. Studies typically find that only some (usually between 10% and 40%) of sampled individuals diagnosed as autistic exhibit any particular marker under study.

Throughout these efforts, Kanner's original observations of the severe problems of social interaction have remained the basis for all schemes of diagnosis. But, during the past 40 years, interest has moved away from direct investigation of the nature of social impairment in autism. First, attempts were made to explain the clinical picture in terms of parental (emotional) influence (Bettelheim, 1967). These views are maintained in some areas in clinical practice, and appear in some current theorizing about autism (Tinbergen & Tinbergen, 1983). Then attention focused on language deficits (Bartak & Rutter, 1976; Bartak, Rutter, & Cox, 1975, 1977), on cognitive functioning (Frith, 1970; Hermelin & O'Connor, 1970; Waterhouse & Fein, 1982, 1984), and on neurological dysfunctions hypothesized to underlie cognitive deficits (Ornitz, 1974; Rimland, 1964).

The field has now circled back to consider in detail the social impairment of autistic individuals (Denckla, 1986). Some investigators currently argue that the basis for the social impairment that defines autism is a neurological deficit. This abnormality is variously construed, but is generally thought to give rise to social deficits either directly (Fein, Pennington, Markowitz, Braverman, & Waterhouse, 1986; Wing & Gould, 1979) or indirectly, through mechanisms of impaired attention that lead to dysfunction in the ability to attend to complex social events (Courchesne, 1987; Damasio & Maurer, 1978; Howlin, 1986; Mundy, Sigman, Ungerer, & Sherman, 1985). The nature of social impairment is also viewed differently by various authors. Impaired social imagination (Wing, 1982), impaired social cognition (Hobson, 1987), impaired concepts concerning other people's inner thoughts or feelings (Baron-Cohen, Leslie, & Frith, 1985, 1986), impaired social attention (Mundy *et al.*, 1985), and impaired social play (Sherman, Shapiro, & Glassman, 1983), have all been identified as key problems for autism.

At the same time that the social impairments of autism have taken center stage in much recent research, controversy continues about whether autism exists as a specific disorder (i.e., whether it has either a specific etiology, as in Down syndrome, or a specific focus of pathology, as in cerebellar ataxia), or whether it even exists as a separate syndrome (i.e., a set of features that reliably cluster together, regardless of the cause).

The formulation of the syndrome of autism has been and continues to be problematic, for a number of reasons. Six specific problems are considered in this chapter. First, because most definitions of autism include language impairments and stereotypies as well as social impairments, the syndrome has fuzzy boundaries with mental retardation that is not related to Down syndrome, with severe developmental language delay, and with the generically defined category of (PDD) (American Psychiatric Association, 1980, 1987). Historically, there have also been concerns with the possible blurred boundary between childhood autism and adult schizophrenia—a concern that has been reinforced by current reports of autistic children becoming schizophrenic as they develop (Green *et al.*, 1984; Petty, Ornitz, Michelman, & Zimmerman, 1984; Rumsey, Andreason, & Rapoport, 1986).

Second, among individuals diagnosed as autistic, both the heterogeneity of developmental–behavioral patterns and of presumptive etiology are very great, and empirical studies have failed to find a unifying marker at any level of exploration.

Third, five essential requirements for drawing brain–behavior inferences that have been posited by the philosopher Barbara von Eckardt (1986) cannot be met by any of the current theoretical models that postulate a mechanism to unify the syndrome.

Fourth, efforts to determine subgroups with the syndrome, though promising, face the dangerous prospect of claiming validity for artifactual groupings.

Fifth, the current return to focus on the specific aspects of social impairment in autism runs the risk of attempting external validity on the basis of a tautology.

Finally, and perhaps most disheartening for the researcher, the claim that each case of brain damage is unique (Caramazza, 1984) cannot be adequately rebutted by any autism research done to date.

The present chapter considers each of these six problems with the identity of autism in turn. One caveat is that the following discussions are not meant to encompass an exhaustive review of relevant publications. Research reviewed here has been selected as illustrative of the issues raised in current findings and projects.

PROBLEM 1: FUZZY BOUNDARIES

"Fuzzy set theory" was developed as a mathematical model to describe relationships between categories in cases where the categorized groups do not have clear absolute feature boundaries separating them from each other (Zadeh, 1965). Membership in a "fuzzy set" is assumed to vary on a continuum for each feature that is proposed as part of the category descriptors. Therefore an individual's inclusion in a category is not absolute, but a matter of degree.

"Degree," in turn, may depend on the relative number of features present in the individual. In autism, for example, degree could be indexed as the presence of relatively more or fewer of the DSM-IIIR criteria for autistic disorder, beyond the minimum required for a diagnosis. "Degree" of group membership may also depend on the relative intensity of expression of each particular feature. For example, self-biting may be on a continuum of severity from biting one's own cuticles off from time to time to constant full-mouth biting of several parts of one's own body. The former puts the feature outside PDD; the latter may allow a diagnosis of PDD or autistic disorder.

In a set of interviews with 22 U.S. clinicians and researchers concerned with child psychopathology, each of whom had published at least one recent article on PDD, it was the unanimous response that autism, childhood-onset PDD, and atypical PDD fall into one difficult-to-distinguish diagnostic domain (Waterhouse, Fein, Nath, & Snyder, 1987). This was also the general consensus of a research round-table forum at the 1985 meeting of the American Academy of Child Psychiatry.

Not only impressions from clinical practice, but also the findings of empirical research, suggest that the boundaries of the autistic syndrome are ill defined. There are three areas where borderlines are blurred: etiology; behavioral features; and the relationship of autism to wider categories of childhood disorders.

Fuzzy Boundaries of Etiologically Defined Syndromes

It is by now clear that the syndrome of autism can arise in individuals who have a wide variety of identifiable physical disorders, and these disorders in turn suggest a presumptive etiology for the autistic behavior in each of those individuals (Coleman & Gillberg, 1985). The boundary problem, however, is not that the syndrome can be the outcome of a variety of etiological agents. Rather, it is that for each given etiological agent across individuals subject to that agent, a shaded and dimensional spectrum of behaviors emerges, instead of a distinct and categorical spectrum. Moreover, within the group of individuals sharing an etiology those individuals identified as autistic will occupy some section of that associated behavioral spectrum, and that section in turn will widely overlap the behavioral spectrum occupied by individuals not diagnosed as autistic.

Fragile X syndrome is a good case in point. Individuals identified as having fragile X are often identified as mildly retarded, severely retarded, or autistic. Behaviors such as social aloofness that are part of the diagnostic criteria for autism are among the spectrum of behaviors associated with fragile X. It is unclear whether there is any qualitative or quantitative difference in social aloofness for autistic individuals with or without fragile X (Fisch et al., 1986; Hagerman, Jackson,

Levitas, Rimland, & Braden, 1986). In one response to the diagnostic dilemmas caused by the existence of this fuzzy boundary, some have suggested that there are so few cases of autism associated with fragile X that the issue is trivial (Goldfine *et al.*, 1985); others have claimed that there may be mistaken diagnoses of autism associated with fragile X.

These arguments do not really deal with the difficulties (Fisch *et al.*, 1986). The following facts must be accounted for: (1) the presence of similar symptom groups in fragile-X-positive and fragile-X-negative individuals; (2) the presence of shared behaviors (such as digit biting) in fragile-X-positive males who can and cannot be diagnosed as autistic; and (3) the presence or absence of autistic features of behavior in fragile-X-positive males. The issue cannot be dismissed simply by claiming that the problem is a small one. The within- and across-etiology complex "mix-and-match" sharing of a spectrum of behavioral disorders, of which fragile X and autism provide only one example, suggests that autism cannot be viewed even as a unitary behavioral syndrome.

Fuzzy Boundaries of Syndromes Sharing Behavioral Features

Although formal definitions of diagnostic entities (such as those of DSM-III) seem to have clear boundaries, in clinical practice and research work these distinctions are far from clear. Freeman, Ritvo, and Schroth (1984), using their own behavior observation system, found that there was a great deal of overlap in observed behaviors between mentally retarded and autistic children. The number of behaviors investigated was sizeable, as was the observed behavioral overlap. The authors concluded that the data could be interpreted to mean that diagnosis should not be based on these behaviors, and, furthermore, that autistic individuals should be subgrouped by mental age level.

In an epidemiological study undertaken in one geographical area, Wing and Gould (1979) found that half of all severely retarded children were socially impaired, whether or not they fitted Kanner's descriptions of the autistic syndrome. They pointed out that "the most notable feature of the association between mental retardation and social impairment . . . was the positive correlation between severity of retardation and the proportion of children who were socially impaired. Furthermore, the lower the level of intelligence, the more likely it was that the social impairment would take the form of aloofness and indifference" (p. 26). Wing and Gould also reported that, within their samples, children with a history typical of autism as defined by Kanner and Eisenberg (1956) comprised approximately 10% of the samples with an IQ range below 50. Conversely, a variety of reports indicates that about one-half of individuals diagnosed as autistic have IQs below 50, and only about one-third or fewer are in the normal range (IQs of 70 or above).

It has been suggested that high-functioning autistic people form a separate group from those who are also mentally retarded (Bartak & Rutter, 1976). However, attempts to validate this have not been successful (Prior, 1979). Epidemiological studies do not support a sharp behavioral distinction (Wing, 1988). It is probably often true that children with higher IQs who are diagnosed as having autistic disorder may have a generally better prognosis than do positively diagnosed children with lower IQs (Lockyer & Rutter, 1970; Rutter & Lockyer, 1967). However, this finding does not support the notion that there are two IQ-separable subgroups of individuals within the autistic spectrum; it only suggests that being in the top half of the IQ distribution is beneficial for later outcome. Burd, Fisher, Knowlton, and Kerbeshian (1987) have recently argued that hyperlexia is a marker for improved outcome in PDD. These "signs"—higher IQ, hyperlexia—may simply be emblematic of the fact that a particular child's system has experienced less "damage" and/or has greater self-righting tendencies during development. Unconstrained skills, such as those that may underlie hyperlexia and splinter skills in cognition, may be indexing a more general failure of meshing of systems in development.

More importantly, higher versus lower IQ cannot yet be identified as separating out mental retardation from the "pure" disorder of autsim. Given what is known about brain structure interrelationships, brain development, and the complex reaction of the human brain to various insults, it is extremely unlikely that a simple additive formula (autism plus mental retardation vs. autism minus mental retardation) obtains.

Another issue for the additivity model is that if "pure autism" as social impairment were hypothesized to be a specific deficit in some isolable cortical or subcortical ability to express and experience "social intelligence" or "social cognition" (Baron-Cohen, 1985; Rutter, 1983), then it would seem likely that such social disability would have a more complex distribution than simple additivity. Allowing for genetic, traumatic, and medical illness etiologies, first, there should be many more "mild" cases than are currently diagnosed; second, a continuum of social impairment should operate independently of imapirment to other processes. Casting a wider net in research, and reaching a better understanding of sociability in development, may help answer this modeling question.

In addition to the problem of the relationship between autism and mental retardation, there is also a difficulty in defining the boundary with severe developmental language disorder (DLD). Hallmark features of autism include problems with perception and production of speech. Paul and Cohen (1984) reviewed a sample of adolescents who had been diagnosed as having DLD with atypical features and found that the behavioral development of children in this sample would support a diagnosis of autism. Another ongoing study of two groups of preschool children—one group diagnosed as having DLD and another group diagnosed as autistic—has already revealed a subsample of children whose initial diagnosis of DLD has given way to a diagnosis of autism or PDD, and vice versa (Waterhouse, Wing, Allen, Fein, & Rapin, 1987).

The features that create the fuzzy boundary between a diagnosis of DLD and a diagnosis of autism include a range of language disability—from complete absence of speech, to severe dysfluency of single-word speech and impaired comprehension, to language development that is essentially normal but delayed in most domains. Children with a primary diagnosis of DLD also may show echolalia and/ or prosodic impairment, both of which are thought to be hallmark features of the language impairment of autism (Waterhouse, Wing, *et al.*, 1987).

The ultimate appeal to one diagnosis or another is based on the clinical features of impairment in social relatedness. However, here too specific features may be problematic, as some DLD children also have aberrant social relatedness, which would allow them to be diagnosed as having autistic features of interactive behavior.

Fuzzy Boundaries of More Inclusive Syndromes

In the 40-year history of the syndrome of autism, identification of autistic individuals as separate from some larger, more inclusive group of children (in the past, this larger group would have been termed "psychotic" and is now referred to as having PDD) has remained a persistent difficulty. This problem is sufficiently extensive that clinical groupings and empirical groupings are often not consonant within the same population.

Recently, for example (Dahl, Cohen, & Provence, 1986), it was found that 62 of 86 children with a diagnosis of PDD were diagnosable as having infantile autism. When a statistical clustering solution was applied, 44 of the 86 PDD children were identified as sharing a cluster of features. Only 36 of the 44 in that cluster had had a diagnosis prior to 30 months of age, and from reading the report it may be assumed (though it is not clearly stated as such) that of the 36 identified as having been diagnosed before 30 months and sharing a cluster of features, some were not part of the original 62 identified as autistic by clinical means.

Although the authors of this report argue that these findings suggest empirical support for the notion of the entity of autism per se, if fewer than 36 of 62 in fact are empirically identified as forming a group out of the original sample, then the overlap between clinical and empirical groupings is not great. Therefore, these findings do not support the notion of a clear syndrome identity. Most important to note is the fact that the authors see the clustering solutions they obtained as suggesting a continuum of severity, wherein "at one end were those clusters of children with little impairment of functioning and in whom the disorder was confined to the disruption of little more than one aspect of the child's development; at the other end were those clusters of children in whom many aspects of functioning were impaired" (Dahl *et al.*, 1986, p. 177).

Earlier in our own research, two of us (Waterhouse & Fein, 1982, 1984) found that of 102 PDD children, the subset of those who could be identified as autistic showed no significant difference in language and cognitive skills from the other PDD children. Furthermore, the same group of children followed longitudinally showed no significant difference in cognitive and linguistic development from the other PDD children across a period of 5 years. In fact, "comparisons of age and test score correlations, comparisons of cross-sequential means, and trends for means for diagnostic groups and normal controls suggested developmental delay for all skills at all ages" (Waterhouse & Fein, 1984, 236). This delay was seen identically in the subsample positively diagnosed as autistic, as well as in the larger sample of children who could be identified as having PDD. In the Camberwell epidemiological study (Wing, 1988), the autistic continuum was not simple, but had identifiable subgroups along its extent. The most common profile found in the epidemiological study comprised individuals who were socially aloof, were severely or profoundly retarded with no areas of better skills (apart from independent mobility), and exhibited only simple (not complex) repetitive routines. The age-specific prevalence of this subgroup was 6.9 per 10,000, compared with 4.9 for Kanner's syndrome defined on two criteria and 2.0 defined on five criteria. It was the most stable clinical picture over time and place, but has never been named as a syndrome (Wing, 1988).

In the epidemiological study conducted by one of us (Wing, 1982, 1988; Wing & Gould, 1979), it was found that making a diagnostic division between autistic and nonautistic individuals using Kanner and Eisenberg's (1956) criteria was not the most cogent way to address subgroup characteristics. In fact,

> clustering of the social, language, and behavioral abnormalities and the evidence from the psychological and medical data provided support for the main division into socially impaired and sociable though severely retarded groups. . . . [T]he social impairment subgroups [three in number] did not differ significantly on the speech and behavioral abnormalities associated with typical autism, but were significantly differentiated on other cognitive and behavioral measures, and on presence of associated organic conditions. However, the distribution of the variables among the subgroups suggested that they formed a continuum of severity rather than discrete entities. (Wing & Gould, 1979, pp. 25–26)

Furthermore, Wing and Gould found that grouping by severity of social impairment showed an important relationship to etiology, whereas grouping by a history of typical autism as defined by Kanner did not.

Taken together, the three types of boundary problems discussed here—cross-diagnostic spread of symptoms associated with a single etiological agent; the sharing of diagnostic features such as language delay and intellectual retardation across syndromes; and the lack of consistent or significant empirical distinctions between autistic individuals and other socially impaired children who have primary diagnoses other than autism—remain as serious issues that are not consistent with belief in the separate identity of typical autism, either as a syndrome or as a discrete specific disorder.

PROBLEM 2: HETEROGENEITY WITHIN
AUTISTIC POPULATIONS

As Kanner reported in 1973 in a follow-up of his original 11 cases, the outcome for children initially diagnosed as autistic varies so widely as to "invite serious curiosities about the departures from the initial likeness ranging all the way from complete deterioration to a combination of occupational adequacy with limited though superficially smooth social adjustment" (Kanner, 1973, p. 186). Kanner's response to his own findings was to suggest that treatment programs may have a lot to do with outcome. More recent work (e.g., Rutter, 1983) has shown that outcome is positively correlated with IQ level, though this by no means accounts for all the variation. A majority of autistic individuals studied in follow-up do show some improvement in social behavior over time (Howlin, 1986). Even within groups of those individuals who show poor outcome for social behavior or cognitive skills or both, the nature of this poor outcome is quite variable. Similarly, among those who show improved social skills and continuing improvement or plateau in cognitive skills, there is again a continuum of improvement, ranging from the rare near-normal functioning in adulthood to the odd but acceptably adaptive adjustment for many who are judged as having achieved a successful outcome.

A variety of conditions have been found to be associated with autism. Sex-linked patterns of inheritance, including fragile X, have been described (Brown *et al.*, 1982); others have argued for an autosomal recessive pattern of inheritance (Ritvo *et al.*, 1985). Studies of perinatal events suggest that there is a higher-than-expected number of risk factors involved for infants who later are diagnosed as autistic (Tsai, 1987; Waterhouse & Fein, 1983). Torrey, Hersh, and McCabe (1975) found that midtrimester bleeding was significantly associated with autism. Biochemical studies of autistic individuals show a mixed picture, suggesting problems in the serotonergic and dopaminergic systems (Coleman & Gillberg, 1985). Certain diseases (e.g., rubella) and metabolic diseases (e.g., phenylketonuria, purine disorder, and lactic acidosis) have also been found to be associated with the autistic syndrome. (Coleman & Gillberg, 1985). In fact, nearly every marker studied suggests some abnormality, and it is a rare marker that does not show up as a suggestive or presumptive etiology for this syndrome for at least some subset of patients seen or tested.

There is also wide variability in cognitive functioning, in language skills, and even in social functioning (Howlin, 1986; Lord, 1984). Even the autistic aloofness, which is identified as the hallmark of the syndrome and is used as a diagnostic feature in all systems of diagnosis, is itself quite variable, and may change with increasing age and in different environments (Wing, 1988; Wing & Gould, 1979).

The fact that populations of positively diagnosed autistic individuals are so various in so many domains is often ascribed to problems with diagnostic systems themselves (Parks, 1983) or to the improper use of diagnostic systems in research or clinical settings (Cohen *et al.*, 1978; Meehl, 1986). Despite these claims, it is unlikely that improper employment of diagnostic schemes is a major factor in the heterogeneity in autistic samples. Evidence suggests that even with the most stringent subject selection criteria, heterogeneity will necessarily exist, because the essential conceptualization of the syndrome itself involves the inclusion of many different sorts of children who may have many different sorts of neurological deficits. Thus, despite the hopefulness engendered by the presumably ever-increasing focus on diagnostic precision and proper use of diagnosis within studies, samples of children positively diagnosed will continue to exhibit a range of etiologies and varying patterns of development, as well as different sets of skills and disabilities in cognition and language development.

PROBLEM 3: BRAIN–BEHAVIOR LINKS

Along with the shifting trends in behavioral research, there has been a consistent background of research for biological markers in autism. Those that have so far been investigated fail to bind the group together. Although work continues, it has become clear to most researchers that such markers are unlikely to serve as a firm index for the entire syndrome or even the majority of cases within the syndrome (Coleman & Gillberg, 1985).

Because of the inability to unify or validate the syndrome on the basis of either biological or behavioral elements, some workers are now focusing on the possibility that an abnormality in a specific brain–behavior mechanism is the common link. The hypothesis here is that autism is a specific disorder because of a specific identifiable locus of pathology, even if this may be caused by many different gross causes.

In looking at critical limitations associated with drawing brain–behavior inferences concerning behavioral pathology, von Eckardt (1986) has generated the following list of requirements:

1. Pathology outlined must be correctly interpreted as a failure of some specific and well-understood behavioral function.
2. Normal parameters of the specific behavior should be thoroughly understood *a priori*.
3. There should be a good model of the normal functional path for brain–behavior connections leading to the specific behavior (in which the pathology has been noted).
4. A specific deficit in this modeled pathway should be hypothesized as the source for the behavioral impairment.
5. There should be no better competing explanation for the phenomenon of impairment.

These are stringent requirements indeed, and much of neuropsychology and neuropsychiatric research would fail if set against von Eckardt's standards. Certainly the theories concerning brain–behavior links that have centered on the autistic syndrome cannot meet any of the five criteria set by von Eckardt.

If, for example, we assume that failure of social attention is the key problem in autism and is produced by a specifically localized brain pathology, then we would have to face the following:

1. We do not yet understand the system of normal social attention and its relationship to social cognition, essential attachment, general sociability, personality, and the like (Seyfarth, 1987).
2. We do not understand the development of social attention nor do we have a functional analysis of the elements that contribute to social attention, although we do know something about the elements involved in making up social attachment (Bretherton & Waters, 1985).
3. We do have models (Damasio & Van Hoesen, 1983) that theorize a limbic system basis for emotion and sociability, but these models do not outline the mechanism by which social attention per se is engendered.
4. Electrophysiological and anatomical studies suggest multiple sites of dysfunction or damage for different autistic individuals.
5. Whether or not a particular brain–behavior link to explain autistic pathology is superior to competing explanations cannot yet be judged, because all models presently fail to meet the preceding four stringent requirements.

One of the most fully articulated models is that provided by Courchesne (1987; Courchesne, Yeung-Courchesne, Press, Hesselink, & Jernigan, 1988). This author's argument is that an autistic individual's nervous system is full of "static" and has a kind of "off–on" quality of fluctuations. Courchesne believes that interference in the functioning of mechanisms of attention in autistic individuals will interrupt processes necessary for storing and retrieving information; yet, on occasion, fragments of awareness may be more extended, allowing autistic individuals to build narrow channels of knowledge by means of an "off-and-on again" process. It is Courchesne's contention that certain kinds of information about the world can be learned piecemeal (in an "off-and-on again" fashion), but that other things, such as knowledge about social situations and language, cannot be built up in this fragmented way. He also argues that strong emotional states within autistic individuals may provide enough arousal for other neural systems to override interfering processes and again allow more attention. More than one neural system may be responsible for this, including reticular, thalamic, or cortical systems. He further argues that problems in the basic neurotransmitter systems may be responsible for disrupting neural activation, thus impairing attention in autistic individuals.

When von Eckardt's requirements are applied to Courchesne's model, its limitations become evident. First, we do not yet know what the relationship is between attention and social relatedness. Second, we do not really understand the developmental parameters of attention and social relatedness. Third, we do not yet have a consistent model of a particular pathway that would lead us to understand a specific deficit. Thus Courchesne, like Damasio and Maurer (1978) and others, in the face of this lack of essential knowledge, is forced to hypothesize many systems and many possible pathways.

This is not to argue that theoretical models should not be attempted; they may serve heuristic functions. However, until the brain–behavior links for normal social attention and social relatedness are better understood, the issue of specifying neurological impairment will remain an open question. It should be noted that Courchesne's model is one of many that have been hypothesized in the past 10 years and is probably closer than most to meeting von Eckardt's requirements.

PROBLEM 4: FINDING SUBGROUPS

In the epidemiological study mentioned previously, Wing and Gould (1979) examined all retarded children (IQs below 50) without exceptions, plus any children with IQs of 50 and above (no upper limit) who had deficits in social interaction, impairment of language, or stereotyped activities. A variety of behavioral, psychological, and medical data was gathered on each child. They then attempted to find a classification system that would be reliable and clinically useful, using traditional psychiatric syndrome delineation or aspects of current behavior. They found that classifying children by the quality of their social interaction gave more significant differences on behavioral, psychological, and medical variables than did classifying by diagnostic categories. Their social categorization is given below.

1. *Social aloofness* covered very severe impairment of social interaction. Some of the children with this behavior were aloof and indifferent in all situations. Others would make approaches to obtain things they wanted, but returned to aloofness once the need was gratified. Some liked simple physical contact with adults, such as cuddling, tickling, or games of chasing, but had no interest in the purely social aspects of the contact. The social indifference was especially marked toward other children, as compared with adults.

2. *Passive interaction* described the behavior of children who did not make social contact spontaneously, but who amiably accepted approaches and did not resist if other children dragged them into games. Some of these children were liked by their classmates because they could be used as babies in a game of mothers and fathers or as patients for doctors and nurses. They would remain in their allotted role as long as the other children were playing, but would wander off at the end of the game unless redirected by their peers.

3. *Active but odd interaction* included children who did make spontaneous social approaches, mostly to adults but also to other children. Their behavior was

inappropriate because it was undertaken mainly to indulge some repetitive, idio-syncratic preoccupation. They had no interest in, and no feeling for, the needs and ideas of others. They did not modify their speech or behavior to adapt to others, but continued to pursue their own topics of favorite activities even in the face of active discouragement. They tended to pester other people and were some-times rejected by their peers because of their peculiar behavior. For this reason they were less socially acceptable than the "passive" group.

4. *Appropriate interaction* covered those whose social interactions were ap-propriate for their mental age. They enjoyed social contact for its own sake with adults and with other children. They used eye contact, facial expression, and gesture to indicate interest and to try to join in conversation as best they could.

The first three groups were, collectively, classified as "socially impaired."

Another attempt at empirical subclassification was made by Siegel, Anders, Ciaranello, Bienenstock, and Kraemer (1986). Subjects in this study were 35 males and 11 females who had previous diagnoses of early infantile autism or residual state autism. This sample included children who did not meet DSM-III criteria for autism (infantile or residual state). They performed a three-step operation: they (1) identified observational variables that discriminated among different children in their sample; (2) established behavioral profiles for each child; and (3) per-formed a cluster analysis of children based on similarity of behavioral profiles. A four-group solution was selected. Group 1 was most typically autistic, with perseve-rative sensory–motor play and noncommunicative language. Group 2 was the most retarded, had motor difficulties, and was generally nonverbal. Group 3 showed bizarre ideation, was more communicative, and was least retarded. Group 4 was anxious and negativistic and actively avoided social contact. Group differences in parent-reported behaviors, pre- and perinatal events, and developmental mile-stones provided some external validation.

A similar cluster-analytic approach was employed by Sherman *et al.* (1983). Children were grouped on the basis of a total behavior checklist score, a global severity rating, and IQ. A four-cluster solution produced adequate within-group homogeneity with regard to behavioral symptomatology and severity, but left a range of IQ within each group. Further subdivisions were necessary to produce homogeneity in levels of retardation. This may suggest a relative independence of behavioral severity and intellectual level. Play and language variables were used for external validation. Symbolic ability differentiated the groups, and from Sher-man *et al.*'s data seemed more correlated with behavior totals and behavior sever-ity than with IQ. This supports a relationship between sociability and symbolic activity not attributable to cognitive level. Thus, these findings run counter to those considered earlier regarding IQ and social deficit.

The problem with all such methods is that the groupings may be artifactual. The artifact may be one stemming from the developmental level of the children or from the nature of the grouping methods themselves. Siegel (personal com-munication, 1986) has preliminary findings to suggest that her subgroups change with developmental change in the children. Cohen (1987) has reported that Wing and Gould's (1979) social impairment groups reflect in part developmental level (with aloof children being relatively more delayed than passive children, and passive children being more delayed than active but odd children).

In terms of methodological artifact, the clustering systems do create groups of children with shared features, but the variables that have been indexed may not include those most clinically salient for identifying a disease or disorder entity, or even a meaningful clinical picture (e.g., if a cluster solution does not take "autistic aloofness" in as a variable). Nevertheless, one important point that should be considered is that the larger the sample and the more clinical information that can be involved in the analysis, the less likely it will be that groups formed are unsatisfactory because they are artifactual. Moreover, the use of clinically significant variables as checks on empirical validity of groups can help to distinguish artifactual groups. Still better would be the finding that distinct outcomes and distinct etiologies aggregate by subgroups discovered.

PROBLEM 5: SOCIAL IMPAIRMENT FEATURES

Recently, in the return to social impairment in autism as the research focus of the field, there have been several suggestions as to the key underlying impairment associated with problems in social relatedness. We (Fein et al., 1986) have argued for the general position that social impairment in autism is likely to be caused by a variety of neuropsychological deficits.

Recently, others have hypothesized that some quite specific mechanisms may be to blame. Hobson (1987) argues that person perception any perception of the emotional meaning of social events are the key deficits. Baron-Cohen et al. (1985) argue that autistic children fail to develop a "theory" of the mind of others—something that Leslie has postulated develops in young normal children by the age of 2. Mundy et al. (1985) have argued that joint social attention to a task is the heart of impaired social relatedness in autistic children.

Each of these studies is unique and fascinating and helps draw attention to the issue of social relatedness. However, the inferences that may be drawn from them are strictly limited. In each case, the study samples were small, and the socially impaired subjects were limited to those diagnosed as "classically" autistic. Single points of behavior were used to support complex theories of the nature of social impairment. Without considerably more evidence, it cannot yet be concluded that any of these models accounts for social impairment in all people diagnosed as autistic. Furthermore, even if one of the hypotheses is proved to be correct for individuals diagnosed as autistic, it would still remain to be seen whether the same model applies to people who are socially impaired but not diagnosed as autistic. This question is relevant not only to social impairment originating from birth or in early life, but also to abnormality of social interaction of later onset (e.g., that resulting from trauma to the brain, schizophrenia in adult life, or dementia such as that seen in Alzheimer disease).

PROBLEM 6: THE UNIQUENESS OF EACH CASE

Caramazza (1984) has claimed that inferring functional cognitive lesions is never theory-neutral. He argues that inferring the brain–behavior link requires separate theories of behavior, of psychological functioning, and of neurological functioning, as well as a theory of the integration of behavioral, psychological, and neurological functioning. In his view, most cases of brain damage are better approached as single-case studies in which details of function in different domains can help to suggest the possible specific deficits in the individual concerned.

Caramazza's claims have been greeted with a considerable degree of skepticism (Caplan, 1986). It is hard to say whether all the criticism is based on an impartial notion of what is cogent and possible, or whether in fact it is simply disagreeable for people in the field to consider that each case may be a law unto itself. It is much more satisfying to find general laws and general principles than it is to argue that various accidents in nature combine to generate a variability that is difficult or perhaps even impossible to cattegorize.

In the literature on autism, various forms of the Caramazza hypothesis coexist with the contrary belief that a unifying element for the disorder will eventually be identified. It may be that the elusiveness of the putative biological or behavioral marker for the syndrome drives individuals in the field to new areas that they hope may permit the identification of the ultimate unifying element. Kuhn, in his book *The Structure of Scientific Revolutions* (1970), argues that a paradigm will receive increasingly "fanatical" attention, to the point at which there is a transition that could be likened to the notion of old wine in new bottles. In the field of autism, this transition may be taking the form of a search for subgroups within populations diagnosed as autistic or PDD; the same quest for a unitary basis for autism will reappear as a quest for the unity of the subgroups of autism.

It may be that reasonable and significant subgroups associated with a marker providing external validation will be found. However, it is also possible that there will prove to be nearly as many categories or subgroups as there are individuals identified as autistic or PDD.

Caramazza's notions might be reformulated as advice for autism researchers: Go out and explore in great detail the most interesting cases of social impairment available. Although many may consider the return to the "clinical" study of individual cases a retrograde step for the field, this so-to-speak "microscopic" approach could be of great value, especially if linked with "macroscopic" epidemiological studies wherein ascertainment of a whole population is based on some specified parameters of social impairment. If "microscopic" analysis of cases permits understanding of specific brain–behavior links in an individual, and if the brain–behavior links can be understood in relationship to the distribution of associated behaviors in the larger population, then the disorders these individuals have can be understood adequately, independently of syndrome identity.

Most research to date does not support the existence of a specific syndrome of typical autism. The special quality that makes the type of young child described by Kanner instantly recognizable to those with experience in the field is the combination of social impairment, in the form of aloofness and indifference to others, with absorption in meaningless and repetitive activities, good visual–spatial skills or rote memory, and an attractive physical appearance. Plausible though it may seem to suggest that this is a separate condition, results from studies indicate that the characteristic behaviors are each part of a continuum of abnormalities with no sharp borderlines, and that they can be caused by a wide range of etiologies. The features of Kanner's so-called "syndrome" may occur together from time to time, simply because the various gross etiologies that can produce social impairment can also affect a variety of other brain functions. It may be chance combinations of factors that determine the final patterns of skills or impairments, of which the picture described by Kanner is only one example among the many that include social impairment.

As an alternative to concentrating upon "typical autism," a more fruitful approach may be to examine the behavioral abnormalities, especially the crucial one of social impairment, across the whole autistic spectrum. Epidemiological surveys, investigations of selected samples, and individual case studies directed to the full range of related conditions would, over time, reveal continuities and discontinuities within the variables investigated and permit the definition of valid subgroups (if such really do exist). This type of approach would remove the limitations imposed by the automatic acceptance of syndromes defined before current methods of neurological, psychological, and epidemiological examination were developed.

References

American Psychiatric Association. (1980). *Diagnostic and statistical manual of mental disorders* (3rd ed.). Washington, DC: Author.

American Psychiatric Association. (1987). *Diagnostic and statistical manual of mental disorders* (3rd ed., rev.). Washington, DC: Author.

Baron-Cohen, S. (1985). *Social cognition and pretend play in autism*. Unpublished doctoral dissertation, University of London.

Baron-Cohen, S., Leslie, A. M., & Frith, U. (1985). Does the autistic child have a "theory of mind"? *Cognition, 21*, 37–46.

Baron-Cohen, S., Leslie, A. M., & Frith, U. (1986). Mechanical, behavioural and intentional understanding of picture stories in autistic children. *British Journal of Developmental Psychology, 4*, 113–125.

Bartak, L., & Rutter, M. (1976). Differences between mentally retarded and normally intelligent autistic children. *Journal of Autism and Childhood Schizophrenia, 6*(2), 109–120.

Bartak, L., Rutter, M., & Cox, A. (1975). A comparative study of infantile autism and specific developmental receptive language disorders: I. The children. *British Journal of Psychiatry, 126*, 127–145.

Bartak, L., Rutter, M., & Cox, A. (1977). A comparative study of infantile autism and specific developmental receptive language disorders: III. Discriminate function analysis. *Journal of Autism and Childhood Schizophrenia, 7*, 383–396.

Bettelheim, B. (1967). *The empty fortress: Infantile autism and the birth of the self.* New York: Free Press.

Bretherton, I., & Waters, E. (Eds.). (1985). *Growing points of attachment theory and research.* Chicago: University of Chicago Press.

Brown, W. T., Jenkins, E. C., Friedman, E., Brooks, J., Wisniewski, K., Raguthu, S., & French, J. (1982). Autism is associated with the fragile X syndrome. *Journal of Autism and Developmental Disorders, 12,* 303–308.

Burd, L., Fisher, W., Knowlton, D., & Kerbeshian, J. (1987). Hyperlexia: A marker for improvement in children with pervasive developmental disorder? *Journal of the American Academy of Child Psychiatry, 26*(3), 407–412.

Caplan, D. (Chair). (1986, June). *Inferring normal cognitive function from pathological cases.* Symposium conducted at the annual meeting of the Society for Philosophy and Psychology, Johns Hopkins University, Baltimore.

Caramazza, A. (1984). The logic of neuropsychological research and the problem of patient classification in aphasia. *Brain and Language, 21,* 9–20.

Cohen, D. J. (1987, April 25). *Autism and pervasive developmental disorder: Behavioral and biological studies and their relevance for intervention.* Invited address to the meeting of the Society for Research in Child Development, Baltimore.

Cohen, D. J., Caparulo, B. K., Gold, J. R., Waldo, M. C., Shaywitz, B. A., Ruttenberg, B. A., & Rimland, B. (1978). Clinical assessment and behavior rating scales for pervasively disturbed children. *Journal of the American Academy of Child and Adolescent Psychiatry, 17,* 589–603.

Coleman, M., & Gillberg, G. (1985). *The biology of the autistic syndromes.* New York: Praeger.

Courchesne, E. (1987). A neurophysiological view of autism. In E. Schopler & G. Mesibov (Eds.), *Neurobiological issues in autism* (pp. 285–324). New York: Plenum.

Courchesne, E., Yeung-Courchesne, R., Press, G. A., Hesselink, M. D., & Jernigan, T. L. (1988). Hypoplasia of cerebellar vermal lobules VI and VII in autism. *New England Journal of Medicine, 318,* 1349–1354.

Dahl, E. K., Cohen, D. J., & Provence, S. (1986). Clinical and multi-variate approaches to nosology of pervasive developmental disorders. *Journal of the American Academy of Child Psychiatry, 25,* 170–180.

Damasio, A. R., & Maurer, R. (1978). A neurological model for childhood autism. *Archives of Neurology, 35,* 777–786.

Damasio, A. R., & Van Hoesen, G. W. (1983). Emotional disturbances associated with focal lesions of the limbic frontal lobe. In K. M. Heilman & P. Satz (Eds.), *Neuropsychology of human emotion* (pp. 85–110). New York: Guilford Press.

Denckla, M. (1986). New diagnostic criteria for autism and related behavioral disorders: Guidelines for research protocols. *Journal of the American Academy of Child Psychiatry, 25*(2), 221–224.

Fein, D., Pennington, B., Markowitz, P., Braverman, M., & Waterhouse, L. (1986). Toward a neuropsychological model of infantile autism: Are the social dificits primary? *Journal of the American Academy of Child Psychiatry, 25*(2), 198–212.

Fisch, G. S., Cohen, I. L., Wolf, E. G., Brown, W. T., Jenkins, E. C., & Gross, A. (1986). Autism and the fragile X syndrome. *American Journal of Psychiatry, 143,* 71–73.

Freeman, B. J., Ritvo, E. R., & Schroth, P. C. (1984). Behavior assessment of the syndrome of autism: Behavior observation system. *Journal of the American Academy of Child Psychiatry, 23*(5), 588–594.

Frith, U. (1970). Studies of pattern detection in normal and autistic children: I. Immediate recall of auditory sequences. *Journal of Abnormal Psychology, 76,* 413–420.

Goldfine, P. E., McPherson, P. M., Heath, G. A., Hardesty, V. A., Beauregard, L. J., & Gordon, B. (1985). Association of fragile X syndrome with autism. *American Journal of Psychiatry, 142,* 108–110.

Green, W. H., Campbell, M., Hardesty, A. S., Grega, D. M., Padron-Gayol, M., Shell, J., & Erlenmeyer-Kimling, L. (1984). A comparison of schizophrenic and autistic children. *Journal of the American Academy of Child Psychiatry, 23*(4), 399–409.

Hagerman, R. J., Jackson, A. W., Levitas, A., Rimland, B., & Braden, M. (1986). An analysis of autism in fifty males with the fragile X syndrome. *American Journal of Medical Genetics, 23*, 359–374.

Hermelin, B., & O'Connor, N. (1970). *Psychological experiments with autistic children.* Oxford: Pergamon Press.

Hobson, P. (1987). Commentary and explanation: Social cognition in autism. In M. Sigman & L. Waterhouse (Chairs), *Social cognition in autism.* Symposium conducted at the meeting of the Society for Research in Child Development, Baltimore.

Howlin, P. (1986). An overview of social behavior in autism. In E. Schopler & G. B. Mesibov (Eds.), *Social behavior in autism* (pp. 103–131). New York: Plenum.

Kanner, L. (1943). Autistic disturbances of affective contact. *The Nervous Child, 2*, 217–250.

Kanner, L. (1973). *Childhood psychosis: Initial studies and new insights.* Washington, DC: V. H. Winston.

Kanner, L., & Eisenberg, L. (1956). Early infantile autism: 1943–1955. *American Journal of Orthopsychiatry, 26*, 55–65.

Kuhn, T. S. (1970). *The structure of scientific revolutions.* Chicago: University of Chicago Press.

Lockyer, L., & Rutter, M. (1970). A five to fifteen year follow-up of infantile psychosis: IV. Patterns of cognitive ability. *British Journal of Social and Clinical Psychology, 9*, 152–163.

Lord, C. (1984). The development of peer relations in children with autism. In F. J. Morrison, C. Lord, & D. P. Keating (Eds.), *Advances in applied developmental psychology* (pp. 165–229). New York: Academic Press.

Meehl, P. E. (1986). Diagnostic taxa as open concepts: Metatheoretical and statistical questions about reliability and construct validity in the grand strategy of nosological revision. In T. Millon & G. L. Klerman (Eds.), *Contemporary directions in psychopathology: Toward the DSM-IV* (pp. 215–232). New York: Guilford Press.

Mundy, P., Sigman, M., Ungerer, J., & Sherman, T. (1985, April). *Defining the deficits of autism.* Poster presentation at the meeting of the Society for Research in Child Development, Toronto.

Ornitz, E. M. (1974). The modulation of sensory input and motor output in autistic children. *Journal of Autism and Developmental Disorders, 4*, 197–218.

Parks, S. (1983). The assessment of autistic children: A selective review of available instruments. *Journal of Autism and Developmental Disorders, 13*, 255–268.

Paul, R., & Cohen, D. J. (1984). Outcomes of severe disorders of language acquisition. *Journal of Autism and Developmental Disorders, 14*, 405–422.

Petty, L. K., Ornitz, E. M., Michelman, D. D., & Zimmerman, E. G. (1984). Autistic children who become schizophrenic. *Archives of General Psychiatry, 41*, 129–135.

Prior, M. (1979). Cognitive abilities and disabilities in infantile autism: A review. *Journal of Abnormal Child Psychology, 7*, 359–380.

Rimland, B. (1964). *Infantile autism.* New York: Appleton-Century-Crofts.

Ritvo, E. R., & Freeman, B. J. (1977). National Autistic Society definition of the syndrome of autism. *Journal of Pediatric Psychology, 4*, 146–148.

Ritvo, E. R., Spence, M. A., Freeman, B. J., Mason-Brothers, A. M., Mo, A., & Marazita, M. L. (1985). Evidence for autosomal recessive inheritance in 46 families with multiple incidences of autism. *American Journal of Psychiatry, 142*, 187–192.

Rumsey, J. M., Andreasen, N. C., & Rapoport, J. L. (1986). Thought, language, communication, and affective flattening in autistic adults. *Archives of General Psychiatry, 43*, 771–777.

Rutter, M. (1972). Childhood schizophrenia reconsidered. *Journal of Autism and Childhood Schizophrenia, 2*, 315–338.

Rutter, M. (1983). Cognitive deficits in the pathogenesis of autism. *Journal of Child Psychology and Psychiatry, 24*, 513–531.

Rutter, M., & Lockyer, L. (1967). A five to fifteen year followup study of infantile psychosis: I. Description of the sample. *British Journal of Psychiatry, 113*, 1169–1182.

Seyfarth, R. (1987, January 19). *Social relationships and social cognition in primates.* Paper presented at the University of Pennsylvania Symposium on Brain and Behavior, Philadelphia.

Sherman, M., Shapiro, T., & Glassman, M. (1983). Play and language in developmentally disordered preschoolers: a new approach to classification. *Journal of the American Academy of Child Psychiatry*, 22, 511–524.

Siegel, B., Anders, T., Ciaranello, R. O., Bienenstock, B., & Kraemer, H. C. (1986). Empirically derived subclassification of the autistic syndrome. *Journal of Autism and Developmental Disorders*, 16, 275–293.

Tinbergen, N., & Tinbergen, E. A. (1983). *Autistic children: New hope for a cure*. London: Allen & Unwin.

Torrey, E. F., Hersh, S. P., & McCabe, K. D. (1975). Early childhood psychosis and bleeding during pregnancy: A prospective study of gravid women and their offspring. *Journal of Autism and Childhood Schizophrenia*, 5, 287–297.

Tsai, L. Y. (1987). Pre-, peri- and neonatal factors in autism. In E. Schopler & G. Mesibov (Eds.), *Neurobiological issues in autism* (pp. 180–191). New York: Plenum.

von Eckardt, B. (1986, June). Criteria for brain–behavior models. In D. Caplan (Chair), *Inferring normal cognitive function from pathological cases*. Symposium conducted at the annual meeting of the Society for Philosophy and Psychology, Johns Hopkins University, Baltimore.

Waterhouse, L., & Fein, D. (1982). Language skills in developmentally disabled children. *Brain and Language*, 15, 307–333.

Waterhouse, L., & Fein, D. (1983, May). *Perinatal factors and cognition in PDD*. Paper presented at the meeting of the American Association for Advancement of Science, New York.

Waterhouse, L., & Fein, D. (1984). Developmental trends in cognitive skills for children diagnosed as autistic and schizophrenic. *Child Development*, 55, 312–336.

Waterhouse, L., Fein, D., Nath, J., & Snyder, D. (1987). Pervasive developmental disorders and schizophrenia occurring in childhood: A review of critical commentary. In G. Tischler (Ed.), *Diagnosis and classification in psychiatry: A critical appraisal of DSM III* (pp. 335–368). New York: Cambridge University Press.

Waterhouse, L., Wing, L., Allen, D., Fein, D., & Rapin, I. (1987, April). *DLD and Autism: A large sample study*. Paper presented at the Association for All Speech Impaired Children First International Conference, Reading, England.

Wing, L. (1982, November). *Infantile autism*. Paper presented at the Swedish Medical Council seminar, Gothenburg, Sweden.

Wing, L. (1988). The continuum of autistic characteristics. In E. Schopler & G. Mesibov (Eds.), *Diagnosis and assessment in autism*. New York: Plenum.

Wing, L., & Gould, J. (1979). Severe impairments of social interaction and associated abnormalities in children: Epidemiology and classificaiton. *Journal of Autism and Developmental Disorders*, 9, 11–29.

World Health Organization (1978). *Mental disorders: Glossary and guide to their classification in accordance with the ninth revision of the International Classification of Diseases*. Geneva: Author.

World Health Organization (in press). *Mental disorders: Glossary and guide to their classification in accordance with the tenth revision of the International Classification of Diseases*. Geneva: Author.

Zadeh, L. A. (1965). Fuzzy sets. *Information and Control*, 8, 338–353.

CHAPTER 12

Enhancing Language and Communication in Autism

From Theory to Practice

BARRY M. PRIZANT

Emma Pendleton Bradley Hospital, East Providence, Rhode Island
Brown University Program in Medicine

AMY M. WETHERBY

Florida State University

INTRODUCTION

Most educational and treatment programs currently serving individuals with autism cite the development of language and social communication as a major objective (Rutter, 1985). For persons with autism, the level of communicative competence achieved is closely related to the development of social behavior (Garfin & Lord, 1986) and measures of outcome (Lotter, 1978). Furthermore, there is preliminary evidence that the development of communicative abilities is directly related to the reduction of socially unacceptable and aberrant behavior (Carr & Durand, 1985; Smith, 1985), a significant problem for many persons with autism. Thus, communicative competence may be a primary determinant of the extent to which an individual with autism may be able to participate in daily activities and routines in his or her school, home, and community.

Although few would argue about the importance of the goal of enhancing communication, approaches to working toward this general goal have varied greatly. In some instances, different approaches appear to be diametrically opposed in reference to the selection of specific objectives (e.g., compliance vs. active initiation) and the application of procedures to reach stated objectives. Differences in the practice of communication enhancement appear to derive from or reflect differences in underlying theories, beliefs, and/or philosophies regarding the nature of autism, the nature of language and communication, the developmental process of learning to communicate, and the role played by all individuals involved in the process (e.g., the person with autism, teachers, clincians, caregivers, siblings, etc.).

In this chapter, we scrutinize the relationship between theory and practice in enhancing communication for autistic individuals. We support the position that approaches to communication enhancement must be rooted in a sound theoretical or philosophical framework. Otherwise, clinical attempts will be haphazard, unsystematic, ineffective, or inefficient, and may be frustrating and confusing for all persons involved. The discussion begins with an overview of how theories have shaped understandings of social-communicative problems in autism and how these theories have influenced communication assessment and intervention practices. Following this discussion, approaches to communication assessment and enhancement based on current literature on normal social-communicative development are considered.

TYPES OF THEORIES

For the purposes of this discussion, the term "theory" refers to "a belief, policy, or procedure proposed or followed as the basis of action" (*Webster's Dictionary*, 1981, p. 1200). Theories may be formal, such as Skinner's (1957) account of verbal behavior, or informal, such as an educator's or clinician's beliefs about how children learn language, based upon previous experience rather than reference to available literature. In reality, all educators and clinicians bring some theory or underlying philosophy to bear on their work with autistic persons, whether it is based on years of hypothesis testing or grounded in a specific research and theoretical literature.

In general, types of theories affecting communication assessment and enhancement fall into three categories:

1. Theories about the development of communication and language and applicability of these theories to autistic persons.
2. Theories about the role of the learner and the environment in communication development.
3. Theories about the nature of autism and the effect of the concomitant impairment(s) on communicative growth.

Theories about the Nature of Language and Communication Development

The development of language and communication involves a complex interplay of emerging abilities in social, affective, cognitive, and linguistic domains (Bates, 1979). The burgeoning literature in social, communicative, and cognitive development provides a theoretical foundation both for understanding communication problems and for implementing effective and developmentally appropriate interventions. Sameroff (1987) has stated that "unless one understands how development proceeds, there is little basis for attempts to alter it, either through prevention or intervention programs" (p. 274).

Numerous theories have been proposed to account for the normal development and use of language and communication in children. The three major theoretical categories are behavioral, cognitive/psycholinguistic, and pragmatic/social-interactive (Duchan, 1984). Behavioral theory is nondevelopmental in nature; that is, it is based on general models of learning, and not on research in child language development. Cognitive/psycholinguistic and pragmatic/social-interactive theories have emerged out of proposed models of development, as well as cross-sectional and longitudinal investigations of language and communication development.

More specifically, a behavioral account of speech and language development was provided by Skinner (1957). Skinner saw environmental variables as playing the major role in development; in his view, children's production and imitation of sounds are gradually shaped into recognizable speech through reinforcement of successive approximations. In this account, the child learning to speak is considered to be a passive participant. Skinner did not make reference to cognitive variables or unobservable processes (e.g., rule induction), because observable behavior was the focus of inquiry.

Cognitive/psycholinguistic theories emerged in the 1960s and 1970s and described children as active participants in the language learning process. These theories attempted to account for how children develop internalized knowledge regarding language structure, and the relationships between language forms and meanings expressed through language (Bloom, 1970; R. Brown, 1973; Chomsky, 1968). Cognitive/psycholinguistic theories have also stressed the relationships between language and communication development and other dimensions of cognitive development, especially those discussed by Piaget (1954). In general, these theories emphasized that speech and language acquisition are not results of direct teaching by caregivers, but result from children "discovering" language by observing and interacting with others. Although social experiences were acknowledged to influence the learning process, the clear focus of these theories was on the acquisition of cognitive (nonsocial) knowledge believed to be related to language.

Finally, pragmatic/social-interactive theories of the 1970s and 1980s have placed great emphasis on the role of social experiences. Social interaction in the first year of life is seen as providing the foundation for later language and communication development. Children are viewed as active participants who learn to affect the behavior and attitudes of others through active signaling, and gradually learn to use more sophisticated and conventional means to communicate through these interactions. The quality and nature of the contexts in which interaction occurs are considered to have a great influence on the successful acquisition of language and communicative behavior. Thus, proponents of pragmatic theory state that development can only be understood by analysis of the interactive context, not simply by focusing solely on the child or caregivers. The reader is referred to Duchan (1984), Muma (1986), and Snyder and Lindstedt (1985) for further discussion of these and related theories.

Because autism is a developmental disorder, information on normal language and communication development offers an organizational framework for the assessment and intervention of language and communication. The current developmental literature provides a rich source of information applicable to clinical practice and offers more than merely a guideline for sequencing communication objectives. This section provides an overview of some of the major issues in the pragmatic and cognitive/psycholinguistic developmental language literature that influence clinical practice, with a discussion of how these not only can contribute to our understanding of communication problems in autism, but also can provide a strong conceptual basis for improving the effectiveness and efficiency of intervention with autistic individuals.

A Matter of Timing

Developmental principles may help to explain the wide discrepancies between linguistic and nonlinguistic abilities and between social and nonsocial abilities that are characteristic of persons with autism. The typically scattered profile may be explained by the accelerated and protracted development of skills requisite for normal communication (Cairns, 1986; Wetherby, 1985). The particular combination of skills and experiences available to the autistic person is not seen at any point in normal development and leads to distinct patterns and strategies for communicating because of the interplay among the available components.

The autism literature consistently describes development in autism as "deviant," rather than as merely "delayed"; this implies that autistic children develop abilities in a sequence and manner different from those of normal children. However, it may be the relative timing of emergence of skills that is unique, and not merely the sequence of development. Many of the behaviors displayed by autistic children that have been considered "deviant" or "aberrant" may be better understood and even considered legitimate and functional when the combination of skills available to the child is considered from a developmental perspective. Furthermore, normal developmental progressions within specific domains may still be applicable in planning intervention; however, they must be used flexibly.

Developmental Progressions

Developmental theorists have been describing sequences, phases, stages, or progressions in the development of specific skills within cognitive, social-communicative, and linguistic domains for many years (e.g., Bates, 1976; R. Brown, 1973; Bruner, 1975, 1978; Piaget, 1952, 1954; Sander, 1962). Because of the developmental interaction of these domains, knowledge about developmental progressions is critical to understanding the communicative impairments in autism.

In order to utilize a developmental approach in communication assessment and enhancement, clinicians must be knowledgeable about normal developmental progressions. This information can provide a frame of reference for understanding developmental discrepancies across social-cognitive abilities and the specific language-related domains of phonology, morphology, syntax, semantics, and pragmatics (Tager-Flusberg, 1981). However, clinicians must be careful not to apply developmental information too rigidly. A distinction must be made between working with a developmental model and teaching according to a developmental checklist. Bruner (1983) noted that a developmental model stipulates that an individual's understanding of information or acquisition of skills will be framed by the level of intellectual operations or cognitive development reached. Too rigid an interpretation of a developmental model has resulted in "readiness models," which indicate that a certain level of cognitive ability or development *must* be reached in order for an individual to learn certain skills or information. Donnellan and Kilman (1986) noted that this misinterpretation has resulted in inappropriate teaching practices with autistic children, in which so-called "readiness skills" may be targeted for extended time periods.

Developmental Underpinnings

A major theme that appears in the developmental literature is the mutual interaction and interdependence of cognition and social knowledge in development (Cicchetti & Pogge-Hesse, 1981; Emde, 1980; Piaget, 1954; Saarni, 1978). This intimate relationship is reflected in the recent development of the field of social cognition, which refers to the way individuals perceive, interact with, and organize knowledge about other people (Sherrod & Lamb, 1981). Communication lies at the interface of cognition and affect, and thus may be considered a window into the child's social cognition (Saarni, 1978).

Evidence is available from a variety of sources that certain social, cognitive, and communicative skills are correlates to the emergence of words (Bates, 1979; Piaget, 1954; Snyder, 1984; Steckol & Leonard, 1981). Specific component skills that have been identified include tool use or means–ends behavior, communicative intent or social causality, imitation, and functional object use. These foundation skills contribute to the child's ability to use words communicatively and to learn conventional meanings of words.

Several studies have examined these foundation skills in autistic children in relation to language acquisition. Developmental level of imitation and symbolic play have been found to be deficient and related to language level (Curcio, 1978; Dawson & Adams, 1984; Hammes & Langdell, 1981; McHale, Simeonsson, Marcus, & Olley, 1980; Shapiro, Huebner, & Campbell, 1974; Sigman & Ungerer, 1984; Wetherby & Prutting, 1984; Wing, Gould, Yeates, & Brierley, 1977). Curcio (1978) found that causality and means–ends behavior were related to communicative abilities of nonverbal autistic subjects. Wetherby and Prutting (1984) found that autistic subjects at prelinguistic and early language levels showed better performance in tool use and combinatorial play and poorer performance in symbolic play than normal subjects matched for language level. They suggested that their autistic subjects' propensity for the use of communication to regulate others' behavior and deficiency in the use of communication to attract and direct another's attention may be related to the differential timing of acquisition of these cognitive-social skills.

The recent application of developmental theory to the pattern of behaviors seen in the autistic population suggests that the language and communication impairments reflect underlying impairments in social cognition. Based on this premise, intervention should address the underlying problem, and not merely the surface behavior. In other words, clinicians should consider a child's social-cognitive capacity for learning language and focus on strengthening the social-cognitive underpinnings of language that may be lagging behind. To teach speech or language without consideration for the social-communicative bases for using these tools seems counterintuitive and counterproductive. For example, Lovaas's (1977) inability to teach communicative speech to all his subjects and the massive number of teaching trials needed for many subjects may have resulted from the fact that these developmental issues were not considered. The potential for true progress in communicative growth may only be increased if the foundation skills are present.

Individual Variation in Strategy

Psycholinguistic approaches of the 1960s and early 1970s focused on identifying similar language patterns across children. More recently, the child language literature has shifted focus to exploring individual variation in communication development, and, more specifically, variation in language-learning strategies or styles (Nelson, 1981). Several dichotomous strategies of language development and use have been identified, such as "referential–expressive" development (Nelson, 1973), "intonation–word" learning (Dore, 1974), "nominal–pronominal" strategies (Bloom, Hood, & Lightbown, 1974), and "analytic–gestalt" learning (Peters, 1983). Thus, the lesson of the past decade has been that normal children may approach and successfully accomplish the task of learning language in more than one way. Differences in learning strategies have been explained by many factors that contribute to the child's individual makeup, including heredity, cerebral hemispheric organization, cognitive style, and the language-learning environment. Bates (1979) proposed that variations in the relative timing of the emergence of cognitive abilities may lead to differences in language-learning strategies.

Similar principles may be operating in contributing to the language-learning strategies of the autistic child. Prizant (1982, 1983b) proposed that autistic children use a gestalt strategy in early language learning by imitating unanalyzed chunks or multiword units of speech and subsequently breaking down these units into meaningful segments. He suggested that for many verbal autistic children, language acquisition progresses from the predominant use of echolalia with little evidence of comprehension or communicative intent to the use of echolalia for a variety of communicative functions, later followed by a decrease in echolalia ac-companied by an increase in spontaneous utterances. The use of pronoun re-versals and stereotypic utterances, as well as the insistence on certain verbal rou-tines, may reflect a gestalt strategy.

Prizant (1983b) proposed that language learning by autistic children may rep-resent an extreme form of the gestalt style that has been identified in normal children (Peters, 1983). It is intriguing to speculate why a large proportion of autistic children utilize a gestalt strategy to learn language. Dawson, Finley, Phil-lips, and Galpert (1986) hypothesized that early in language development, autistic children "may tend to rely heavily on those cognitive strategies associated with the right hemisphere" (p. 1452). In a similar vein, Wetherby (1984) noted that "some autistic children may be using the gestalt processing abilities of the right hemi-sphere as a heuristic means to induce the rules of language" (p. 28). Both Dawson *et al.* (1986) and Wetherby (1984) suggested that a shift from right- to left-hemi-sphere processing of speech and language may occur in development, possibly accounting for the shift from gestalt to analytic style of language acquisition as discussed by Prizant (1983b). However, a gestalt style has also been observed in some children without social impairments (Nelson, 1981). Many relevant ques-tions regarding the mutual influence of social and cognitive impairments in au-tism have yet to be addressed (Shah & Wing, 1986). It is likely that the observa-tion and identification of language-learning strategies used by autistic children can provide guidelines for intervention approaches. An understanding of these strate-gies may serve to provide specific direction for enhancing language. This issue is expanded upon in the final section of this chapter.

Relationship between Language Comprehension and Production

The traditional position on the relationship between language comprehension and production in normal children is that comprehension precedes production. How-ever, studies of normal children's comprehension and production of vocabulary (Goldin-Meadow, Seligman, & Gelman, 1976; Huttenlocher, 1974; Snyder, Bates, & Bretherton, 1981) and subject–object constructions (Chapman & Miller, 1975) indicate that comprehension does not always precede or surpass production. The contemporary position is that comprehension and production proceed through similar developmental sequences, but that the developmental discrepancy between them varies across children and at different points in development (Bloom & Lahey, 1978; McLean & Snyder-McLean, 1978; Musselwhite & St. Louis, 1982; Owens, 1984).

Bloom and Lahey (1978) suggested that waiting to teach production of a particular word, concept, or rule until comprehension has developed is not a prudent clinical practice. The few training studies that have been done have found that training comprehension does not transfer to production skills (Guess & Baer, 1973; Miller, Cuvo, & Borakove, 1977), but that training production does transfer to comprehension (Miller *et al.*, 1977). Furthermore, normal and language-impaired children have been found to produce words that they do not comprehend (see Leonard *et al.*, 1982). Although further research is needed to explore this relationship, it seems warranted to conclude from the evidence to date that language comprehension and production should be targeted concurrently or that language production should be the primary focus of intervention.

In summary, it is our contention that educators and clinicians can be most effective in enhancing language and communicative ability by judiciously applying knowledge of normal communication development, based on the current theoretical and research literature.

Theories about the Role of the Child and the Language-Learning Environment in Communication Development

Current developmental theories emphasize the child's active, constructive role in conceptually structuring, mastering, and making sense of the environment (Piaget, 1954; Sherrod & Lamb, 1981). Sameroff (1987) has discussed models of longitudinal development based on considerations of both the child and environment, and the nature of the role each plays (i.e., active vs. passive). Sameroff indicates that developmental growth is

> never a function of the individual taken alone or the experiential context taken alone. Behavioral competencies are a product of the combination of an individual and his or her experiences. To predict outcome, a singular focus on characteristics of the individual . . . will be misleading. What needs to be added is an analysis and assessment of the experiences available . . . (p. 275)

Three of the models discussed by Sameroff that are applicable to an analysis of communication enhancement efforts are "passive person–active environment," "active person–passive environment," and "active person–active environment." In the first model, "passive person–active environment," Sameroff includes "approaches to behavior modification in which the conditioner actively structures the input . . . but where the person is assumed to make no contribution to the outcome independent of experience" (p. 273). The behavioral notions of "reinforcing properties of a stimulus" or a child's behavior "being under stimulus control" exemplify the environmental rather than person focus of this model.

The second model, "active individual–passive environment," is most descriptive of psycholinguistic and cognitivist approaches where the individual is seen as an active hypothesis tester and constructor of experience, with little emphasis on the nature or quality of environmental experiences. According to Sameroff, Chomskian and Piagetian theories fall under this category. Both Chomsky and Piaget have been criticized for overlooking the significant influence of the quality of environmental experience, especially linguistic, social, and communicative experience, in influencing linguistic and cognitive growth.

Finally, the last model—"active person–active environment"—is exemplified by the "transactional model" of Sameroff and Chandler (1975), which stipulates that

> developmental outcomes are not a product of the initial characteristics of the child or the context or even their combination. . . . [They] are the result of interplay between child and context over time, in which the state of one impacts on the next state of the other in a continuous dynamic process. (Sameroff, 1987, p. 274)

Many contemporary approaches to communication enhancement fall within this third model, including the transactional model described by McLean and Snyder-McLean (1978), the interactionist approach described by Bloom and Lahey (1978) and Fey (1986), and the functionalistic perspective described by Muma (1986).

The distinction between the "active person–active environment" model and the "passive person–active environment" model is paralleled by Bloom and Lahey's (1978) and Fey's (1986) discussion of how clinicians and educators view their role as interventionists. They noted that a "facilitator" of communicative competence acknowledges the active role of the child in learning. In this model, the clinician's or educator's responsibility is to structure opportunities for learning and to react actively and flexibly to the child's actions or communicative attempts. Great emphasis is placed on individual differences in children and their strategies and current means of communication (Duchan, 1983). This information helps to guide efforts in identifying goals and objectives for communication enhancement. In contrast, the "passive person–active environment" model dictates that the "trainer" is responsible for determining what is to be learned, how it is to be learned, and what behaviors or responses are judged to be acceptable or unacceptable. The often-noted goal of training "compliance" is exemplary of this model. In our experience, this latter model often results in lack of initiation, cue dependency, and problems in generalization.

Recognizing these problems, behavioral interventionists (Halle, 1984; Hart, 1985; Peck, 1985) have begun to apply an "active person–active environment" model to communication enhancement, acknowledging the significance of a child's motivation and strategies in learning, as well as the dangers of approaches that rely too much on external control and do not consider individual differences in children.

Theories about the Nature of Autism

Theories about the nature of the autistic syndrome may have a significant impact on strategies to enhance communication ability. Various theories have been formulated from two different approaches to the study of autism: first, attempts to identify the primary and/or most significant deficits that are presumed to impair communication development; and second, efforts to describe how persons with autism learn, which address profiles of learning strengths and weaknesses.

The first approach identifies primary deficits or pathology that may account for a wide range of symptomatology. Specific examples are as diverse as theories of stimulus overselectivity (Koegel, Egel, & Dunlap, 1980), social avoidance (Tinbergen & Tinbergen, 1983), problems in sensory integration (Ayres, 1979), or an inability to maintain stable states of arousal to sensory stimuli (Delacato, 1974). Practitioners of this type of approach suggest that remediation of primary deficits should have a positive impact on communication, because communication deficits are believed to be secondary to these problems.

The second type of approach places greater emphasis on profiles of ability and disability in determining communication problems and developing approaches to enhance communication ability. It has been documented repeatedly that persons with autism demonstrate relative abilities in rote memory (including memory for and adherence to activity routines), visual–spatial and configurational judgment, and, in some cases, specific musical skills (Hermelin & O'Connor, 1970; Prior, 1979; Prizant, 1983b; Rimland, 1978). Relative disabilities are in communication development, social skills, symbolization, and the ability to express emotions in a conventional manner and understand the emotions and intentions of others (Fein, Pennington, Markowitz, Braverman, & Waterhouse, 1986; Hobson, Chapter 2, this volume; Mundy & Sigman, Chapter 1, this volume; Ricks & Wing, 1975). In general, strengths lie in knowledge about the inanimate (nonsocial) world (i.e., objects, spatial orientation, sequences of events), and weaknesses lie in knowledge of people, interpersonal interaction, and social conventions. It also has been suggested that for persons with autism, the processing of nontransient information, such as that presented through the visual modality (e.g., visual display), is easier than processing of transient, "rapidly fading" information, such as the auditory signals comprising speech (Prizant & Schuler, 1987b).

A reconciliation of the differing approaches (i.e., primary-deficit debates and theories of abilities and disabilities) is now emerging in the literature. Current conceptualizations of the autistic syndrome emphasize the centrality of impairments in social and communicative behaviors (Cohen, Paul, & Volkmar, 1986; Dawson & Galpert, 1986; Denckla, 1986; Fein *et al.*, 1986), based on developmental information. There is now general agreement that the language impairments specific to autism are not primary, but are secondary to impairments within cognitive and social domains (Fein *et al.*, 1986; Rutter, 1983). Most current definitions of the syndrome emphasize impairments in social communication, not just in speech or language (American Psychiatric Association, 1987; Denckla, 1986; Rutter, 1978). The study of social-cognitive, linguistic, and communication impairments has demonstrated that what differentiates the autistic child from the specific language-impaired child and from the nonautistic mentally retarded child is the specific developmental pattern of abilities and disabilities across communicative, social-cognitive, and non-social-cognitive domains.

These recent changes in theory indicate that efforts to understand and enhance communication in autism *must* be guided by addressing the learning strengths of autistic persons. Furthermore, specific symptomatology, especially so-called "deviant" behavior and patterns of language use, should be understood in refer-ence to the learning style discussed above, rather than simply dismissed as inap-propriate and bizarre (Prizant, 1983b). Efforts to enhance communication must take into account how persons with autism learn to communicate. Because such learning may not reflect normal patterns and profiles of communication and social development (Prizant, 1983b; Wetherby, 1986), goals and procedures may have to accommodate such differences.

IMPLICATIONS FOR COMMUNICATION ASSESSMENT AND ENHANCEMENT

It is beyond the scope and purpose of this chapter to present a comprehensive discussion on communication assessment and enhancement (see Fay & Schuler, 1980; Prizant & Schuler, 1987a, 1987b; Prizant & Wetherby, 1985; Rutter, 1985; Schuler & Prizant, 1987). However, we continue to traverse the bridge between theory and practice by reconsidering how current information about normal so-cial-communicative development, about the transactional process affecting com-municative growth, and about the nature of autism is beginning to affect both communication assessment and enhancement efforts.

Applying Normal Developmental Information

Over the past decade, theory and research on normal social–communicative de-velopment have provided the foundation for assessment and communication en-hancement for language-impaired children (Bloom & Lahey, 1978; McLean & Snyder-McLean, 1978; Schiefelbusch & Bricker, 1981). Only recently has this literature begun to have an effect on programs for persons with autism and other severe handicaps. For many years, approaches based upon Skinner's (1957) ac-count of verbal behavior dominated the literature on language training for persons with autism and severe handicaps (Bryen & Joyce, 1985), as exemplified by Lo-vaas's (1977, 1981) programs. Many authors following behavioral theory either did not consider the emerging literature on language and communication devel-opment, due to their belief that such development could be explained by basic tenets of traditional learning theory, or dismissed developmental theories because of the belief that they could not be applied to populations that were not develop-ing normally. Although significant differences remain between so-called behav-ioral and developmental approaches to enhancing communication, a constructive dialogue has begun that has resulted in a theoretical sharing and cross-fertilization of these models. For further discussion, the reader is referred to Carr (1985), Fey (1986), Koegel and Johnson (Chapter 13, this volume), Lord (1985b), Duchan (1984), and Donnellan and Kilman (1986). As we see it, the most significant contributions of this recent developmental literature to communication assessment and enhancement are based on the following principles.

*Preverbal Communication as a Precursor to
Verbal Communication*

Communication development involves continuity from preverbal communication through linguistic communication, and the development of preverbal communication is a necessary precursor to the development of the intentional use of language to communicate (Bates, 1976; Harding, 1984; Harding & Golinkoff, 1979). This basic tenet holds for children with autism as well as for other children with or without disabilities (Prizant & Wetherby, 1985). Thus, for assessment purposes, it is incumbent upon clinicians to develop a communicative profile for an individual, based on the specific communicative intents expressed and the means used to express specific intents, whether verbal, vocal, gestural, or combinations thereof (Prizant & Schuler, 1987b; Prizant & Wetherby, 1985; Wetherby & Prizant, in press). An individual's strategies and abilities in communication, and the ways in which they vary across situational contexts, need to be delineated. Thus, the focus is on current competence and ability, rather than simply on listing absent behaviors that need to be developed and/or prioritizing so-called "deficits" for eradication (Prizant, 1983b).

Within a developmental approach, communicative growth may be conceptualized as bidimensional (McLean, Snyder-McLean, Jacobs, & Rowland, 1981; Prizant & Wetherby, 1985). The vertical dimension involves movement from less sophisticated and less conventional means of communication to more sophisticated, conventional, and explicit means, based loosely on patterns of normal development. For example, vertical growth may involve movement from the use of idiosyncratic or unconventional communicative means (e.g., idiosyncratic gestures, physical manipulation) to more sophisticated and conventional means (e.g., conventional gestures, use of a communication board) to express the same intents. Movement from prelinguistic to emerging language stages and beyond also reflects vertical growth.

The notion of developmental continuity from preverbal to verbal levels, one aspect of vertical development, has led to an understanding that communicative intent should be a primary focus of communication enhancement efforts, and that nonspeech communication is a legitimate goal for many persons. The recent use of augmentative communication systems with autistic persons (see Kiernan, 1983, and Schuler, 1985, for reviews) is predicated largely on the understanding that for many nonverbal or minimally verbal individuals, an immediate goal may not be speech but any socially acceptable means of expressing intent, which may provide the necessary scaffolding for later language development. With a careful description of current levels of intentional communication, enhancement efforts may then focus on movement to more sophisticated means of expressing intent. For example, a child who consistently uses physical manipulation to request objects or actions may be taught to use gestures, simple signs, or pictures to accomplish the same goals.

Horizontal growth, which involves expansion of expressive repertoire at specific levels of development, is also an integral part of the development of communicative competence. However, it is not enough to address only the forms used to express specific meanings. Other language- and communication-related abilities must be taken into account. Expansion may be targeted for areas as diverse as a child's use of different gestural complexes (Bates, 1979), pictures on a communication board, spoken vocabulary, a variety of semantic relations expressed in two- to three-word utterances, or range of functions or intents expressed (e.g., requests, protests, comments).

Communicative Competence as the Outcome
of Synergistic Development

The development of communicative competence is the outcome of synergistic development in social, cognitive, communicative, and linguistic domains. Traditionally, behavioral approaches to language training were concerned primarily with teaching speech or other surface forms, with little consideration given to conceptual underpinnings and social use of communicative acts (Bryen & Joyce, 1985; Carr, 1985). With a narrow, nondevelopmental focus on form, and an apparent unawareness of the applicability of emerging literature on normal language acquisition, advocates of these approaches did not consider social and cognitive foundations for language acquisition and use. Bryen and Joyce (1985) reviewed 43 language intervention studies with autistic and severely handicapped individuals from the 1970s and found that only 16.2% considered social factors; consideration of specific cognitive factors ranged from 0% (means–ends skills) to a high of 11.6% (symbolic functioning). Similarly, they found that clinicians who began to use nonspeech communication systems with nonverbal individuals rarely considered social and cognitive factors. Assessments were relegated to collecting baseline data on the presence or absence of various aspects of linguistic form (e.g., repertoire of speech sounds, expressive and receptive vocabulary, presence or absence of specific grammatical forms, etc.). Without a framework for understanding the complexities and interdependencies in development, efforts to teach language targeted isolated behaviors for intervention, with the underlying assumption being that training sound production (through imitation) would result in "words," and "sentences" would result from training children to combine "words." Although Skinner's (1957) theory of the development of verbal behavior no longer is considered a credible explanation of language development, researchers and clinicians have clung to this model in their efforts to train speech (Lovaas, 1977, 1981).

Recent approaches to assessment and intervention are now concerned with examining a child's communicative profile in reference to specific emerging social and cognitive capacities found to be related to communicative development. In fact, this literature has provided greater insight into the very nature of autism by identifying profiles of discrepancies among emerging abilities in communicative, social-cognitive, cognitive, and social-affective domains (Cohen *et al.*, 1986; Fein *et al.*, 1986; Wetherby & Prutting, 1984).

In reference to communication enhancement, a child's developmental profile (i.e., social, cognitive, and communicative) provides important information for clinical decision making. For example, decisions regarding the introduction of nonspeech communication systems are derived from a child's developmental profile, based on measures of expressive and receptive language, vocal and gestural imitation, communicative intent, and social and nonsocial means–ends behavior. However, the inflexible use of decision-making rules should be avoided (Schuler, 1985). Furthermore, because the most severe impairments in autism involve social-cognitive and social-affective realms of development (Denckla, 1986; Fein *et al.*, 1986), communication enhancement efforts need to be framed by social and affective contexts appropriate to a child's developmental level (Dawson & Galpert, 1986). Dawson and Adams (1984) found that they were able to increase social responsiveness, quality of play, and gaze behavior in autistic children who were "low imitators" by imitating their behavior rather than presenting developmentally discrepant models for imitation. The significance of these findings is that the early development of imitation may provide young children with a strategy for further social and communicative growth, and that such development can be stimulated in intensive "naturalistic" play interactions. Because imitation provides a context for learning about and sharing social, cognitive, and affective experiences (Dawson & Galpert, 1986; Prizant, 1986; Uzgiris, 1981), progress in this area could enhance development in many domains.

For older and/or higher-functioning individuals, it is important to target linguistic forms (e.g., spoken, signed written words and phrases) that not only will have an impact on everyday independent functioning, but also are within the developmental range of linguistic and conceptual capacities of an individual. Many persons with autism are quite adept at memorizing and rotely reproducing linguistic forms (either written, signed, or spoken); however, this strategy may not result in the development of an internalized rule-governed system. Unfortunately, these "splinter skills" may not be realized as functional in an individual's life unless equal emphasis is placed on the meanings or conceptual underpinnings of such forms, and how they may be used in interacting with others (Prizant & Schuler, 1987b). This information can only be obtained by considering the relative profile of abilities and disabilities in cognitive, social, and linguistic domains.

Developmental theory also provides specific guidelines for selecting a sequence of language and communicative forms appropriate to an individual's linguistic and cognitive capacities. Behavioral language treatment programs often violate normal developmental progressions. For example, Lovaas (1977) suggested teaching yes–no to encode affirmation–denial (e.g., "Is this an X?") without considering teaching yes–no to encode acceptance–rejection (e.g., "Do you want X?")—a progression that contradicts normal developmental patterns (Bloom, 1970). Similar problems have been noted in the training of pronouns (Fay, 1979). Normal patterns of linguistic and communication development typically reflect a gradual increase in linguistic and cognitive complexity (R. Brown, 1973). This would suggest that developmentally earlier forms and meanings should be targeted first to provide a foundation for later development.

Recently, Carr (1985) and Donnellan and Kilman (1986) have claimed that the best communication-enhancing practices at present wed teaching technology ("how to teach") contributed primarily by behavioral theory with content ("what to teach") contributed by developmental approaches. These authors add that so-called functional approaches (L. Brown et al., 1979) to communication enhance-ment, which emphasizes the relevance of communicative acts to a child's life, have emerged largely from the behavioral literature, although developmentalists have also addressed this issue in detail (Holland, 1975).

The Importance of a Systemic Approach

In a developmental model, attempts are made to understand how a child's behav-ior "fits into" developing social, cognitive, and communicative competencies. The approach is systemic, rather than one of isolated components. In a developmental approach, all behavior is viewed in reference to a child's growing capacity across developmental domains. One contribution in this area is the application of the developmental concept of communicative intent to understanding both conven-tional and unconventional communicative behaviors in autism (Prizant & Weth-erby, 1985, 1987). Recent analyses of communicative intent and function (Prizant & Duchan, 1981; Prizant & Rydell, 1984; Wetherby & Prutting, 1984) have not only identified communicative intent underlying behaviors previously considered to be socially unacceptable and aberrant, but have also pointed out the need to understand such behavior in reference to developing social, cognitive, and com-municative capacities. Thus, assessment is concerned with the varied means a child may use to communicate intent, whether verbal or preverbal, conventional or unconventional. In fact, Wetherby (1986) and Wetherby and Prutting (1984) have noted that the developmental sophistication of certain communicative means may be different for different intents (e.g., words for requests, and self-injurious behavior for protest or rejection).

Within this framework, communication enhancement efforts are concerned primarily with helping a child to acquire conventional means to express intents, with continuing movement toward the use of more sophisticated forms. This issue is relevant for those communicating at prelinguistic levels as well as at emerging language levels. Possibly due to the pervasive impairments in social cognition, and more specifically in imitation and joint referencing (Mundy & Sigman, Chapter 1, this volume), the communication attempts of individuals with autism are often idiosyncratic and not easily readable. In a developmental approach the two gen-eral tasks are, first, to understand an individual's relative levels of functioning in communicative and social-cognitive domains; and, second, to help the individual acquire more conventional means to communicate, emphasizing the conceptual and social-cognitive "meanings" encoded by the communicative acts.

Applying Pragmatic/Social-Interactive Theory

Pragmatic theory (Bates, 1976), or social-interactive theory (Duchan, 1984), "asks how people negotiate interactions with one another" (Duchan, 1984, p. 66). As discussed earlier, recent developmental literature in communication has used pragmatic constructs in attempting to describe the processes and sequences in children's acquisition of social-communicative competence. Behaviorally oriented researchers have also applied pragmatic constructs to communication of autistic children, although these approaches have been largely nondevelopmental (Carr, 1985).

The essence of pragmatic theory is that the unit of analysis is the interaction between two or more people. This research and theoretical literature, which has emerged over the past decade, has addressed three major areas relative to children's emerging communicative competence: communicative intent and function; discourse and conversational behavior; and language adjustments and social-linguistic sensitivity. These areas are now discussed in reference to assessment and communication enhancement for persons with autism.

Within pragmatic theory, the recent emphasis on communicative intention and function highlights the fact that children learn to communicate to get things done (Halliday, 1975). In communication assessment, the challenge for the educator or clinician is to give a clear description of a child's ability to influence others, regardless of the means used. Functional analyses of behavioral approaches (Carr & Durand, 1985; Donnellan, Mirenda, Mesaros, & Fassbender, 1984; Skinner, 1957) have focused on the effects of behavioral acts and not on the child's intentions. A truly pragmatic approach takes into account both a child's intentions and the functions served by behavioral acts (Duchan, 1987; Prizant & Wetherby, 1985; Wetherby & Prizant, in press). Documentation of a child's current ability to express a range of intentions provides a foundation for enhancing communication.

Communicative intent can only be inferred by observing behavior across situational contexts. Pragmatic theory has emphasized the need for clinicians and educators to respond to inferred intent, thus providing natural reinforcement. That is, what should be reinforcing to a child's communicative efforts is the child's realizing the impact of his or her efforts. Thus, current approaches encourage clinicians and educators to impute intent to the behavior of children who are at early stages of communicative intentionality, or whose communicative attempts are less conventional and therefore less readable (Dunst & Lowe, 1986; Schuler & Prizant, 1987). Recent pragmatic literature (Harding, 1984) suggests that young children learn how to communicate intentionally by observing others reacting to their behavior *as if* it was intentionally communicative.

Pragmatic theory also acknowledges the active role of the child in hypothesis testing about communicative interactions and what makes interactions work (Duchan, 1984). Thus, if responses to a child's communicative efforts are clear, consistent, and true to the content and intent expressed, it is more likely that the child will learn about the most effective way he or she is able to express specific intents successfully, or, if necessary, will adjust his or her means to communicate to be more effective.

The developmental literature on discourse and conversation emphasizes that successful communication involves reciprocity and mutual negotiation. Communication assessment and enhancement efforts should, first, determine the extent to which an individual is aware of and can participate in both initiator and respondent roles in communication; and second, determine the most appropriate approaches for helping an individual progress in such knowledge.

Because early taking of turns may provide the foundation for later conversational abilities (Bruner, 1975), current approaches emphasize the active involvement of even very young and lower-functioning individuals at developmentally appropriate levels (Dawson & Galpert, 1986). For older individuals or those with greater communicative competencies, greater emphasis is placed on language use and adherence to conventions of conversation, including strategies to initiate, maintain, and terminate conversations and repair communicative breakdowns (Lapidus, 1985; Prizant & Schuler, 1987a). A major problem resulting from past discrete trial communication training in autism has been the resulting lack of initiation and cue-dependent responding of the persons receiving training (Bryen & Joyce, 1985; Carr, 1985; Prizant & Schuler, 1987b).

The more recent focus on encouraging children to initiate more and to take a more active role in communicating should result in the acquisition of greater knowledge of the reciprocal nature of conversation (Dawson & Galpert, 1986; Mirenda & Donnellan, 1986). Mirenda and Donnellan (1986) found that the use of a "facilitative" versus a "directive" style with autistic and mentally retarded adolescents resulted in higher rates of student-initiated interactions, asking of questions, and initiation of conversational topics. The facilitative style was defined by a high level of adult responsiveness to student initiations. Peck (1985) studied eight severely handicapped students with autism and/or mental retardation and found that "substantial increases in the social communicative behavior of children . . . [were] achieved . . . when teacher interaction style [was] modified to afford more opportunities for student initiation and control of social interactions" (p. 191). Peck added that the teachers had no difficulty in shifting to a more "facilitative" style and in arranging social-communicative opportunities after the basic principles were described and modeled for them. Tiegerman and Primavera (1984), Dawson and Adams (1984), and Dawson and Lewy (Chapter 3, this volume) found that facilitative strategies increased the use of communicative eye gaze in autistic subjects. Such studies are beginning to provide empirical support for the applicability of basic developmental principles regarding social interaction and pragmatic theory.

The third major area of pragmatic theory and research is that of language adjustments and social-linguistic sensitivity. This literature has identified two relevant dimensions for communication assessment and enhancement: first, the need for individuals with autism to be able to make judgments about and adapt to the shifting demands of different communicative situations; and, second, the need for persons communicating with autistic persons to adjust their language and style of social interaction to help facilitate successful interactions.

In communication assessment, it is essential to observe an individual across different situations to determine whether and how communicative abilities vary with different cointeractants. If significant discrepancies are noted, attempts should be made to determine the sources of communicative breakdowns in reference to both the types of interactions that occur and the features of situations that may preclude successful communicative exchanges. For example, persons with autism tend to do better in structured and predictable interactions than in novel and unfamiliar situations (Clark & Rutter, 1981; Ferrara & Hill, 1980). The use of caregivers and other informants (e.g., teachers, siblings, etc.) as essential partners in this process is of great importance. Recently, instruments have been developed to help gather information regarding communicative abilities across situational and interpersonal contexts (Lapidus, 1985; Theimer, Schuler, & Perillo, 1985).

In communication enhancement, the ability to adjust language use and communicative style is important for participating appropriately in school, home, and community contexts. For individuals communicating through nonspeech means or at earlier prelinguistic levels of communication, a goal of communication enhancement is the acquisition of the ability to "shift codes," whether it involves using more than one nonspeech system (e.g., sign language for school and home, communication board for community) or, for more competent communicators, learning rules of politeness and "conversational scripts" for specific types of interactions (e.g., talking on the telephone, addressing unfamiliar people). The more recent emphasis on functional approaches (Donnellan & Kilman, 1986) and facilitative styles has placed greater emphasis on language and communication enhancement in varied and natural contexts, requiring communicative adjustments. Role playing of frequently recurring social-interactive routines has been utilized to help foster this ability (Donnellan & Kilman, 1986; Lapidus, 1985).

The significant language comprehension deficits of autistic persons have been discussed extensively (Lord, 1985a; Ricks & Wing, 1975). For individuals at lower cognitive levels, problems may include an inability to acquire any meaning from speech, whereas problems for individuals functioning at higher cognitive and linguistic levels typically include literal and concrete interpretations of language. Ability to participate in communicative interactions depends upon understanding the social and conceptual meanings of verbal and nonverbal communication. Thus, successful communicative exchanges are more likely when verbal and nonverbal communication is adjusted to an individual's level of comprehension. Assessment of comprehension through formal and informal testing, as well as observation in natural environments, helps to determine approximate developmental levels of comprehension of both verbal and nonverbal communication. Communication directed toward persons with autism can then be adjusted accordingly. This is especially crucial for echolalic individuals, who may give a spurious picture of linguistic competence (Prizant, 1983a). Specific suggestions for adjusting verbal and nonverbal communication are discussed in detail by Prizant and Schuler (1987a).

Traditional behavioral language treatment programs used with autistic children often target receptive language objectives before expressive language objectives. In addition, comprehension is usually taught in a discrimination paradigm devoid of contextual cues and natural motivations to respond, which is counter to the way in which normal children develop comprehension (see Lord, 1985a). Thus, this approach needs to be reconsidered in light of current developmental theory and research. This is particularly pertinent to autistic children because of motivational and attentional problems faced during discrimination-training procedures. Furthermore, because echolalia is common, many verbal autistic children may be able to repeat and produce utterances for a communicative purpose, although they may not comprehend the individual components. Developmental relationships between comprehension and production indicate alternative approaches. The reader is referred to Lord (1985a) for an in-depth discussion of the application of developmental strategies to assessing and facilitating comprehension to autistic children.

Pragmatic/social-interactive theory has probably had the most significant impact on recent trends in communication enhancement for both nondevelopmentalists (Carr, 1985; Hart, 1985) and developmentalists (Dawson & Galpert, 1986; Lord, 1985a; Prizant & Wetherby, 1985). It also has provided a common working language for neobehaviorists, developmentalists, and functionalists, which should result in the continuing dissolution of theoretical boundaries.

Applying Information about the Nature and Symptomatology of the Autistic Syndrome

The recent recategorization of autism as a lifelong developmental disability has provided the impetus for clinicians and researchers to understand autism from a developmental perspective. As discussed earlier, research exploring normal development in social-cognitive and communicative domains has helped to elucidate the characteristics and patterns of abilities and disabilities in autism. With a greater understanding of the syndrome, clinicians are beginning to apply this information to communication assessment and intervention. The primary impact is occurring in several areas: developing understanding of specific symptomatology associated with autism; developing understanding of speech and language characteristics in autism; acknowledging the need to capitalize on autistic individuals' relative strengths; and, finally, constructing models of development in autism that may be the most appropriate standards of reference for assessing communicative growth.

Developing Understanding of Specific Unconventional Behaviors

The words "bizarre," "deviant," and "aberrant" have come to be all too familiar to persons who work and live with autistic individuals. What these descriptors imply is that the behavior observed is often difficult to understand by reference to behavior of normally developing children and other children with disabilities. The range of specific behaviors may be as diverse as repetitive motility patterns (e.g., rocking, hand flapping), use of socially unacceptable means to communicate intent (e.g., aggression, self-injurious behavior), and characteristics of speech and language (e.g., immediate and delayed echolalia, perseverative speech, and metaphorical language). The recent application of various research methodologies, including behavioral, pragmatic, and psycholinguistic, has provided a greater understanding of seemingly difficult-to-understand behavior (Duchan, 1985). For example, there has been a major shift in how disruptive, aggressive, and self-injurious behavior is now viewed (Carr & Durand, 1985). Early conceptualizations of autism as a behavior disorder or emotional disturbance justified efforts to extinguish many of these behaviors, with few attempts to understand dynamics of the behaviors relative to their functions in different situational contexts.

With more recent conceptualizations of autism, such behavior is viewed as secondary to the more basic social-cognitive and communicative impairments (Cohen *et al.*, 1986). Current theory and research is indicating that many of these behaviors can be better understood if they are viewed as an inevitable outcome of pervasive social-cognitive and communicative impairments (Carr & Durand, 1985; Donnellan *et al.*, 1984; Prizant, 1983b; Schuler & Prizant, 1987; Wetherby & Prutting, 1984). In assessment, clinicians and educators are now attempting to understand situational determinants of behavior across contexts and the functions that such behavior may serve for the individuals involved. In communication enhancement, the emphasis is now on altering or adapting environments to preclude the occurence of aberrant behavior, or on replacing/modifying such behavior with more socially acceptable means that may serve the same functions. These approaches recognize the legitimacy of the child's behavior relative to learning profiles, with an emphasis on building competence rather then simply decreasing behavior.

Developing Understanding of Speech and Language Characteristics

Specific changes have occurred in the way speech and language characteristics are viewed. For example, the work of Prizant and colleagues (Prizant, 1983b; Prizant & Duchan, 1981; Prizant & Rydell, 1984; Schuler & Prizant, 1985) on immediate and delayed echolalia has identified the need to understand such behavior along the continua of intentionality, conventionality, and communicativeness. Thus, assessments need to determine the range of different functional forms of echolalia and the degree of intentionality underlying these forms. With greater insight into an individual's pattern of echolalic behavior, appropriate strategies for communication enhancement may be derived (Prizant, 1983a). Similarly, Hurtig, Ensrud, and Tomblin (1982) have identified specific functions of incessant questioning, a frequently noted "problem behavior" of persons with autism. They found that in approximately 50% of their observations of autistic individuals, incessant questioning was used as an effort to establish contact with others rather than to request information. Hurtig *et al.*'s findings are easily understood if one considers the difficulty autistic persons have in learning appropriate social conventions of conversation. For both echolalic forms and incessant questioning, communication enhancement efforts have shifted to acknowledging the functions that those forms may serve and helping the individuals involved to acquire more conventional means of expressing the same intent.

Capitalizing on Relative Strengths

Increasing knowledge of autism has also led to strategies in communication assessment and enhancement that attempt to capitalize on specific abilities. One relative strength in autism, visual–spatial ability, has had a significant impact on communication enhancement. Information may be presented through the visual–spatial modality, using pictures, picture symbols, and/or written words either as primary means of communication or as an augmentation to spoken language. Mirenda (1985) provided specific suggestions for constructing pictorial communication systems, based on the premise that many persons with autism are more effective in processing information visually than auditorally. Prizant and Schuler (1987a) have also recommended the use of pictures and written words to help individuals with autism understand abstract temporal concepts, including past and future events. Many educational programs currently use "picture schedules" to help children anticipate events and develop a concept of daily routines. For those individuals who have particular difficulty dealing with unpredictable change, concretizing the abstractions of temporal structure may allow the individuals to have greater control by helping them to anticipate changes in routine, and if possible, to select among alternative activities. Clinical experience suggests that visual–spatial representation of time fosters conceptual understandings of life routines, resulting in increased motivation and capacity to communicate about the "not-here-and-now."

　　Recently, supported employment programs (e.g., Community Services for Autistic Citizens [CSAC], Rockville, Maryland) have demonstrated the efficacy of focusing in on learning strengths. In the CSAC program, formerly institutionalized persons with autism are placed in a variety of vocational settings involving structured tasks that demand good visual–spatial skills (e.g., sorting library books, collating and binding in printing shops, etc.) (Juhrs, 1985). Anecdotal accounts of the use of musical skills to foster motivation and even provide employment (e.g., piano tuning) pervade the literature on autism (Rimland, 1978). Thus, the exploitation of relative abilities is applicable to activities for daily living and to acquisition of vocational skills, as well as to enhancement of communication. Assessment should identify patterns of relative abilities and disabilities to help in setting goals for communication and independent living.

Constructing Models of Development

Finally, researchers and clinicians are beginning to construct models of development in autism that may be used as standards of reference for communication assessment and enhancement. For example, Wetherby (1986) has described an "ontogeny of communicative functions" in autism that may be qualitatively different from that of normal children and other language-impaired children. She noted that children with autism first communicate for behavioral regulation, a relatively nonsocial purpose for communicating. Later in development, the general functions of attracting another's attention to self and directing another's attention to an object or event may emerge in respective order. For normal and other language-impaired children, a wide range of communicative functions is typically observed in the early development of intentional communication (Wetherby & Prizant, in press; Wollner, 1983). The specific pattern observed in autism may be understood in reference to the nature of the social-cognitive impairment. That is, more social forms of communication are more difficult to acquire because the end goal is social sharing, whereas less social forms having a goal of behavioral regulation (e.g., requesting, protesting) may be easier to acquire.

Prizant's (1983b) proposed model of language development in autism, based on gestalt styles observed in other children, has specific implications for assessment and communication enhancement. In noting that the great majority of individuals with autism who speak either are echolalic or were echolalic in development (Prizant, 1983a), he suggested that a gestalt style may be the primary strategy by which autistic individuals acquire a linguistic system. As noted earlier, this style of language acquisition involves early memorization and repetition of language "chunks" (immediate and delayed echolalia), with subsequent analysis and segmentation of these unanalyzed forms to help form the foundation of a more creative and rule-governed linguistic system. Based upon this model, Prizant (1983a) and Prizant and Schuler (1987a) have suggested specific guidelines for assessment and communication enhancement that address the proposed developmental sequence of language acquisition. For example, assessment of progress in language development should take into account movement from gestalt forms (i.e., echolalia) to creative, generative language. Language intervention should help individuals "break the linguistic code" through reduction and simplication of gestalt forms, while acknowledging the functions that such forms may serve. Clearly, longitudinal research is needed to validate hypotheses about proposed developmental models in autism and to stimulate new hypotheses about the course of development in various domains and interrelationships among these domains.

CONCLUSIONS AND FUTURE DIRECTIONS

Since 1980, communication assessment and enhancement for persons with autism has been greatly influenced by the application of various theoretical models and research methodologies emerging largely from the developmental literature. This is in distinct contrast to the predominance in the 1970s of theory and procedures emerging from traditional behaviorism. This recent influx of information has provided a greater understanding of the autistic syndrome and, more specifically, of problems in social interaction and communication. However, empirical validation of the current application of this knowledge is needed. As noted earlier, these data are beginning to emerge.

Some of the most challenging applications of theory to practice still remain. For example, recent research has focused on the affective and emotional dimensions of autism (Prizant & Schaechter, 1988) and has demonstrated pervasive impairments in the ability of persons with autism to understand others' emotional states (Hobson, 1986 and Chapter 2, this volume) and the often subtle signals associated with affective communication (Hermelin & O'Connor, 1985). The extent to which new insights and research findings such as these can be applied to education and treatment remains to be seen. What seems to be clear, however, is that autistic persons and their families are the beneficiaries of increased efforts to tie theory to practice.

References

American Psychiatric Association. (1987). *Diagnostic and statistical manual of mental disorders* (3rd ed.—rev.). Washington, DC: Author.

Ayres, A. J. (1979). *Sensory integration and the child.* Los Angeles: Western Psychological Services.

Bates, E. (1976). *Language and context: The acquisition of pragmatics.* New York: Academic Press.

Bates, E. (1979). On the evolution and development of symbols. In E. Bates. T. Benigni, I. Bretherton, L. Camaioni, & V. Voltera (Eds.), *The emergence of symbols: Cognition and communication in infancy* (pp. 1–32). New York: Academic Press.

Bloom, L. (1970). *Language development: Form and function in emerging grammars.* Cambridge, MA: MIT Press.

Bloom, L., Hood, L., & Lightbown, P. (1974). Imitation in language development: If, when, and why. *Cognitive Psychology, 6,* 380–420.

Bloom, L., & Lahey, M. (1978). *Language development and language disorders.* New York: Wiley.

Brown, L., Branston, M., Hamre-Nietupski, S., Pumpian, I., Certo, N., & Gruenewald, L. (1979). A strategy for developing chronological age-appropriate and functional curricular content for severely handicapped adolescents and adults. *Journal of Special Education, 13,* 81–90.

Brown, R. (1973). *A first language: The early stages.* Cambridge, MA: Harvard University Press.

Bruner, J. (1975). The ontogenesis of speech acts. *Journal of Child Language, 2,* 1–19.

Bruner, J. (1978). From communication to language: A psychological perspective. In I. Markova (Ed.), *The social context of language* (pp. 17–48). Chichester, England: Wiley.

Bruner, J. (1983). *In search of mind: Essays in autobiography.* New York: Basic Books.

Bryen, D., & Joyce, D. (1985). Language intervention with the severely handicapped: A decade of research. *Journal of Special Education, 19,* 7–39.

Cairns, R. (1986). Social development: Recent theoretical trends and relevance for autism. In E. Schopler & G. Mesibov (Eds.), *Social behavior in autism* (pp. 15–33). New York: Plenum.

Carr, E. (1985). Behavioral approaches to language and communication. In E. Schopler & G. Mesibov (Ed.), *Communication problems in autism* (pp. 37–57). New York: Plenum.

Carr, E., & Durand, V. M. (1985). The social-communicative basis of severe behavior problems in children. In S. Reiss & R. Bootzin (Eds.), *Theoretical issues in behavior therapy* (pp. 219–254). New York: Academic Press.

Chapman, R., & Miller, J. (1975). Word order in early two and three word utterances: Does production precede comprehension? *Journal of Speech and Hearing Research, 18*, 355–371.

Chomsky, N. (1968). *Language and mind.* New York: Harcourt Brace Jovanovich.

Cicchetti, D., & Pogge-Hesse, P. (1981). The relation between emotion and cognition in infant development. In M. Lamb & L. Sherrod (Eds.), *Infant social cognition: Empirical and theoretical considerations* (pp. 205–272). Hillsdale, NJ: Erlbaum.

Clark, P., & Rutter, M. (1981). Autistic children's responses to structure and interpersonal demands. *Journal of Autism and Developmental Disorders, 11*, 201–217.

Cohen, D. J., Paul, R., & Volkmar, F. R. (1986). Issues in the classification of pervasive and other developmental disorders: Towards DSM IV. *Journal of the American Academy of Child Psychiatry, 25*, 213–220.

Curcio, F. (1978). Sensorimotor functioning and communication in mute autistic children. *Journal of Autism and Childhood Schizophrenia, 8*, 181–189.

Dawson, G., & Adams, A. (1984). Imitation and social responsiveness in autistic children. *Journal of Abnormal Child Psychology, 12*, 209–226.

Dawson, G., Finley, C., Phillips, S., & Galpert, L. (1986). Hemispheric specialization and the language abilities of autistic children. *Child Development, 57*, 1440–1453.

Dawson, G., & Galpert, L. (1986). A developmental model for facilitating the social behavior of autistic children. In E. Schopler & G. Mesibov (Eds.), *Social behavior in autism* (237–261). New York: Plenum.

Delacato, C. (1974). *The ultimate stranger: The autistic child.* Garden City, NY: Doubleday.

Denckla, M. B. (1986). New diagnostic criteria for autism and related behavioral disorders: Guidelines for research protocols. *Journal of the American Academy of Child Psychiatry, 25*, 221–224.

Donnellan, A., & Kilman, E. (1986). Behavioral approaches to social skill development in autism: Strengths, misapplications and alternatives. In E. Schopler & G. Mesibov (Eds.), *Social behavior in autism* (pp. 213–235). New York: Plenum.

Donnellan, A., Mirenda, P., Mesaros, R., & Fassbender, L. (1984). Analyzing the communicative functions of aberrant behavior. *Journal of the Association for Persons with Severe Handicaps, 9*, 201–212.

Dore, J. (1974). A pragmatic description of early language development. *Journal of Psycholinguistic Research, 3*, 343–350.

Duchan, J. (1983). Autistic children are noninteractive: Or so we say. *Seminars in Speech and Language, 4*, 63–78.

Duchan, J. (1984). Clinical interactions with autistic children: The role of theory. *Topics in Language Disorders, 4*, 62–71.

Duchan, J. (1985). Autistic behavior: Deviant or different. *Australian Journal of Human Communication Disorders, 13*, 3–8.

Duchan, J. (1987). Functionalism: A perspective on autistic communication. In D. Cohen & A. Donnellan (Eds.), *Handbook of autism and pervasive developmental disorders* (pp. 703–709). New York: Wiley.

Dunst, C., & Lowe, L. (1986). From reflex to symbol: Describing, explaining and fostering communicative competence. *Augmentative and Alternative Communication, 2*, 11–18.

Emde, R. N. (1980). Toward a psychoanalytic theory of affect. In S. Greenspan & G. Pollock (Eds.), *The course of life: Psychoanalytic contributions toward understanding personality development. Vol. 1. Infancy and early childhood* (U.S. DHHS Publication No. 80-786, pp. 63–112). Washington, DC: U.S. Government Printing Office.

Fay, W. (1979). Personal pronouns and the autistic child. *Journal of Autism and Developmental Disorders, 9*, 247–260.

Fay, W., & Schuler, A. L. (1980). *Emerging language in autistic children*. Baltimore: University Park Press.

Fein, D., Pennington, D., Markowitz, P., Braverman, M., & Waterhouse, L. (1986). Toward a neuropsychological model of infantile autism: Are the social deficits primary? *Journal of the American Academy of Child Psychiatry, 25,* 198–212.

Ferrara, C., & Hill, S. (1980). The responsiveness of autistic children to the predictability of social and nonsocial toys. *Journal of Autism and Developmental Disorders, 10,* 51–57.

Fey, M. (1986). *Language intervention with young children*. San Diego: College-Hill Press.

Garfin, D., & Lord, C. (1986). Communication as a social problem in autism. In E. Schopler & G. Mesibov (Eds.), *Social behavior in autism* (pp. 133–152) New York: Plenum.

Goldin-Meadow, S., Seligman, M., & Gelman, R. (1976). Language in the two-year old: Receptive and productive stages. *Cognition, 4,* 189–202.

Guess, D., & Baer, D. (1973). An analysis of individual differences in generalization between receptive and productive language in retarded children. *Journal of Applied Behavior Analysis, 6,* 311–329.

Halle, J. (1984). Arranging the natural environment to occasion language: Giving severely language delayed children reasons to communicate. *Seminars in Speech and Language, 5,* 185–199.

Halliday, M. (1975). *Learning how to mean: Explorations in the development of language*. London: Edward Arnold.

Hammes, J., & Langdell, T. (1981). Precursors of symbol formation and childhood autism. *Journal of Autism and Developmental Disorders, 11,* 331–346.

Harding, C. (1984). Acting with intention: A framework for examining the development of the intention to communicate. In L. Feagans, C. Garvey, & R. Golinkoff (Eds.), *The origins and growth of communication* (pp. 123–135). Norwood, NJ: Ablex.

Harding, C., & Golinkoff, R. (1979). The origins of intentional vocalizations in prelinguistic infants. *Child Development, 50,* 33–40.

Hart, B. (1985). Naturalistic language training techniques. In S. Warren & A. Rogers-Warren (Eds.), *Teaching functional language* (pp. 63–88). Baltimore: University Park Press

Hermelin, B. & O'Connor, N. (1970). *Psychological experiments with autistic children*. Oxford: Pergamon Press.

Hermelin, B., & O'Connor, N. (1985). Logico-affective states and nonverbal language. In E. Schopler & G. Mesibov (Eds.), *Communication problems in autism* (pp. 283–310). New York: Plenum.

Hobson, P. (1986). The autistic child's appraisal of expression of emotion. *Journal of Child Psychology and Psychiatry, 27,* 321–342.

Holland, A. (1975). Language therapy for children: Some thoughts on context and content. *Journal of Speech and Hearing Disorders, 40,* 514–523.

Hurtig, R., Ensrud, S., & Tomblin, J. (1982). The communicative function of question production in autistic children. *Journal of Autism and Developmental Disorders, 12,* 57–69.

Huttenlocher, J. (1974). The origins of language comprehension. In R. L. Solso (Ed.), *Theories in cognitive psychology* (pp. 331–368). Hillsdale, NJ: Erlbaum.

Juhrs, P. (1985, May). *Supported employment program for adults with autism*. Paper presented at the conference Enhancing the Community Presence and Participation of Persons with Autism, Worcester, MA.

Kiernan, C. (1983). The use of nonvocal communication techniques with autistic individuals. *Journal of Child Psychology and Psychiatry, 24,* 339–376.

Koegel, R., Egel, A. & Dunlap, G. (1980). Learning characteristics of autistic children. In W. Sailor, B. Wilcox, & L. Brown (Eds.), *Methods of instruction for severely handicapped students*. Baltimore: Paul H. Brookes.

Lapidus, D. (1985). *Developing communication and language skills in autism*. Unpublished manual.

Leonard, L., Schwartz, R. G., Chapman, K., Rowan, L., Prelock, P., Terrell, B., Weiss, A. L., & Messick, C. (1982). Early lexical acquisition in children with specific language impairment. *Journal of Speech and Hearing Research, 25,* 554–564.

Lord, C. (1985a). Autism and the comprehension of language. In E. Schopler & G. Mesibov (Eds.), *Communication problems in autism* (pp. 257–281). New York: Plenum.

Lord, C. (1985b). Contribution of behavioral approaches to language and communication of persons with autism. In E. Schopler & G. Mesibov (Eds.), *Communication problems in autism* (59–68). New York: Plenum.

Lotter, V. (1978). Follow-up studies. In M. Rutter & E. Schopler (Eds.), *Autism: A reappraisal of concepts and treatment* (475–495). New York: Plenum.

Lovaas, O. (1977). *The autistic child: Language development through behavior modification.* New York: Wiley.

Lovaas, O. (1981). *Teaching developmentally disabled children: The "me" book.* Baltimore: University Park Press.

McHale, S., Simeonsson, R., Marcus, L., & Olley, J. (1980). The social and symbolic quality of autistic children's communication. *Journal of Autism and Developmental Disorders, 10,* 299–310.

McLean, J., & Snyder-McLean, L. (1978). *A transactional approach to early language training.* Columbus, OH: Charles E. Merrill.

McLean, J., Snyder-McLean, L., Jacobs, P., & Rowland, C. (1981). *Process oriented educational programming for the severely–profoundly handicapped adolescent.* Parsons: University of Kansas, Bureau of Research.

Mirenda, P. (1985). Designing pictorial communication systems for physically able-bodied students with severe handicaps. *Augmentative and Alternative Communication, 1,* 58–64.

Mirenda, P., & Donnellan, A. (1986). Effects of adult interactions style on conversational behavior in students with severe communication problems. *Language, Speech and Hearing Services in the Schools, 17,* 126–141.

Miller, M., Cuvo, A., & Borakove, L. (1977). Teaching naming of coin values—comprehension before production versus production alone. *Journal of Applied Behavior Analysis, 10,* 735–736.

Muma, J. (1986). *Language acquisition: A functionalistic perspective.* Austin, TX: Pro-Ed.

Musselwhite, C., & St. Louis, K. (1982). *Communication programming for the severely handicapped: Vocal and nonvocal strategies.* San Diego: College-Hill Press.

Nelson, K. (1973). Structure and strategy in learning to talk. *Monographs of the Society for Research in Child Development, 38,* (1–2, Serial No. 149).

Nelson, K. (1981). Individual differences in language development: Implications for development and language. *Developmental Psychology, 17,* 170–187.

Owens, R. (1984). *Language development: An introduction.* Columbus, OH: Charles E. Merrill.

Peck, C. (1985). Increasing opportunities for social control by children with autism and severe handicaps: Effects on student behavior and perceived classroom climate. *Journal of the Association for Persons with Severe Handicaps, 4,* 183–193.

Peters, A. (1983). *The units of language acquisition.* Cambridge, England: Cambridge University Press.

Piaget, J. (1952). *The origins of intelligence in children.* New York: International Universities Press.

Piaget, J. (1954). *The construction of reality in the child.* New York: Basic Books.

Prior, M. (1979). Cognitive abilities and disabilities in autism: A review. *Journal of Abnormal Child Psychology, 2,* 357–380.

Prizant, B. M. (1982). Gestalt processing and gestalt language in autism. *Topics in Language Disorders, 3,* 16–23.

Prizant, B. M. (1983a). Echolalia in autism: Assessment and intervention. *Seminars in Speech and Language, 4,* 63–78.

Prizant, B. M. (1983b). Language acquisition and communicative behavior in autism: Toward an understanding of the "whole" of it. *Journal of Speech and Hearing Disorders, 48,* 296–307.

Prizant, B. M. (1986, August). *Social relatedness and severely communicatively impaired children.* Paper presented at the Third Sino-American Symposium on Communicative Disorders, Taipei, Taiwan.

Prizant, B. M., & Duchan, J. (1981). The functions of immediate echolalia in autistic children. *Journal of Speech and Hearing Disorders, 46,* 241–249.

Prizant, B. M., & Rydell, P. J. (1984). An analysis of the functions of delayed echolalia in autistic children. *Journal of Speech and Hearing Research, 27,* 183–192.

Prizant, B. M., & Schaechter, B. T. (1988). *Autism: The emotional and social dimensions.* Boston: Exceptional Parent Press.

Prizant, B. M., & Schuler, A. L. (1987a). Facilitating communication: Language approaches. In D. Cohen & A. Donnellan (Eds.), *Handbook of autism and pervasive developmental disorders* (316–332). New York: Wiley.

Prizant, B. M., & Schuler, A. L. (1987b). Facilitating communication: Theoretical foundations. In D. Cohen & A. Donnellan (Eds.), *Handbook of autism and pervasive developmental disorders* (pp. 289–300). New York: Wiley.

Prizant, B. M., & Wetherby, A. M. (1985). Intentional communicative behavior of children with autism: Theoretical and practical issues. *Australian Journal of Human Communication Disorders, 13,* 21–59.

Prizant, B. M., & Wetherby, A. M. (1987). Communicative intent: A framework for understanding social–communicative behavior in autism. *Journal of the American Academy of Child Psychiatry, 26,* 472–479.

Ricks, D., & Wing, L. (1975). Language, communication and the use of symbols in normal and autistic children. *Journal of Autism and Childhood Schizophrenia, 5,* 191–221.

Rimland, B. (1978, August). Inside the mind of the autistic savant. *Psychology Today,* pp. 69–80.

Rutter, M. (1978). Language disorder and infantile autism. In M. Rutter & E. Schopler (Eds.), *Autism: A reappraisal of concepts and treatment* (pp. 85–104). New York: Plenum.

Rutter, M. (1983). Cognitive deficits in the pathogenesis of autism. *Journal of Child Psychology and Psychiatry, 24,* 513–531.

Rutter, M. (1985). The treatment of autistic children. *Journal of Child Psychology and Psychiatry, 26,* 193–214.

Saarni, C. (1978). Cognitive and communicative features of emotional experience, or do you show what you think you feel? In M. Lewis & L. Rosenblum (Eds.), *The development of affect* (pp. 361–375). New York: Plenum.

Sameroff, A. (1987). The social context of development. In N. Eisenberg (Ed.), *Contemporary topics in developmental psychology* (pp. 273–291). New York: Wiley.

Sameroff, A., & Chandler, M. J. (1975). Reproductive risk and the continuum of caretaking causality. In F. Horowitz, M. Hetherington, F. Scarr-Salapatek, & G. Siegel (Eds.), *Review of child development research* (Vol. 4, pp. 187–244). Chicago: University of Chicago Press.

Sander, L. (1962). Issues in early mother–child interaction. *Journal of the American Academy of Child Psychiatry, 1,* 141–166.

Schiefelbusch, R., & Bricker, D. (Eds.). (1981). *Early language: Assessment and intervention.* Baltimore: University Park Press.

Schuler, A. L. (1985). Selecting augmentative communication systems on the basis of current means and functions. *Australian Journal of Human Communication Disorders, 13,* 102–120.

Schuler, A. L., & Prizant, B. M. (1985). Echolalia. In E. Schopler & G. Mesibov (Eds.), *Communication problems in autism* (pp. 163–184). New York: Plenum.

Schuler, A. L., & Prizant, B. M. (1987). Facilitating communication: Prelanguage approaches. In D. Cohen & A. Donnellan (Eds.), *Handbook of autism and pervasive developmental disorders* (p. 301–315). New York: Plenum.

Shah, A., & Wing, L. (1986). Cognitive impairments and social behavior in autism. In E. Schopler & G. Mesibov (Eds.), *Social behavior in autism.* New York: Plenum.

Shapiro, P., Huebner, H. & Campbell, M. (1974). Language behavior and hierarchic integration in a psychotic child. *Journal of Autism and Child Schizophrenia, 4,* 71–90.

Sherrod, L., & Lamb, M. (1981). Infant social cognition: An introduction. In M. Lamb & L. Sherrod (Eds.), *Infant social cognition: Empirical and theoretical considerations* (pp. 1–10). Hillsdale, NJ: Erlbaum.

Sigman, M., & Ungerer, J. (1984). Cognitive and language skills in autistic, mentally retarded and normal children. *Developmental Psychology, 20,* 293–302.

Skinner, B. F. (1957). Verbal behavior New York: Appleton-Century-Crofts.

Smith, M. (1985). Managing the aggressive and self-injurious behavior of adults disabled by autism. *Journal of the Association for Persons with Severe Handicaps, 4,* 228–232.

Snyder, L. (1984). Communicative competence in children with delayed language development. In R. Schiefelbusch & J. Pickar (Eds.), *The acquisition of communicative competence* (pp. 423–478). Baltimore: University Park Press.

Snyder, L., Bates, E., & Bretherton, I. (1981). Content and context in early lexical development. *Journal of Speech and Hearing Disorders, 24,* 262–268.

Snyder, L., & Lindstedt, D. (1985). Models of child language development. In E. Schopler & G. Mesibov (Eds.), *Communication problems in autism* (pp. 17–35). New York: Plenum.

Steckol, K., & Leonard, L. (1981). Sensorimotor development and the use of prelinguistic performatives. *Journal of Speech and Hearing Disorders, 24,* 262–268.

Tager-Flusberg, H. (1981). On the nature of linguistic functioning in early infantile autism. *Journal of Autism and Developmental Disorders, 2,* 45–56.

Theimer, R., Schuler, A. L., & Perillo, C. (1985). *The family's contribution to social competence: A parent guide for children with autism and severe handicaps.* Santa Barbara, CA: Special Education Research Institute.

Tiegerman, E., & Primavera, L. (1984). Imitating the autistic child: Facilitating communicative gaze behavior. *Journal of Autism and Developmental Disorders, 14,* 27–38.

Tinbergen, N., & Tinbergen, E. (1983). *Autistic children: New hope for a cure.* London: Allen & Unwin.

Uzgiris, I. (1981). Experience in the social context: Imitation and play. In R. Schiefelbusch & D. Bricker (Eds.), *Early language: Acquisition and intervention* (pp. 141–168). Baltimore: University Park Press.

Webster's Dictionary. (1981). Springfield, MA: G. & C Merriam.

Wetherby, A. M. (1984). Possible neurolinguistic breakdown in autistic children. *Topics in Language Disorders, 4,* 19–33.

Wetherby, A. M. (1985). Speech and language disorders in children: An overview. In J. Darby (Ed.), *Speech and language evaluations in neurology: Childhood disorders* (pp. 3–32). New York: Grune & Stratton.

Wetherby, A. M. (1986). Ontogeny of communicative functions in autism. *Journal of Autism and Developmental Disorders, 15,* 295–315.

Wetherby, A. M., & Prizant, B. M. (in press). The expression of communicative intent: Assessment guidelines. *Seminars in Speech and Language.*

Wetherby, A. M., & Prutting, C. (1984). Profiles of communicative and cognitive–social abilities in autistic children. *Journal of Speech and Research, 27,* 364–377.

Wing, L., Gould, J., Yeates, S., & Brierley, L. (1977). Symbolic play in severely mentally retarded and in autistic children. *Journal of Child Psychology and Psychiatry, 18,* 167–178.

Wollner, S. (1983). Communicating intent: How well do language impaired children do? *Topics in Language Disorders, 4,* 1–14.

CHAPTER 13

Motivating Language Use in Autistic Children

ROBERT L. KOEGEL
JEAN JOHNSON
University of California at Santa Barbara

INTRODUCTION

The difficulties demonstrated by autistic children in using language effectively in their natural environments is one of the major characteristics of autism (Kanner, 1946; Rutter, 1978; Schopler & Mesibov, 1985). Although the language abilities and characteristics of autistic children differ widely, most of these children show deficits in pragmatic aspects of language use (Alpert & Rogers-Warren, 1985; Tager-Flusberg, 1981; Wetherby & Prutting, 1984). Many factors influence the likelihood that autistic children will use language in their natural environments, including their general level of linguistic and language abilities, the degree of generalization of specific skills to varied environments, and the learning histories that have been established by the children within specific environments. A great deal of observation and research has taken place in the areas of language development in autistic children (Fay & Schuler, 1980; Lovaas, 1977; Schopler & Mesibov, 1985), generalization of language skills (Carr, 1985; McGee, Krantz, Mason, & McClannahan, 1983; Neef, Walters, & Egel, 1984), the description of language functions in autistic children (Prizant & Duchan, 1981; Prizant & Rydell, 1984; Wetherby & Prutting, 1984), and the maintenance of responsiveness in autistic children through "motivational" techniques (Dunlap, 1984; Dunlap & Koegel, 1980a; Egel, 1980; Koegel & Egel, 1979). Knowledge developed in these areas has recently suggested improved approaches for motivating language use by autistic children, using "natural language-teaching" techniques (Koegel, O'Dell, & Koegel, 1987).

Because autistic children may generally exhibit little motivation to communicate, the type of language stimulation program referred to above emphasizes language use in naturalistic contexts to achieve environmental ends. The focus of the treatment is to motivate language use in natural contexts, by incorporating various procedural qualities that have been demonstrated to facilitate both motivation and generalization in autistic children.

310

THE IMPORTANCE OF MOTIVATION

The natural language-teaching activities were originally designed to help promote language learning and language use with autistic children who had especially severe language impairments (Koegel, O'Dell, & Koegel, 1987). The children were preverbal, resisted most forms of language and other therapy, showed especially weak motivation to communicate and interact, and showed especially high levels of disruptive and/or self-stimulatory activities that interfered with all aspects of training. In other words, these were children who cried when they saw their therapist or therapy room; who used screams, shrieks, and gestures to indicate their needs; and who typically responded once only, or not at all, to training stimuli when they were provided. Typically, most of the language-teaching lesson was spent in subduing inappropriate behaviors and trying to promote even the simplest vocal or verbal response.

For these children, it became apparent that a severe language handicap was interacting with a severe *motivational* handicap (see also Alpert & Rogers-Warren, 1985). These children often ended up not attempting to respond verbally at all, and would resort to a wide variety of disruptive behaviors in order to avoid the perceived difficulties of the language tasks (cf. Carr, Newsom, & Binkoff, 1980; Plummer, Baer, & LeBlanc, 1977).

THE NATURAL LANGUAGE-TEACHING PARADIGM

Thus, for these children, various "motivational" treatment components were incorporated into a more traditional language treatment format in order to increase the amount and spontaneity of language use. These components were intended to (1) emphasize naturalistic and functional language use; and (2) incorporate "motivational" teaching techniques for children who show special resistance to social interaction and communication.

Activities

The treatment is conducted within the context of naturally occurring activities or naturalistic planned activities that can provide a wide variety of action and object words (see also Halle, Baer, & Spradlin, 1981; Hart, 1985; Hart & Risley, 1975; McGee *et al.*, 1983; McGee, Krantz, & McClannahan, 1985; Neef *et al.*, 1984; Rogers-Warren & Warren, 1980). The program capitalizes as much as possible on the favored or preferred activities in which the child demonstrates an interest (see Hart, 1985; Koegel, Dyer, & Bell, 1987).

The activities are chosen to incorporate highly motivating stimuli such as the following: (1) simple mechanical toys that can be operated by the child to produce sensory reinforcers such as music or action (e.g., a clown that pops up when a button is pressed); (2) interesting stimuli that can be presented within the context of a "communicative temptation" (e.g., a toy rattling inside a box that the child cannot open without help, or a favored food that is eaten in front of the child without any being specifically offered) (Wetherby, 1985); and (3) sensory stimuli such as sand, rice, or water that can be manipulated and may hold fascination for some autistic children. Activities can be anything—rolling balls, stacking blocks, playing music, sifting flour, making or eating lunch, and so on. The key to the activity is that it must *itself* provide access to or be a reinforcing activity (Bloom & Lahey, 1978; Halle, Alpert, & Anderson, 1984; Hart, 1980; Koegel & Williams, 1980; Saunders & Sailor, 1979; Williams, Koegel, & Egel, 1981). Therefore, for this type of program, the choice of the activity follows guidelines similar to general reinforcement principles: Specifically, reinforcing activities, which, like reinforcers, are idiosyncratic and individualized (Dunlap & Egel, 1982; Premack, 1959). Therefore, we choose activities that provide an adequate language stimulus (i.e., in most cases, an adequate variety of words can be said about the activities) and that are very reinforcing for the client. One indication that an activity is reinforcing for a child is the child's engaging (or attempting to engage) in that activity during free time without prompts or suggestions to do so.

Motivational Components

The following sections of the chapter are intended to highlight the basic motivational principles that are at the core of the natural language-teaching paradigm. These include (1) capitalizing on opportunities to respond for natural reinforcers; (2) reinforcing verbal attempts to respond to tasks; (3) varying tasks; and (4) taking turns and sharing control over activities. These language-stimulating techniques are superimposed upon more traditional procedures of presenting instructions, prompts, and reinforcement in discrete trials (cf. Koegel, Russo, & Rincover, 1977; Koegel & Schreibman, 1982), which are embedded within naturalistic interactions in a variety of the child's chosen activities (see also Hart, 1985).

Capitalizing on Opportunities to Respond for Natural Reinforcers

When autistic children are present in a natural environment, they typically may not use language in a manner that is successful in achieving their desired ends. They do, however, often achieve desired ends using nonverbal communicative behaviors. For instance, autistic children have been observed to take an adult's hand and lead the adult to a desired object or activity (cf. Carr & Kologinsky, 1983; Olley, 1985; Wetherby & Prutting, 1984). The children may also simply obtain the object or access to the activity on their own, without asking another person, thus avoiding the difficult task of communication (Koegel, Dyer, & Bell, 1987). Alternatively, an autistic person may exhibit a disruptive or inappropriate behavior to obtain access to reinforcing events (Carr & Durand, 1985; Carr *et al.*, 1980; Horner & Budd, 1985; Olley, 1985). These types of behaviors are typically seen when a child reaches and whines for a glass of juice (Spradlin & Siegel, 1982) or exhibits aggressive or self-injurious behaviors to terminate an undesirable task (Carr *et al.*, 1980).

In each of these examples, the autistic individual can be seen to achieve an environmental end while circumventing the need to communicate verbally in an appropriate fashion. In order to motivate appropriate language use, the natural language-teaching paradigm capitalizes upon these opportunities to highlight the important notion of *functional* communication.

These language-stimulating activities emphasize functional communication in several ways. Importantly, objects and activities are present in the environment that are reinforcing to the client, or that provide access to reinforcers (see Hart & Risley, 1974, 1975, 1980). When the natural environment is "salted" with desirable and/or interesting objects and activities, the likelihood that the autistic child will attempt to obtain one of the stimuli is increased (Carr, 1985). In this natural language treatment paradigm, all self-initiated nonverbal or verbal responses made by the child in order to obtain access to a reinforcer are conceptualized as an opportunity for the child to use appropriate verbal language to obtain the desired reinforcer (Halle *et al.*, 1984).

The natural language-teaching paradigm often capitalizes on these inherently motivating opportunities by interrupting the child during the act of obtaining the reinforcer in order to prompt a verbal response from the child. Following the verbal response about the object or activity, the child is reinforced with the same object or activity that was requested.

These procedures incorporate several principles and methods of language training that have individually been experimentally tested. For example, functional relationships between the language response and the reinforcer are emphasized by providing the object requested as the reinforcer (see Halle *et al.*, 1984; Hart & Risley, 1983; Rogers-Warren & Warren, 1980; Wetherby, 1985). Koegel and Williams (1980) demonstrated that acquisition is facilitated when the access to a reinforcer is functionally related to the target response. In addition, Goetz, Gee, and Sailor (1985) investigated the response interruption strategy, in which children were interrupted at specific points in the execution of a task and asked to communicate (using picture books) in order to resume the task. Although the exact parameters of such an interruption strategy may vary (e.g., identification of the optimum time or place for an interruption), these authors suggested that, at least under some conditions, maintenance of an ongoing event may be an even more powerful motivational consequence than the access to an event in supporting communicative behavior.

Therefore, one component of the natural language-teaching paradigm consists of certain timely interruptions of the child's ongoing activities to prevent their completion until the child makes a verbal request or comment about the activity. Each statement is followed by a further period for the child to continue engaging in the ongoing activity. This approach is loosely based on the "Premack principle" (Premack, 1959) in psychology, which roughly states that a high-occurrence behavior (the ongoing activity) can reinforce a low-occurrence behavior (requesting or commenting about the ongoing activity) when there is a contingent relationship between the two (see also Alpert & Rogers-Warren, 1985; Halle *et al.*, 1984). Thus, strategically interrupting the child's preferred activities and requiring verbalization prior to allowing the child to continue the activity teaches the child not only that verbal responses can provide access to reinforcers, but also that not using speech will restrict access to those reinforcers.

Reinforcing Verbal Attempts to Respond

Another aspect of the natural language-teaching paradigm that was designed to increase and maintain the child's motivation to continue responding is to provide reinforcement for verbal attempts to respond to tasks (Dunlap & Egel, 1982; Koegel & Egel, 1979; Koegel, O'Dell, & Dunlap, 1988; Spradlin & Siegel, 1982). This approach provides for reinforcement of the desire or willingness to communicate, apart from the "correct" nature of the response.

With many autistic children, reinforcing verbal attempts to respond to task stimuli can be the most powerful motivational technique for supporting initial verbal responsiveness to language-learning tasks. Koegel and Mentis (1985) discussed several important aspects of responding in autistic children that may contribute to the power of reinforcing verbal attempts. These authors reviewed literature suggesting that repeated failure experiences due to the severity of the autism handicap may result in depressed motivation, impaired performance, and increased task avoidance. Furthermore, repeated attempts that are unsuccessful and therefore go unrewarded may lead to conditions of "learned helplessness" (Miller & Seligman, 1975; Overmeir & Seligman, 1967; Seligman & Maier, 1967), in which the autistic child begins to perceive responding and reinforcement as independent. This could result in decreased response initiations and greater difficulty in learning subsequent response–reinforcer relationships (Koegel & Mentis, 1985; Miller & Seligman, 1975).

Behaviors resembling those seen in learned helplessness have been observed in autistic children. For example, Koegel and Egel (1979) reported that persistent failure experiences on a learning task appeared to produce a decrease in subsequent response initiations and failure to acquire the response in three autistic children. However, when the children were prompted and rewarded for correctly completing the tasks, their attempts to respond to the task in new and creative ways increased in frequency, and their motivation (as reflected on a rating scale measure of enthusiasm, interest, and happiness) also improved.

Not only does prompting correct completion of a task produce increases in the attempts to complete the task, but the corollary also appears to be true. That is, reinforcing attempts to communicate also seems to produce further increases in correct responding. Koegel *et al.* (1988) compared the effects of two conditions of reinforcement on the level of correct verbal responding on language-learning tasks. The experiment compared a traditional motor shaping contingency that provided reinforcement for successive motor speech approximations to a target response, with a "motivation" contingency that provided reinforcement for *any verbal attempt* to respond to the communicative task. The data indicated that not only were the children more enthusiastic, happier, and better behaved when their therapists used the reinforcement-for-verbal-attempts contingency, but they also produced more correct responses than when their motor speech behavior was being carefully and systematically shaped by reinforcing successive motor speech approximations. Therefore, this procedure of reinforcing speech attempts is incorporated into the natural language-teaching paradigm, and is considered to be one of the major advancements of this technique over traditional approaches. The procedure of reinforcing verbal attempts to respond also helps to underline the difference between teaching *language* and teaching *language use*. By reinforcing attempts to communicate, one is strengthening the probability that the child will attempt to communicate, as a greater priority than the actual form of the response.

However, the form of the response remains a priority (albeit a lower one) as well. We can improve the form of the response (e.g., "b" → "ba" → "ball" → "roll ball"), following familiar principles of prompting, shaping, and chaining, utilized at strategic points of especially strong responding on the child's part. However, when the form of the response is not improving, the child is reinforced for the effort as long as he or she has demonstrated an attempt to communicate verbally. This promotes the child's responding for longer periods, which provides further opportunities to improve the form of the response through techniques such as shaping (Koegel & Egel, 1979). The exact method of programming shaping and chaining within the reinforcement of verbal attempts is still in need of research in order to identify the optimal parameters. However, at this point it appears as if the motivational factors involved in reinforcing verbal attempts are more important than those involved in shaping the form of the motor speech responses per se.

Varying Tasks

Task variation is an important component of the natural language-teaching activities for a variety of reasons. Importantly, varying tasks has been shown to increase autistic children's motivation to respond to tasks. In addition, the concept of task variation may provide further benefits in the areas of generalization; moreover, when used in conjunction with functional communication, varying the task necessarily results in varied reinforcers, which have also been shown to improve acquisition in autistic children (Egel, 1980).

The relationship between task variation and appropriate responding was explored by Dunlap and Koegel (1980a). These authors found that autistic children involved in a wide variety of learning tasks responded more favorably when their therapists presented a variety of tasks randomly intermixed together during a teaching session than when the therapists presented the same tasks in a blocked series of trials (i.e., first all of the trials for task 1, then all of the trials for task 2, etc.). These results were reflected both in measures of correct responding on the tasks and in measures of the children's enthusiasm, interest, and general behavior during the lessons. Thus, the experiment indicated that learning and affect were facilitated by varying the tasks during instructional presentation. Subsequent research indicated that the facilitative effects of task variation on acquisition were greatly enhanced when the tasks that were interspersed with acquisition tasks were *previously acquired* tasks (i.e., *maintenance* tasks). Simply put, varying trials on new learning tasks with trials of previously learned tasks improves correct responding and positive motivation to learn in autistic children (Dunlap, 1984; L. K. Koegel & Koegel, 1986).

The natural language-teaching activities incorporate task variation as a major component. This is accomplished by incorporating a wide variety of stimulus items into the language-learning sessions in the contexts of the motivational activities described earlier. Task variation can be introduced in many ways (cf. Dunlap & Koegel, 1980b). One way is to vary the instructional objective within a given activity. For example, in the context of playing with a toy truck, language objectives such as action words (e.g., "push," "fast," "go," "roll") and attribute words (e.g., those pertaining to color, size, quantity, and composition) can be interspersed. Given that some of these concepts may have been previously acquired (e.g., "go," "red"), they can be interspersed with acquisition tasks (such as "metal" vs. "wood" composition) to help maintain the child's motivation to keep responding in the newer tasks in the language-learning session. Task variation can also be emphasized by limiting the amount of instructional time devoted to a particular activity. That is, as the child begins to lose interest in an activity, or as the number of different things to say about an activity declines, the therapist can remove the activity and begin a new one. Thus, within the language-learning sessions, the therapist can rapidly vary activities and the learning tasks within an activity, making sure to incorporate maintenance tasks with acquisition tasks. The presentation of learning stimuli in this manner helps to maintain the child's motivation during the language-learning sessions.

Task variation (a motivational component of the natural language-teaching activities) can be easily coupled with the use of multiple exemplars, a major variable influencing generalization (Stokes & Baer, 1977). That is, the therapist can present a wide variety of words that can be used with a given activity; can incorporate different activities for which the same word might be applied, so that the child can learn about the naturalistic array of multiple exemplars of a word; and can provide multiple verbal responses to make about a given activity. Similarly, the strategy of general case programming teaches an exemplar of each type of variation the child is expected to encounter in executing a specific task in the natural community (Horner, Sprague, & Wilcox, 1982). This procedure has been demonstrated to be extremely effective in promoting generalization to untrained stimuli (Horner, McDonnell, & Bellamy, 1985). Thus, the strategy of teaching multiple exemplars attempts to adequately represent the range of variation and consistency expected within members and nonmembers of a naturally occurring stimulus class.

The use of multiple exemplars is complementary to the principle of task variation discussed earlier. Within a natural language-teaching paradigm, the two principles are emphasized within the choice of activities to which the child is given access as a reinforcer for using verbal language. For instance, activities are chosen to represent multiple exemplars of a linguistic class: Trucks can go, they can roll, they can be big, they can be red; balls can also roll, and can be big and can be red. But balls can also bounce, and toy rabbits can bounce, and autistic children can bounce if they like. If these kinds of activities are rapidly varied within the verbal language-learning session, the child can benefit from both the use of task variation and the use of multiple exemplars simultaneously.

When access to these widely varying and interesting activities is dependent upon the child's appropriate attempted use of verbal language as described by the principles of functional communication, the language-stimulating activities can also be shown to provide a wide array of *varying reinforcers* as a consequence of verbal responding. That is, the child is rewarded by access to a reinforcing object or event as a consequence for appropriate verbal attempts to respond to the language tasks. Each time the task or activity is varied, the appropriate language response also varies. The reinforcer is functionally related to the language response, such that when the child says "roll," the ball is rolled, and when the child says "bounce," the ball is bounced. Interestingly, it has been shown that the presentation of varied reinforcing stimuli produces faster acquisition and better motivation than the presentation of repetitive reinforcing stimuli (Egel, 1980, 1981).

Sharing Control and Taking Turns

In addition to the difficulties autistic children demonstrate in learning and applying linguistic abilities, marked deficits have also been noted in the pragmatic aspects governing language use (Baltaxe, 1977; Carr, 1985; Tager-Flusberg, 1981). These deficits may be exhibited in the limited functions evidenced by some autistic children when compared to normal children (Wetherby & Prutting, 1984). Pragmatic deficits have also been evidenced as a "lack of to and fro chatter" (Rutter, 1978, p. 149). The apparent lack of reciprocity typically continues to a great extent into adolescence and adulthood (Dewey & Everard, 1974).

These types of difficulties in language use in context argue strongly for a modification of language-learning contexts in order that the child may receive exposure to and instruction in *taking appropriate conversational turns* and using language to direct instructional activities (cf. Lieven, 1976; MacDonald, 1985).

Taking conversational turns can at first be imposed by the therapist by using the response interruption strategy discussed previously, in which the therapist's timely interruption of the child's ongoing activity provides the stimulus for the child to take a conversational turn. The therapist can prompt the child to take the turn if necessary, by asking the child a question regarding the activity or the child's desire regarding the activity. The therapist can then take turns, in order to model appropriate verbal and nonverbal responses for the child to imitate (cf. Halle *et al.*, 1984). The turn-taking procedures constitute both the context and the desired outcome of the activities (cf. Bricker & Schiefelbush, 1984), providing the child with exposure to and experience with some of the pragmatic aspects of communicative interactions.

The turn-taking format facilitates *shared control* over the teaching interactions by the teacher and the child. Wetherby (1985) has also proposed that the nature of language intervention interactions should be planned so that the child assumes not only the role of respondent, but also that of initiator. Wetherby (1985) believes that communicative interactions should center around an activity of mutual interest and shared attention (see also Alpert & Rogers-Warren, 1985; Hart, 1985). The emphasis on the turn-taking format allows the child opportunities to direct the interactions, emphasizing further the pragmatic aspects of employing language to direct environmental events and activities. In normal infants, the contingent feedback provided by adults to the infants' signals appears to be instrumental in fostering the development of communication, as it increases the infants' ability to control the environment (Bricker & Schiefelbush, 1984). The natural language-teaching program likewise provides contingent feedback to the autistic child by placing an emphasis on responding to the child's desires about the activity and allowing the child to direct the activity while prompting and reinforcing appropriate attempts to communicate those desires (Holland, 1975; Koegel, Dyer, & Bell, 1987; Johnston, 1982; Snow, 1976; Turner, 1978). Thus, a child who exhibits inappropriate behavior every time a particular unfavored task is presented is not granted a reprieve from the task, but is instead prompted to use appropriate *verbal* responses or requests to direct the activity and/or to choose a different one. As long as the child uses appropriate communication and behavior, the activities may be directed by the child, with the therapist providing systematic interruption (stimulus for child to speak) and resumption or initiation (reinforcer for speaking) of the child's chosen activity. Such shared control over the selection of the specific stimulus materials used to teach a task results in improved social behavior, improved learning, and reductions in off-task behavior (Dyer, 1985; Koegel, Dyer, & Bell, 1987). For example, Koegel, Dyer, and Bell (1987) noted that autistic and other severely handicapped children exhibit severe social avoidance behavior when adults attempt to engage them in adult-directed activities without considering the children's preferred activities. Therefore, they conducted an investigation to assess whether the type of activity (a child-preferred activity vs. an activity that was arbitrarily determined by an adult) engaged in during an interaction would be correlated with the amount of social avoidance behavior such children exhibit.

The results of the experiment revealed a negative correlation between child-preferred activities and social avoidance behavior. That is, the autistic children were *not* socially unresponsive when they were engaged in child-preferred and child-directed activities. Additional analyses revealed that (1) social avoidance behavior could be manipulated within a reversal design, and predictably decreased when the children were prompted to initiate child-preferred activities; and (2) these procedures could be employed to teach children to initiate child-preferred activities in community settings, resulting in reductions in social avoidance responses even after the therapist's prompts were completely removed. These data suggest that the manipulation of shared control variables may have a large influence on the degree of social unresponsiveness that is evidenced by autistic and other severely handicapped children in different social contexts.

EFFECTIVENESS OF THE PARADIGM

Clinical Testing

The components utilized within the natural language-teaching paradim described above were experimentally tested by Koegel, O'Dell, and Koegel (1987). This experiment compared the natural language-teaching paradigm to a heretofore state-of-the-art language treatment package, employing massed trials in a one-to-one clinic format in which the child was expected to respond to clinician-directed stimulus items and was then reinforced with powerful primary or secondary reinforcers for "good talking." Specifically, within a multiple-baseline design, treatment was first conducted in a baseline condition with trials presented serially in a traditional analogue clinical format, in which the therapist presented instructions, prompts, and reinforcers for correct responses. Then these variables were manipulated in the natural language-teaching condition, such that (1) stimulus items were selected by the child, resulting in functional and varied stimulus materials; (2) natural reinforcers were employed; (3) communicative attempts were also reinforced; and (4) trials were conducted within natural interchanges. Treatment and generalization data demonstrated that manipulation of these variables resulted in broadly generalized treatment gains, with increases both in imitative responding and in spontaneous speech across many environmental contexts.

These results concur with current formulations and research data in the fields of psycholinguistic and behavioral language treatment, which suggest that language treatment contexts can be expected to influence the generalization of language treatment gains as reflected by the client's use of language in natural settings (Costello, 1982; Hart, 1985; Spradlin & Siegel, 1982). For many reasons, it appears that treatment contexts that most closely resemble natural linguistic contexts may improve generalization to natural settings (Carr, 1985; Halle *et al.*, 1984; Hart, 1985; Hart & Risley, 1980; Neef *et al.*, 1985; McGee *et al.*, 1983). For example, Hart and Risley (1974, 1980, 1983), developed incidental-teaching techniques with a language-handicapped preschool population. They reported that teaching techniques that capitalized on the children's interest in their environment—teaching trials were conducted only after the children initiated interaction in some manner, and the children were reinforced with access to the natural reinforcers in which they had demonstrated interest—produced more generalized language learning that was successfully employed with new persons and in new settings. Incidental-teaching techniques have also been used with autistic children and youths. This incidental teaching involves the systematic use of naturally occurring discriminative stimuli, varied adult prompts, and functional reinforcers within the context of child initiated teaching episodes. McGee *et al.* (1983) employed a modified incidental-teaching procedure to teach receptive labeling tasks to two autistic youths in the context of naturalistic, functional lunch-making procedures conducted in a group home. Their results indicated that the naturalistic teaching context and functional reinforcement procedures facilitated generalization to the experimental generalization sessions, and also produced dramatic increases in the frequency of spontaneous verbal requests by one subject during family meals, as reported by teaching parents. These authors also noted that incidental-teaching procedures could maximize the benefits of community-based treatment for autistic children by embedding language teaching into other teaching activities, such as meal preparation, leisure activities, and self-care skills. Thus, evidence is beginning to accumulate that incidental or naturalistic teaching can increase generalized language use in severely language-handicapped children.

Parent Training

Very often, parents of severely language-handicapped children desire to become involved in their children's language program. In addition, many researchers have advocated such involvement because parents can accompany their children in many settings and have access to naturally reinforcing activities that can present opportunities for language teaching (Halle *et al.*, 1984). It is desirable for both the child and the parent to maximize the effectiveness of language lessons by embedding them in naturally occurring reinforcing contexts. The parent can capitalize on the natural curriculum generated by the child's interest in the environment (Spradlin & Siegel, 1982), and the child appears to benefit in terms of generalization of language use in other contexts. Our preliminary data on training parents to utilize a natural language-teaching program suggest that (1) the parents learn to use these techniques much faster than traditional techniques; (2) the parents enjoy using the techniques; (3) the children learn much more language with these techniques; and (4) the children use their language more spontaneously and in more environmental contexts (see Koegel, Koegel, & O'Neill, in press).

It is expected that parent training could help to maximize language learning and use in other ways as well. For instance, Halle *et al.* (1981) demonstrated that adults present in a handicapped child's environment very often "pre-empt" the child's use of language by anticipating his or her needs. When adults were taught to delay the provision of reinforcers, or of materials required to engage in or complete reinforcing activities, handicapped children were more likely to attempt to request those reinforcers using a response that could then be shaped into appropriate verbal requests. After participation in a delay procedure, the children's increases in verbal requests showed a generalized increase to untrained situations. These results were replicated with autistic children by Charlop, Schreibman, and Thibodeau (1985), who employed the time-delay procedure to transfer stimulus control over the vocalizations of autistic children from verbal stimuli (e.g., an adult saying "What is this?" or "What do you want?"), to a nonverbal stimulus (i.e., the desired object). Their results confirmed that the time-delay procedure was effective in facilitating spontaneous and generalized requesting behavior by autistic children over untrained settings, people, situations, and objects. Thus, if parents can also be taught to delay their prompts until the children initiate responses, the spontaneity of language use should be expected to increase. Important in this regard is research reported by Horner, Williams, and Knobbe (1985), which indicated that opportunity to use target behaviors in natural environments had a significant influence on the subsequent maintenance of those responses. That is, target behaviors that handicapped students had little opportunity to perform in their natural environments were not maintained a year after treatment. In contrast, target behaviors that the students had many opportunities to perform were more likely to be maintained for long durations into the future. These two lines of research emphasize the importance of teaching parents to recognize opportunities for teaching and to maximize those opportunities by using delay procedures, so that children are expected to use language frequently in order to obtain reinforcers and reinforcing activities in their natural environments.

SUMMARY

Autistic children characteristically exhibit profound handicaps in learning and applying language in a flexible and generalized manner. This primary linguistic disorder is often exacerbated by learning experiences that result in low motivation to learn and use language in natural contexts. However, when specific motivational components are combined with traditional language-learning approaches within a natural language-teaching paradigm, benefits for autistic children include increases in motivation, learning, and generalization of language abilities. When parents can be included in helping to provide the therapy, it is expected that further benefits in motivating language use by autistic children in naturalistic contexts will be realized.

Acknowledgments

Preparation of this chapter was supported in part by U.S. Public Health Service Research Grant Nos. MH28210 and MH28231 from the National Institute of Mental Health,

U.S. Department of Education, Special Education Program Contract No. 300-82-0362, and NIDRR Cooperative Agreement No. G0087C0234. Special appreciation is expressed to Mary O'Dell, Jean Bramer, and Karen Kozloff for their valuable input in developing the procedures described in this chapter.

References

Alpert, C. L., & Rogers-Warren, A. K. (1985). Communication in autistic persons: Characteristics and intervention. In S. F. Warren & A. K. Rogers-Warren (Eds.), *Teaching functional language* (pp. 123–155). Baltimore: University Park Press.

Baltaxe, C. A. M. (1977). Pragmatic deficits in the language of autistic adolescents. *Journal of Pediatric Psychology, 2,* 176–180.

Bloom, L., & Lahey, M. (1978). *Language development and language disorders.* New York: Wiley.

Bricker, D., & Schiefelbush, R. L. (1984). Infants at risk. In L. McCormick & R. L. Schiefelbush (Eds.), *Early language intervention* (pp. 243–266). Columbus, OH: Charles E. Merrill.

Carr, E. G. (1985). Behavioral approaches to language and communication. In E. Schopler & G. Mesibov (Eds.), *Communication problems in autism* (pp. 37–57). New York: Plenum.

Carr, E. G., & Durand, V. M. (1985). Reducing behavior problems through functional communication training. *Journal of Applied Behavior Analysis, 18,* 111–126.

Carr, E. G., & Kologinsky, E. (1983). Acquisition of sign language by autistic children: II. Spontaneity and generalization effects. *Journal of Applied Behavior Analysis, 16,* 297–314.

Carr, E. G., Newsom, C. D., & Binkoff, J. (1980). Escape as a factor in the aggressive behavior of two retarded children. *Journal of Applied Behavior Analysis, 13,* 101–112.

Charlop, M. H., Schreibman, L., & Thibodeau, M. G. (1985). Increasing spontaneous verbal responding in autistic children using a time delay procedure. *Journal of Applied Behavior Analysis, 18,* 208–214.

Costello, J. M. (1982, April). *Generalization in the treatment of language disorders.* Paper presented at the National Language Intervention Conference, Omaha, NE.

Dewey, M. A., & Everard, M. P. (1974). The near-normal autistic adolescent. *Journal of Autism and Childhood Schizophrenia, 4,* 348–364.

Dunlap, G. (1984). The influence of task variation and maintenance tasks on the learning and affect of autistic children. *Journal of Experimental Child Psychology, 37,* 41–64.

Dunlap, G., & Egel, A. L. (1982). Motivational techniques. In R. L. Koegel, A. Rincover, & A. L. Egel (Eds.), *Educating and understanding autistic children* (pp. 106–126). San Diego: College-Hill Press.

Dunlap, G., & Koegel, R. L. (1980a). Motivating autistic children through stimulus variation. *Journal of Applied Behavior Analysis, 13,* 619–627.

Dunlap, G., & Koegel, R. L. (1980b). Programming the delivery of instruction of autistic children. In B. Wilcox & A. Thompson (Eds.), *Critical issues in educating autistic children* (pp. 89–117). Washington, DC: U.S. Department of Education, Office of Special Education.

Dyer, K. (1985). *The competition of stereotyped behavior with external reinforcers in autistic children.* Unpublished doctoral dissertation, University of California at Santa Barbara.

Egel, A. L. (1980). The effects of constant versus varied reinforcer presentation on responding by autistic children. *Journal of Experimental Child Psychology, 30,* 455–463.

Egel, A. L. (1981). Reinforcer variation: Implications for motivating developmentally delayed children. *Journal of Applied Behavior Analysis, 14,* 345–350.

Fay, W. H., & Schuler, A. L. (1980). *Emerging language in autistic children.* Baltimore: University Park Press.

Goetz, L., Gee, K., & Sailor, W. (1985). Using a behavior change interruption strategy to teach communication skills to students with servere disabilities. *Journal of the Association for Persons with Severe Handicaps, 10,* 21–30.

Halle, J. W., Alpert, C. L., & Anderson, S. R. (1984). Natural environment language assessment and intervention with severely impaired preschoolers. *Topics in Early Childhood Special Education, 4*, 36–56.

Halle, J. W., Baer, D. M., & Spradlin, J. (1981). Teachers generalized use of delay as a stimulus control procedure to increase language use in handicapped children. *Journal of Applied Behavior Analysis, 14*, 389–409.

Hart, B. M. (1980). Pragmatics and language development. In B. B. Lahey & A. E. Kazdin (Eds.), *Advances in clinical child psychology* (Vol. 3, pp. 383–427). New York: Plenum.

Hart, B. M. (1985). Naturalistic language training techniques. In S. F. Warren & A. K. Rogers-Warren (Eds.), *Teaching functional language* (pp. 63–88). Baltimore: University Park Press.

Hart, B. M., Risley, T. R. (1974). Using preschool material to modify the language of disadvantaged children. *Journal of Applied Behavior Analysis, 7*, 243–256.

Hart, B. M., & Risley, T. R. (1975). Incidental teaching of language in preschool. *Journal of Applied Behavior Analysis, 8*, 411–420.

Hart, B. M., & Risley, T. R. (1980). *In vivo* language intervention: Unanticipated general effects. *Journal of Applied Behavior Analysis, 12*, 407–432.

Hart, B. M., & Risley, T. R. (1983). *How to use incidental teaching procedures.* Lawrence, KS: H & H Enterprises.

Holland, A. (1975). Language therapy for children: Some thoughts on context and content. *Journal of Speech and Hearing Disorders, 40*, 514–523.

Horner, R. H., & Budd, C. M. (1985). Teaching manual sign language to a nonverbal student: Generalization and collateral reduction of maladaptive behavior. *Education and Training of the Mentally Retarded 20*, 39–47.

Horner, R. H., McDonnell, J. J., & Bellamy, G. T. (1985). Teaching generalized skills: General case instruction in simulation and community settings. In R. H. Horner, L. Meyer, & H. D. Fredericks (Eds.), *Education of learners with severe handicaps: Exemplary service strategies* (pp. 289–314). Baltimore: Paul H. Brookes.

Horner, R. H., Sprague, J., & Wilcox, B. (1982). General case programming for community activities. In B. Wilcox & G. T. Bellamy (Eds.), *Design of high school programs for severely handicapped students* (pp. 61–98). Baltimore: Paul H. Brookes.

Horner, R. H., Williams, J. A., & Knobbe, C. A. (1985). The effect of "opportunity to perform" on the maintenance of skills learned by high school students with severe handicaps. *Journal of the Association for Persons with Severe Handicaps, 10*, 172–175.

Johnston, J. (1982). The language disordered child. In N. Lass, J. Northern, D. Yoder, & L. McReynolds (Eds.), *Speech, language and hearing* (Vol. 2, pp. 780–801). Philadelphia: W. B. Saunders.

Kanner, L. (1946). Irrelevant and metaphorical language in early infantile autism. *American Journal of Psychiatry, 103*, 242–245.

Koegel, L. K., & Koegel, R. L. (1986). The effects of interspersed maintenance tasks on academic performance in a severe childhood stroke victim. *Journal of Applied Behavior Analysis, 19*, 425–430.

Koegel, R. L., Dyer, K., & Bell, L. K. (1987). The influence of child-preferred activities on autistic children's social behavior. *Journal of Applied Behavior Analysis, 20*, 243–252.

Koegel, R. L., & Egel, A. L. (1979). Motivating autistic children. *Journal of Abnormal Psychology, 88*, 418–426.

Koegel, R. L., Koegel, L. K., & O'Neill, R. E. (in press). Generalization in the treatment of autism. In L. McReynolds & J. Spradlin (Eds.), *Generalization strategies in the treatment of communication disorders.* Ontario: B. C. Decker.

Koegel, R. L., & Mentis, M. (1985). Motivation in childhood autism: Can they or won't they? *Journal of Child Psychology and Psychiatry, 26*, 185–191.

Koegel, R. L., O'Dell, M. C., & Dunlap, G. (1988). Producing speech use in nonverbal autistic children by reinforcing attempts. *Journal of Autism and Developmental Disorders, 18*.

Koegel, R. L., O'Dell, M. C., & Koegel, L. K. (1987). A natural language teaching paradigm for nonverbal autistic children. *Journal of Autism and Developmental Disorders, 17*, 187–200.

Koegel, R. L., Russo, D. C., & Rincover, A. (1977). Assessing and training teachers in the generalized use of behavior modification with autistic children. *Journal of Applied Behavior Analysis, 10*, 197–205.

Koegel, R. L., & Schreibman, L. (1982). *How to teach autistic and other severely handicapped children.* Lawrence, KS: H & H Enterprises.

Koegel, R. L., & Williams, J. A. (1980). Direct vs. indirect response–reinforcer relationships in teaching autistic children. *Journal of Abnormal Child Psychology, 8*, 537–547.

Lieven, E. V. M. (1976). Turn-taking and pragmatics: Two issues in early child language. In R. N. Campbell, & P. T. Smith (Eds.), *Recent advances in the psychology of language* (pp. 215–236). New York: Plenum.

Lovaas, O. I. (1977). *The autistic child: Language development through behavior modification.* New York: Irvington.

MacDonald, J. D. (1985). Language through conversation: A model for intervention with language delayed persons. In S. F. Warren & A. K. Rogers-Warren (Eds.), *Teaching functional language* (pp. 89–122). Baltimore: University Park Press.

McGee, G. G., Krantz, P. J., Mason, D., & McClannahan, L. E. (1983). A modified incidental teaching procedure for autistic youth: Acquisition and generalization of receptive object labels. *Journal of Applied Behavior Analysis, 16*, 329–338.

McGee, G. G., Krantz, P. J., & McClannahan, L. E. (1985). Comparison of incidental teaching and discrete trial teaching of prepositions to autistic children. *Journal of Applied Behavior Analysis, 18*, 17–31.

Miller, W. R., & Seligman, M. E. P. (1975). Depression and learned helplessness in man. *Journal of Experimental Psychology, 84*, 228–238.

Neef, N. A., Walters, J., & Egel, A. L. (1984). Establishing generative yes/no responses in developmentally disabled children. *Journal of Applied Behavior Analysis, 17*, 453–460.

Olley, J. G. (1985). Social aspects of communication in children with autism. In E. Schopler & G. Mesibov (Eds.), *Communication problems in autism* (pp. 311–329). New York: Plenum.

Overmier, O. B., & Seligman, M. E. P. (1967). Effects of inescapable shock upon subsequent escape and avoidance learning. *Journal of Comparative and Physiological Psychology, 63*, 28–33.

Plummer, S., Baer, D. M., & LeBlanc, J. M. (1977). Functional considerations in the use of procedural time-out and an effective alternative. *Journal of Applied Behavior Analysis, 10*, 689–705.

Premack, D. (1959). Toward empirical behavior laws: I. Positive reinforcement. *Psychological Review, 66*, 219–233.

Prizant, B. M., & Duchan, J. F. (1981). The functions of immediate echolalia in autistic children. *Journal of Speech and Hearing Disorders, 46*, 241–249.

Prizant, B. M., & Rydell, P. (1984). An analysis of the functions of delayed echolalia in autistic children. *Journal of Speech and Hearing Research, 27*, 183–192.

Rogers-Warren, A., & Warren, S. F. (1980). Mands for verbalization: Facilitating the display of newly trained language in children. *Behavior Modification, 4*, 361–382.

Rutter, M. (1978). Diagnosis and definition of childhood autism. *Journal of Autism and Childhood Schizophrenia, 8*, 139–161.

Saunders, K., & Sailor, W. (1979). A comparison of three strategies of reinforcement on two-choice language problems with severely retarded children. *AAESPH Review, 4*, 323–333.

Schopler, E., & Mesibov, G. (Eds.). (1985). *Communication problems in autism.* New York: Plenum.

Seligman, M. E. P., & Maier, S. F. (1967). Failure to escape traumatic shock. *Journal of Experimental Psychology, 74*, 1–9.

Snow, C. E. (1976). The conversational context of language acquisition. In R. N. Campbell & P. T. Smith (Eds.), *Recent advances in the psychology of language* (pp. 253–269). New York: Plenum.

Spradlin, J. E., & Siegel, G. M. (1982). Language training in natural and clinical environments. *Journal of Speech and Hearing Disorders, 47*, 2–6.

Stokes, T. F., & Baer, D. M. (1977). An implicit technology of generalization. *Journal of Applied Behavior Analysis, 10*, 349–367.

Tager-Flusberg, H. (1981). On the nature of linguistic functioning in early infantile autism. *Journal of Autism and Developmental Disorders, 11*, 45–56.

Turner, B. L. (1978). *The effects of choice of stimulus materials on interest in the remediation process and the generalized use of language training.* Unpublished master's thesis, University of California at Santa Barbara.

Wetherby, A. M. (1985). Speech and language disorders in children: An overview. In J. K. Darby (Ed.), *Speech and language evaluation in neurology: Childhood disorders* (pp. 3–32). New York: Grune & Stratton.

Wetherby, A. M., & Prutting, C. A. (1984). Profiles of communicative and cognitive–social abilities in autistic children. *Journal of Speech and Hearing Research, 27*, 364–377.

Williams, J. A., Koegel, R. L., & Egel, A. L. (1981). Response reinforcement relationships and improved learning in autistic children. *Journal of Applied Behavior Analysis, 14*, 53–60.

CHAPTER 14

Methodological and Theoretical Issues in Studying Peer-Directed Behavior and Autism

CATHERINE LORD
JOYCE MAGILL
University of Alberta/Glenrose Rehabilitation Hospital

Children with autism have typically been described as having particularly marked deficits in peer interaction (Rutter & Schopler, 1988; Wing, 1976). Though most autistic children's social skills with adults improve as they grow older, interactions with other children and with adolescent age-mates remain significantly impaired (Baltaxe & Simmons, 1983; Cantwell, Baker, & Rutter, 1977). The nature and specificity of these deficits are important for both clinical and theoretical reasons.

The contrast between social skills exhibited by autistic children with adults and those exhibited with peers provides a starting point to look more closely at the nature of the social deficit in autism. Studying peer interactions directly, particularly in developmental contexts, can provide insights into relationships between and among basic social skills (e.g., eye contact), higher-order social skills (e.g., the development of friendships), language and communication abilities, affective development, cognitive strengths and deficits, and the effects of familiarity and experience. Because all of these factors contribute or have the potential to contribute to how a child with autism interacts with peers, it becomes possible and necessary to consider each of them in turn, when evaluating the quality and quantity of social interactions in autism.

The aim of this chapter is to consider some of the methodological and theoretical issues that have arisen from studies on peer interactions by autistic children that we have carried out in the last few years. In particular, we address methodological issues in studying a low-frequency behavior (i.e., spontaneous social interaction in autistic children) and the problem of defining a child's intent to participate in social interaction when the child has limited communication and social skills. Our objective is to discuss issues that routinely arise in carrying out this sort of research, as exemplified in our own work and that of others. Since all of the studies referred to are clinical in nature, we also hope to provide some suggestions for designing clinical programs related to social development in autistic persons.

ISSUES IN STUDYING LOW-FREQUENCY BEHAVIORS

Assessing Frequency of Interaction

Although parents and professionals working with autistic persons have consistently described autistic children as having few spontaneous interactions with other children in everyday environments (Howlin, 1986; Rutter, 1978), this statement has received surprisingly little direct documentation. Strain and Cooke (1976) reported few interactions shown by a small number of autistic children integrated into a regular kindergarten. Of the interactions that occurred, most were seen as quite negative. Rutter and Bartak (1973) attempted to observe the number of spontaneous peer interactions shown by children with autism in three types of educational settings, but found interactions to be so few in all three that statistical comparisons were inappropriate. Lord and Hopkins (Lord, 1984; Lord & Hopkins, 1986) observed autistic children grouped with two other classmates during 15 minutes of free play in their classrooms. They found that out of six autistic children, none interacted for more than 2 minutes, with a modal interaction time of *zero* 15-second intervals. Another study of spontaneous communication (O'Neill & Lord, 1982) in six verbal, moderately retarded autistic children included two 6-hour observations at school and two 3-hour home observations. Peer-directed communicative acts (each of which were estimated to take less than 5 *seconds*) at school ranged from 0 to 37, and sibling-directed communicative acts at home ranged from 0 to 65 during these time periods. All of the communications at school and home were made by the same three children.

Although it is generally assumed that these very low rates of peer interaction are specific to autism, only a few studies have included control groups. Attwood, Frith, and Hermelin (1988) compared the amount of time interacting on the playground of high- and low-functioning autistic adolescents to IQ- and chronological-age-matched adolescents with Down syndrome and normally developing preschool children. The children were all in schools segregated by diagnosis and intellectual level. When compared to the controls, the autistic group showed significantly less interaction.

Over two summers, in the context of integrated 1- and 2-week day camps for nonretarded autistic, nonautistic behavior-disordered, and normally developing children, observations were made of the amount of time children in each diagnostic group spent interacting with other children during free play (Lord, in press). In both younger (ages 6–11 years) and older (ages 12–19 years) children's day camps during both summers, the autistic children always spent less time interacting—and, in fact, less time doing anything purposeful during unstructured periods—than the normally developing children. For example, in one study, the

autistic children spent an average of about 55% of their free-play time not interacting, compared to 31% for the behavior-disordered children and 21% for the
normally developing children.

A follow-up of these studies (Magill, 1987) involved observations of the initiations made by children in the three diagnostic groups during another series of
1-week day camps. The initial aim of this follow-up was not to evaluate the frequency of interactions, but rather to observe (both directly and with videotape
recordings) the *quality* of approaches made by autistic, behavior-disordered, and
normally developing groups, while holding constant the number of initiations
observed for each child. However, there were such marked differences among the
groups that it was impossible to equate number of initiations across diagnostic
groups. Two autistic children (out of 11), in more than 60 minutes of observation
spaced over a week, produced only 2 spontaneous approaches, as compared to an
average of 7–12 initiations by the other autistic children and the children in other
diagnostic groups during 14 minutes of observation.

Interpreting Low Rates of Interaction

There are many reasons, both "real" and methodological, that might account for
the low rates of peer interaction typically attributed to autistic children. Below,
three of these reasons—lack of opportunity to interact, lack of familiarity and
experience, and lack of basic social skills—are discussed. Implications for further
research and intervention follow.

Lack of Opportunity to Interact

One of the problems in interpreting the meaning of low-frequency peer interaction is that a number of factors could potentially contribute to it. In many cases,
children with autism are geographically isolated from normally developing children at school. Their failure to interact with *each other*, as in the Attwood *et al.*
(1988), Lord (1984), and Rutter and Bartak (1973) studies, may be seen as the
inability to deal with the double disadvantage of their own social deficits and those
of their autistic classmates. Also, educational philosophies and structures in school
often do not encourage spontaneous interactions among children.

Yet, if the appropriate peers for autistic children are not other autistic children, who are proper "peers"? That is, who are the peers who provide the most
appropriate opportunity for an autistic child to interact?

Highly variable profiles of skill in autism make matching on more than one
variable almost impossible. For example, it is not clear that placing autistic children with nonhandicapped children of equivalent nonverbal mental age provides
the same context for peer interaction as placing normally developing children with
age-mates, if the autistic children are less verbal and significantly older than their

playmates. However, matching on nonverbal mental age, chronological age, *and* verbal skills is often simply not possible. Decisions have to be made that mean compromising some aspect of "equivalence," which in turn requires making a value judgment as to the most important variables in defining either a "peer" or a potential friend (Lord, 1984). This is particularly important in clinical research, where standard practice may dictate matching on nonverbal IQ or language age, but where similarities in height, interests, or rowdiness may actually be more important equivalents for potential friends than standardized test scores.

Lack of Familiarity and Experience

Autistic children in segregated educational programs may seldom interact with nonhandicapped children (other than perhaps siblings). Thus, their interactions with nonhandicapped children may be confounded by unfamiliarity with specific peers and lack of experience in "peer" situations in general. In fact, when placed in dyads with unfamiliar schoolmates, autistic children interacted less and stayed farther away from the unfamiliar nonhandicapped peers than they did from autistic classmates (Lord, 1984).

From a more positive perspective, several studies have shown increases in the amount of interaction in a classroom group (McHale, 1983) and in dyads (Lord, 1984; Lord & Hopkins, 1986) between autistic and nonhandicapped playmates as a function of time spent together, without direct instruction or specific programming. These gains are not surprising, given similar effects of familiarity for nonhandicapped children, especially those of preschool age (Doyle, Connolly, & Rivest, 1980; Holmberg, 1980). Autistic children who are strongly influenced by familiarity may be showing responsiveness to a "normal" social variable, but in ways that differ from the responses of other children. It is thus important to know whether the behaviors that differentiate autistic children from others are general in nature or a particular response to a variable such as lack of familiarity. Lack of experience in specific situations, as opposed to lack of familiarity with particular children, may also be a significant variable in any study in which autistic children are put in a situation they have encountered less frequently than other children.

Our day camp data allowed us to compare the effects of familiarity gained over 1- and 2-week sessions across diagnostic and age groups. For day camps during both years, increases in interaction over time were greatest for all ages of autistic children, with the youngest groups of nonhandicapped and behavior-disordered children (ages 6–8 years) also showing significant amounts of change (Lord, in press). Interactions increased both between autistic youngsters and other autistic children and between them and nonhandicapped children. Changes did not seem to be related to whether the autistic children had been in day camp before, suggesting a fairly specific effect of familiarity rather than a more general effect of experience.

Lack of Basic Social Skills

It is often assumed that even if they were given repeated opportunities to be with familiar, appropriately selected peers, autistic children would still interact less than other children. This low rate of interaction is often explicitly or implicitly thought to be related to deficits in basic social skills. That is, autistic children are assumed not to interact because they lack the prerequisite communicative skills (i.e., eye contact, social language) to do so. This may be the case. However, the reverse may also be true: It may be possible to account for what appear to be deficits in specific social behaviors by an extremely low rate of interaction.

For example, in a recent paper by Attwood *et al.* (1988), autistic children, when they were interacting, used instrumental gestures at the same rate as other children. However, autistic children produced a far lower absolute number of gestures, presumably because they spent so little time interacting. This finding is particularly important, since any count of isolated social behaviors is likely to be reduced in frequency, at least in part because the overall rate of social interaction itself is so low. Thus, although it may be tempting to conclude that because autistic children do not communicate nonverbally (i.e., using gestures) as much as do other children, they have few interactions, the reverse may be equally true. That is, a child who has very few interactions has few appropriate contexts for nonverbal communication, and so may be limited in opportunities to use the communication skills he or she does possess. The same may be true for use of language. Many nonverbal behaviors are used primarily, at least by adults, to modify language (Jaffe, 1977) rather than to substitute for it. Someone who talks a great deal is more likely to gesture than someone who is silent.

Thus, the finding that an autistic child does not gesture may be accounted for by his or her rare use of language, rather than seen as a specific deficit. Theoretically, one could test this proposition further by comparing the production of gesture in autistic children to nonautistic severely language-impaired children (which is what Attwood and colleagues did with mentally handicapped children). In fact, social interaction (linguistic or not), at least in studies to date, has generally been much less frequent in autistic groups than in comparison groups (Rutter & Bartak, 1973). In addition, autistic children have generally been found to show more *severe* language deficits than other groups, so that unless children are matched on pragmatic performance, differences in nonverbal behaviors due to language use cannot be ruled out completely.

Implications for Further Research

Although results from no single study are conclusive, the available studies as a whole seem to suggest two conclusions about the absolute frequency of interactions between autistic youngsters and other children. First, when compared to control groups, autistic children show a lower rate of interaction with peers in natural settings than do normally developing or some behavior-disordered children (Attwood *et al.*, 1988; Lord, in press). Second, familiarity and perhaps experience have a significant effect on the amount of interaction that takes place, at least between school-age autistic children and nonhandicapped children (Lord, 1984; Lord & Hopkins, 1986; McHale, 1983). It is possible that in some cases, the effect of familiarity is even greater for interactions involving autistic children than for other children (Lord, in press).

Three additional comments are in order. First, though the combined evidence is convincing, no single study controlled *all* of the relevant variables. That is, no study compared autistic children's interactions with familiar, nonhandicapped peers to the interactions of matched controls in the same setting. The day camp studies came closest to this goal, but even then one could argue that although familiarity with the other children was controlled (i.e., all the children were unfamiliar), the autistic children had less experience in a group setting than the normally developing children (although this was also the case for the IQ-matched behavior-disordered children). Since the social experiences of many children with autism and other developmental and psychiatric disorders are limited, finding a setting for observation of interactions with nonhandicapped peers that is equivalent in experience across diagnostic groups can be very difficult. Home observations of interactions with siblings might be one way to address this issue, but would introduce other confounding factors.

Second, since familiarity and experience have an effect on the *amount* of social behavior of autistic children, careful controls must be instituted when observing such interactions. To place youngsters with autism in a new type of interaction (with which they have had little experience) and to reach conclusions from this interaction about their general social deficits is not appropriate. Furthermore, results from the dyad studies (Hopkins & Lord, 1982; Lord, 1984; Lord & Hopkins, 1986) and the day camp studies (Lord, in press) showed increases in amount of interaction continuing into the second and sometimes third week of daily interactions, even with no specific intervention. Thus, very brief baseline observations (used before some kind of formal treatment is introduced) are not sufficient to rule out effects of familiarity in accounting for "treatment effects."

Third, increases in the amount of interaction that occurred with familiarity between autistic and nonhandicapped children may have been due to changes in the behavior of the nonhandicapped children. Results from the dyad studies suggest that, in part, this was the case, at least for the particular circumstance where nonhandicapped children were explicitly recruited to "help autistic children learn to play" (Lord, 1984; Lord & Hopkins, 1986). Over the course of 2 weeks of daily 15-minute dyadic interactions with autistic children, 10- to 12-year-old nonhandicapped children consistently came to make more initiations and to use more objects and other nonverbal modes of communication with their autistic partners than they had before. In turn, over time, all of the autistic children in the study responded to an increased percentage of initiations. However, only a few autistic children increased *their* level of initiation. Thus, familiarity affected both nonhandicapped children and autistic children, but in different ways. This finding is not surprising, particularly since in this case the "tasks" presented to the two diagnostic groups were somewhat different. However, it illustrates the need to consider the meaning of such concepts as "familiarity" separately for autistic children and any controls within a particular study. This finding also illustrates a point to be discussed later: namely, the need to treat responsiveness as a separate dimension of social skill from initiation.

Structure and Amount of Interaction

Besides familiarity and experience, other factors have been shown to affect the amount of social interaction autistic children exhibit with other children. Each of these factors has to do with "structure," operationally defined here as the extent to which clear expectations for behavior are communicated. Children made more communicative attempts (although not necessarily directed to peers) in a teacher-directed storytelling session than in less structured groups (McHale, Simeonsson, Marcus, & Olley, 1980). Direct prompts to interact made by teachers to autistic preschool children were also shown to increase both the rate of initiation and response when compared to peer-initiated approaches (Odom & Strain, 1986).

Similarly, numerous studies have shown that peers tutored in advance to initiate, to persist in initiating, and to reinforce the actions of autistic children can produce relatively high rates of interaction with autistic children almost immediately (Lord, 1984; Ragland, Kerr, & Strain, 1978; Strain, Kerr, & Ragland, 1979). The responsiveness of autistic children to such "trained" playmates has been found to generalize to unfamiliar nonhandicapped children trained on the same skills, and to be maintained over at least several weeks. However, little generalization to interactions with "untrained" peers occurred. In fact, there was some indication that autistic children who learned to interact with highly intrusive "trained" peers subsequently had less interaction with "untrained" children than they would have had if simply exposed to untrained children in the first place (Lord, 1984).

Exactly how "structure" increases social interaction is not clear. By simplifying the behavior of the partner, "structure" may act to reduce the cognitive demands on autistic children, which could conceivably make them more comfortable and hence responsive (Lord, 1984), and/or to "free up" their attention or processing capacity so that they can better cope with social "input" (Brownell, 1986). In a recent study (Dewey, Lord, & Magill, 1988), autistic, behavior-disordered, and normally developing children were presented with a variety of materials in dyads with normally developing children. The materials were intended to vary in the structure they provided for play. For example, two sets of materials were designed to elicit functional play: colored sand and colored water, both with a variety of containers. The children were given no particular instructions as to what to do with these materials. Materials for dramatic play included dress-up clothes, musical instruments, hair spray, and makeup with mirrors, so that the children could play at being punk rock stars. There were also materials for construction (i.e., various types of bricks and blocks) and standard table games, such as air hockey and board games. Dependent variables consisted of seven subjective rating scales based on work by Sroufe and colleagues (Pancake & Sroufe, 1984) and designed to rate qualitative aspects of peer interaction.

Type of material affected almost every aspect of the interaction rated for children in all diagnostic groups. For example, the symmetry of the interaction was highest (i.e., closest to being equal between partners) with the least structured materials (i.e., the colored water and the colored sand). However, the children were rated as having the most fun and being the most involved during games, the most traditionally structured of any of the tasks. Social play was rated as being most complex during games and a construction task, and least complex during play with dramatic and functional materials (Dewey *et al.*, 1988).

Very basic deficits in social skills (such as joint attention) have been hypothesized as underlying the social limitations of children with autism (Mundy & Sigman, Chapter 1, this volume; Mundy, Sigman, Ungerer, & Sherman, 1986). Structure may also act to increase interaction by helping a child to compensate for these deficits. An autistic child may be able to join in working on a very structured task with other children, and thus can join in the interaction without having to determine on his or her own the focus of the other children's attention or to coordinate his or her behavior with that of the other children except around object use. Of course, this assumes that the task is within the range of skill and comprehension of the autistic child. If the cognitive demands of the task are high, then the effect may actually be the reverse.

In summary, increases in the amount of social interaction of autistic children have been linked to increased structure provided by adult direction, peer training, or selection of tasks. These factors may operate by reducing the need for appropriate basic social behaviors, particularly joint attention and initiation, and/or by providing shared, clearly defined tasks. Thus, besides familiarity and experience, structure also appears as a significant variable that must be considered in the study of social deficits in autism. Higher-order social factors must be considered as well. For example, autistic children may communicate their emotions less expressively not only because they have difficulties in emotional expression, but also because they do not have the same emotional attachments or friendships with their peers as one would expect in other children (and so have no one to communicate these feelings to), or because they do not feel exactly the same emotions in the first place. Neither "top-down" nor "bottom-up" theories can be easily rejected.

THE CONCEPT OF INTENTION

Defining a "Spontaneous" Initiation

We have discussed the difficulty in deciding which comes first—deficits in specific communicative behaviors, low rates of interaction, or lack of higher-order relationships. Trying to define when an autistic person produces a truly spontaneous social overture with intent to initiate is in some ways an even more circular process.

In particular, over the last few years, we have been interested in studying the initiations made by autistic children and adolescents. Our focus has been on peer-directed behavior, but our interest is more generally in overtures that do not have an object-getting or environmental goal, but seem to be social in motivation. Earlier research suggested that in autistic children, the short-term and long-term development of the ability and motivation to make spontaneous social approaches to peers was quite separate in many ways from changes in responses to the acts of other children (Lord, 1984). Although many factors have been shown to affect the responsiveness of autistic children, few of these same measures resulted in changes in the rate or quality of initiations to peers. In fact, generally, the rate of spontaneous initiation was so low that only global judgments or anecdotal comments could be made to describe the nature of these behaviors.

However, a discussion of initiations depends greatly on one's definition of them. For example, even a simple decision as to the time necessary between two behaviors for the second action to be treated as an initiation rather than a response to the first behavior has significant implications. Strain (1983) required only a 3-second interval between behaviors and found "initiations" occurring at a much higher rate than either Schafer, Egel, and Neef (1984), who used a 10-second interval, or Lord and Hopkins (1986), who used a 15-second interval. Of course, there were other differences in definition as well. However, though the difference between 3 seconds and 15 seconds sounds minor, the social implications are quite marked (Jaffe, 1977).

Similarly, in a recent paper, Odom and Strain (1986) found that autistic children in a teacher-antecedent condition, in which a teacher prompted them to initiate to another child, made more overtures than autistic children in a peer initiation condition, where the teacher prompted the peer. To be considered is whether the "approaches" of the autistic children in the teacher-antecedent condition were in fact initiations or whether they were child *responses* to *teacher* initiations.

Attributing the Intent to Initiate

An even more complex question in any serious attempt to define "initiation" is that of intent. Following Asher (1983), we have used in our definition of an initiation the imperfect criteria of spontaneity, observability, and a change in ongoing behavior. Thus, to be considered an initiation, a child's action has to be a *spontaneous* (defined by time and lack of prompting; see below), *observable* attempt *to begin an interaction* with another child. However, a subjective decision is clearly required as to whether or not the child *intends* to begin an interaction.

Decisions as to whether or not an initiation has occurred have been made with high reliability (Lord, 1984; Magill, 1987). However, this reliability has been achieved by deliberately specifying behaviors that are necessary to meet the research criteria for an initiation. At the same time, other criteria in attributing an attempt to initiate could be equally if not more valid. Let us consider some examples below.

Cazden (1977) proposed that to conclude that a child has intent to communicate requires co-occurring behavioral features that are observable and differentiable from other behaviors and to which a communicative intent can be attributed. Harding and Golinkoff (1979) suggested even more specific criteria for very young children. That is, intent to communicate regarding an object can be assumed in a prelinguistic child when the child (1) looks directly at the recipient; (2) gestures or looks at an object; (3) persists in this behavior until the "goal" is reached; *and* (4) terminates this behavior once the "goal" is reached.

The case of a child attempting to communicate about an object is a relatively clear one, because manipulation of the object can be observed somewhat more easily than more idiosyncratic, often fleeting social behaviors involving only persons. "Distal" communicative acts (including speech and variation of eye gaze) are more easily characterized in terms of intent than "proximal" ones (e.g., shifts in posture). In part, this may be because actions that take place over space include a component of getting attention that is often more easily observable to a third party than those where attention is already jointly directed.

Implications of a Particular Definition of Intent

As noted earlier, the aim in our research was to study the *quality* of such initiations, rather than the quantity. Thus, the concept of initiations needed to be operationalized to include those overtures that were not necessarily "perfect in form," but did seem to indicate intent. On the other hand, we did not want to attribute intent where it did not exist. Some minimal criteria for observable behaviors were necessary in order to obtain reliability across observers.

Our working definition of an initiation was a deliberate, observable attempt to begin an interaction (Asher, 1983), as characterized by *at least two* of any of the following behaviors (Magill, 1987; Magill & Lord, 1988):

1. Overt, whole-body movement toward the recipient (i.e., approach).
2. Looking at recipient.
3. Looking at object related to the presumably intended activity.
4. Use of object directed toward the recipient (e.g., showing).
5. Smiling.
6. Gesture.
7. Speech directed to recipient (if speech included a specific reference to an initiation, this was the only behavior considered to be sufficient on its

own to score as an initiation, without requiring another of the behaviors above).

In this context, except for speech, it was felt that any isolated incidence of the behaviors above could not be judged as a sufficient indication of *deliberate* intent to communicate.

Initiations were coded through direct observation, and then codings were confirmed (and the duration of the interaction was measured) by watching videotapes the same day. A random list of children's names across the three diagnostic groups was used to target individual children, who were then observed in free play at the day camp until they made an initiation, or for up to 7 minutes if they did not. Following 20 seconds of no interaction, as soon as a child gave any indication that he or she might make an overture to another child, the child's behavior was coded on-line until he or she received a response from the "recipient" or stopped the overture. Behaviors were coded in sequence as they changed, except that there was no attempt made to place in order behaviors that occurred within 3-second intervals. Direction of gaze (at recipient, at object, or away) was always coded. Other behaviors were marked only as they occurred. Thus, one entry of an initiation might consist of "L3VO" to describe a child who, while looking at a ball (L3), bounced it toward another child (O) and called out "Catch!" (V). The child's behavior preceding the initiation that received a response would also have been coded. For example, if this child first directed his or her gaze to the other child (L1), then looked away and bounced the ball (L2), this would be coded as L1; L2; and then L3VO as the initiation. Using these procedures, after substantial practice, we were able to reach and maintain at least 90% reliability for the occurrence of initiation and the behaviors of which it consisted.

The results were not what was expected. Though developmental differences between younger (ages 6–11 years) and older (ages 12–18 years) children were found, there were *no* simple differences between diagnostic groups (autistic, behavior-disordered, and normally developing children matched on sex and verbal mental age). There were no group differences in the use of any *single* communicative behavior, including direction of gaze, use of speech, or use of gesture alone or in combination with other behaviors. There were also no group differences in the use of multiple or coordinated overtures, which we defined as looking at the recipient plus two other behaviors (Mueller & Brenner, 1977).

Of autistic children's initiations, 33% resulted in ongoing interactions, compared to 42% of behavior-disordered children's approaches and 60% of normally developing children's overtures. Autistic children were more likely to receive no response at all (i.e., for 23% of their initiations) and more likely to be involved in an interaction that ended less than 30 seconds after it started (i.e., 41% of initiations), compared to the normally developing children (14% no response, 26% terminated). Like the autistic children, the behavior-disordered children had a high rate of terminations (46%), but a much lower rate of no response (11%).

Clearly, there *were* problems for the autistic children in getting an interaction started and sustaining it once it had begun. Whether these differences were due to factors other than how the children went about initiation (such as what they did once they were interacting), or whether they were due to factors that we did not measure in the initiation, cannot be determined from these data.

In part, the failure to find differences in the number and type of social behaviors used by the autistic children to initiate was related to variability in the nonhandicapped and behavior-disordered children that was greater than expected (e.g., only 76% and 55%, respectively, of their overtures involved eye contact with the recipient, compared to 63% for autistic children). Small sample sizes may have exacerbated difficulties with variability. However, this finding also serves as a reminder that care must be taken when basing definitions of an overture on an idealized conception of what is "normal."

In studying the initiations of autistic children, the difficulties occur not so much when the children's behavior meets the criteria described above as when it does not. The low rates of spontaneous initiations found in observations of most youngsters with autism have already been discussed. However, on the basis of Harding and Golinkoff's (1979) criteria, the obvious question is whether, if one is using this or a similar definition of "intent," the low rate is due to a lack of communicative intent or to specific deficits in the ability to communicate that intent to the *observer*, as well as to the recipient of the action.

For example, deficits in particular social behaviors could account for a somewhat reduced rate of initiation. Specifically, according to Harding and Golinkoff's (1979) criteria for attributing intent, "overtures" made without eye contact would not be classified as acts with communicative intent. This would be the case even if the failure to use direct gaze was not specific to people or people's faces, but rather a general tendency for autistic children to use peripheral vision or not to look at anything in particular (Mirenda, Donnellan, & Yoder, 1983).

The initiation/day camp study described earlier provides some evidence against the notion that lack of eye contact accounted for artificially low rates of initiation, because overtures without eye contact could be categorized as initiations on the basis of other criteria. In fact, no simple difference in the use of gaze during initiations was found between autistic youngsters and matched controls. However, as noted earlier, the definition of "direction of gaze" may have been so broad as to miss subtleties of eye contact apparent to the actual recipient of the initiation. Thus, although it can be stated that low rates of initiation were not due to differences in direction of gaze, it cannot be stated that no subtle differences in looking at faces differentiated autistic from other groups of children.

A second possibility is that autistic children, rather than lacking communicative intent, produce fewer different social behaviors when making initiations, both overall and at any specific time, and so fail to gesture, vocalize, or vary direction of gaze (to objects or goals) along with eye contact. Again, this would result in actions that may be intended communicatively not being coded as such by criteria such as ours or Harding and Golinkoff's (1979). Research with nonhandicapped infants and toddlers has indicated that the use of multiple communicative acts is a skill that gradually develops over the first few years of life (Brownell, 1986; Eckerman, 1979). Thus, delays in this ability in autistic children might coincide with delays in related skills such as language comprehension, without ever requiring any assumption of deviance (Wing & Gold, 1979).

Given the floor set by the criteria of two behaviors necessary to be called an initiation, no differences in the number of behaviors used per initiation or the number of initiations composed of more than two behaviors were found in our observations of spontaneous initiations of high-functioning, school-age autistic children. However, results might be quite different for younger and/or lower-functioning children.

The opposite problem can also arise. That is, if the operational definition of initiation is set too specifically, then only "high-quality" initiations will be noted. For example, one may erroneously conclude that there are differences in the rate of interaction but not quality, because "low-quality" interactions have been excluded from the count. Consider a child who may intend to initiate interactions by asking repeated questions (e.g., "Is Atlanta in Georgia?", "Did Humpty Dumpty fall off the wall?"). According to many coding paradigms, the child would *not* be scored as initiating if these comments are not directed at anyone in particular, and are not accompanied by changes in eye gaze, gesture, or whole-body approaches. If this child is only scored as initiating when he or she is socially appropriate, he or she may seem indiscriminable from a nonhandicapped child, except for number of initiations.

In fact, though this explanation may be true in part, there is some evidence that it does not completely explain the lack of differences between autistic children and other children in quality of initiation. In our research, during the same free-play periods during which initiations were observed, other observers coded on a 10-second basis, how, where, and with whom each child spent his or her time (Lord, in press). Using these codes, a conglomerate score of "hovering" was generated, which consisted of intervals during which a child was within 6 feet of another child, watching or imitating him or her, but not interacting. Gottman (1977) suggested that hovering is typical of rejected or neglected children identified within normal groups. One might expect high-functioning autistic children to show similar behaviors. One might also speculate that, if the autistic children were producing a high number of incomplete initiations, they might be coded as "hovering" more often than other groups. In fact, the autistic children, as a group and as individuals, were less likely to spend time "hovering" than children in either of the other groups.

Another possibility is that our coding system was not fine enough to discriminate overtures that felt different to the recipients because the categories that were coded were not sufficiently specific, or the description of sequences or timing of behaviors was not sufficiently detailed. One suggestive result emerged during an assessment of which behaviors accompanied different directions of gaze in greetings made by children in the three diagnostic groups. Autistic youngsters were most likely to look directly at another child as they walked toward him or her and least likely to look at the other child when they spoke. This was the reverse of the relationship between direction of gaze and language or approaches for the two other groups. It may be differences of this sort—in relationships between nonverbal behaviors and language—that may provide the best discrimination between older, higher-functioning autistic children and others, in contrast to comparisons of specific isolated behaviors.

Similarly, earlier studies indicated that moderately retarded school-age autistic children had particular difficulty coordinating eye contact and gestures with their vocalizations, which resulted in even quite appropriate simple verbalizations being ineffective in eliciting responses from age-matched peers (Lord, 1984; Lord & Hopkins, 1986). However, although this lack of or poor coordination among social behaviors might be interpreted by people in everyday circumstances as a lack of intent, it would not have accounted completely for low rates of initiation, because even very poorly or unusually coordinated actions would still have been coded under our system.

On the other hand, a lack of coordination among behaviors may have been one factor in the lower rate of *response* that the autistic children received from other children to their overtures. Scoville (1979) has recently argued that the most straightforward method of determining intent is to observe the response of the "recipient." This is, in fact, what the differences in percentage of ongoing interaction represent. However, difficulties in initiating are then confounded with the particular expectations and perceptions of the recipient.

Lack of Communicative Intent versus Alternative Explanations

Lack of communicative intent is one explanation for the underlying cause of limited peer relations in autistic children. An alternative explanation focuses on deficits in the ability to communicate that intent, through specific social behaviors in isolation or in coordination. Of course, in reality, this is not an either–or decision. As discussed earlier, social deficits may well exist on numerous levels (see Lord & Garfin, 1986).

Results from a related study of greetings, also carried out at the day camps using the same groups of subjects, are relevant to this point (Magill, 1987; Magill & Lord, 1988). In this study, a situation was devised so that observations could be made and coded on the spot (using a similar system to that of the initiation study) and videotapes could be made of how autistic, behavior-disordered, and nonhandicapped children behaved when encountering their camp counselors for the first time in the morning on two different days. Each counselor followed a set protocol, so that the initial onus for getting the counselor's attention and initiating a greeting was on the children. If the child did not greet the counselor, the counselor proceeded through a rehearsed series of behaviors that included looking at the child, smiling, and eventually vocalizing. Two sets of instructions were given to the children and counterbalanced over the two days: (1) The children were explicitly told to "go say hi to [counselor's name] in your club room," and (2) they were told only to go to the club room.

In this context, group differences both for categorical data by individual subjects and for means *were* found in the extent to which children used multiple actions in their greetings. Group differences also appeared in how far into their protocol the counselors were required to proceed before the children produced a greeting. There were also differences between diagnostic groups in smiling, but no differences in direction of gaze. Differences in whether or not a vocalization occurred were not possible to assess, because the protocol continued until all children vocalized or made a clear greeting in some other way. Gestures such as waving would have been sufficient without language, but this situation never occurred.

In this study, because the goal of the subjects' action (i.e., producing a greeting) was made explicit (at least in one condition), the *behavioral* component (i.e., the need for two behaviors) could be eliminated from the criteria for attributing intention. Thus, the arbitrary "floor" that had been necessary in the study of spontaneous initiation was avoided. Whether it was this factor that accounted for the differences in findings between the greetings study and the spontaneous initiation study in the use of multiple behaviors, or whether it was other differences in context, we do not know.

Two other characteristics of intentional communication that relate to the coordination and use of multiple behaviors are ritualization and underlying differentiation. "Ritualization" (Prizant & Wetherby, 1985) is the idea that social behaviors are gradually modified into socially acceptable, conventional rituals, such as looking someone in the eye, saying "Hello," and offering a hand to shake upon introduction. It is easier to attribute communicative intent to a child who uses highly conventional rituals in social occasions than to a child whose behavior is idiosyncratic. Research has shown that autistic children may use a variety of actions, including self-stimulatory behavior, delayed echolalia, and even self-injurious behavior, to get or maintain attention. Whether these behaviors are used with communicative intent depends on the individual and on one's definition of communicative intent, but, to the extent that they are different from conventional, ritualized forms of initiation, they become difficult to interpret. In our day camp data, we were surprised, especially during the study of spontaneous initiations, by how often the behaviors of the normally developing children were *not* ritualized. Rather, the behavior of the normally developing children seemed to reflect a large number of factors in the immediate and long-term contexts. Greetings were more conventional, especially for the autistic children, than were peer-directed initiations, but still showed more variability than we had expected.

"Differentiation" refers to context-dependent changes in social behaviors. Thus, the intent to communicate is more easily attributed when a child uses different behaviors on different occasions than when he or she is limited to a few types of multipurpose actions (e.g., a newborn whose most frequent behavior, social or otherwise, is to cry or kick). There is some evidence to suggest that as individuals, youngsters with autism have more limited repertoires of social or communicative behavior than other children (Attwood *et al.*, 1988). Again, what is not clear is whether these limits are intrinsic to the children or whether they have to do with the kinds of situations they experience or with cognitive factors that affect the meanings different social encounters have for them (Baron-Cohen, Leslie, & Frith, 1986).

Another consideration in attributing communicative intent has been the child's behavior when he or she receives no response. Various authors have argued that communicative intent can be inferred when a child persists in the behavior until he or she gets a response (Harding & Golinkoff, 1979; Prizant & Wetherby, 1985). Similarly, if the child modifies the behavior when he or she does not receive a response and terminates the behavior when he or she does receive one, intent (to get a response at least) is more easily inferred. It is on the basis of such contingencies that intent (at least to get attention) has been attributed to behavior such as self-injury or self-stimulation (Lovaas, Schaefer, & Simmons, 1965). Research with learning-disabled children (Wollner, 1983) has shown them to be equally persistent when faced with no response but less skilled at modifying their behaviors than other children.

Persistence and the ability to modify one's behaviors are both valuable skills. They are skills that may well differentiate autistic children from other children. However, it also seems important to remember that the current significance of these skills lies in their effect on the *observers'* ability to infer intention, not in any necessary relationship between them and the *capacity* for communicative intent. That is, a child may well make an attempt to communicate with intent, but then for other reasons may fail to persist in this attempt or fail to try alternative strategies to reach his or her goal. The failure to persist or modify does not *necessarily* imply a lack of intent, even though the act of persisting or modifying makes the attribution of intent easier.

A final variable in considering lack of communicative intent as an explanation for low rates of peer initiation is the possibility that at least some autistic children are less motivated in general than other children (Ferster, 1961). Thus, a lack of intent to communicate would be part of a more general lack of intent to do anything. Although this seems unlikely to be true for *all* autistic children, some data from the free-play observations during the day camps support this notion to some extent. Autistic children were consistently more likely than other children to do absolutely nothing, as well as to engage in very simple, "functional" play (e.g., tapping things, ripping the pages of a book) (Lord, in press). In fact, the autistic children were as discriminable from other children by how they spent their nonsocial time as by how they interacted. It is worth noting that these were higher-functioning autistic children (with mean IQs close to 90), and were matched to the other groups on verbal mental age, so these deficits were not due to low intelligence.

Similarly, in another study of dyads that always included one nonhandicapped and either an autistic, a behavior-disordered, or a nonhandicapped child, autistic children were more often characterized by low involvement in both social and nonsocial play than either of the other two groups (Dewey et al., 1988). For some autistic children, who produce far lower rates of any sort of meaningful behavior than other children, then a lack of communicative behavior might be seen as part of a more general deficit in cognition, attention, and/or motivation, rather than as a specific deficit in social or communication skills. However, it seems unlikely that this general statement will hold true for all autistic children.

CONCLUSIONS

The purpose of this chapter has been to discuss some of the theoretical and methodological issues involved in studies of spontaneous social behavior of autistic youngsters, particularly with peers. The focus has been on issues that arise in studying a low-frequency behavior and questions concerning how to define intent to interact in this socially deficient population.

One of the underlying themes throughout this chapter has been the relative ease of showing autistic children to be "worse" or to have fewer social behaviors than other children. Developmental or possibly treatment-related increases in behaviors are also relatively easy to identify, compared to the process of beginning to discern where the deficits truly lie. The need to use both "bottom-up" strategies of asking how deficits in very specific social skills (e.g., joint attention) might contribute to overall impairment, and "top-down" strategies of asking how general deficits in personal relations or cognition might be reflected in specific social skills (Attwood et al., 1988; Baron-Cohen et al., 1986; Hobson, Chapter 2, this volume), has been stressed.

In addition, a certain degree of common sense seems in order. Given the very low absolute numbers of occurrences of behaviors in many studies (see Attwood et al., 1988; O'Neill & Lord, 1982; Ungerer & Sigman, 1981), one has to be careful not to attribute qualitative differences to what are differences between very small numbers. As fellow researchers, we can respect the amount of work that has gone into accumulating such data. We can acknowledge that these data probably reflect a much greater proportion of autistic children's total behavior than more traditional studies of nonhandicapped children. On the other hand, very small numbers have inherent problems with reliability. If autistic children are only rarely interacting or communicating, it seems worth wondering what they are doing the remainder of the time, as well as analyzing what they do when they do interact.

Altogether, these findings suggest the need for a model of social functioning in autism that includes recognition of both "bottom-up" and "top-down" effects and the transactional nature of social relationships (Lord, in press). There is also a need for constant awareness of the influence of factors other than the targeted social skills, which may range from highly related but slightly different aspects of development (such as emotional growth and social cognition) to theoretically unrelated behaviors that still may have major social consequences (such as self-stim-ulatory behavior, noise level, or odd intonation patterns). Knowledge both of in-dividual social features and of how they interact is gradually accumulating, though it sometimes feels as if the more we learn the more we need to know. On the other hand, the practical offshoots of such research are invaluable. In the mean-while, they are sufficient to sustain interest in understanding the nature of the deficits that underlie the limited peer relations in autism.

References

Asher, S. R. (1983). Social competence and peer status: Recent advances and future directions. *Child Development, 54*, 1427–1434.

Attwood, A., Frith, U., & Hermelin, B. (1988). The understanding and use of interpersonal gesture by autistic and Down's syndrome children. *Journal of Autism and Developmental Disorders, 18*, 241–258.

Baltaxe, C. A. M., & Simmons, J. Q. (1983). Communication deficits in the adolescent and adult autistic. *Seminars in Speech and Language, 4*, 27–42.

Baron-Cohen, S., Leslie, N. M., & Frith, U. (1986). Mechanical behavioral and intentional under-standing of picture stories in autistic children. *British Journal of Developmental Psychology, 4*, 113–125.

Brownell, C. A. (1986). Convergent developments: Cognitive-developmental correlates of growth in infant/toddler peer skills. *Child Development, 57*, 275–286.

Cantwell, D. P., Baker, L., & Rutter, M. (1977). Families of autistic and dysphasic children: II. Mothers' speech to the children. *Journal of Autism and Childhood Schizophrenia, 7*, 313–317.

Cazden, C. B. (1977). The question of intent. In M. Lewis & L. A. Rosenblum (Eds.), *Interaction, conversation and the development of language* (pp. 309–313). New York: Wiley.

Dewey, D., Lord, C., & Magill, J. (1988). Qualitative assessment of the effect of play materials in dyadic peer interactions of children with autism. *Canadian Journal of Psychology, 42*, 242–260.

Doyle, A. B., Connolly, J., & Rivest, L. P. (1980). The effect of playmate familiarity on the social interactions of young children. *Child Development, 51*, 217–223.

Eckerman, C. O. (1979). The human infant in social interaction. In R. B. Cairns (Ed.), *Social interaction: Methods, analysis and illustrations*. Hillsdale, NJ: Erlbaum.

Ferster, C. B. (1961). Positive reinforcement and behavioral deficits of autistic children. *Child Development, 32*, 437–447.

Gottman, J. M. (1977). Toward a definition of social isolation in children. *Child Development, 48*, 513–517.

Harding, C., & Golinkoff, R. M. (1979). The origins of intentional vocalizations in prelinguistic infants. *Child Development, 50*, 33–40.

Holmberg, M. C. (1980). The development of social interchange patterns from 12 to 24 months. *Child Development, 51*, 448–456.

Hopkins, J. M., & Lord, C. (1982). The social behavior of autistic children with younger and same-age nonhandicapped peers. In D. Park (Ed.), *Proceedings from the international meetings of the National Society for Autistic Children* (pp. 83–84). Boston: National Society for Autistic Children.

Howlin, P. (1986). An overview of social behavior in autism. In E. Schopler & G. Mesibov (Eds.), *Social behavior in autism* (pp. 103–132). New York: Plenum.

Jaffe, J. (1977). Markovian communication rhythms: Their biological significance. In M. Lewis & L. A. Rosenblum (Eds.), *Interaction, conversation and the development of language* (pp. 319–325.) New York: Wiley.

Lord, C. (1984). The development of peer relations in children with autism. In F. J. Morrison, C. Lord & D. P. Keating (Eds.), *Applied developmental psychology* (pp. 165–229). New York: Academic Press.

Lord, C. (in press). Treatment of communication and social deficits in adolescents with autism. In R. J. McMahon & R. D. Peters (Eds.), *Behavior disorders of adolescence: Research, intervention, and policy in clinical and school settings.* New York: Plenum.

Lord, C., & Garfin, D. (1986). Facilitating peer-directed communication in autistic children and adolescents. *Australian Journal of Human Communication Disorders, 14,* 33–49.

Lord, C., & Hopkins, J. M. (1986). The social behavior of autistic children with younger and same age nonhandicapped peers. *Journal of Autism and Developmental Disorders, 16,* 449–462.

Lovaas, O. I., Schaefer, B., & Simmons, J. O. (1965). Experimental studies in childhood schizophrenia. *Journal of Experimental Research and Personality, 1,* 99–109.

Magill, J. (1987). *The nature of social deficits of children with autism.* Unpublished doctoral dissertation, University of Alberta.

Magill, J., & Lord, C. (1988). *An observational study of greetings of autistic, behavior-disordered and normally developing children.* Manuscript submitted for publication.

McHale, S. M. (1983). Social interactions of autistic and non-handicapped children during free play. *American Journal of Orthopsychiatry, 53,* 81–91.

McHale, S. M., Simeonsson, R. J., Marcus, L. M., & Olley, J. G. (1980). The social and symbolic quality of autistic children's communication. *Journal of Autism and Developmental Disorders, 10,* 299–310.

Mirenda, P. L., Donnellan, A. M., & Yoder, D. E. (1983). Gaze behavior: A new look at an old problem. *Journal of Autism and Developmental Disorders, 13,* 397–410.

Mueller, E., & Brenner, J. (1977). The origins of social skills and interaction among playgroup toddlers. *Child Development, 48,* 854–861.

Mundy, P., Sigman, M., Ungerer, J., & Sherman, T. (1986). Defining the contribution of nonverbal communication measures. *Journal of Child Psychology and Psychiatry, 27,* 657–669.

Odom, S. L., & Strain, P. S. (1986). Comparison of peer-initiation and teacher antecedent interventions for promoting reciprocal social interaction of autistic preschoolers. *Journal of Applied Behavior Analysis, 19,* 59–71.

O'Neill, P. I., & Lord, C. (1982). Functional and semantic characteristics of child-directed speech of autistic children. In D. Park (Ed.), *Proceedings from the international meetings of the National Society for Autistic Children* (pp. 79–82). Boston: National Society for Autistic Children.

Pancake, V. R., & Sroufe, L. A. (1984, July). *Qualitative assessment of dyadic peer-relationships in preschool: A new system of rating scales.* Paper presented at the 2nd International Conference on Interpersonal Relationships, Madison, WI.

Prizant, R. M., & Wetherby, A. M. (1985). Intentional communicative behavior of children with autism: Theoretical and practical issues. *Australian Journal of Human Communication Disorders, 13,* 21–59.

Ragland, E. V., Kerr, M. M., & Strain, P. S. (1978). Effects of social initiations on the behavior of withdrawn autistic children. *Behavior Modification, 2,* 565–578.

Rutter, M. (1978). Diagosis and definition. In M. Rutter & E. Schopler (Eds.), *Autism: A reappraisal of concepts and treatment* (pp. 1–26). New York: Plenum.

Rutter, M., & Bartak, L. (1973). Special educational treatment of autistic children: A comparative study. II. Follow-up findings and implications for services. *Journal of Child Psychology and Psychiatry, 14,* 241–270.

Rutter, M., & Schopler, E. (1988). Autism and pervasive developmental disorders. In M. Rutter, A. H. Tuma, & I. S. Lann (Eds.), *Assessment and diagnosis in child psychopathology* (pp. 408–434). New York: Guilford Press.

Schafer, M. S., Egel, A. L., & Neef, N. A. (1984). Training mildly handicapped peers to facilitate in the social interaction skills of autistic children. *Journal of Applied Behavior Analysis, 17,* 461–476.

Scoville, R. (1979). Development of the intention to communicate: The eye of the beholder. In L. Feagans, C. Garvey, R. Golinkoff, M. T. Greenberg, C. Harding, & J. N. Bohannon (Eds.), *The origins and growth of communication* (pp. 109–135). Norwood, NJ: Ablex.

Strain, P. S. (1983). Identification of social skill curriculum targets for severely handicapped children in mainstream preschools. *Applied Research in Mental Retardation, 4,* 369–382.

Strain, P. S., & Cooke, T. P. (1976). An observational investigation of two elementary-age autistic children during free play. *Psychology in the Schools, 13,* 82–91.

Strain, P. S., Kerr, M. M., & Ragland, E. V. (1979). Effects of peer-mediated social initiations and promoting/reinforcement procedures on the social behavior of autistic children. *Journal of Autism and Developmental Disorders, 9,* 41–54.

Ungerer, J. A., & Sigman, M. (1981). Symbolic and language comprehension in autistic children. *Journal of the American Academy of Child Psychiatry, 20,* 318–337.

Wing, L. (1976). Diagnosis, clinical description, and prognosis. In L. Wing (Ed.), *Early childhood autism* (pp. 15–64). Oxford: Pergamon Press.

Wing, L., & Gould, J. (1979). Severe impairments of social interaction and associated abnormalities in children: Epidemiology and classification. *Journal of Autism and Developmental Disorders, 9,* 11–29.

Wollner, S. G. (1983). Communicating intentions: How well do language-impaired children do? *Topics in Language Disorders, 4,* 1–14.

CHAPTER 15

Preschool Curriculum for Children with Autism
Addressing Early Social Skills

J. GREGORY OLLEY
SUSAN E. STEVENSON
The Groden Center, Inc., Providence, Rhode Island

Interest in autism has shown a growth spurt in recent years. Growth is evident not only in interest, but also in research, services, and public awareness. Much about autism remains unknown, but the importance of several factors has become clearer.

All definitions of autism stress difficulties in social behavior and related problems in communication. Research and practice point to the importance of teaching social and communication skills in school. This chapter reviews approaches to teaching social and related skills to young children, emphasizing curricula that have received support from research and have been demonstrated to be effective. The effective elements of these curricula, as well as the areas of unsolved problems, point to important conclusions and to areas for further research.

WHAT IS MEANT BY "SOCIAL SKILLS"?

The social unresponsiveness and difficulties in relating to others that Kanner (1943) described are part of a larger picture of pervasive social deficits. Virtually all practical skills have a social component. Therefore, it is important to view social skills as a consideration that cuts across all curricular areas. Many descriptions of curricula include individual social behaviors, such as responding to one's name, looking at others, and shaking hands, but skills taught in isolation seldom generalize to natural contexts.

In order to avoid this problem, one may define "social skills" broadly as all of those behaviors needed to be successful in the presence of others or to affect the behavior of others. Crucial behaviors in interaction with others include following social rules, taking cues from others, initiating interaction, and responding appropriately. Important skills that affect the likelihood of others' being social include grooming, hygiene, posture, and facial expression. Such a broad definition overlaps with language or communication and includes the related skill of good judgment. It is a common comment of teachers and parents that children with autism have many skills that they do not use. When the social elements are taught as part of all skills, they can be applied more effectively when they are needed.

WHAT IS MEANT BY "CURRICULUM"?

When the term "curriculum" is used in regular education, it typically refers to a clearly specified and sequenced description of the information to be taught. Specific curricula usually address traditional academic areas, as well as such topics as the arts and physical education. Disagreement about curriculum is probably as old as the field of education, but setting curricular priorities for children who have severe problems in so many areas of learning and behavior is especially difficult.

By the very nature of autism, one would expect that teaching social behavior should be a prominent part of any curriculum. In fact, when Itard described his first curriculum for Victor, the Wild Boy of Aveyron, three of his first five goals were social (Itard, 1894/1962). The educational progress of the last 100 years has confirmed Itard's wisdom. Social behavior is still regarded as very important, but only very recently has research helped to refine curricula for children with autism.

CONSIDERATIONS IN DEVELOPING A
SOCIAL SKILLS CURRICULUM

The development of curricula for early social skills that involve appropriate observing, responding to, and affecting one's environment has been influenced by several viewpoints. The viewpoints are not mutually exclusive, but do stress different considerations in approaching curriculum development. These considerations include (1) developmental principles of normal child growth, (2) learning characteristics of children with autism, (3) environmental components affecting learning and performance, and (4) social validity of curriculum targets.

Understanding Normal Child Development

The sequence in which skills are acquired in normal child development has been a major influence on curriculum for young children (Powell, 1982), including children with severe handicaps (Mori & Neisworth, 1983). In this approach, it is assumed that children with learning problems benefit from following the normal sequence, although their progress may be slow. The developmental approach is a strong theme in preschool curricula for children who have autism and severe handicaps. During the younger years, the discrepancy is small between the skills of children with and without handicaps. The normal developmental sequence provides a logical guide for curriculum.

Most preschool assessment instruments are based upon normal development, and the results of such assessment—the areas of skill deficit—help in the devising of an individualized curriculum. This developmental approach based on objective assessment should result in a well-structured and clearly defined instructional plan.

In recent years, clinicians have begun to examine additional factors to guide them in curriculum planning. These considerations include (1) the individual learning characteristics of children with handicaps (e.g., primary sensory channels used to learn, stimulus overselectivity); (2) the environments and social contexts in which skills are taught and used (e.g., the expectations and cues found in classrooms, home, and community); and (3) the relevance of the curriculum targets (e.g., how useful particular skills are to the child presently and in the future). One of the primary considerations for curricula, in addition to developmental principles, is an understanding of the unique way in which children with autism learn and respond.

Learning Characteristics of Children with Autism

The unusual learning characteristics of children with autism have been noted by researchers representing both behavioral (e.g., Koegel, Rincover, & Egel, 1982) and cognitive-developmental viewpoints (e.g., Lord & O'Neill, 1980). These writers emphasize the importance of a careful assessment of each child's strengths and weaknesses in order to plan an individualized curriculum.

Some examples of areas in which the authors cited above found children with autism to have most difficulty include generalization, imitation, modeling, communication, symbolic representation, and means–ends relationships. The children's relative strengths include rote memory and understanding of physical and spatial properties. Children with this pattern of abilities will clearly have difficulty learning social skills. The abstract and inconsistent nature of social rules presents special problems to children whose strengths are in concrete and visible tasks.

The literature on the nature of autism is extensive, but perhaps one example can illustrate the importance of this information for curriculum development. This example is research on stimulus overselectivity (reviewed by Cook, Anderson, & Rincover, 1982). Learning in both social and nonsocial settings requires attention to complex, multiple stimuli. It requires one to attend to certain relevant pieces of information and to ignore irrelevant stimuli. Children with autism tend to rely rather stubbornly on certain idiosyncratic (and usually irrelevant) cues while ignoring relevant stimuli. The results are persistent patterns of incorrect responses. This problem is quite noticeable in response to social cues, which are complex and often ambiguous. Children who show stimulus overselectivity require a curriculum that makes social cues more obvious and salient and that teaches basic social rules in a consistent manner.

Teaching for Specific Environments

Another consideration in developing a preschool social skills curriculum is the environment that a child is expected to understand and participate in effectively. The previously described considerations have addressed more general guidelines and strategies in curricula. Because one of the characteristics of autism is difficulty in generalizing skills to new situations, clinicians are finding that they must teach specific skills required in particular environments.

To do so, the first step is to observe normally developing young children in preschool, kindergarten, or first grade to determine which social behaviors are essential for success. Children with autism usually lack these crucial skills, and this information can form the basis for an individualized curriculum.

Tremblay, Strain, Hendrickson, and Shores (1980, 1981) used this approach and concluded that assessing children's social behavior in natural settings is more efficient than trying to predetermine social skill priorities. This emphasis in curriculum development identifies and teaches skills known to be needed in each child's school environment. An extension of this approach is to teach to the criteria of the "next educational environment."

Vincent *et al.* (1980) noted that if the goal for early education is to decrease children's later placement in segregated special education, then the curriculum should address skills that are expected of the children in the next least restrictive environment. With this approach, children in the future environment (i.e., kindergarten) are observed, and the social skills of children considered successful are identified and compared to those of children who are less successful in the classroom. Skills are identified as critical when they are performed by the successful group and not by the group with less adaptive behaviors. As before, the children with autism are assessed in relation to this set of skills, and a curriculum is formed around the children's performance discrepancies. Finally, the instructional strategy is to create an environment that closely approximates the next less restrictive setting.

This approach to curriculum development generally leads to identification of skills that are more functionally relevant for the learner. It also allows the learner more time to acquire needed skills before being expected to use them independently. The emphasis on future environments should complement teaching skills needed in current integrated environments (e.g., preschool, home, community).

A final consideration in developing a social skills curriculum goes beyond the identification of specific skills and addresses the issue of the quality or social validity of the instructional targets. In addition to examining skills relevant to the classroom, decisions should be made regarding the skills' cultural relevance outside of the school.

The Social Validity of a Curriculum

Two considerations emerge regarding the assessment and development of social competence in individuals. First, are the curriculum targets judged to be critical or to have a significant social impact by parents, teachers, siblings, peers, and community (Odom & McConnell, 1985)? Second, are the natural social components (i.e., interaction, cues, correction procedures, and consequences) of skills identified that help children sustain positive social behavior (Meyer, McQuarter, & Kiski, 1985)?

Addressing these issues requires additional steps in planning a curriculum. For example, Meyer *et al.* (1985) have determined the social validity of activities by judging their degree of normalization. Concerns in normalization include age-appropriateness, integration, acceptability/attractiveness, flexibility, degree of supervision, longitudinal application, caregiver preferences, and multiple applications. The social skill targets and activities that are identified from this process of assessment are those that are most valued in the child's world, and are thus likely to have great social impact.

Integration of Approaches

Each of the considerations described above suggests a method to define the content of a social skill curriculum. However, they are not necessarily exclusive of one another. Donnellan and Kilman (1986) discussed the importance of integrating approaches to curriculum development to achieve a balance in the important aspects of each theory. Environmental considerations identify content that will be functional for children in specific settings. Developmental theory helps us organize that content into appropriate instructional sequences. Our knowledge of characteristics of autism guides us in developing curriculum that is most interesting and effective. Evaluating the social impact of the content leads to greater validity and social support for the curriculum.

There may be other considerations to be examined when planning a preschool curriculum for children with autism. For instance, in Strain, Odom, and McConnell's (1984) discussion of effectiveness of curriculum, they included the factors noted above, as well as the physical setting, the sex of the target child, the social responsiveness of the peers, and the effects particular behaviors have on them. Once identified, these considerations are organized by translating them into specific curriculum targets that will guide the teacher in planning instructional activities. The targets then define the scope and sequence of the curriculum.

SOCIAL SKILLS CURRICULUM TARGETS

Stowitschek and Powell (1981) analyzed 75 instructional programs that had been published to teach social skills to children with handicaps. Their findings indicated that (1) only a few had behaviorally stated objectives, (2) selected targets were seldom supported by empirical evidence, (3) less than half of the material involved interactions between peers, and (4) over half of the materials focused on skills other than social interaction. This evidence suggests the need to re-evaluate our social skills programs to identify targets that have been demonstrated to be effective in positively influencing others' behaviors and attitudes. The remainder of this section describes social skill targets for preschool children with autism that have emerged from the literature and that are appropriate in light of the factors listed above.

Reducing Problem Behavior

In addition to deficits in social skills, many young children with autism have high rates of inappropriate behavior that interfere with the acquisition of new skills. One approach to social skill development is to eliminate or reduce problem behavior before trying to teach appropriate behavior.

One of the earliest empirical reports of a behavioral treatment of a child with autism is that of "Dicky" (Wolf, Risley, Johnston, Harris, & Allen, 1967; Wolf, Risley, & Meese, 1964). Dicky's treatment began at the age of 3½ and combined the reduction of problem behaviors, such as tantrums, self-injury, and aggression, with the teaching of appropriate social behavior. For instance, Dicky was taught to "pat" other children in his nursery school class instead of pinching them (Wolf *et al.*, 1967). In the last published report of Dicky's progress at age 13 (Nedelman & Sulzbacher, 1972), he was in a regular junior high school class, making good academic and social progress.

Also beginning in the early 1960s, Ivar Lovaas at UCLA conducted a series of studies in which interfering behaviors were punished and appropriate social behaviors reinforced (Lovaas, 1968). In this same vein, two later studies used mild punishment to suppress self-stimulation, and social behavior increased without specific instruction or reinforcement (Koegel & Covert, 1972; Koegel, Firestone, Kramme, & Dunlap, 1974). Recent applications of this approach have combined the suppression of self-stimulation with intensive teaching of social behavior (Epstein, Taubman, & Lovaas, 1985).

A question that arises here is the role that problem behaviors of children with autism play in developing social skills. In a study of mainstreaming a preschool girl with autism, Russo and Koegel (1977) targeted the reduction of the girl's self-stimulation. This behavior was targeted for change because of the wishes of school officials. Strain (1983b) based priorities for behavior change on an analysis of the social status of children with and without handicaps. This analysis indicated that negative behavior resulted in a negative evaluation of children by their peers. This social validity consideration may draw us to the conclusion that reducing maladaptive behaviors of children with autism is a target demanded by peers if the children are to have positive interactions.

Deciding whether to target a problem behavior for reduction, which problems to target, and which methods to use is a complex process. Evans and Meyer (1985) have described a decision model that emphasizes nonaversive strategies and many aspects of the child's ecology. This guide to setting priorities is a helpful balance between the need to reduce excess behavior and the need to build new skills.

Play

Preschool children spend the majority of their time engaged in some form of play. Children learn many early developmental skills from play, such as object classification, means–ends concepts, spatial relationships, speech, gross and fine motor manipulation, and so on. Unfortunately, children with autism almost always have difficulty playing appropriately. Their play may be characterized by nonsocial object fixation or rituals and by isolation from others. Though they may learn various properties of objects, their play typically remains solitary, with social behavior restricted to some onlooking or parallel play (Federlein, Lessen-Firestone, & Elliott, 1982).

Play is also the activity in which interaction with others, particularly peers, occurs most frequently. Many studies have been conducted recently to identify elements of play and the types of play that most frequently result in positive interactions between peers. Finally, environmental variables such as teacher involvement and types of toys have been investigated for their effects on interactions during play.

In 1980, Tremblay *et al.* analyzed the type of play activities that high-rate social interactors engaged in, compared to low-rate social interactors. Following observations of the children's play, activities were categorized into six areas: (1) fantasy, (2) cooperative, (3) game, (4) isolate, (5) parallel, and (6) observer. Results indicated that children with low rates of interaction engaged in more isolate and observer activity, and children with high interaction rates engaged in more cooperative and fantasy activity. For both groups of children, positive interactions occurred most frequently during cooperative and fantasy play. This finding suggested to the authors appropriate activity contexts in which to teach specific play behaviors. The authors also suggested the importance of parallel and onlooker activities as prerequisites or developmental precursors to the later development of interactive behaviors.

Tremblay *et al.* (1981) went on to assess the specific social initiations and responses of normally developing preschool children in an effort to target behaviors for intervention with socially withdrawn children. Their results indicated that peers responded most positively to motor/gestural initiations, including rough-and-tumble play, sharing, assistance, and affection. The verbal/vocal initiations of questions and play organizers were also successful in gaining positive peer responses. Selection of these behaviors as treatment targets for preschoolers with autism may both increase their social skills and raise their sociometric status with their nonhandicapped peers.

As discussed previously, social skills do not occur in isolation. Strain (1983b) emphasized the reciprocal nature of social exchanges and the need to teach effective social responding and initiating. In this study, analysis of the observational data indicated that children who were more positively responsive to social initiations were also higher in sociometric status. Because children with autism frequently respond to others in a negative manner, an important target for these individuals is positive responding.

Environmental events also affect children's play. Interactions may be more likely to occur when particular elements of the environment are manipulated. Selection of toys is important, since they are usually the focus of play. Social toys such as blocks, balls, and puppets have been found to encourage more social interactions than isolate toys such as books, art supplies, and puzzles (Beckman & Kohl, 1984). Teacher behavior also influences children's play with peers. Romanczyk, Diament, Goren, Trunell, and Harris (1975) demonstrated that social play of autistic children could be increased through a passive shaping procedure in a small-group instructional format. The procedure involved moving a child next to another child and placing the target child's hand on the toy the other child was playing with. Shores, Hester, and Strain (1976) found that the most frequent child–child interactions occurred when the teacher structured a sociodramatic play activity but then remained uninvolved in its action. Odom and Strain (1984a) suggested arranging the physical features of the environment so that areas are small and defined, density of children is increased, and materials are prominently displayed and limited in number to facilitate social behavior among peers. These various features of the environment should be analyzed to help select play targets for young children within the social context.

Imitation

Researchers have noted for several years that children with autism are deficient in the imitation skills that characterize early social interaction and learning (e.g., DeMyer *et al.*, 1972; Lovaas, 1968). Furthermore, children with the poorest imitation skills also tend to be very deficient in other social skills (Dawson & Adams, 1984). This finding has influenced treatment efforts from a behavioral perspective for many years, and recently has been the stimulus for treatment from a developmental viewpoint as well.

In several early behavioral studies (e.g., Lovaas, Berberich, Perloff, & Schaeffer, 1966; Risley & Wolf, 1967), young children with autism were taught "generalized imitation." That is, the children were prompted to imitate an adult, and behavior performed in imitation was reinforced. Children learned to do what adults did in the highly structured teaching settings, and this strategy has been extensively used to teach speech (Lovaas, 1977). Although this approach has been very effective in teaching some children to interact with adults, it is only a beginning step toward interacting in natural social situations (Carr, 1982). The early studies demonstrating generalized imitation were criticized for leading to rather robot-like speech and social behavior.

Peck, Apolloni, Cooke, and Raver (1978) taught mentally retarded preschoolers to imitate the play of their nonhandicapped peers through prompting and social reinforcement (i.e., praise, hugs). In this more natural setting, using social rather than food reinforcers, imitation of play not only increased but occurred spontaneously in generalization sessions with no adults present. Many preschools that use peers to help children with autism and other handicaps are based on the premise that imitation will take place and will lead to natural social reinforcers that will facilitate generalization. (See examples described at the end of this chapter.)

More recently, several studies taking a developmental viewpoint have shown that being imitated by an adult is a particularly effective form of social reinforcement for some young children with autism. Rather that teaching children to imitate, Tiegerman and Primavera (1981) imitated the object manipulations of children during free play. They found that imitating the manipulations and the objects used led to increased object manipulation by the children.

In a follow-up study, Tiegerman and Primavera (1984) found that imitation of the object manipulation of six preschool-age autistic children led to increased frequency and duration of eye contact. Dawson and Adams (1984) also imitated the actions of preschool children with autism and found that for children with low levels of imitative ability, this approach was more effective than modeling toy play in eliciting social behavior. Children with higher levels of imitative ability were more social overall, but simultaneous imitation had no more effect than modeling in facilitating their social behavior. Although there is no research on the use of this strategy in classrooms or other natural environments, imitation of children may be an effective way to increase overall social attentiveness. It is an easy, readily available, positive consequence that can be used by adults and peers to facilitate the social behavior of even low-functioning children.

Classroom Readiness Skills

In the Vincent *et al.* (1980) description of curriculum development through identification of criteria in the next educational environment, the authors discussed skills that are required of children in kindergarten classrooms. Their premise was that while specific skills (e.g., shape and color discrimination, classification, counting, alphabet recognition, etc.) are typical screening items for determining kindergarten placement, special educators should not assume that attainment of these skills will make a child successful in the classroom. Instead, a child's acquisition of self-control or awareness of social rules may be more important to academic success.

By analyzing social environments, one can begin to identify behaviors that demonstrate this social awareness and responsiveness. The skills discussed by Vincent *et al.* (1980) include turn taking, quiet sitting, listening to directions, attending, volunteering, and complying. Although these skills are considered within a structured, academic context, they can also be applied to play behavior. When children take turns, attend to each other's actions, contribute, and respond to others' suggestions, play becomes more successful for the participants, and the participants become more reinforcing to each other.

Social Routines

We have discussed the problems that children with autism have in using many of the skills they have learned when those skills are taught in isolation or out of an environmental context. Neel *et al.* (1983) have described the concept of social routines as an alternative approach. An example of a routine is lunch. This activity involves many discrete skills, such as getting to the table, finding the right chair, passing food, and so on. The routine occurs in a predictable sequence, and each discrete activity cues the next event. Neel *et al.*'s rationale for teaching whole routines rather than discrete skills involves two important components: (1) It focuses on the critical effects of behaviors, and (2) the instructional targets and contexts come from the children's environments.

Teaching social skills as part of a whole routine can be a powerful strategy, because the children achieve a perceptible outcome from their actions. The approach also gains effectiveness for children with autism, because routines are consistent and reliable for them. When several different routines are taught for a particular outcome, children can be more flexible in their responses to contextual changes. Finally, because the children achieve an immediate effect, the behavior that leads to maintenance of the routine is reinforced.

Component Behaviors of Social Skills

A natural extension to teaching skills through social routines involves the identification of stimuli and consequences of the environments that are the components of the routine. Meyer *et al.* (1985) have identified 11 critical components of social interactions that require judgments and responses to natural cues and consequences. Several of the components are (1) initiating/gaining entry, (2) following rules/routines, (3) reinforcing and consequating others, (4) attending to relevant situation cues, and (5) exiting.

For children to become more independent in interacting with their environment, they must be able to recognize or perceive the natural stimuli that cue them to engage in a particular behavior or routine. Once a routine has been initiated, other stimuli and consequences serve to chain behaviors in the routine.

Finally, recognizing when and how to terminate the behavior/routine is a critical component of social independence.

Our role as educators is to help children recognize the cues for them to initiate, sustain, and terminate behaviors/routines/ This may involve (1) adapting the environment (e.g., through exaggerating particular stimuli) to make the natural cues and consequences more perceptible or meaningful to children with autism, or (2) teaching the discrimination of relevant stimuli (e.g., facial expressions). It may also involve helping children understand and make judgments about the cues and consequences of the environments and their ability to have some social control over them.

GENERALIZATION

The demonstrated gains in social skills by preschool children with autism have almost always been seriously limited by their failure to generalize. Most typically, social behavior learned in one setting does not occur in other settings. Skills learned in the presence of certain children or adults are not used in the presence of other people. Behavior learned at one time seems lost or forgotten a short time later if the exact conditions of training are not present.

All of these are examples of failures in stimulus generalization. Response generalization is a similar, difficult problem. A student may learn one response and use it consistently, but when a somewhat different response is called for, generalization does not occur.

In a thorough and up-to-date review of problems and strategies in generalization, Stokes and Osnes (1986) identified three broad classes of strategies for facilitating the generalization of social skills in all children. These three approaches are (1) to take advantage of natural communities of reinforcement, (2) to train diversely, and (3) to incorporate functional mediators.

Natural Reinforcement

Although the reinforcement that is naturally available is seldom effective in teaching and maintaining social behavior for children with autism, careful planning can help children to experience more natural consequences and can make the reinforcers more salient. The suggestions made by Stokes and Osnes (1986) include teaching more functional skills and modifying environments to ensure that children will experience natural consequences for social acts.

For example, most functional behaviors lead to natural consequences. People who dress and groom themselves appropriately receive social approaches from others. People who work and travel and who refrain from self-stimulatory behavior are able to enjoy a full life in the community. Those without such skills are likely to lead restricted lives.

Children with autism often have a double problem in learning from natural consequences. They emit a low level of social behavior, and therefore do not experience natural reinforcers as often as other children do. In addition, social reinforcers are, by their nature, not concrete and are delivered on an irregular schedule. Thus, children with the cognitive deficits associated with autism fail to understand social contingencies and find the consequences of social acts not to be reinforcing (Fein, Pennington, Markowitz, Braverman, & Waterhouse, 1986). Effective use of natural reinforcement for children with autism is an important but largely unexplored area.

Training Diversely

If children learn social skills under a variety of conditions, they are more likely to use their skills when confronted with new conditions (Handleman & Harris, 1983). Stokes and Osnes (1986) pointed out the need to teach several appropriate social responses in several settings. They also emphasized "loose teaching," a condition in which antecedents and consequences are presented in a less predictable manner to approximate the conditions of natural social life. Under such conditions, unprompted generalization may occur and be reinforced.

Successful teaching of children with autism has usually been carried out under highly structured and predictable settings. "Teaching loosely" without confusing the child is a challenging task that has not been adequately studied. However, the use of multiple settings has been an effective approach demonstrated with elementary-age autistic children by Handleman and Harris (1983).

Functional Mediators

If one knows which stimuli are used by the child to discriminate conditions for using social skills, these "discriminative stimuli" can be offered in many settings or with many people, thereby aiding generalization. The most obvious discriminative stimulus is the teacher, but it is not practical or desirable for teachers to accompany their students in all social situations. If materials (e.g., a special toy) or peers are effective stimuli for social behavior, they may be helpful in mediating generalization. The toy or the peer can be present and signal social behavior in new settings or at later times. This strategy takes advantage of autistic children's insistence on sameness or familiarity. If a child goes shopping, meets a new person, or encounters a new task, the presence of a familiar social mediator may cue the child to respond appropriately. Of course, identifying such effective mediators and applying them in natural social settings are areas in which much research is needed.

The most effective mediators are those under the control of the child. J. Groden, Baron, and Groden (1984) have strongly argued for teaching procedures such as relaxation and covert conditioning to children with autism as tools for self-control. These approaches have not been studied systematically with pre-school children with autism, but they offer great promise, because the mediator is controlled by the child rather than the teacher. Children who have learned to relax cue themselves in new settings and with new people and are able to control behaviors that interfere with social interaction.

Adult relaxation procedures have been adapted for autistic children (Cautela & Groden, 1978). For instance, children are taught first to tighten and then to relax gross motor movements (e.g., arms, legs), then fine motor responses (e.g., forehead). Shaping of responses and initial physical prompting may be used.

A related approach to self-control is covert conditioning (Cautela, 1982). After children have learned to relax, they are taught to imagine that they are engaged in appropriate behavior and that they experience a positive consequence. These imagery scenes are rehearsed frequently and can serve as a mediator to aid gen-eralization of self-control. J. Groden (1982) used these procedures to increase social interaction in adolescents with autism, and J. Groden and Cautela (1984) had similar success with school-age children with mental retardation. Relaxation was one component of the successful treatment of a preschool child with autism in a case study by G. Groden, Domingue, Chesnick, Groden, and Baron (1983). Although most of the clinical application of self-control procedures has been with older children (Browder & Shapiro, 1985; G. Groden & Baron, 1988), and self-control is a difficult goal even for normal preschoolers, early training in self-control is worthy of emphasis for most children.

Use of Peers

The most effective and practical strategy for applying the Stokes and Osnes (1986) suggestions (natural reinforcement, diverse training, and functional mediators) has been the use of peers. Two studies by Strain (1983a, 1984) have demonstrated generalization of play skills by preschool children with autism when a nonhandi-capped peer was used to train the skills and the generalization setting involved nonhandicapped playmates.

The reason for this success is evident within the Stokes and Osnes (1986) framework. When autistic children emit social behaviors in the presence of non-handicapped peers, natural reinforcers follow. That is, the peers respond, and the social episode continues. In play settings made up only of children with autism, social behaviors are typically ignored by peers and are thus extinguished.

Both of Strain's studies (1983a, 1984) demonstrated the effectiveness of a 7-year-old boy as a peer trainer for preschool autistic children and the generalization of play skills to an integrated setting (handicapped and nonhandicapped children present). In both studies, generalization did not occur in segregated (handicapped-only) settings. The second of these studies (Strain, 1984) extended the findings by placing children with autism in a play group in which all of the nonhandicapped peers were trained to make social initiations. In this condition, the level of positive social interactions by children with autism approximated that of nonhandicapped children.

These studies demonstrate that generalization of social skills can be accomplished, but even careful efforts to program for generalization are unlikely to be successful in segregated groups of children with autism or other deficits in social skills (Odom & Strain, 1984b). This evidence is supportive of the trend toward integration that has been growing throughout this decade.

CURRICULA FOR SOCIAL SKILLS

The research and theory on social skills development described above have led to several curricula for young children with autism and other problems involving social deficits. Although they have somewhat different emphases, each has application for some young children with autism.

Social Competence Intervention Package for Preschool Youngsters

The research on teaching social skills to handicapped preschool children at George Peabody College of Vanderbilt University led to a curriculum called Social Competence Intervention Package for Preschool Youngsters (SCIPPY; Day, Powell, & Stowitschek, 1980). This curriculum is intended for all children who have low rates of social interaction. It consists of 20 activity cards that describe the activities and give peers ideas for teaching three important play skills; play organizing, sharing, and assisting. Teaching can be done by directly prompting and praising children or by teaching peers to prompt and praise the three skills in handicapped children.

SCIPPY uses play as the format for teaching social skills. The activities are developmentally sequenced and are based upon play skills empirically shown to be effective. Field testing showed that the curriculum is an effective means to increase prompting and praising of play in both teachers and peers (Day, Fox, Shores, Lindeman, & Stowitschek, 1983; Day, Powell, Dy-Lin, & Stowitschek, 1982). This package is not primarily designed for children with autism, but it is based on sound principles that could be used effectively, especially with higher-functioning children who have some interest in play activities and materials. It is simple enough for nonhandicapped peers to learn easily, and it provides a practical system for data collection for each activity.

Jowonio: The Learning Place

Research and theory on the normal sequence of social and cognitive development influenced the curriculum for Jowonio: The Learning Place, an integrated preschool in Syracuse, New York (Knoblock, 1982). The presence of nonhandicapped children enables young children with autism to interact with good models and to participate in the normal sequence of socialization from awareness of others to cooperative play. Play is viewed as a crucial experience in developing social, language, cognitive, and independence skills. The curriculum also includes affective skills, such as recognizing, labeling, and responding appropriately to emotions (e.g., fear, anger) and developing a positive self-concept.

Much of the evaluation of Jowonio has been subjective, but, in addition, observational data have shown increased social skills and interaction with peers over time, and sociometric approaches have indicated an encouraging level of acceptance of the children with autism by their "typical" classmates (Knoblock, 1982).

Young Autism Project

In 1970, Ivar Lovaas at UCLA began an extensive research and treatment program for children with autism who were under 4 years old. The project has continued to this date, and in the most recent report, Lovaas (1987) described the outcome for 19 children in an intensive treatment condition and 40 children who received less intensive treatment.

The curriculum was described earlier by Lovaas (1981). In the first phase, it emphasizes prompting and reinforcement of appropriate social behavior and mild punishment to reduce self-stimulation and aggression, as well as teaching compliance, imitation, and toy play. As soon as feasible, parents are trained to provide treatment at home, and a combination of parents and graduate student therapists provide treatment for virtually all waking hours. As the program progresses, the curriculum includes language and interactive play skills taught in preschool groups and community settings. As the children approach school age, academic skills are added to the curriculum.

In addition to behavioral teaching of basic skills, Lovaas (1987) has incorporated other elements shown to be effective. He involves parents in the treatment program, places children in preschools with nonhandicapped peers, emphasizes school survival skills, and continues intensive treatment as long as children continue to require help in school.

The 19 children in the intensive treatment group studied by Lovaas (1987) showed impressive outcomes. Almost half (9) successfully completed first grade with no special help and achieved scores on IQ tests and other measures indicating normal intellectual and educational skills. By school age, another 8 children had shown some progress but were still considered mildly retarded and required special education services. The remaining 2 children continued to have clear signs of autism and severe retardation. In the less intensive treatment group, only 1 of 40 children achieved regular school placement and test scores in the normal range.

The intensive treatment provided by Lovaas would be difficult to offer on a large scale, but it does provide encouragement that a curriculum emphasizing social skills at a young age can have a great impact on many children with autism.

Learning Experiences . . . An Alternative Program for Preschoolers and Parents

The last curriculum to be discussed here is Learning Experiences . . . An Alternative Program for Preschoolers and Parents (LEAP). For a more comprehensive description of LEAP, the reader is directed to an article by Hoyson, Jamieson, and Strain (1984). LEAP is a model demonstration preschool program associated with the University of Pittsburgh. Its services include classroom instruction for 3 hours every weekday for behaviorally handicapped ("autistic-like") and normally developing children. At the time of the 1984 article, 13 nonhandicapped children and 6 handicapped children had participated in the program. Twelve children were in the classroom at one time, 6 with "autistic-like" behaviors (behavior disorders and mild to severe cognitive impairments) and 6 who were normally developing. A critical feature of LEAP is its requirement of parent involvement and training.

The conceptual model of LEAP is built around three assumptions: (1) Curriculum targets must focus on functional skills needed in the children's next settings (home, school, community); (2) gains will be maintained through the active involvement of parents, teachers, and peers; and (3) precise planning, implementation, and evaluation of each activity will lead to improved education. Its curriculum model focuses on group instruction as the primary instructional arrangement, because it can provide more opportunities for learning and social interaction with peers, results in greater efficiency in child learning and teacher time, and is the format more often used in less restrictive environments. Although instruction is given in groups, objectives are highly individualized to the developmental levels of the children.

Teaching objectives are developed through frequent assessments of each child. Assessment is conducted using the Learning Accomplishment Profile (LAP; LeMay, Griffin, & Sanford, 1977), and objectives are selected that are midway between the basal level and ceiling in each of the LAP's eight skill areas. These include fine motor manipulation, fine motor writing, language comprehension, language expression, cognitive counting, cognitive matching, gross motor object movement, and gross motor body movement. For children with behavioral handicaps, objectives are chosen that are needed for successful participation in classroom, home, and community settings. This approach to curriculum development accomplishes the difficult task of integrating the developmental and environmental approaches. It assesses a child on a standardized sequence of developmental skills, but targets only those skills that will be useful to the child in the next environments. Because parents, teachers, and peers are involved in the process, the social validity of the selected skills is emphasized.

LEAP has been innovative in providing a comprehensive guide to serving children with autism in a mainstream preschool. Through its research on social skill targets and interventions, we have learned much about designing and implementing a social skills curriculum for these children. For specific information on outcome data from this project, see Strain, Jamieson, and Hoyson (1986).

CONCLUSION

Increased research in teaching social skills to young children with autism has produced substantial new knowledge and theory, impressive demonstrations of effective curriculum, and promising areas that will require further research. The curricula that have been effective in teaching social skills have had some common elements:

1. Curricula that have successfully prepared young children for the social demands of school have included the skills needed in typical classrooms and have taught these functional skills in a manner that is individualized for the developmental level of each child.

2. Effective programs have taught social skills in settings where children with autism can interact with nonhandicapped peers, thus gaining more practice in social routines, more natural reinforcement for their efforts, more exposure to good models (or peers trained to encourage social interaction), and more opportunities to generalize their skills.

3. The programs showing the most dramatic results (Lovaas, 1987; Strain *et al.*, 1986) used a behavioral strategy in which individualized social skill targets were integrated into the total curriculum and taught explicitly, using prompting and reinforcement.

In a recent review, Simeonsson, Olley, and Rosenthal (1987) found only three studies that evaluated comprehensive preschool programs for children with autism using empirical data and scientific methods. The three were those of Fenske, Zalenski, Krantz, and McClannahan (1985), Lovaas (1987), and Strain *et al.* (1986). All of these programs used a behavioral approach. One cannot conclude that other approaches are not also effective; however, no comparable evaluations of nonbehavioral programs have been published.

Much research on curriculum remains to be done, but intensive programs that include these elements beginning at an early age offer much hope for improving social skills. Such an improvement would be a large early step toward improved adult functioning for people with autism.

References

Beckman, P. J., & Kohl, F. L. (1984). The effects of social and isolate toys on the interactions and play of integrated and nonintegrated groups of preschoolers. *Education and Training of the Mentally Retarded, 19,* 169–174.

Browder, D. M., & Shapiro, E. S. (1985). Applications of self-management to individuals with severe handicaps: A review. *Journal of the Association for Persons with Severe Handicaps, 10,* 200–208.

Carr, E. G. (1982). Sign language. In R. L. Koegel, A. Rincover, & A. L. Egel (Eds.), *Educating and understanding autistic children* (pp. 142–157). San Diego: College-Hill Press.

Cautela, J. R. (1982).Covert conditioning with children. *Journal of Behavior Therapy and Experimental Psychiatry, 13,* 209–214.

Cautela, J. R., & Groden, J. (1978). *Relaxation: A comprehensive manual for adults, children, and children with special needs.* Champaign, IL: Research Press.

Cook, A.R., Anderson, N., & Rincover, A. (1982). Stimulus overselectivity and stimulus control: Problems and strategies. In R. L. Koegel, A. Rincover, & A. Egel (Eds.), *Educating and understanding autistic children* (pp. 90–105). San Diego: College-Hill Press.

Dawson, G., & Adams, A. (1984). Imitation and social responsiveness in autistic children. *Journal of Abnormal Child Psychology, 12,* 209–226.

Day, R. M., Fox, J. J., Shores, R. E., Lindeman, D. P., & Stowitschek, J. J. (1983). The Social Competence Intervention Project: Developing educational procedures for teaching social interaction skills to handicapped children. *Behavioral Disorders, 8,* 120–127.

Day, R. M., Powell, T. H., Dy-Lin, E. B., & Stowitschek, J. J. (1982). An evaluation of the effects of a social interaction training package on mentally handicapped preschool children. *Education and Training of the Mentally Retarded, 17,* 125–130.

Day, R. M., Powell, T. H., & Stowitschek, J. J. (1980). *SCIPPY: Social Competence Intervention Package for Preschool Youngsters.* Nashville, TN: Social Competence Intervention Project, Vanderbilt University.

DeMyer, M. K., Alpern, G. D., Barton, S., DeMyer, W. E., Churchill, D. W., Hingtgen, J. N., Bryson, C. Q., Pontius, W., & Kimberlin, C. (1972). Imitation in autistic, early schizophrenic, and nonpsychotic subnormal children. *Journal of Autism and Childhood Schizophrenia, 2,* 264–287.

Donnellan, A. M., & Kilman, B. A. (1986). Behavioral approaches to social skill development in autism: Strengths, misapplications, and alternatives. In E. Schopler & G. B. Mesibov (Eds.), *Social behavior in autism* (pp. 213–236). New York: Plenum.

Epstein, L. J., Taubman, M. T., & Lovaas, O. I. (1985). Changes in self-stimulatory behaviors with treatment. *Journal of Abnormal Child Psychology, 13,* 281–294.

Evans, I. M., & Meyer, L. H. (1985). *An educative approach to behavior problems: A practical decision model for interventions with severely handicapped learners.* Baltimore: Paul H. Brookes.

Federlein, A. C., Lessen-Firestone, J., & Elliott, S. (1982). Special education preschoolers: Evaluating their play. *Early Child Development and Care, 9*(3–4), 245–254.

Fein, D., Pennington, B., Markowitz, P., Braverman, M., & Waterhouse, L. (1986). Towards a neuropsychological model of infantile autism: Are the social deficits primary? *Journal of the American Academy of Child Psychiatry, 25,* 198–212.

Fenske, E. C., Zalenski, S., Krantz, P. J., & McClannahan, L. E. (1985). Age at intervention and treatment outcome for autistic children in a comprehensive intervention program. *Analysis and Intervention in Developmental Disabilities, 5,* 49–58.

Groden, G., & Baron, M. G. (Eds.). (1988). *Autism: Strategies for change.* New York: Gardner Press.

Groden, G., Domingue, D., Chesnick, M., Groden, J., & Baron, G. (1983). Early intervention with autistic children: A case presentation with pre-program, program and follow-up data. *Psychological Reports, 53,* 713–722.

Groden, J. (1982). *Procedures to increase social interaction among autistic adolescents: A multiple baseline analysis.* Unpublished doctoral dissertation, Boston College.

Groden, J., Baron, G., & Groden, G. (1984). The need for the development of self-control procedures with the autistic population. In *Proceedings 1984: Annual meeting and conference of NSAC, The National Society for Children and Adults with Autism* (pp. 198–220). Washington, DC: National Society for Children and Adults with Autism.

Groden, J., & Cautela, J. R. (1984). Use of imagery procedures with students labeled "trainable retarded." *Psychological Reports, 54,* 595–605.

Handleman, J. S., & Harris, S. L. (1983). Generalization across instructional settings by autistic children. *Child and Family Behavior Therapy, 5,* 73–83.

Hoyson, M., Jamieson, B., & Strain, P. S. (1984). Individualized group instruction of normally developing and autistic-like children: The LEAP curriculum model. *Journal of the Division for Early Childhood, 8,* 157–172.

Itard, J. (1962). *The wild boy of Aveyron* (G. Humphrey & M. Humphrey, Trans.). New York: Appleton-Century-Crofts. (Original work published 1894)

Kanner, L. (1943). Autistic disturbances of affective contact. *The Nervous Child, 2,* 217–250.

Knoblock, P. (1982). *Teaching and mainstreaming autistic children.* Denver, CO: Love.

Koegel, R. L., & Covert, A. (1972). The relationship of self-stimulation to learning in autistic children. *Journal of Applied Behavior Analysis, 5,* 381–388.

Koegel, R. L., Firestone, P. B., Kramme, K. W., & Dunlap, G. (1974). Increasing spontaneous play by suppressing self-stimulation in autistic children. *Journal of Applied Behavior Analysis, 7,* 521–528.

Koegel, R. L., Rincover, A., & Egel, A. L. (Eds.). (1982). *Educating and understanding autistic children.* San Diego: College-Hill Press.

LeMay, D., Griffin, P., & Sanford, A. (1977). *Learning Accomplishment Profile—diagnostic edition.* Chapel Hill, NC: Chapel Hill Training–Outreach Project.

Lord, C., & O'Neill, P. J. (1980). A developmental–behavioral model for the prescriptive evaluation of autistic and severely socially impaired children. In B. Wilcox & A. Thompson (Eds.), *Critical issues in educating autistic children and youth* (pp. 24–52). Washington, DC: U.S. Department of Education, Office of Special Education.

Lovaas, O. I. (1968). Some studies on the treatment of childhood schizophrenia. In J. M. Shlien (Ed.), *Research in psychotherapy* (Vol. 3, pp. 103–121). Washington, DC: American Psychological Association.

Lovaas, O. I. (1977). *The autistic child: Language development through behavior modification.* New York: Irvington.

Lovaas, O. I. (1981). *Teaching developmentally disabled children: The ME book.* Baltimore: University Park Press.

Lovaas, O. I. (1987). Behavioral treatment and normal educational and intellectual functioning in young autistic children. *Journal of Consulting and Clinical Psychology, 55,* 3–9.

Lovaas, O. I., Berberich, J. P., Perloff, B. F., & Schaeffer, B. (1966). Acquisition of imitative speech in schizophrenic children. *Science, 151,* 705–707.

Meyer, L. H., McQuarter, R. J., & Kishi, G. S. (1985). Assessing and teaching social interaction skills. In S. Stainback & W. Stainback (Eds.), *Integration of students with severe handicaps into regular schools* (pp. 66–86). Reston, VA: Council for Exceptional Children.

Mori, A., & Neisworth, J. T. (1983). Curricula in early childhood education: Some generic and special considerations. *Topics in Early Childhood Special Education, 2*(4), 1–8.

Nedelman, D., & Sulzbacher, S. I. (1972). Dicky at 13 years of age: A long-term success following early application of operant conditioning procedures. In G. Semb (Ed.), *Behavior analysis and education* (pp. 3–10). Lawrence: University of Kansas, Department of Human Development.

Neel, R. S., Billingsley, F. F., McCarty, F., Symonds, D., Lambert, C., Lewis-Smith, N., & Hanashiro, R. (1983). *Teaching autistic children: A functional curriculum approach.* Seattle: University of Washington.

Odom, S. L., & McConnell, S. R. (1985). A performance-based conceptualization of social competence of handicapped preschool children: Implications for assessment. *Topics in Early Childhood Special Education, 4*(4), 1–19.

Odom, S. L., & Strain, P. S. (1984a). Classroom-based social skills instruction for severely handicapped preschool children. *Topics in Early Childhood Special Education, 4*(3), 97–116.

Odom, S. L., & Strain, P. S. (1984b). Peer-mediated approaches to promoting children's social interaction: A review. *American Journal of Orthopsychiatry, 54*, 544–577.

Peck, C. A., Apolloni, T., Cook, T. P., & Raver, S. A. (1978). Teaching retarded preschoolers to imitate the free-play behavior of nonretarded classmates: Trained and generalized effects. *Journal of Special Education, 12*, 195–207.

Powell, J. V. (1982). A field-based approach to the validation of behavioral competencies for young children. In N. Nir-Janiv, B. Spodek, & D. Steg (Eds.), *Early childhood education: An international perspective* (pp. 505–512). New York: Plenum.

Risley, T. R., & Wolf, M. M. (1967). Establishing functional speech in echolalic children. *Behaviour Research and Therapy, 5*, 73–88.

Romanczyk, R. G., Diament, C., Goren, E. R., Trunell, G., & Harris, S. L. (1975). Increasing isolate and social play in severely disturbed children: Intervention and postintervention effectiveness. *Journal of Autism and Childhood Schizophrenia, 5*, 57–70.

Russo, D., & Koegel, R. (1977). A method of integrating the autistic child into a normal public school classroom. *Journal of Applied Behavior Analysis, 10*, 579–590.

Shores, R. E., Hester, P., & Strain, P. S. (1976). The effects of amount and type of teacher–child interaction in child–child interaction during free play. *Psychology in the Schools, 13*, 171–175.

Simeonsson, R. J., Olley, J. G., & Rosenthal, S. L. (1987). Early intervention for children with autism. In M. J. Guralnick & F. C. Bennett (Eds.), *The effectiveness of early intervention for at-risk and handicapped children* (pp. 275–296). New York: Academic Press.

Stokes, T. F., & Osnes, P. G. (1986). Programming the generalization of children's social behavior. In P. S. Strain, M. J. Guralnick, & H. M. Walker (Eds.), *Children's social behavior: Development, assessment, and modification* (pp. 407–443). New York: Academic Press.

Stowitschek, J. J., & Powell, T. H. (1981). Materials for teaching social skills to handicapped children: An analytic review. *Journal of Special Education Technology, 4*, 40–49.

Strain, P. S. (1983a). Generalization of autistic children's social behavior change: Effects of developmentally integrated and segregated settings. *Analysis and Intervention in Developmental Disabilities, 3*, 23–34.

Strain, P. S. (1983b). Identification of social skill curriculum targets for severely handicapped children in mainstream preschools. *Applied Research in Mental Retardation, 4*, 369–382.

Strain, P. S. (1984). Social interactions of handicapped preschoolers in developmentally integrated and segregated settings: A study of generalization effects. In T. Field, J. L. Rooparine, & M. Segal (Eds.), *Friendships in normal and handicapped children* (pp. 187–207). Norwood, NJ: Ablex.

Strain, P. S., Jamieson, B. J., & Hoyson, M. H. (1986). Learning Experiences . . . An Alternative Program for Preschoolers and Parents: A comprehensive service system for mainstreaming of autistic-like preschoolers. In C. J. Meisel (Ed.), *Mainstreaming handicapped children: Outcomes, controversies, and new directions* (pp. 251–269). Hillsdale, NJ: Erlbaum.

Strain, P. S., Odom, S. L., & McConnell, S. (1984). Promoting social reciprocity of exceptional children: Identification, target behavior selection, and intervention. *Remedial and Special Education, 5*(1), 21–28.

Tiegerman, E., & Primavera, L. (1981). Object manipulation: An interactional strategy with autistic children. *Journal of Autism and Developmental Disorders, 11*, 427–438.

Tiegerman, E., & Primavera, L. H. (1984). Imitating the autistic child: Facilitating communicative gaze behavior. *Journal of Autism and Developmental Disorders, 14*, 27–38.

Tremblay, A., Strain, P. S., Hendrickson, J. M., & Shores, R. E. (1980). The activity context of preschool children's social interactions: A comparison of high and low social interactors. *Psychology in the Schools, 17,* 380–385.

Tremblay, A., Strain, P. S., Hendrickson, J. M., & Shores, R. E. (1981). Social interactions of normal preschool children: Using normative data for subject and target behavior selection. *Behavior Modification, 5,* 237–253.

Vincent, L. J., Salisbury, C., Walter, G., Brown, P., Gruenewald, L. J., & Powers, J. (1980). Program evaluation and curriculum development in early childhood/special education: Criteria of the next environment. In W. Sailor, B. Wilcox, & L. Brown (Eds.), *Methods of instruction for severely handicapped students* (pp. 303–328). Baltimore: Paul H. Brookes.

Wolf, M , Risley, T., Johnston, M., Harris, F., & Allen, E. (1967). Application of operant conditioning procedures to the behavior problems of an autistic child: A follow-up and extension. *Behaviour Research and Therapy, 5,* 103–111.

Wolf, M. M., Risley, T. R., & Mees, H. L. (1964). Application of operant conditioning procedures to the behavior problems of an autistic child. *Behaviour Research and Therapy, 1,* 305–312.

CHAPTER 16

Diagnosis and Treatment of Adolescents and Adults with Autism

MARY E. VAN BOURGONDIEN
GARY B. MESIBOV
University of North Carolina at Chapel Hill

As autistic children grow into adolescence and adulthood, they begin to face many of the same issues and conflicts as normally developing youngsters. Adolescence is a time when individuals must become independent from their families; develop and expand on their interpersonal relationships; and resolve issues concerning their identity by moving into special vocational, recreational, and leisure areas. Obviously, their handicaps make these issues somewhat different for autistic people than for their nonhandicapped peers, but no less difficult, complicated, or important. In order for them to develop the skills required to achieve these adolescent developmental milestones, special diagnostic, assessment, and intervention strategies are required. The purpose of this chapter is to describe the approaches and strategies that are being developed for this age group.

DIAGNOSIS

General Considerations

Although many people use the terms "diagnosis" and "assessment" interchangeably, because they usually occur together, these terms actually refer to different parts of the process when families bring a child with a problem to a clinic. The diagnostic part of the process is the determination of autism. It is the diagnosis that identifies the child as autistic and suggests that the child has characteristics similar to those of others with the same designation. The purpose of diagnosis is generally for administrative and research groupings. Assessment also occurs during a child's initial evaluation, although it continues beyond that point as well. Assessment is the process of defining an individual's strengths, weaknesses, and needs from a variety of perspectives. The purpose of assessment is to develop appropriate individualized programs and to continue evaluating their effectiveness. The as-

367

sessment process emphasizes how autistic people are unique and different from one another.

Although the main purpose of a diagnosis is to establish appropriate groupings, this process does have some implications for treatment and for the families involved. First, a diagnostic label like "autism" can be extremely helpful for families. It suggests that their children have an identifiable and therefore somewhat comprehensible condition that professionals have seen before and know something about. Given the generally accepted concept of autism as a developmental problem, the label also suggests that parents have not caused the disability, which helps relieve them of the enormous guilt that is often associated with children experiencing problems. Finally, the designation of a label ends the first phase of coping with a handicap that most parents of handicapped children go through. Most families are not able to mobilize themselves to seek appropriate treatment until they know what is wrong with their children. The label "autistic" frees the families to begin important remediation efforts.

Although the assessment process has the most implications for treatment, an accurate diagnosis of autism can also have treatment implications. First, accurately identifying autistic people can teach us about the fundamental nature of the disability through observation and research. Accurate diagnostic techniques have enabled researchers to follow autistic people as they have grown older and have demonstrated their increasing sociability. The more we have observed autistic adolescents and adults, the more we have realized the variability of their social deficits and the wide spectrum of people who can be considered autistic. This has had a significant effect on the identification and subsequent treatment of younger autistic people.

Accurate diagnosis can also have more direct treatment implications. Although this diagnostic category does not suggest a specific intervention, as do many forms of medical diagnoses, there are important implications in the differential diagnosis of mental retardation with or without autism or of autism versus schizophrenia. Although individuals in all of these groups will benefit from a structured, individualized, and psychoeducationally oriented environment, those diagnosed as autistic will benefit from the services of professionals trained in this disability who understand their communicative and social deficits, their difficulties in understanding subtle cues, and their tendencies to respond less to social reinforcements. The diagnosis also suggests that they will be less likely to benefit from verbally oriented treatment strategies, even if they have some verbal ability.

In diagnosing adolescents and adults, our first assumption has always been that anyone diagnosed as autistic in childhood continues to be so as an adult, even though changes and considerable improvement may have occurred. This is consistent with most current definitions of autism, suggesting that it is pervasive and lifelong, and that these clients frequently improve though rarely are cured (Lotter, 1978). This approach also acknowledges that autism is easier to diagnose in younger children because the characteristics of this disability tend to vary and become more idiosyncratic as the youngsters grow older (Schopler & Mesibov,

1983). Diagnostic instruments that have been developed for younger children need to be re-examined and adapted in order to ensure their reliability and validity with adolescents and adults.

Use of the Childhood Autism Rating Scale with Adolescents and Adults

The major diagnostic instrument used within the Treatment and Education of Autistic and Related Communication Handicapped CHildren (TEACCH) program in North Carolina has been the Childhood Autism Rating Scale (CARS; Schopler, Reichler, DeVellis, & Daly, 1980). Based on data from autistic children in the TEACCH program over the past decade, the CARS has been recently revised (Schopler, Reichler, & Renner, 1986), and the new version has excellent reliability and validity. Like the earlier version, the revised CARS is easy to administer without substantial training or experience. Items rated on the CARS include the following: Relating to People; Imitation; Emotional Response; Body Use; Object Use; Adaptation to Change; Visual Response; Listening Response; Taste, Smell, and Touch Response and Use; Fear or Nervousness; Verbal Communication; Nonverbal Communication; Activity Level; Consistency of Intellectual Response; and General Impressions. Each of these 15 items is rated on a scale of 1–4, so that the total score range is from 15 to 60. The cutoff scores are as follows: nonautistic, 15–29.5; mildly to moderately autistic, 30–36.5; severely autistic, 37–60. Recent efforts have been designed to adapt this instrument for use with adolescents and adults.

As indicated earlier, in adapting the CARS for adolescents and adults, the first assumption is that any child diagnosed as autistic retains that diagnosis for the rest of his or her life. Therefore, adolescents and adults who were diagnosed as autistic as younger children pose no particular diagnostic difficulties. The problem comes when one must make a diagnostic decision about an adolescent or adult who did not have an earlier diagnosis of autism. To evaluate the effectiveness of the CARS with this group, we examined CARS data for autistic youngsters in our program who had been diagnosed as autistic before age 10 and then re-evaluated after age 13. We were able to locate 59 such children in our program. This represented an excellent group for verifying the CARS, because we were confident in their early diagnosis (prior to age 10) and had CARS scores for them as adolescents and adults as well.

Examination of the data showed that the average CARS total score decreased by 2.2 points over time. In other words, the average score for these clients after age 13 was 2.2 points lower than their average CARS score as younger children. The overwhelming majority of subjects showed a drop in their CARS scores. Given the cutoff scores and the fact that most autistic people score within the 20–40 range, this 2.2 drop represents both a statistically significant and a clinically significant change. The significant drop suggests that these children, though still autistic, show those characteristics to a lesser extent after adolescence.

Considering this change, we then adjusted the CARS cutoff for mild to moderate autism by 2 points, from 30 to 28. (Our previous use of the CARS required a score of 30 for a client to be diagnosed as autistic.) Using 28 as a cutoff, we then evaluated the adolescent scores of these youngsters to see how many of them would still be diagnosed as autistic if we had no data available on them as youngsters. With this revised cutoff, 92% of these youngsters would still be diagnosed as autistic and only 8% would be misdiagnosed. This suggests that, with a slight modification, the CARS is a reasonable diagnostic instrument for adolescents and adults with autism.

Our research on the CARS has also investigated several observational techniques. When we began our work on this instrument with younger children, ratings were made while they were working on our assessment instrument, the Psychoeducational Profile (PEP; see below). Since then we have learned that the CARS is more flexible and can be rated while a child, adolescent, or adult is engaged in a variety of tasks. The CARS has been administered while children have been involved with the PEP or Adolescent and Adult Psychoeducational Profile (AAPEP), a measure of communication, vocational functioning, and social functioning designed for autistic adolescents and adults (see below). The CARS has also been used while an autistic individual is involved in less standardized situations, such as during a classroom observation or home visit. We have also reliably scored the CARS based on parent report or a client's history in a comprehensive chart. An important advantage of the CARS is that it gives reliable information about adolescents and adults, based on observations in a variety of settings or parental report.

ASSESSMENT

As described earlier, the purpose of assessment is for individualized education and behavioral management. Diagnosis examines common characteristics in autistic individuals, whereas assessment looks at the aspects that make each person an individual in order to develop appropriate individualized intervention plans. Historically, assessment with autistic children has been difficult because of their generally high activity levels and unwillingness to participate in the testing process. However, our TEACCH program has developed an instrument for younger children called the PEP (Schopler & Reichler, 1979; mentioned above), which maximizes their strengths and interests. The PEP has been successful in assessing children who had frequently been described as "untestable" by other programs using other assessment instruments.

The AAPEP (Mesibov, Schopler, & Schaffer, 1984; also mentioned above) has been developed as our adolescent and adult counterpart to the PEP. This instrument was designed along similar lines, using strategies consistent with the

PEP. For example, the AAPEP utilizes the "pass–emerge–fail" scoring system that was originally developed for the PEP. The "emerge" rating is the critical concept in this system; it is assigned when an individual has some knowledge of what is required but lacks the skill necessary for complete mastery and understanding. Emerging skills are the most amenable to improvement through instruction, so a major focus of our assessment efforts is to identify these emerging skills.

Administration of the AAPEP is also similar to that of the PEP, in that it allows the examiner the flexibility necessary for working with autistic students. The examiner is permitted to teach new skills, as well as to adjust the materials and presentation techniques as necessary, and still be within the standardization guidelines. This flexibility is very important in assessing the skills of autistic individuals, who, because of their communication deficits, may not understand what they are being asked to do until someone demonstrates the task for them. Examiner flexibility provides more information about the skill acquisition process, which is essential if one is to make practical recommendations for autistic youngsters.

As on the PEP, verbal language is minimized on the AAPEP, and little emphasis is placed on speed. These modifications are designed to minimize the deficits frequently observed in autistic people, so that their skills can be accurately identified. Visual models and cues are used extensively instead of verbal language to provide information and instruction.

Finally, the AAPEP is geared to lower-functioning, less verbally oriented autistic clients. This group is generally more difficult to assess and has fewer other assessment options available. Those higher-functioning clients who are not appropriate for the AAPEP will generally be able to respond to other assessment instruments.

Although the AAPEP is similar to the PEP in many ways, because it is also designed primarily for autistic clients, there are several significant ways in which the two tests differ. First, the AAPEP is not as developmental as the PEP. The PEP items are arranged in a developmental sequence, so that the examiner is able to derive an estimate of the child's developmental age level in a given area. The AAPEP, however, is a criterion-referenced test. The skills assessed on this scale relate to successful adult functioning in a vocational or residential setting and are not designed to correspond to a developmental progression. Although an understanding of developmental levels is important for working with all handicapped children, they do not have the same meaning as clients get older. For example, a 20-year-old person with a mental age of 6 is quite different from a 10-year-old with the same mental age. A second change is the addition of Home and School/Work scales to the AAPEP. The Home and School/Work scales include many of the same items and dimensions as the Direct Observation scale and are administered through parent or teacher interviews. These were added because autistic people often respond to specific environments, which makes it important to look at their skills across situations.

The final difference between the AAPEP and the PEP is in the actual skills that are measured. An important reason for developing the AAPEP was that the skills we emphasize with older children and adults are quite different from those that are most productive in working with preadolescents. Therefore, while the PEP measures Imitation, Perception, Fine Motor, Gross Motor, Eye–Hand Integration, Cognitive Performance, and Cognitive Verbal, the AAPEP measures skills more important for adolescents and adults, including Vocational Skills, Independent Functioning, Leisure Skills, Vocational Behavior, Functional Communication, and Interpersonal Behavior.

In order to assess the reliability and validity of the AAPEP, 60 adolescents and adults functioning within the moderate to severe range of mental retardation were selected for our study. Of this group, 30 were diagnosed as autistic and 30 were diagnosed as having mental retardation without autism. The diagnoses were based on observations of the individuals during clinic evaluations and on family history data. These diagnoses were corroborated by using the CARS. On this measurement, all individuals in the autistic group had scores above 28, and all of the members of the nonautistic group had scores below 25. The average chronological age of the participants was 20 years, 4 months, and the average IQ was 41.2. As expected, the only significant difference between these groups was in their CARS scores measuring autistic characteristics.

Interrater reliability was determined by having a research assistant observe 15 assessments and score them independently of the examiner. The percentage of agreement between the research assistant and the examiner on each individual item constituted the reliability score. Table 16-1 shows the reliability for the 15 clients evaluated. Reliability seems quite acceptable, with the single exception of Interpersonal Behavior on both the Direct Observation and School/Work scales. These categories have therefore been reworked to clarify the scoring of those items.

External validity is the extent to which a test measures what it was designed to measure. Traditionally, it is determined by correlating results obtained on a new test with those obtained on existing instruments. Unfortunately, there are no existing instruments for assessing autistic adolescents or adults who are functioning intellectually in the moderately to severely retarded range. Therefore, it was decided to focus on the main goal of this test in order to develop an appropriate strategy for determining validity.

Because the main goal of the AAPEP is to generate recommendations that will be helpful for each individual client, we decided to correlate recommendations developed from this test with those already in use. Existing recommendations were taken from the Individual Education Plans (IEPs) for school-age clients and from the Individual Habilitation Plans (IHPs) for adults. A summary paragraph was written on each client, and then the five recommendations from the IEPs (or IHPs) were randomly mixed with five recommendations generated from the AAPEP. Each set of 10 recommendations was presented to two professionals with extensive experience with adolescents and adults, one from the TEACCH program and one associated with community-based services for developmentally handicapped adults. Raters were blind to the source of each recommendation (IEP, IHP, or AAPEP) and were asked to rank them on a 5-point scale as to their degree of helpfulness for working with that client in a community-based setting.

TABLE 16-1. AAPEP Reliability Data

	R		
	Autistic	Control	Total
AAPEP total	.845	.872	.865
Direct Observation	.844	.931	.879
Vocational Skills	.809	.917	.851
Independent Functioning	.950	.955	.952
Leisure Skills	.896	.899	.897
Vocational Behavior	.783	1.000	.855
Functional Communication	.851	.850	.873
Interpersonal Behavior	.438	.920	.679
Home	.820	.817	.843
Vocational Skills	.884	.751	.855
Independent Functioning	.898	.875	.910
Leisure Skills	.670	.749	.740
Vocational Behavior	.854	.879	.875
Functional Communication	.719	.930	.840
Interpersonal Behavior	.754	.793	.799
School/Work	.831	.882	.862
Vocational Skills	.981	.881	.939
Independent Functioning	.762	.892	.822
Leisure Skills	.800	.844	.850
Vocational Behavior	.786	1.000	.856
Functional Communication	.929	.921	.927
Interpersonal Behavior	.583	.921	.738

The main validity measure was the comparison of the AAPEP test recommendations with those already in use in the clients' IEPs or IHPs. Data analyses revealed a main effect of recommendation source, with the AAPEP-generated recommendations being superior. There was no effect of group, so that the recommendations were equally helpful for both autistic and nonautistic clients. However, there was a significant group × recommendation source interaction, suggesting that the effect was greater for autistic clients. Therefore, although the superiority of the AAPEP recommendations was greater for the autistic group, they were generally more helpful than the IEPs and IHPs for both of the groups in this study.

TREATMENT AREAS

Once an appropriate diagnostic evaluation and assessment have been completed, the next and most important phase is the development of appropriate individualized treatment programs. As indicated earlier, the PEP and AAPEP have been designed specifically to facilitate this phase by examining relevant areas for program planning by identifying emerging skills. The major treatment areas targeted for autistic adolescents and adults include communication, social relationships, behavior management, leisure skills, and vocational skills, all with a special emphasis on functional skills to increase independence.

Communication training with nonverbal autistic adolescents and adults emphasizes the development of alternative communications systems. Sign language, picture cards, and word card systems, as well as a variety of related techniques, have been effective with this population (Bonvillian & Nelson, 1976; Lancioni, 1983; LaVigna, 1977; Prizant & Wetherby, Chapter 12, this volume). Determining which approach is best for a given individual will depend on his or her functioning level and unique strengths and weaknesses. It is especially important to match the functional communication system to the client's developmental level. For example, many have used sign language for nonverbal autistic adults without realizing its complexity and the complex skills required to utilize this system productively. For many of these clients, a more appropriate communication system might be picture cards.

For more verbal autistic individuals, the focus of communication training is usually to make their language more social and appropriate. Although many higher-functioning clients can talk, their statements are frequently meaningless to independent observers. Efforts to make their language more meaningful, communicative, and social should be a major focus of intervention efforts.

Socially, one observes considerable improvement as autistic children grow from childhood through adolescence and adulthood (Ando & Yoshimura, 1979; Mesibov, 1983; Schopler & Mesibov, 1983). As adolescents and young adults, many show an interest in other people but still lack the skills to initiate and maintain interactions, let alone friendships (Rutter, 1970). Even though these social deficits continue to be among the most salient and distinguishing features of the autism syndrome, few programs have been targeted specifically at improving these skills.

Several programs have been developed more recently that are designed to increase the interactions and verbal communication skills of autistic people (McGee, Krantz, & McClannahan, 1984; Ragland, Kerr, & Strain, 1978). A more comprehensive approach to social skills training has been developed by Mesibov (1984, 1986) and Lord (1984; see also Lord & Magill, Chapter 14, this volume). These programs apply some of the well-documented cognitive social skills training models to the teaching of social behaviors to clients with autism, targeting their lack of interaction, difficulties in understanding social rules, attention deficits, and communication problems. They also emphasize more positive aspects of social interactions and are designed to teach autistic people that social interactions can be positive and rewarding.

Behavior management programs for adolescents and adults with autism have been influenced by current research suggesting that many behavior problems decrease as autistic people grow older. Current research suggests that overactivity, ritualistic and compulsive behaviors, and aggression all decrease with age (Ando & Yoshimura, 1979; Mesibov & Shea, 1980; Rutter, 1970; Rutter, Greenfield, &

Lockyer, 1967). Although aggressive and self-injurious behaviors decrease with age, they remain the most common targets of behavioral interventions for adolescents and adults (Carr, 1981; Favell, 1977, 1983; Foxx & Azrin, 1972; Hughes & Davis, 1980). They are of greater concern because of their more devastating effect when exhibited by physically mature individuals. Part of the current trend toward increasing independence means that autistic individuals are likely to be living in more normalized settings, where aggressive behaviors may result in termination of employment or recreational opportunities.

Probably the greatest change in current treatment programs is seen in the new emphasis on developing leisure and vocational skills. These new trends have had the greatest impact on work with adolescents and adults, because they are so close to moving into environments where these skills will be required. The ability to amuse oneself in appropriate ways has far-reaching effects on the life of an autistic person and those around him or her. Entry into and continued placement in vocational programs or group homes can be influenced by an individual's ability to occupy himself or herself during breaks (Wehman, 1977), or the individual's ability to use free time appropriately (Kraus, 1978). In addition to decreasing boredom and increasing morale, the ability to make constructive use of free leisure time also decreases the likelihood of behavior problems and makes management of the autistic person easier (Akerley, 1984; Wehman, 1977). Overall, an autistic adult's ability to function successfully in a community-based program is enhanced by the presence of recreational and leisure skills (Mesibov, 1983; Wehman, 1983). However, the most compelling reason for teaching adolescents and adults leisure and recreational skills is that, once acquired, these skills and interests truly enrich their lives.

Unfortunately, during late adolescence, when autistic individuals become more interested in interacting with others during their free time, the structures for facilitating these interactions—primarily public school programs—are no longer available. Therefore, autistic adolescents and adults need to find and function in the relatively unstructured recreational activities that exist in the community. Most successful leisure skills training programs emphasize the development of specific skills (e.g., bowling), as well as accompanying social and communication skills (Kraus, 1978; Mesibov, 1984; Wuerch & Voeltz, 1981).

Since the 1973 amendments to the Rehabilitation Act were passed, there has been increasing emphasis on providing vocational rehabilitation services to a wide variety of severely handicapped people. The goals of these programs are usually to teach handicapped individuals the vocational skills and behaviors necessary for them to function in less restrictive settings. These settings range from work–activity centers for the most severely handicapped people to competitive employment for those who are more capable. For individuals with autism, vocational training must emphasize the development of appropriate work habits or behaviors much more than specific job skills. Learning how to work for long periods of time and dealing with changes in routine are typically more difficult for autistic adolescents and adults than the specific job skills a task requires.

TREATMENT STRATEGIES

There are many similarities between the approaches used with autistic children and those with adolescents and adults. Task analysis, systematic training, and behavior modification techniques are as applicable to the teaching of vocational skills as to the teaching of academic skills (Bellamy, Sheehan, Horner, & Boles, 1980; Gold, 1976; Wehman & Hill, 1981). The Jay Nolan Center (LaVigna, 1983) is an example of an adult program that uses operant reinforcement, developmental programming, and intensive data collection techniques to teach a wide variety of vocational and independence skills to autistic adolescents and adults.

Simplifying tasks and increasing structure are additional techniques proven equally effective with autistic children, adolescents, and adults (Schopler, Brehm, Kinsbourne, & Reichler, 1971; Schopler & Mesibov, 1983). Behavior problems such as aggression are frequently responses to situations that are confusing or beyond the capabilities of the autistic person. Simplifying tasks and clarifying expectations reduce confusion and frequently lead to improvements in behavior (Carr, 1981).

Although there are many similarities between the principles and techniques used in teaching autistic children and adults, there are also some significant differences. Reinforcement and time out are still employed as autistic people become older, but what is reinforcing varies and the feasibility of time-out procedures changes. Autistic adults usually respond to a more varied array of reinforcers. Their increased interest in people and social events make the use of social reinforcers more viable (Mesibov, 1983). Allowing clients to engage in limited amounts of sensory stimulation (Favell, 1983; Rincover, Cook, Peoples, & Packard, 1979) has also been shown to be a potent reinforcer. As in all differential reinforcement programs, it is essential that rewards for appropriate behavior be more intense and enjoyable than consequences of inappropriate responses.

As autistic individuals mature, there is an increased emphasis on the use of positive interventions as opposed to punishment (Favell, 1983). An important reason for this shift is the difficulty in administering negative procedures with physically mature adults. In addition, it has been reported that negative procedures can lead to increases in aggression, which can have severe consequences with large autistic adolescents and adults (Foxx & Azrin, 1972; Hughes & Davis, 1980).

In spite of these current trends, some situations still suggest the need for some form of punishment if positive techniques alone are not effective. Time out from positive enforcement is the most frequently used punishment, which involves removing an individual from a reinforcing situation. If the situation from which the individual is being removed is not more reinforcing than the time-out area, the technique will not be effective, and can in fact increase negative behaviors. Time-out procedures have included holding a client's hands (Repp & Dietz, 1974), removing him or her from a group (Porterfield, Herbert-Jackson, & Risley, 1976), physical restraint (Vukelich & Hake, 1971), and total isolation (Wahler & Foxx, 1980) among others.

Another change in treatment strategies is the increased use of a combination of one-to-one training with group experiences. The adolescent and adult training program sponsored by Division TEACCH in North Carolina (Mesibov, 1984, 1986) has employed a training model for social, recreational, and vocational skills that uses nonhandicapped peers, as well as a combination of one-to-one and group training. New skills are first introduced in one-to-one sessions with the clients and then practiced in larger groups that include both handicapped and nonhandicapped individuals. The autistic clients play a major role in planning group activities. Professionals working with severely handicapped clients have also found that providing them with opportunities to choose among a variety of interesting activities is essential in both maintaining morale and avoiding potential behavior problems (Favell & Cannon, 1976; LeLaurin & Risley, 1972).

TREATMENT ISSUES

Normalization

Along with an increasing emphasis on the development of functional skills in order to maximize independent functioning with age, there is an increasing expectation for normalization. The normalization principle (Wolfensberger, 1972) states that programming should be community-based in as "normal" a setting as possible, utilizing age-appropriate materials and nonhandicapped peers. Three programs exemplifying community-based models for serving the needs of autistic adolescents and adults are Division TEACCH, the Jay Nolan Center, and Community Services for Autistic Citizens (CSAC).

Division TEACCH is the most comprehensive statewide program serving autistic people in the United States. The TEACCH program's model includes individualized diagnostic assessment, work with parents, and a comprehensive service network including day and residential programs. This model for serving autistic children has been expanded with equal success to meet the needs of adolescents and young adults with autism since the late 1970s. The special needs of older clients brought about the development of the AAPEP (Mesibov *et al.*, 1984). As described earlier, this diagnostic tool is helpful in determining appropriate goals and intervention strategies in the areas of Vocational Skills, Vocational Behaviors, Leisure Skills, Independent Functioning, Functional Communication, and Interpersonal Behavior. The treatment programs offered to adolescents/young adults and their families emphasize the development of these skills in the least restrictive environments. The program includes classrooms for autistic adolescents, group homes, and clinics for outpatient diagnostic evaluations and treatment. One-to-one training in the actual vocational or social setting is stressed. The social skills training programs include nonhandicapped peers and involve age-appropriate recreational and social activities.

CSAC is located in Rockville, Maryland (Juhrs, 1987). CSAC provides a

wide variety of community-based services, including a classroom, residential programs, and a vocational training program. The major goal of CSAC is to facilitate
deinstitutionalization of autistic people. The CSAC vocational training program
exemplifies the desired outcome of the normalization principle at work. It has
shown that individuals with autism can succeed in supported employment situations when provided with appropriate supervision. Each trainee has a fully trained,
nonhandicapped job counselor who works in the job setting to provide training
and take care of any problems related to the disability. In addition to the vocational skills, the trainer also helps the individual to learn the other related skills
that are necessary to maintain the position (e.g., how to get into work, how to
deal with schedule changes, how to behave with coworkers). In conjunction with
the vocational programs, CSAC also operates residential facilities where individuals with autism can live in a supervised apartment setting. For those individuals
who are not ready for supported employment, CSAC has a classroom program
designed to help them acquire the necessary prevocational skills.

The Jay Nolan Center in southern California (LaVigna, 1983) also epito-
mizes the successful application of the normalization principle. The program includes residential units, vocational training, and family support services for those
individuals living at home. Both the living units and the training programs are
designed to fit in with the community, and to provide the autistic individual with
age-appropriate work and leisure activities. Developmental programming and operant reinforcement techniques are utilized to maximize the productivity and independence of the autistic clients. Parent advocacy is also an instrumental part of
this program.

The data generated by these three programs provide much of the existing
documentation on the overall effectiveness of community-based training programs
(Juhrs, 1987; LaVigna, 1983; Mesibov, Schopler, & Sloan, 1983). There is some
additional support for the efficacy of the normalization principle. For example,
language training is much more effective and meaningful when it occurs in the
natural setting (Beisley & Tsai, 1983; Goetz, Schuler, & Sailor, 1979; Watson,
1985). Special attention has also been given to the development of leisure skills
in normal settings. Appropriate leisure and recreational skills increase the likelihood that a handicapped adult will be able to function successfully in a normal
setting (Kraus, 1978).

A number of authors have stressed the importance of using a variety of age-
appropriate materials in both work and leisure activities (Wehman, 1977, 1983;
Wuerch & Voeltz, 1981). The use of age-appropriate activities increases the likelihood that the individual can be integrated into existing community programs. It
also affects the morale of the autistic individual who is trying to become more
grown-up and independent. Handicapped individuals have the same need for variety in their daily activities as do nonhandicapped adults (Favell & Cannon,
1976; LeLaurin & Risley, 1972).

Approaches that stress the importance of the normalization principle have
not been without their problems. Natural settings, such as competitive employ-

ment opportunities or even workshops designed for mentally retarded individuals, are frequently not able to tolerate the unusual behaviors displayed by an autistic individual.

Although there is general agreement among professionals that many normalized experiences are helpful for most autistic individuals, there is less agreement about the extent to which this principle is to be followed. Some believe that virtually all experiences should be in "normal" settings with age-appropriate materials and nonhandicapped individuals (LaVigna, 1983). Others would argue that sometimes the environmental changes that decrease confusion and provide the structure needed by some autistic people are less feasible in certain community settings (Mesibov, 1976). They suggest that the normalization process can sometimes lead well-meaning professionals to ignore environments that may ultimately be in the best interests of their clients.

Benhaven and Bittersweet Farms are two residential programs that follow the normalization process in general, but have made certain major adaptations to better meet the individualized needs of the autistic clients they serve. Benhaven is a day and residential school community in New Haven, Connecticut, that offers a continuum of services for children and adults. Within its own physical boundaries, Benhaven offers a variety of environments—urban, suburban, school, workshop, residence, and farm (Lettick, 1983). Bittersweet Farms is a comprehensive living and working environment for 15 autistic adults. The autistic adults work as partners with the staff in doing housework, growing and preparing their own food, caring for farm animals, maintaining the property, and making and selling crafts (Kay, Koch, Cafiero, & Klein, 1986). The vocational emphasis is on teaching skills that relate to the daily needs of food, shelter and clothing. Both of these programs offer experiences to address the vocational, recreational, and social needs of their clients. Although both programs allow for some interaction with others outside the program, they are both generally self-contained environments. This allows for more integration among the vocational, recreational, and residential parts of the programs than is typical in community settings, where vocational and residential programs are physically separated and run by different people. In addition, the sheltered nature of these programs makes it possible for the individual to be given more independence than is always possible in programs in the mainstream.

Changes in Community Resources

The late teens and early 20s are the times when most offspring and their families expect that they will become increasingly independent of each other. Unfortunately, for many autistic individuals, this process is reversed. Instead of spending less time with their families, these individuals may actually be at home *more* often, due to lack of jobs or appropriate day programs. Most autistic adults will continue to need some degree of supervision and support, but there are fewer options open to them as they get older. The responsibility often falls back on the family to provide the needed structure and supervision.

By law, schools are responsible for providing services to address the academic, communicative, and social needs of school-aged children. These educational settings often provide additional assistance to autistic children and their families. Teachers and school counselors often assist parents in advocating programs to meet the needs of their offspring. School personnel can also be a source of support to the parents. The fact that they have the children 6 hours a day is in itself a major source of relief to parents of younger children.

However, when autistic youngsters reach the age of 18 (or in some states 21), they are no longer eligible for public school services. In most places, there are no equivalent community programs that provide the training or support these young adults require.

The needs of autistic adults are many. When they complete high school, few autistic individuals (or nonautistic individuals, for that matter) have the skills required to obtain and succeed in competitive employment situations. They need to learn both vocational skills and the behaviors necessary to succeed in working environments. As discussed earlier, most vocational rehabilitation and sheltered employment programs are designed to meet the needs of mentally retarded individuals, and are not always flexible enough to address the needs of handicapped persons with autism.

It is ironic that as autistic individuals become more interested in social and recreational pursuits, the major nonfamily source of these experiences ends. There is a tremendous gap between the structured social interactions of the school day and the very loosely structured recreational options available in most communities. Very few autistic adults have the skills required to take advantage of these community programs.

Families often find even more limited support services for their needs. The advocacy, counseling, and respite services offered by schools and other community agencies for the families of younger autistic persons are greatly diminished for the families of adults.

With the exception of the handful of programs mentioned earlier in the chapter, there are very few community living situations or appropriate residential programs available to autistic adults. DeMyer (1979) estimated that 75% of autistic adults will at some time require residential care. With variable success, some autistic individuals have been placed in group homes for the mentally retarded. Many more wind up in state mental institutions.

Clearly, there is a need for a wide variety of resources for autistic adolescents and adults. Programs are just starting to be developed to meet some of the vocational and social needs of these individuals. Professionals need to continue to explore ways of maximizing the acquisition of the functional skills that will lead to increased independent functioning in these individuals. A continuum of living situations and work opportunities will need to be developed to address the wide discrepancies in skills among autistic individuals. The greatest challenge for those in the field will be to balance the desire for normalization with the structure necessary to minimize confusion and unnecessary stress.

Changes in Concerns of Parents and Families

Parents of younger autistic children frequently feel stressed and frustrated by their children's developmental problems (Marcus, 1977). As times goes on, the demands on these families increase, and they often begin to feel burned out (Bristol & Schopler, 1984). These families of adults with autism must continue to serve as the main advocates for their offspring throughout their lives. As the children grow older and the parents are less able to care for them, a major concern becomes the lack of appropriate community-based or residential programs (Cantwell & Baker, 1984; DeMyer, 1979). The lack of services, coupled with the continued limitations in their offspring's ability to function independently, puts a heavy burden on these families. Autistic individuals' physical development during adolescence also brings additional stresses and concerns for their families. DeMyer (1979) and Cantwell and Baker (1984) have found that families have a difficult time dealing with the sexual development of their handicapped children. Autistic adolescents' social limitations often leave them without appropriate means of reducing the frustrations that result from sexual tensions (DeMyer, 1979). The release of these sexual tensions through physical activity and masturbation can create difficulties for their families in dealing with their children, as well as with the reactions of others to these behaviors. The increased size and strength of these youngsters make aggressive behavior a major concern for their families as well.

All of the issues surrounding autistic individuals' physical growth without commensurate skill development or appropriate services increase families' concerns at a time when they are becoming fatigued rather than energized (Harris & Powers, 1984). These families need continued support and assistance from professionals to deal with the day-to-day stresses, and also to advocate and develop the services that will be needed when these parents can no longer care for their handicapped children (DeMyer & Goldberg, 1983).

Implications for the Treatment of Children with Autism

The knowledge gained from learning more about how autism affects the lives of autistic individuals and their families as they get older has led to some changes in how professionals view and work with younger autistic children. Increased knowledge about adolescent and adult development has led to changes in treatment goals as well as strategies.

One important change has been a new emphasis on teaching practical skills that will lead to increased independence. In addition, the development of functional communication skills, prevocational behaviors, and social and leisure skills has been integrated into the school day in most autistic children's educational programs. The emphasis has even affected early intervention and preschool programs (Nay, 1984). Teachers who work with autistic adolescents and adults have found that it is never too early to begin preparing autistic individuals for the future. With individuals with autism, it is very difficult to break routines that have been going on for years, so it is important from the first educational experience to be thinking about why one is teaching a particular skill and how it will affect a child's ability to be independent and to get along with others in the future.

Difficulties in dealing with change, as well as problems in generalizing what is learned to new situations, have led teachers to begin speculating about their children's eventual living situations and employment sites. More and more, these teachers observe actual workshops, group homes, or prospective competitive employment settings to enable them to adapt their educational programming to meet their students' eventual needs.

Sex education and more general social skills training are also becoming important parts of most educational curricula. The importance of recreational and leisure skills for successful adult outcomes has been recognized of late (Mesibov, 1983). Concerns about the generalization of these skills have led to more training in natural environments. Field trips to restaurants, stores, and community recreational sites are becoming accepted parts of many special education curricula.

Another important shift that has been stimulated by work with autistic adolescents and adults is in the area of behavior management. Behaviors that are considered "cute" or minimally disruptive in young children (e.g., touching others) are often not tolerated in physically mature adults. Aggressive behaviors occurring infrequently in young children are not nearly as disturbing as the same behaviors in 180-pound adults. Seeing how difficult these behaviors can be to manage in adults and the impact they can have on an autistic individual's ability to succeed in vocational or residential programs has forced professionals to address these problems more directly at much younger ages.

SUMMARY AND CONCLUSION

Autistic adolescents and adults have presented new challenges for families and professionals who are concerned about their current and future development. As they face many of the same issues that normally developing individuals encounter, the autistic individuals want to become more adept and independent in their interpersonal, vocational, recreational, and leisure pursuits. Diagnostic, assessment, and intervention strategies are beginning to be developed that take into account the changes occurring in clinical presentation and educational objectives as autistic individuals mature. Future research and clinical efforts need to address the need for greater variety, availability, and flexibility in services for autistic adolescents and adults.

References

Akerley, M. (1984). Developmental changes in families with autistic children: A parent's perspective. In E. Schopler & G. Mesibov (Eds.), *The effects of autism on the family* (pp. 85–97). New York: Plenum.

Ando, H., & Yoshimura, I. (1979). Effects of age on communication skill levels and prevalence of maladaptive behaviors in autistic and mentally retarded children. *Journal of Autism and Developmental Disorders, 9,* 83–93.

Beisler, J. M., & Tsai, L. (1983). A pragmatic approach to increase expressive language skills in young autistic children. *Journal of Autism and Developmental Disorders, 13,* 287–303.

Bellamy, T., Sheehan, M., Horner, R., & Boles, S. (1980). Community programs for severely handicapped adults: An analysis. *Journal of the Association for the Severely Handicapped, 5,* 307–324.

Bonvillian, J., & Nelson, K. (1976). Sign language acquisition in a mute autistic boy. *Journal of Speech and Hearing Disorders, 41,* 339–347.

Bristol, M., & Schopler, E. (1984). A developmental perspective on stress and coping in families of autistic children. In J. Blacher (Ed.), *Families of severely handicapped children* (pp. 91–134). New York: Academic Press.

Cantwell, D., & Baker, L. (1984). Research concerning families of children with autism. In E. Schopler & G. Mesibov (Eds.), *The effects of autism on the family* (pp. 41–63). New York: Plenum.

Carr, E. G. (1981, July). *Analysis and remediation of severe behavior problems.* Paper presented at the meeting of the National Society for Children and Adults with Autism, Boston.

DeMyer, M. K. (1979). *Parents and children in autism.* Washington, DC: V. H. Winston.

DeMyer, M. K., & Goldberg, P. (1983). Family needs of the autistic adolescent. In E. Schopler & G. Mesibov (Eds.), *Autism in adolescents and adults* (pp. 225–250). New York: Plenum.

Favell, J. E. (1977). *The power of positive reinforcement: A handbook of behavior modification.* Springfield, IL: Charles C Thomas.

Favell, J. E. (1983). The management of aggressive behavior. In E. Schopler & G. B. Mesibov (Eds.), *Autism in adolescents and adults* (pp. 187–222). New York: Plenum.

Favell, J. E., & Cannon, P. (1976). Evaluation of entertainment materials for severely retarded persons. *American Journal of Mental Deficiency, 81,* 357–361.

Foxx, R. M., & Azrin, N. H. (1972). Restitution: A method of eliminating aggressive–disruptive behaviour of retarded and brain-damaged patients. *Behaviour Research and Therapy, 1,* 305–312.

Goetz, L., Schuler, A., & Sailor, W. (1979). Teaching functional speech to the severely handicapped: Current issues. *Journal of Autism and Developmental Disorders, 9,* 325–344.

Gold, M. (1976). Task analysis of a complex assembly task by the retarded blind. *Exceptional Children, 43,* 78–87.

Harris, S., & Powers, M. (1984). Behavior therapists look at the impact of an autistic child on the family system. In E. Schopler & G. Mesibov (Eds.), *The effects of autism on the family* (pp. 207–224). New York: Plenum.

Hughes, H., & Davis, R. (1980). Treatment of aggressive behavior: The effects of EMG response discrimination biofeedback training. *Journal of Autism and Developmental Disorders, 10,* 193–202.

Juhrs, P. D. (1987, January). *Supported employment for persons with autism.* Paper presented at the North Carolina Conference on Vocational Alternatives for Youth and Adults with Developmental Disabilities, Durham, NC.

Kay, B. R., Koch, J., Cafiero, J., & Klein, L. (1986). *The Bittersweet Farms way.* Unpublished manuscript.

Kraus, R. (1978). *Therapeutic recreation service: Principles and practices.* Philadelphia: W. B. Saunders.

Lancioni, G. (1983). Using pictorial representatives as communication means with low functioning children. *Journal of Autism and Developmental Disorders, 13*, 87–105.

LaVigna, G. W. (1977). Communication training in mute autistic adolescents using the written word. *Journal of Autism and Childhood Schizophrenia, 7*, 135–150.

LaVigna, G. W. (1983). The Jay Nolan Center: A community-based program. In E. Schopler & G. Mesibov (Eds.), *Autism in adolescents and adults* (pp. 381–410). New York: Plenum.

Lettick, A. L. (1983). Benhaven. In E. Schopler & G. Mesibov (Eds.), *Autism in adolescents and adults* (pp. 355–380). New York: Plenum.

LeLaurin, K., & Risley, T. R. (1972). The organization of day care environments: "Zone" versus "man to man" staff assignments. *Journal of Applied Behavior Analysis, 5*, 225–232.

Lord, C. (1984, July). *A developmental approach to social training for young autistic children.* Paper presented at the annual meeting of the National Society for Children and Adults with Autism, San Antonio, TX.

Lotter, V. (1978). Follow-up studies. In M. Rutter & E. Schopler (Eds.), *Autism: A reappraisal of concepts and treatment* (pp. 475–495). New York: Plenum.

Marcus, L. (1977). Patterns of coping in families of psychotic children. *American Journal of Orthopsychiatry, 47*, 383–399.

McGee, G. G., Krantz, P. J., & McClannahan, L. E. (1984). Conversational skills for autistic adolescents: Teaching assertiveness in naturalistic game settings. *Journal of Autism and Developmental Disorders, 14*, 319–330.

Mesibov, G. B. (1976). Implications of the normalization principle for psychotic children. *Journal of Autism and Childhood Schizophrenia, 6*, 360–377.

Mesibov, G. B. (1983). Current perspectives and issues in autism and adolescence. In E. Schopler & G. Mesibov (Eds.), *Autism in adolescents and adults* (pp. 37–53). New York: Plenum.

Mesibov, G. B. (1984). Social skills training with verbal autistic adolescents and adults: A program model. *Journal of Autism and Developmental Disorders, 14*, 395–404.

Mesibov, G. B. (1986). A cognitive program for teaching social behaviors to verbal autistic adolescents and adults. In E. Schopler & G. B. Mesibov (Eds.), *Social behavior in autism* (pp. 265–283). New York: Plenum.

Mesibov, G. B., Schopler, E., & Schaffer, B. (1984). *Adolescent and Adult Psychoeducational Profile.* Hillsborough, NC: Orange Industries.

Mesibov, G. B., Schopler, E., & Sloan, G. (1983). Service development for adolescents and adults in North Carolina's TEACCH program. In E. Schopler & G. Mesibov (Eds.), *Autism in adolescents and adults* (pp. 411–432). New York: Plenum.

Mesibov, G. B., & Shea (1980, March). *Social and interpersonal problems of autistic adolescents and adults.* Paper presented at the meeting of the Southeastern Psychological Association, Washington, DC.

Nay, D. (1984). A change in perspective. *TEACCHer's report.* (Available from Division TEACCH, University of North Carolina at Chapel Hill, 310 Medical School Wing E, 222H, Chapel Hill, NC 27514)

Porterfield, J. K., Herbert-Jackson, E., & Risley, T. R. (1976). Contingent observation: An effective and acceptable procedure for reducing disruptive behaviors in young children in group settings. *Journal of Applied Behavior Analysis, 9*, 55–64.

Ragland, E. U., Kerr, M. M., & Strain, P. S. (1978). Effects of peer social initiation on the behavior of withdrawn autistic children. *Behavior Modification, 2*, 565–578.

Repp, A. C., & Dietz, S. M. (1974). Reducing aggressive and self-injurious behavior of institutionalized retarded children through reinforcement of other behaviors. *Journal of Applied Behavior Analysis, 7*, 313–325.

Rincover, A., Cook, R., Peoples, A., & Packard, D. (1979). Sensory extinction and sensory reinforcement principles for programming multiple adaptive behavior change. *Journal of Applied Behavior Analysis, 12*, 221–233.

Rutter, M. (1970). Autistic children: Infancy to adulthood. *Seminars in Psychiatry, 2*, 435–450.

Rutter, M., Greenfeld, D., & Lockyer, L. (1967). A five to fifteen year follow-up study of infantile psychosis: II. Social and behavioral outcome. *British Journal of Psychology, 113,* 1169–1182.

Schopler, E., Brehm, S., Kinsbourne, M., & Reichler, R. J. (1971). The effects of treatment structure on development in autistic children. *Archives of General Psychiatry, 24,* 415–421.

Schopler, E., & Mesibov, G. B. (Eds.). (1983). *Autism in adolescents and adults.* New York: Plenum.

Schopler, E., & Reichler, R. J. (1979). *Individualized assessment and treatment for autistic and developmentally disabled children: Psychoeducational profile.* Baltimore: University Park Press.

Schopler, E., Reichler, R. J., & Renner, B. R. (1986). *The Childhood Autism Rating Scale (CARS).* New York: Irvington.

Schopler, E., Reichler, R. J., DeVellis, R. F., & Daly, K. (1980). Toward objective classification of childhood autism: Childhood Autism Rating Scale (CARS). *Journal of Autism and Developmental Disorders, 10,* 91–103.

Vukelich, R., & Hake, D. (1971). Reduction of dangerously aggressive behavior in a severely retarded resident through a combination of positive reinforcement procedures. *Journal of Applied Behavior Analysis, 4,* 215–225.

Wahler, R. G., & Foxx, J. J. (1980). Solitary toy play and time-out: A family treatment package for children with aggressive and oppositional behavior. *Journal of Applied Behavior Analysis, 13,* 23–29.

Watson, L. R. (1985). The TEACCH communication curriculum. In E. Schopler & G. B. Mesibov (Eds.), *Communication problems in autism* (pp. 187–206). New York: Plenum.

Wehman, P. (1977). *Helping the mentally retarded acquire play skills.* Springfield, IL: Charles C Thomas.

Wehman, P. (1983). Recreation and leisure needs: A community integration approach. In E. Schopler & G. Mesibov (Eds.), *Autism in adolescents and adults* (pp. 111–132). New York: Plenum.

Wehman, P., & Hill, J. (1981). Competitive employment for moderately and severely handicapped individuals. *Exceptional Children, 47,* 338–345.

Wolfensberger, W. (1972). *The principle of normalization in human services.* Toronto: National Institute on Mental Retardation.

Wuerch, B., & Voeltz, L. (1981). *The ho'onanea program: A leisure curriculum component for severely handicapped children and youth.* Unpublished manuscript, University of Hawaii Department of Special Education.

CHAPTER 17

Pharmacological Treatment of Autistic Children

VANJA A. HOLM
CHRISTOPHER K. VARLEY
University of Washington

INTRODUCTION

Children with autism present physicians with a challenge to "do something." A common response is to reach for the prescription pad. Sedatives come readily to mind when one is faced with an uncontrollable, agitated youngster. Indeed, hypnotic medications were probably the earliest pharmacological treatment given to children with autism (Fish, 1976).

In the early 1960s, antipsychotic medications revolutionized the management of adult psychoses (Greenblatt, Solomon, Evans, & Brooks, 1985). It was soon noticed that the childhood psychoses did not respond as well to these medications, confirming the notion that developmental psychiatric disorders are fundamentally different from adult mental illness. Still, investigations of new antipsychotic drugs and antidepressants continue in children with autism.

The effect of stimulant medication on behavior in children was first described in the 1930s by Bradley (Bradley, 1937), but stimulants did not become widely used for this purpose until the 1970s (Krager & Safer, 1974). They have been promoted in the treatment of childhood hyperactivity, now called attention deficit disorder (ADD). It seemed logical to assume that these drugs might also calm children with autism, and this assumption has been investigated by several researchers.

Fenfluramine has received much attention during the last few years as a specific drug for autism. Recently, there has been much interest in the use of naltrexone, an opiate antagonist, in autism. Theoretical rationales have been proposed for the use of nutritional intervention. Finally, anticonvulsants are often prescribed for seizure disorders in children with autism, and their effect on the autism needs to be considered.

This chapter provides a review of present knowledge of the usefulness—or lack thereof—of these agents in autism.

GENERAL COMMENTS

Before we discuss specific pharmacological and nutritional agents, some general comments on studies in autism are in order.

Particularly in older studies, there are problems with the definition of patient populations. Historically, infantile autism, childhood schizophrenia, and other serious psychopathological states of childhood were not discriminated. This diagnostic heterogeneity makes it difficult to interpret outcome. Furthermore, many early studies were anecdotal in nature. Without control groups, commonly accepted statistical practices could not be employed. In appropriate controlled studies, other issues need to be considered. Are the measuring tools used appropriate? In the presence of results that are statistically significant, has an appreciable change for the better been accomplished in the lives of the autistic children or their families? If meaningful improvement is obtained, are there substantial side effects? Are the beneficial effects sustained over time?

SEDATIVES

The sedative–hypnotic group of medications was probably the earliest psychopharmacological treatment given to children with autism. These medications have not been subjected to systematic studies. In an early report (Fish, 1960), diphenhydramine (Benadryl) was determined to be the most effective of the mild sedatives. There are anecdotal reports on the utility of sedative hypnotics for transient sleep disturbances in autistic children. Sedatives for sleep disturbance generally should not be prescribed for periods greater than 2 weeks, because rapid development of tolerance to these medications is a well-described phenomenon (Jaffe, 1970). In addition, there is a risk of paradoxical excitatory responses with barbiturate medications, also seen occasionally with benzodiazepines such as diazepam (Valium) and chlordiazepoxide (Librium).

STIMULANTS

In the United States and Canada, stimulant medications are the most commonly prescribed medications for treatment of behavior disturbances in children. Methylphenidate (Ritalin), dextroamphetamine (Dexedrine), and magnesium pemoline (Cylert) are recognized as efficacious in the treatment of some children with ADD. The primary symptoms in ADD—short attention span, impulsiveness, and distractibility—have been repeatedly demonstrated to be amenable to treatment with drugs in short-term studies (Barkley, 1977; Varley, 1984). The same symptoms are also present in many autistic children as part of the syndrome complex. Therefore, investigations of the effectiveness of these drugs in autistic populations have been undertaken.

Some researchers have demonstrated that stimulant medications have only a mildly positive effect by improving attention, but show clinically and statistically significant increases in stereotypic behavior in autistic children (Campbell, Fish, David, *et al.*, 1972; Campbell *et al.*, 1976). They also describe the emergence of stereotypic behavior in children who previously did not demonstrate such patterns. Amphetamines and other stimulant medications can induce stereotypic behavior in several animal species, including rats, mice, guinea pigs, and monkeys (Fitz-Gerald, 1967; Randrup & Munkvad, 1967). Exacerbation of an underlying psychosis or behavioral disturbance has also been reported with amphetamines and methylphenidate (Fish, 1971). The subject of stimulant drug effect in developmental disorders was reviewed by Aman (1982). The studies he reviewed indicated little or no clinical improvements on stimulant medication, and, using biochemical reasoning, he cited the theoretical negative effects in the autistic population. He concluded that, although attention span problems are present in autistic children, there is no role for the use of stimulants in this population.

Despite these generally negative studies, there are many anecdotal reports of improvement in certain children with autism or related pervasive developmental disorders to stimulant medication. For example, Geller, Guttmacher, and Bleeg (1981) reported that D-amphetamine was effective in reducing some adverse symptoms in children with childhood-onset development disorders. In our clinical experience, an occasional child responds positively to these medications. Consideration for their use might be entertained in a high-functioning autistic child in whom short attention span, distractibility, and excitability are significant symptoms. The available literature suggests, however, that stimulant medications play a limited role at best in the treatment of target symptoms in the child with autism.

NEUROLEPTICS

Of the medication groups to treat individuals with autism, the most widely studied agents have been the neuroleptics. Several reviews of these medications have recently been published (Campbell, 1985; Campbell, Cohen, & Anderson, 1981; DeMyer, Hingtgen, & Jackson, 1981). Although high-dose, low-potency neuroleptics such as chlorpromazine (Thorazine) have been investigated (Campbell, Fish, Korein, *et al.*, 1972), the bulk of the studies have been with low-dose, high-potency neuroleptics, especially haloperidol (Haldol) (Campbell, Anderson, Perry, Green, & Kaplan, 1982).

A sizeable number of studies of the low-dose, high-potency medications have been published from comparatively few laboratories across the United States. Agreement over indications for their use is not uniform (Corbett, 1976; Fish, 1976; Rutter, 1985). To summarize the findings with haloperidol, the use of this drug has been reported to result in improvement in agitation, hyperactivity, aggression, stereotypic behaviors, and affective lability. Less affected are withdrawal behaviors, abnormal interpersonal relationships, and cognitive functioning (Cohen *et al.*, 1980; Ornitz, 1985).

The neuroleptics are, of course, powerful agents. Numerous side effects from these medications have been described. These include sedation, decreased ability to learn, extrapyramidal side effects (fluctuation in muscle tone), akathisia (a sensation of extreme motor restlessness), anticholinergic symptoms (dry mouth, increased pulse rate), hypotension, photosensitivity, and—most worrisome of all—tardive dyskinesia (slow, involuntary motor movements, especially in the mouth and tongue, which can be permanent and untreatable). The risk of an autistic child's developing tardive dyskinesia after long-term use of a neuroleptic agent probably is on the order of 20%, a figure cited as the risk to a general population receiving long-term treatment with neuroleptics (Kane & Smith, 1982).

Although it does appear that some symptoms of autism can be effectively treated with neuroleptic medications, the cost–benefit ratio needs to be carefully evaluated. Even if clinical improvement can be documented, numerous serious side effects of these agents exist. The clinician needs to decide whether placing a child on this medication is worth the potential risk. Children who appear to benefit in some ways from these medications still remain autistic and severely handicapped. Ornitz (1985) has challenged the real clinical efficacy of haloperidol. Anderson *et al.* (1984) reported a significant improvement with no significant side effects in an autistic population treated for 8 weeks. Obviously, tardive dyskinesia or other long-term side effects are unlikely to have emerged in this short-term study. A telling observation in this study was that 36 of 40 children had changes of such positive magnitude that their parents asked that the children be kept on the medication after the study was completed. Thus, there remains considerable ambiguity about the indication for neuroleptics, particularly haloperidol, for long-term use in children with autism.

TRICYCLIC ANTIDEPRESSANTS

The effects of tricyclic antidepressant medications have not been extensively studied in children with autism. In an investigation of imipramine (Tofranil), Campbell, Fish, Shapiro, and Floyd (1971) found that this medication showed many positive effects when compared to amphetamines. About 20% of the children on imipramine showed marked improvement in speech and interpersonal responsivity. This study was compromised by a questionable definition of diagnostic population. Most importantly, three-quarters of the children worsened.

FENFLURAMINE

Background

Fenfluramine hydrochloride is an anorectic drug that has been used for obesity in adults (incidentally, not particularly successfully). It was known that fenfluramine lowers serotonin levels in the brain in animals. Ritvo *et al.* (1970) had noted that blood serotonin levels were increased in some children with autism, and came upon the idea to try fenfluramine in such children. The preliminary findings were encouraging, and their observations in three boys were published by the respected *New England Journal of Medicine* in 1982 (Geller, Ritvo, Freeman, & Yuwiler, 1982).

This paper met with enthusiasm from desperate parents and was widely quoted in the lay literature—a fact that was bemoaned by some professionals working with autistic children (Ruttenberg, 1982). The study has also been criticized on procedural grounds (Field, 1982). The researchers at the University of California at Los Angeles (UCLA), who had made the original observation, received support from the pharmacology firm that makes Pondimin (A. H. Robins Co.), the only commercially available fenfluramine product. The eventual outcome was that several studies on the effect of fenfluramine in children with autism were published.

Studies on Fenfluramine

In all of the fenfluramine studies, the *Diagnostic and Statistical Manual of Mental Disorders*, third edition (DSM-III) definition of autism (American Psychiatric Association, 1980) was used. The amount of fenfluramine given was 1.5 mg/kg in two divided doses. The studies used a variety of measures to evaluate the effect of the medication, including IQ tests, parental observations, and behavioral rating scales. Serotonin levels and platelet counts (platelets are blood cells involved in blood clotting; they contain serotonin) were also obtained.

Research by the UCLA Group

The UCLA group published their findings of treatment with fenfluramine on their first 14 patients in 1983 (Ritvo, Freeman, Geller, & Yuwiler, 1983). The findings were positive. The authors reported that blood serotonin levels fell in all patients after 2 months of medication, both in those with initially high levels and in those with normal levels. The average decrease was 51%. After 4 months on fenfluramine, the blood serotonin level had stabilized at the lower level.

Clinical improvement as measured on the Ritvo–Freeman Real-Life Rating Scale (Freeman, Ritvo, Yokota, & Ritvo, 1986), a test designed specifically to rate behaviors in autism, was observed. Most noteworthy was a significant decrease in abnormal motor behaviors, which was noted in all subjects. The Social and Sensory scales on the same test also showed significant improvement for the mean of the group. The mean Self-Help, Social, and Communication scores on the Alpern–Boll Developmental Profile also improved significantly (Alpern & Boll, 1972). This profile is obtained through parental report. The measurements on these two tests generally tended to reverse after the subjects returned to placebo medication. For many subscales, but not all, the change was significant. Although there were some improvements on IQ testing, these continued into the placebo phase of the study and were felt by the authors to represent test–retest factors.

The research design for this study was a 2-week period of open placebo followed by 1 month of placebo, 4 months of fenfluramine and 2 months of placebo. Although the authors state that this study had a double-blind crossover design, this was not truly so, as three of the investigators were aware of it. Moreover, by the authors' admission, the parents soon became aware of the children's medication status because of the change in their children's behavior.

The same UCLA group later reported on an extension of this study (Ritvo *et al.*, 1984). In the second part of the study, an additional 8-month period of active drug treatment was added, followed by 2 months of placebo. The results were similar to what was reported in the previous publication. On some scales, the clinical improvement previously noted after 4 months of treatment was exceeded after 8 months of treatment. In addition, in this second study the authors found a correlation among good clinical response, initially high verbal IQ, and low blood serotonin concentration.

The Multicenter Study

Several medical centers were enlisted by the UCLA group to participate in a multicenter study on the effect of fenfluramine on children with autism, using the same definition of autism, the same drug dose, and the same evaluation measures used by them (IQ tests, Ritvo–Freeman Real-Life Rating Scale for Autism, and Alpern–Boll Developmental Profile). The authors participated with five patients in that study.

First Phase. The design of the first phase of this study was similar to that of the original UCLA study: 2 weeks of known placebo, 1 month of placebo (instead of 2), 4 months of drug, and 2 months of placebo. One investigator at each center was aware of the drug–placebo schedule, but supposedly did not participate in the dispensing of medication or the assessments.

The results of the first phase of the multicenter study have been published (Ritvo *et al.*, 1986). Nine medical centers contributed to the study, with 81 patients participating. The findings confirm previous reports from the UCLA group and from others using the same study design (August, Raz, & Baird, 1985; August *et al.*, 1984; Stubbs, Budden, Jackson, Terdal, & Ritvo, 1986). Fenfluramine lowered the serotonin level in blood by approximately 50%, and this finding was quite consistent across patients. No serious side effects were encountered. Appetite and weight changes were temporary and manageable.

Monthly parental interviews were conducted, and the parents reported beneficial effects—decreased hyperactivity, increased social responsiveness and attention span, and improved communication. These subjective observations of beneficial effects were generally confirmed by the objective behavioral scales administered. The overall, Motor, Sensory, and Social scales on the Ritvo–Freeman Real-Life

Rating Scale for Autism (Freeman et al., 1986) showed significant improvements. The Affect and Language scales on the same instrument did not. The mean value for the Communication, Self-Help, and overall scales on the Alpern–Boll instrument (Alpern & Boll, 1972) showed significant improvement; the Academic, Social, and Physical Development scales did not. Results on measures of intelligence were less impressive. A mild increase in IQ scores appeared to be a practice effect, as it had a tendency to continue into the last placebo period.

Unfortunately, the report on this comprehensive study provides only summary data and does not answer many pertinent questions about consistencies across subjects, variables that predict good response, and so forth. Instead, clinical response was subjectively rated by the principal investigators at the different centers as follows: 33% of the children were "strong responders" and 15% were "nonresponders"; 52% of the children were rated as "moderate responders." Baseline serotonin concentrations, measured in 35 patients, showed a significant inverse correlation with clinical response categories: They were lowest in the 11 strong responders, next highest in the 20 moderate responders, and highest in the 4 nonresponders. There were no significant correlations between the clinical response categories and any of the test scores. Interestingly, some centers had no strong responders and some had no nonresponders, probably reflecting center bias.

Second Phase. An improved design was used in the second phase of the multicenter study: 1 month of open placebo followed by a double-blind, placebo–drug crossover protocol, with random assignment to initial drug or placebo. None of the investigators at the participating centers was aware of the status of medication versus placebo; thus, this was a true double-blind protocol. The same test data as obtained in the first phase of the study were collected.

At this writing, five papers have been published on subsets of patients in this group. Klykylo, Feldis, O'Grady, Ross, and Halloran (1985) reported that 2 of 10 patients showed clear improvement by parental report and clinic observation, and that 1 additional patient showed some improvement. Test data are not provided in this paper, except for the authors' mentioning that no changes were noted on IQ tests or on the Alpern–Boll Developmental Profile. Confusingly, these authors' findings are included in the report from the first phase of the large multicenter study, which used a different study design (Ritvo et al., 1986).

Ho, Lockitch, Eaves, and Jacobson (1986) compared blood serotonin levels in four groups of children: 13 with autism, 10 who were retarded but nonautistic, 18 with Down syndrome, and a group of normal children of the same age. They report that the Down syndrome children had significantly lower serotonin levels but that there were no differences in the other three groups. Seven autistic boys who were subjects in this study also participated in the second phase of the multicenter study. A decrease in serotonin levels with fenfluramine treatment was observed in all seven of these subjects; in fact, the authors state that this test may be followed as an indication of drug compliance during fenfluramine treatment. These findings are consistent with those of previous studies (August et al., 1984, 1985; Geller et al., 1982; Klykylo et al., 1985; Ritvo et al., 1983, 1984, 1986).

However, Ho and colleagues found no relationship between this phenomenon and clinical drug efficacy. Again, like some other researchers (August *et al.*, 1985; Klykylo *et al.*, 1985), they failed to find improvements in IQ scores. The UCLA group is the only one reporting improved intellectual performance on fenflura-mine (Geller *et al.*, 1982; Ritvo *et al.*, 1983, 1984). This effect was weak in the report of the first phase of the multicenter study (Ritvo *et al.*, 1986).

Ho *et al.* (1986) did report in some detail on several language tests. They observed slight improvement in short-term auditory memory and on some mea-sures of receptive language skills. These findings were variable between subjects, however, and more noticeable in higher-functioning subjects. In contrast to pre-vious reports from the multicenter study, Ho *et al.* (1986) failed to notice consis-tent, uniform subjective improvement in social responsiveness. The numbers were small, however.

A third paper from this phase of the multicenter study reports on the effect of fenfluramine on communication skills in six autistic boys (Beisler, Tsai, & Steifel, 1986). This study showed that fenfluramine did not have any significant effect on communication behaviors (as measured on a variety of standardized tests and in spontaneous speech samples) of these autistic children as a group or as individuals. Our own experience, assessing the communication skills in our five patients, would support this notion (Coggins *et al.*, 1988).

In a separate paper, investigators from the same institution reported a 58% decrease in serotonin levels in this group of children treated with fenfluramine (Beeghly, Kuperman, Perry, Wright, & Tsai, 1987). They also reported that im-provements in behavior could not be demonstrated on the rating instruments em-ployed. Anecdotally, only the parents of the two children with the highest initial serotonin levels noticed behavioral improvements.

In another recent paper, Groden *et al.* (1987) describe four boys and report a reduction in some deviant behaviors and improvement in activity level and attention span.

Our experience also tells us that the physiological effects of fenfluramine are marked enough so that the parents (and probably also the child) can tell when the child is on "the real thing." Interestingly, one of our parents guessed wrong; the discontinuation of fenfluramine resulted in an effect on the child that was per-ceived as more beneficial than its introduction. He was more combative and re-bellious on the fenfluramine, compared to baseline and placebo conditions. At the end of the study, most of the parents chose to continue the medication. We have noted a habituation effect, however—an issue that has not been addressed by the UCLA group or the multicenter study but has been mentioned by Camp-bell, Deutsch, Perry, Wolsky, and Palij (1986). Most of our parents have reported that the beneficial effect seems to wear off after a few months on fenfluramine. Increases in dosage (to what seems safe, compared to acceptable adult levels) have had only moderate success. Eventually all of our parents chose to take their chil-dren off the fenfluramine because of its diminishing efficacy.

Apparently, the data accumulated in the second phase of the multicenter study will not be analyzed together, as, according to the principal investigator, there is too much variation between the kinds of data obtained at the different centers (E. R. Ritvo, personal communication, 1987). This is disappointing, as the direction for data collection was spelled out in detail by the UCLA group and adhered to—at least by us—and faithfully reported to the principal investigator.

Other Studies

Campbell *et al.* (1986) reported on a study of 10 hospitalized children, 7 males and 3 females with a mean age of 4.15 years, who were given fenfluramine in an open trial. A dose of 10 mg/day was given with gradual, individualized increase until positive or untoward effects were noted. Optimal doses were found to be 1.093 to 1.787 mg/kg per day, with a mean of 1.4, similar to the dose used in the multicenter study. Untoward effects were mainly drowsiness and lethargy, but these were not present on optimal dosage. The authors used the Children's Psychiatric Rating Scale (CPRS; National Institute of Mental Health, 1985) and the Clinical Global Impressions (CGI; National Institute of Mental Health, 1985) to assess the effect of fenfluramine on these patients. They reported significant improvement in hyperactivity, withdrawal, negative and uncooperative behavior, and stereotypies. On the CGI, the severity of illness was rated significantly less on fenfluramine. The authors noted, however, that the therapeutic effects of fenfluramine were transient in some children.

Summary

Table 17-1 summarizes the results of published studies to date regarding the effects of fenfluramine on behavior and development in children with autism. The effect of fenfluramine treatment on levels of serotonin has not been included, as there is a clear consensus that blood serotonin levels decrease approximately 50% with treatment. The significance of this finding remains unclear.

Gualtieri (1986) has sounded a strongly worded warning on the use of fenfluramine in autism. His caution that we do not know the long-term effect of *any* drug needs to be remembered. A lengthy editorial correspondence (Gualtieri, 1987; Ritvo *et al.*, 1987) has failed to solve the issue of safety of fenfluramine. The UCLA group and the collaborators from the multicenter study point out that the extensive experience with fenfluramine over a reasonable period of time has been remarkably free of side effects (Ritvo *et al.*, 1987). In his reply, Gualtieri (1987) criticizes the study design and outcome measurements of the fenfluramine studies published so far, cites studies showing neurotoxicity of the drug in animals, and reiterates his concerns about possible adverse long-term effects. His warning cannot be ignored, but may seem overstated to clinicians who have had experience with this drug.

TABLE 17-1. Studies of Fenfluramine Treatment in Austism

Author, date	n	Design	IQ	Social	Language	Motor activity
Geller, Ritvo, Free-man, & Yuwiler (1982)	3	Single subject	+*	+* RLRS	n.a.	n.a.
Ritvo, Freeman, Geller, & Yuwiler (1983)	14	Single-blind	?+	+* RLRS	n.a.	n.a.
Ritvo et al. (1984)	Same as above	Same as above	?+	+* RLRS	+ obs	n.a.
August, Raz, & Baird (1985)	9	Double-blind (?)	=	+ RLRS	n.a.	+ Conners
Klykylo, Feldis, O'Grady, Ross, & Halloran (1985)	10	Double-blind (?) crossover	=	+3/10 obs	n.a.	n.a.
Stubbs, Budden, Jackson, Terdal, & Ritvo (1986)	8	Double-blind (?)	?+	= RLRS	n.s. + Alpern–Boll	+ RLRS
Ho, Lockitch, Eaves, & Jacobson (1986)	7	Double-blind crossover	=	= obs	?+* Several tests	n.a.
Beisler, Tsai, & Steifel (1986)	6	Double-blind crossover	n.a.	n.a.	= Several tests	n.a.
Ritvo et al. (1986)	81	Double-blind	+*	+ RLRS	+* Alpern–Boll	+* RLRS
Groden et al. (1987)	4	Double-blind crossover	=	+ RLRS	n.a.	+ Other

Note. +, positive effect on fenfluramine; +*, positive effect continued into placebo phase; =, no change on fenfluramine; n.a., not available; n.s., nonsignificant; obs, informal observation or parent rating; RLRS, Real-Life Rating Scale (Freeman, Ritvo, Yokota, & Ritvo, 1986); Alpern–Boll, Alpern–Boll Developmental Profile (Alpern & Boll, 1972); Conners, Conners Parent and Teacher Rating Scales (Goyette, Conners, & Ulrich, 1978).

OPIATE ANTAGONISTS

Deutsch (1986) has suggested a rationale for the treatment with opiate antagonists for autism. He described the putative role of endogeneous opioid peptides in the regulation of attention, pain appreciation, affect, and social behavior. Several key symptoms of autism are similar to features seen in opiate addiction (Weizman *et al.*, 1984): insensitivity to pain, decreased socialization, affective lability, and re-petitive stereotypic behavior.

Recently, anecdotal descriptions of the beneficial effects of naltrexone, a po-tent and long-acting opioid antagonist, in children with autism have appeared in the lay literature. Although abstracts from meetings have been published, so far only one carefully designed study is available (Campbell, Adams, Small, McVeigh Tesch, & Curren, 1988). Eight autistic boys with moderate to profound retardation, aged 3.75 to 6.5 years, participated in an open, acute-dose-range tolerance study on the effects of naltrexone. The children's behavior was rated on the CPRS obtained from a semistructured playroom interview, and on the Conners Parent and Teacher Rating Scales (Goyette *et al.*, 1978) obtained in the children's classroom.

Significant improvement was noted in the CPRS Autism factor (underproductive speech, abnormal object relationships, withdrawal, unspontaneous relations to examiner, and stereotypies). The lower dose level (0.5 mg/kg per day given once a week) resulted in tranquilizing effects with less fidgetiness and uncooperative behavior. The highest dose (2.0 mg/kg per day) resulted in strong reduction in stereotypies and significantly increased relatedness to others. Withdrawal was markedly diminished across all three dose levels (a dose of 1 mg/kg per day was also used). Furthermore, the total score on the Conners scale in the classroom was significantly reduced. Extensive laboratory evaluations did not reveal any untoward medical complications. The medical team judged six of the eight children to be responders to naltrexone. With the two nonresponders, the positive changes were weak and of short duration. The authors concluded that their findings require replication with a larger sample, and that efficacy of naltrexone should be critically assessed under double-blind placebo-controlled conditions. One can only hope that such studies are under way.

VITAMINS AND DIET

Nutritional manipulation has emerged as a popular form of treatment for a variety of developmental disorders in children. In autism, the use of megavitamin therapy, especially vitamin B_6, has been proposed as a form of treatment by proponents of orthomolecular psychiatry. Approximately 7.7% of males with autism have been found to have the fragile X syndrome (Brown *et al.*, 1986). Folate, one of the B vitamins, has been tried as a treatment in this disorder, with variable results. Finally, a no-additives type of diet, often referred to as the "Feingold diet" (Feingold, 1975), became popular for hyperactive children some years ago and has followers among those working with children with autism.

Vitamin Therapy

Based upon testimonials collected from parents of 200 children, Rimland (1973) has been promoting treatment with megadoses of vitamins in autism and other severe mental disorders of children for a long time. The vitamin B complex and vitamin C are water-soluble and therefore supposedly innocuous, and have been used in such treatment. According to Rimland (Rimland, Callaway, & Dreyfus, 1978), vitamin B_6 (pyridoxine) eventually turned out to be the key factor in the reported behavioral improvement observed by parents during megavitamin therapy.

Pyridoxine, or vitamin B_6, is an essential vitamin that is a coenzyme in several metabolic reactions. Adequate functioning of the nervous system depends on pyridoxine, for which the minimum daily requirement is 2–4 mg. Pyridoxine dependency is an inborn error of metabolism, which requires very high doses of pyridoxine. These two facts—the importance of pyridoxine to the brain and the need for high doses in dependency syndromes—seem to constitute the rationale for the experimental use of large doses of pyridoxine in children with autism.

In 1978, Rimland *et al.* published a study attempting to look at the question of the effect of pyridoxine in autism in a systematic fashion. A subgroup of 20 children (from Rimland's original group of 200), who, by parental report, seemed to have improved on vitamin B_6 and relapsed on its withdrawal, were identified for this study. Of these 20, 16 participated. The children were already on vitamins, minerals, and perhaps other drugs during the whole study period. Vitamin B_6 (in doses varying from 2.4 to 94.3 mg/kg, alternating with a placebo) was added to the children's usual regimen during two (out of five) study periods of varying length. The results were analyzed by the authors, who judged and rated parent descriptions of the children's behavior.

The authors concluded that the behavior of the children deteriorated significantly during vitamin B_6 withdrawal. However, there are several problems with this conclusion. First and most importantly, if one reanalyzes the data, there is no difference in behavior rating between the two periods when the behavior ratings on all 16 subjects are included. The authors excluded one patient who showed no difference in behavior, with the statement that they had evidence that there had been a mixup and that the child had been on Vitamin B_6 during both periods. Their analysis of the data (with this patient removed) does indicate a difference between the two periods. Second, the children were taking excess pyridoxine all through the study, and the amount of vitamin and the length of time it was given varied between the subjects. Finally, the procedures used to evaluate the results lack objectivity. Considering the many weaknesses of this study, it can hardly be taken as proof that this vitamin improves behavior, even in a very selected group of children with autism.

Encouraged by the findings of Rimland and colleagues, a group of French researchers have been studying the effect of megadoses of pyridoxine and a combination of pyridoxine and magnesium (Mg) in autism. Recently, their results have been published in the English-language literature (Lelord *et al.*, 1981; Martineau, Barthelemy, Garreau, & Lelord, 1985). Severely affected hospitalized children with autism were used in these studies. In their second article (Martineau *et al.*, 1985), they describe an improved research design with 2-week periods when either a vitamin B_6-plus-Mg regimen was compared to Mg alone or to placebo, or B_6 and Mg alone were compared to placebo. Clinical effect was evaluated on a behavior rating scale developed by the authors. A drug-free 2-week baseline was provided before and after the 4-week drug treatment, which had a switchover in the middle. These same authors have also been interested in urinary levels of homovanillic acid (HVA) and auditory and visually evoked potentials on electroencephalographic (EEG) recordings in children with autism. HVA is a metabolite of dopamine, one of the neurotransmitters in the brain; urinary HVA also comes from other sources. Sensory evoked EEG potentials are typically used to assess the intactness of the respective sensory modality.

This French group did not demonstrate any change in autistic symptoms with pyridoxine or Mg alone. Their cautious claim that the combination regimen of pyridoxine and Mg may be of help in autism is not supported after careful reading of the report. In the first trial, behavior improved with the combined vitamin B_6-plus-Mg regimen and improved further with Mg alone; the improvements trends extended into posttreatment baseline. In the comparison of the combined treatment to placebo, the authors report significant changes between before-treatment baseline and treatment, but provide no comparison with the placebo period. In addition, treatment periods were short (2 weeks for each treatment modality), and the behavior scale used is not particularly specific to autism.

The doses of pyridoxine used in these studies were indeed megasized: several hundred up to 1000 mg of vitamin B_6. This vitamin, like other water-soluble vitamins, has been considered safe even in such high doses. A 1983 article in the *New England Journal of Medicine* casts doubt on this assumption, however (Schaumburg *et al.*, 1983). These authors report on seven young adults with severe, long-standing neurological abnormalities following intake of megadoses of pyridoxine. The symptoms slowly improved only after withdrawal of the medication. They issue a strong warning about therapy with megadoses of vitamin B_6 for behavioral disorders.

A small but significant number of boys with autism have been found to have the fragile X syndrome (Brown *et al.*, 1986). The combination of autism and fragile X has been designated "AFRAX" by Swedish researchers (Gillberg, Wahlstrom, Johansson, Tornblom, & Albertson-Wikland, 1986). In cytological studies, a folate-deficient medium is necessary to bring out the chromosomal abnormality in the fragile X condition. This fact led French researchers (Lejune, 1982) to try treatment with this vitamin in boys with fragile X, and their first reports were positive. Recently, well-designed studies have been carried out on the effect of this vitamin in the fragile X syndrome. Many researchers report a decrease, often to zero, of the abnormal fragile X cells in males treated with folate (Froster-Iskenius *et al.*, 1986). Studies of the effects on behavior have shown variable results, however. The largest and probably the best such study (Hagerman *et al.*, 1986) does show behavioral improvement in prepubertal boys with the fragile X condition treated with a reasonable amount of folate (10 mg per day as compared to the recommended daily dose of 1 mg). The one published study on the effect of this vitamin on boys with AFRAX failed to show unequivocal improvement (Gillberg *et al.*, 1986), but only four boys were studied. It is of note that folic acid treatment has been tried and found not to be effective in an *unselected* group of children with autism (Lowe, Cohen, Miller, & Young, 1981).

The Feingold Diet

In a book published in 1975, Feingold wrote about his positive personal experience in treating hyperactive children with an elimination diet that excluded artificial flavors and colors, as well as salicylates (which are present naturally in some fruits) and other additives. Feingold claimed that hyperactive children were allergic to these products and therefore responded to their elimination. The diet became quite popular. It is difficult to adhere to, but not harmful. Eventually, acceptable scientific studies were carried out on the efficacy of this diet in children with common hyperactivity. Early results were equivocal. Several recent studies (Goyette, Conners, Petti, & Curtis, 1978; Harley *et al.*, 1978; Mattes & Gittelman, 1981) have cast serious doubt on its efficacy. These researchers have concluded that the diet at best might be helpful to a selected, very small group of children with hyperactivity.

No studies have been carried out on the effect of this diet on children with autism. We are aware of treatment programs utilizing this diet, which have been accepted with enthusiasm by some parents. Presently, their testimonials are the only support for its use. Other caretakers of children with autism have reasoned that they would rather spend their time and energy in pursuits more likely to be beneficial to the children than a complicated diet.

ANTICONVULSANTS

The relationship between behavior disturbance and anticonvulsant medications has not been studied extensively in autistic children. Many autistic children will develop a seizure disorder by adolescence. The estimated incidence of epilepsy in autism varies. It has been reported to be as high as 75% (Knobloch & Pasamanick, 1975). Others have found an incidence of approximately 40% (Gubbay, Lobascher, & Kingerlee, 1970). Autistic children with seizures are obviously candidates for anticonvulsant medication. Choice of medication depends on seizure type and EEG findings, and is typically not influenced by the diagnosis of autism.

Carbamazepine (Tegretol) has been reported as a medication useful not only in known seizure disorders, but also in lithium-resistant bipolar disturbances and at times in the management of aggression (Ballenger & Post, 1980; Hakola & Laulumaa, 1982). Whether this or other seizure medications have any utility for management of behavioral symptoms in autism is unclear. However, there are situations in which appropriate management of a coexisting seizure disorder might lead to easier-to-manage, more educable children. In our clinical experience, several children who presented with autistic characteristics, severe developmental delay, and explosive behavior turned out to have abnormal EEGs. The level of clinical suspicion of active seizure disorder was not high in these children. Some of them subsequently proved to have significant seizure activity, and institution of anticonvulsant medications not only controlled their seizure disorder, but also made them more amenable to education programs and improved their behavior.

SUMMARY

What emerges from this review is that no medication has unequivocally been demonstrated to alter the course of infantile autism. Judicious use of fenfluramine and haloperidol, at least in the short term, may result in improvement in the symptoms of autism for some children. Naltrexone might turn out to be a useful drug, ameliorating some of the disturbing symptomatology in this condition. Whether there are long-term side effects to these potent medications is not clear. An occasional child may respond to other medications. Where does this leave the clinician in terms of making a therapeutic decision?

Fenfluramine appeared on the horizon in the early 1980s as a promising pharmacological treatment in autism. Not surprisingly, it has not turned out to be the panacea that some anticipated. At the same time, there appears to be a use for this drug in autism. Even if the benefit is temporary, fenfluramine seems to have clinically advantageous effects on some of the most debilitating social symptomatology in some children with autism. And perhaps that is all we can expect from drug treatment in this complex disorder. The overall judgment is that this drug does seem to be safe, but further research and clinical observation are clearly needed on this issue. At the time of this writing, the use of fenfluramine for children with autism has not yet been approved by the Food and Drug Administration. Such approval is anticipated in the near future, however.

In the case of neuroleptic medications, such as haloperidol, debilitating symptoms need to be present before medications can be considered. Appropriate informed consent from patients and their families in terms of potential side effects, and attention to the American Psychiatric Association's guidelines regarding neuroleptic management and the risk of tardive dyskinesia, are essential. Frequent review of medications, with efforts to withdraw them, is necessary. Neuroleptic medication may best be considered at problematic times in the life of an autistic child and his or her family—for example, when periods of combativeness, sleep disturbance, self-injurious behavior, or other behavior disruptions are markedly problematic. Treatment with these drugs may also be considered at times in which children have been demonstrated to be nonresponsive to less invasive procedures, such as appropriate education and parent training.

At the time of this writing, opiate antagonists, such as naltrexone, are experimental drugs in the treatment of autism. Future research will establish if they play a role in the clinical therapy of this condition.

Controversy remains in the area of pharmacological treatment of autism. To date, no medication has been demonstrated to be curative for this chronic and (by definition) lifelong disorder. It seems highly unlikely that such a medication ever will be available. One can be cautiously optimistic, however, that future medications will be developed that have positive effects on selected troublesome behaviors in children with autism. Pharmacological treatment should always be used in conjunction with behavioral therapies, however, never as a substitute for them.

References

Alpern, G. D., & Boll, T. J. (1972). *Developmental Profile II: Manual.* Aspen, CO: Psychological Development.

Aman, M. C. (1982). Stimulant drug effects in developmental disorders and hyperactivity: Toward a resolution of disparate findings. *Journal of Autism and Developmental Disorders, 12,* 385–398.

American Psychiatric Association. (1980). *Diagnostic and statistical manual of mental disorders* (3rd ed.). Washington, DC: Author.

Anderson, L. T., Campbell, M., Grega, D. M., Perry, R., Small, A. M., & Green, W. H. (1984). Haloperidol in the treatment of infantile autism: Effects on learning and behavioral symptoms. *American Journal of Psychiatry, 10,* 1195–1202.

August, G. J., Raz, N., & Baird, T. D. (1985). Brief report: Effects of fenfluramine on behavioral, cognitive, and affective disturbances in autistic children. *Journal of Autism and Developmental Disorders, 15,* 97–107.

August, G. J., Raz, N., Papanicolaou, A. C., Baird, T. D., Hirsh, S. L., & Hsu, L. L. (1984). Fenfluramine treatment in infantile autism: Neurochemical, electrophysiological, and behavioral effects. *Journal of Nervous and Mental Disease, 172,* 604–612.

Ballenger, J. C., & Post, R. M. (1980). Carbamazepine in manic–depressive illness: A new treatment. *American Journal of Psychiatry, 137,* 782–790.

Barkley, R. (1977). A review of stimulant drug research with hyperactive children. *Journal of Child Psychology and Psychiatry, 18,* 137–165.

Beeghly, J. H., Kuperman, S., Perry, P. J., Wright, G. J., & Tsai, L. Y. (1987). Fenfluramine treatment of autism: Relationship of treatment response to blood levels of fenfluramine and norfenfluramine. *Journal of Autism and Developmental Disorders, 17,* 541, 548.

Beisler, J. M., Tsai, L. Y., & Steifel, B. (1986). Brief report: The effects of fenfluramine on communication skills in autistic children. *Journal of Autism and Developmental Disorders, 16,* 227–233.

Bradley, C. (1937). The behavior of children receiving benzedrine. *American Journal of Psychiatry, 94,* 577–585.

Brown, W. T., Jenkins, E. C., Cohen, I. L., Fisch, G. S., Wolf-Schein, E. G., Gross, A., Waterhouse, L., Fein, D., Mason-Brothers, A., Ritvo, E., Ruttenberg, B. A., Bentley, W., & Castells, S. (1986). Fragile X and autism: A multicenter survey. *American Journal of Medical Genetics, 23,* 341–352.

Campbell, M. (1985). Schizophrenic disorders and pervasive developmental disorders/infantile autism. In J. M. Wiener (Ed.), *Diagnosis in psychopharmacology of childhood and adolescent disorders* (pp. 113–150). New York: Wiley.

Campbell, M., Adams, P., Small, A. M., McVeigh Tesch, L., & Curren, E. L. (1988). Naltrexone in infantile autism. *Psychopharmacology Bulletin, 24,* 135, 139.

Campbell, M., Anderson, L. T., Perry, R., Green, W. H., & Kaplan, R. (1982). The effects of haloperidol on learning and behavior in autistic children. *Journal of Autism and Developmental Disorders, 12*(2), 167–175.

Campbell, M., Cohen, I. L., & Anderson, L. T. (1981). Pharmacotherapy for autistic children: A summary of research. *Canadian Journal of Psychiatry, 24*(4), 265–273.

Campbell, M., Deutsch, S. I., Perry, R., Wolsky, B. B., & Palij, M. (1986). Short-term efficacy and safety of fenfluramine in hospitalized preschool-age autistic children: An open study. *Psychopharmacology Bulletin*, 22, 141, 147.

Campbell, M., Fish, B., David, R., Shapiro, P., Collins, P., & Coe, C. (1972). Response to triiodothyronine and dextroamphetamine: A study of preschool schizophrenic children. *Journal of Autism and Childhood Schizophrenia*, 2, 343–358.

Campbell, M., Fish, B., Korein, J., Shapiro, T., Collins, P., & Co, H. C. (1972). Lithium and chlorpromazine controlled crossover study of hyperactive, severely disturbed young children. *Journal of Autism and Childhood Schizophrenia*, 2, 234–263.

Campbell, M., Fish, B., Shapiro, T., & Floyd, A. (1971). Imipramine in preschool autistic and schizophrenic children. *Journal of Autism and Childhood Schizophrenia*, 3, 267–282.

Campbell, M., Small, A. M., Collins, P. J., Friedman, E., David, R., & Genieser, N. (1976). Levodopa and levoamphetamine: A crossover study of young schizophrenic children. *Current Therapeutic Research*, 19, 70–86.

Coggins, T. E., Morisset, C., Krasney, L., Frederickson, R., Holm, V. A., & Rayses, V. (1988). Brief report: Does fenfluramine enhance the cognitive and communicative functioning of autistic children? *Journal of Autism and Developmental Disorders*, 18, 425–437.

Cohen, I. L., Campbell, M., Posner, D., Small, A. M., Triebel, D., & Anderson, L. T. (1980). Behavioral effects of haloperidol in young autistic children: An objective analysis using a within-subjects reversal design. *Journal of the American Academy of Child Psychiatry*, 19(4), 665–677.

Corbett, J. (1976). Medical management. In L. Wing (Ed.), *Early childhood autism: Clinical education and social aspects* (2nd ed., pp. 271–280). Oxford: Pergamon Press.

DeMyer, M. K., Hingtgen, J. N., & Jackson, R. K. (1981). Infantile autism reviewed: A decade of research. *Schizophrenic Bulletin*, 7, 388–451.

Deutsch, C. H., (1986). Rationale for the administration of opiate antagonists in treating infantile autism. *American Journal of Mental Deficiency*, 90(6), 631–635.

Field, M. (1982). Fenfluramine in autism [Letter]. *New England Journal of Medicine*, 307, 1451.

Feingold, B. F. (1975). *Why your child is hyperactive*. New York: Random House.

Fish, B. (1960). Drug therapy in child psychiatry: Pharmacologic aspects. *Comprehensive Psychiatry*, 1, 212–227.

Fish, B. (1971). The "one-child, one-drug" myth of stimulants in hyperkinesis: Importance of diagnostic categories in evaluating treatment. *Archives of General Psychiatry*, 25, 193–203.

Fish, B. (1976). Pharmacotherapy for autistic and schizophrenic children. In E. R. Ritvo (Ed.), *Autism: Diagnosis, current research and management* (pp. 107–120). New York: Spectrum.

Fitz-Gerald, F. (1967). Effects of D-amphetamine upon behavior of young chimpanzees raised under different conditions. In H. Brill & J. Cole (Eds.), *Neuropsychopharmacology* (Vol. 5, pp. 1226–1227). Amsterdam: Elsevier.

Freeman, B. J., Ritvo, E. R., Yokota, A., & Ritvo, A. (1986). A scale for rating symptoms of patients with the syndrome of autism in real life settings. *Journal of the American Academy of Child Psychiatry*, 25, 130–136.

Froster-Iskenius, U., Bodeker, K., Oepen, T., Matthes, R., Piper, U., & Schwinger, E. (1986). Folic acid treatment in males and females with fragile-(X)-syndrome. *American Journal of Medical Genetics*, 23, 273–289.

Geller, B., Guttmacher, L. B., & Bleeg, M. (1981). Coexistence of childhood onset pervasive developmental disorder and attention deficit disorder with hyperactivity. *American Journal of Psychiatry*, 138, 338–389.

Geller, E., Ritvo, E. R., Freeman, B. J., & Yuwiler, A. (1982). Preliminary observations on the effect of fenfluramine on blood serotonin and symptoms in three autistic boys. *New England Journal of Medicine*, 307, 165–167.

Gillberg, C., Whalstrom, J., Johansson, R., Tornblom, M., & Albertson-Wikland, K. (1986). Folic acid as an adjunct in the treatment of children with the autism fragile X syndrome (AFRAX). *Developmental Medicine and Child Neurology*, 28, 624–627.

Goyette, C. H., Conners, C. K., Petti, T. A., & Curtis, L. E. (1978). Effects of artificial colors on hyperactive children: A double-blind challenge study. *Psychopharmacology Bulletin, 14*(2), 39–40.

Goyette, C. H., Conners, C. K., & Ulrich, R. F. (1978). Normative data on revised Conners Parent and Teacher Rating Scales. *Journal of Abnormal Child Psychology, 6*, 221–236.

Greenblatt, M., Solomon, M. H., Evans, A. S., & Brooks, G. W. (1985). *Drugs and social therapy in chronic schizophrenia.* Springfield, IL: Charles C Thomas.

Groden, G., Groden, J., Dondey, M., Zane, T., Pueschel, S. M., & Veliceur, W. (1987). Effects of fenfluramine on the behavior of autistic individuals. *Research in Developmental Disabilities, 8*, 203–211.

Gualtieri, C. T. (1986). Fenfluramine and autism: Careful reappraisal is in order. *Journal of Pediatrics, 103*(3), 417–419.

Gualtieri, C. T. (1987). Reply [Editorial correspondence]. *Journal of Pediatrics, 110*, 159–161.

Gubbay, S. S., Lobascher, M., & Kingerlee, P. A. (1970). A neurological appraisal of autistic children: Results of a Western Australia survey. *Developmental Medicine and Child Neurology, 12*, 422–429.

Hagerman, R. J., Jackson, A. W., Levitas, A., Bracken, M., McBogg, P., Kemper, M., McGravian, L., Berry, R., Matus, I., & Hagerman, P. J. (1986). Oral folic acid versus placebo in the treatment of males with the fragile X syndrome. *American Journal of Medical Genetics, 23*, 241–262.

Hakola, H. A., & Laulumaa, V. A. (1982). Carbamazepine in treatment of violent schizophrenics. *Lancet, i*, 1358.

Harley, J. D., Roy, R. S., Tomasi, L., Eichman, P. L., Matteus, C. G., Chun, R., Cheeland, C. S., & Traisman, E. (1978). Hyperkinesis and food additives: Testing the Feingold hypothesis. *Pediatrics, 61*, 818–826.

Ho, H. H., Lockitch, G., Eaves, L., & Jacobson, B. (1986). Blood serotonin concentrations and fenfluramine therapy in autistic children. *Journal of Pediatrics, 108*, 465–469.

Jaffe, J. H. (1970). Drug addiction and drug abuse. In L. S. Goodman & A. Gilman (Eds.), *The pharmacological basis of therapeutics* (4th ed., pp. 276–313). New York: Macmillan.

Kane, J. M., & Smith, J. M. (1982). Tardive dyskinesia: Prevalence and risk factors, 1959–1979. *Archives of General Psychiatry, 39*, 473–481.

Knobloch, H., & Pasamanick, B. (1975). Some etiologic and prognostic factors in early infantile autism and psychosis. *Pediatrics, 55*, 182–191.

Krager, J. M., & Safer, D. J. (1974). Type and prevalence medication used in the treatment of hyperactive children. *New England Journal of Medicine, 291*, 1118–1121.

Klykylo, W. M., Feldis, D., O'Grady, D., Ross, D. L., & Halloran, C. (1985). Brief report: Clinical effects of fenfluramine in ten autistic subjects. *Journal of Autism and Developmental Disorders, 15*, 417–423.

Lejune, J. (1982). Is the fragile X syndrome amenable to treatment? *Lancet, i*, 273–274.

Lelord, G., Muh, J. P., Barthelemy, C., Martineau, J., Garreau, B., & Callaway, E. (1981). Effects of pyridoxine and magnesium on autistic symptoms: Initial observations. *Journal of Autism and Developmental Disorders, 11*, 219–230.

Lowe, T. L., Cohen, D. J., Miller, S., & Young, J. G. (1981). Folic acid and B12 in autism and neuropsychiatric disturbances of childhood. *Journal of the American Academy of Child Psychiatry, 20*, 104–111.

Martineau, J., Barthelemy, C., Garreau, B., & Lelord, G. (1985). Vitamin B6, magnesium, and combined B6Mg: Therapeutic effects in childhood autism. *Biological Psychiatry, 20*, 467–478.

Mattes, J. A., & Gittelman, R. (1981). Effects of artificial food colorings in children with hyperactive symptoms. *Archives of General Psychiatry, 38*, 714–718.

National Institute of Mental Health. (1985). Special feature: Rating scales and assessment instruments for use in pediatric psychopharmacology research. *Psychopharmacology Bulletin, 21*, 753–770.

Ornitz, E. M. (1985). Should autistic children be treated with haloperidol? *American Journal of PSy-chiatry, 142*(7), 883–884.

Randrup, A., & Munkvad, I. (1967). Stereotyped activities produced by amphetamines in several animal species and man. *Psychopharmacology, 11*, 300–310.

Rimland, B. (1973). High dosage levels of certain vitamins in the treatment of children with severe mental disorders. In D. Hawkins & L. Pauling (Eds.), *Orthomolecular psychiatry* (pp. 513–539). San Francisco: W. H. Freeman.

Rimland, B., Callaway, E., & Dreyfus, P. (1978). The effects of high doses of vitamin B_6 on autistic children: A double-blind crossover study. *American Journal of Psychiatry, 135*, 472–475.

Ritvo, E. R., Freeman, B. J., Geller, E., & Yuwiler, A. (1983). Effects of fenfluramine on 14 outpatients with the syndrome of autism. *Journal of the American Academy of Child Psychiatry, 22*, 549–558.

Ritvo, E. R., Freeman, B. J., Yuwiler, A., Geller, E., Schroth, P., Yokota, A., Mason-Brothers, A., August, G. J., Klykylo, W., Leventhal, B., Lewis, K., Piggott, L., Realmuto, G., Stubbs, E. G., & Umansky, R. (1986). Fenfluramine treatment of autism: UCLA collaborative study of 81 patients at nine medical centers. *Psychopharmacology Bulletin, 22*, 133–140.

Ritvo, E. R., Freeman, B. J., Yuwiler, A., Geller, E., Yokota, A., Schroth, P., & Novak, P. (1984). Study of fenfluramine in outpatients with the syndrome of autism. *Journal of Pediatrics, 105*, 823–828.

Ritvo, E. R., Yuwiler, A., Freeman, B. J., Geller, E., Realmuto, G., Killoran, S. M., Piggott, L. R., Gdowski, C. L., & Fischoff, J. (1987). Reappraisal of "Fenfluramine and autism: Careful reappraisal is in order" [Editorial correspondence]. *Journal of Pediatrics, 110*, 158–159.

Ritvo, E. R., Yuwiler, A., Geller, E., Ornitz, E. M., Saeger, K., & Plotkin, S. (1970). Increased blood serotonin and platelets in early infantile autism. *Archives of General Psychiatry, 23*, 566–572.

Ruttenberg, B. A. (1982). Fenfluramine in autism [Letter]. *New England Journal of Medicine, 307*, 1450–1451.

Rutter, M. (1985). The treatment of autistic children. *Journal of Child Psychology and Psychiatry, 26*(2), 193–214.

Schaumburg, H., Kaplan, J., Windebank, A., Vick, N., Rasmus, S., Pleasure, D., & Brown, M. J. (1983). Sensory neuropathy from pyridoxine abuse: A new megavitamin syndrome. *New England Journal of Medicine, 309*, 445–448.

Stubbs, E. G., Budden, S. S., Jackson, R. H., Terdal, L. G., & Ritvo, E. R. (1986). Effects of fenfluramine on eight outpatients with the syndrome of autism. *Developmental Medicine and Child Neurology, 28*, 229–235.

Varley, C. K. (1984). Attention deficit disorder (the hyperactivity syndrome): A review of selected issues. *Journal of Developmental and Behavioral Pediatrics, 5*, 254–258.

Weizman, R., Weizman, A., Tyano, S., Szekelely, G., Wessman, B. A., & Sarne, Y. (1984). Humoral endorphine blood levels in autistic, schizophrenic, and healthy subjects. *Psychopharmacology, 82*, 368–370.

Index

Abstract ability
    capacity for, development, 27, 28, 35–42
    differential performance, 145, 146
    and emotions, 27, 28
Acoustic startle, 138
Action words, 311
Activation hypothesis, 155, 156, 161–168
Active person–active environment model, 289, 290
Active person–passive environment model, 289, 290
Active social interactions, 274, 275
Additivity model, 268
Adjectives, 100
Adolescent and Adult Psychoeducational Profile (AAPEP), 370–373
Affect, 22–48
    and arousal, 59–62
    autism cause, 22–48
    cognitive impairment cause, 22–48
    nonverbal communication antecedent, 14–16, 24, 25
    right-hemisphere overactivation, 166, 167
    self-recognition relationship, 10–12
    and social deficits, 9–12, 16, 17
    and social development, 3
Affective attunement, 60
Affiliative behaviors, 12–14
AFRAX (autism and fragile X syndrome), 398
Age cues, 85
Age of onset, 176
Aggression
    age-related decrease, 374, 375
    and social skills, 351
Aloofness (see Social aloofness)
Alpern–Boll Developmental Profile, 390
Alpha-blocking method, 147–150
Alternating imitation, 67

Ambiguous meanings, 237, 240, 247, 248
Amphetamines, 387, 388
Amygdala, 195
Analytic language acquisition, 108
Anticonvulsants, 399, 400
Antidepressants, 389
Arizona Articulation Test, 152
Arnold–Chiari type I malformation, 126, 132
Arousal, 49–70 (see also Attention)
    cerebellar hypoplasia, 137–140
    definition, 49n
    homeostatic model, 55
    intervention strategies, 62–70
    novel stimuli, 160, 161
    right-hemisphere overactivation, 164, 165
    and socioemotional impairments, 49–70
Articulation
    brain asymmetry, 152
    verbal autistic children, 97
Assessment, 367, 368, 370–373
Associative learning, 138
Attachment
    arousal relationship, 58, 59
    and social responsiveness, 7
Attention, 49–70 (see also Directed attention; Joint attention)
    cerebellar hypoplasia, 137–140
    imitation facilitation, 64–69
    intervention strategies, 62–70
    limitations, neural hypothesis, 273, 274
    in normal infants, 50–53
    novel stimuli, 159–163
    neural model, 161–168, 273, 274
    physiological correlates, 50–56
    right-hemisphere overactivation, 164, 165
    sensory processing theory, 174–199
    and socioemotional impairments, 49–70
    two-component model, 51

Attention deficit disorder, 387, 388
Auditory evoked response, 158, 159, 182
Auditory stimuli, 156–158
Augmentative communication systems, 293
Autonomic studies, 159–161, 181–183
Autosomal recessive inheritance, 227, 271
Averaged event-related potentials, 163
Aversive response
    and attention, 51, 52
    socioemotional development, 57–62

B

Babbling, 95
Barbiturates, 387
Basal ganglia
    directed attention, 197, 198
    neglect syndromes, 185, 186
Behavioral management
    and developmental progressions, 295, 296
    language training, 292, 295, 296, 300
    programs for, 374, 375
Behavioral theory, 284
Beliefs, 35
Benadryl, 387
Benhaven program, 379
Benzodiazepines, 387
Biological hypothesis
    emotional expression, 24, 25
    limitations, 272, 274
    research trends, 264
    and social deficits, 16, 17, 264
Bittersweet Farms, 379
Blends, facial expression, 61
Blood flow, 160
Brain asymmetry (*see* Laterality)
Brain–behavior theories (*see* Biological hypothesis)
Brain stem
    autism model, 183, 184
    directed attention influence, 190–199
    sensory input, 175–199
Brain stem auditory evoked response
    evaluation, 182
    and neural function, 158, 159, 179, 182
Brain stem reticular formation, 183, 184

Brain systems, 144–172
"Bye-bye" game, 84

C

Caramazza hypothesis, 277
Carbamazepine, 399, 400
Catecholamines, 212
Category knowledge, 79
Causality, 286
Cerebellar cortex, 120–128
Cerebellar hemispheres, 126
Cerebellar nuclei, 121, 122
Cerebellum, 119–143
Cerebral cortex, 144–172
Cerebrospinal fluid 5-HIAA, 213
Chaining, 315
Childhood Autism Rating Scale, 369, 370
Children's Psychiatric Rating Scale, 394
Chlordiazepoxide, 387
Chlorpromazine, 388
Cholinergic mechanisms, 193
Chunking, 250, 251, 287, 303
Cingulate cortex, 194, 195, 197
Cingulectomy, 185
Circadian rhythm, 183
Clinical Global Impressions, 394
Cluster analysis, 275, 276
Cognitive development, 24–32
Cognitive processes, 22–43
    affective and social influence, 22–43
    genetic influences, 231–235
    versus sensory processing theory, 174
    theoretical focus, 4
Cognitive theory, 284
Combinatorial play, 286
Communication board, 294
Communication development, 283–289
Communication training, 374
Communicative competence
    acquisition of, 104–106
    autism thories implication, 292–297
    enchancement of, 282–309
    fenfluramine effect, 393
    preverbal aspects, 293, 294

Communicative intent (*see* Intentional communication)
Community programs, 377–379
Community resources, 379–381
Community Services for Autistic Citizens, 302, 377–379
Comprehension subtest, WISC
  differential performance, 39, 145, 146
  hemispheric asymmetry, 152
Compulsive behavior, 374, 375
Computerized tomography, 179
Conceptual knowledge, 99, 100
Concrete thinking, 36
Congenital rubella, 209, 226
Contextual cues
  communication enhancement, 299, 300
  language teaching, 317, 319
Contrastive stress, 98
Conversational scripts, 299
Conversational turns, 317, 318
Cooperative play, 352
Corpus callosum agenesis, 128, 132
Cortical–limbic–reticular system, 144–172
Cortisol, 218
Courchesne's model, 273, 274
Covert conditioning, 358
Crying, 95
Cue-dependent responding, 298
Cues, 355, 356

D

Dandy–Walker malformation, 128, 132
Day programs, 379
Dentate nucleus, 138
Developmental language disorder, 268, 269
Developmental models
  communication training, 296, 297, 300
  language acquisition, 285, 286
  social behavior, 5
Developmental progressions, 285, 286
Dexamethasone, 218
Dexedrine, 387, 388
Dextroamphetamine, 387, 388
Diagnosis, 367–385
  treatment implications, 368, 369

Diagnostic and Statistical Manual of Mental Disorders (*see* DSM-III; DSM-IIIR)
Diagnostic heterogeneity, 271, 272
Diazepam, 387
Dichotic listening
  brain asymmetry tests, 146–150, 178, 179
  and evoked potential studies, 178, 179
  language relationship, 150
"Dicky," 351
Diet, 396–399
Digit span, 39
Diphenhydramine, 387
Directed attention
  characteristics, 186
  evoked potentials, 181
  model of, 190–199
  and neglect syndromes, 184–186
  neurophysiology, 186–199
  sensory processing theory, 175–199
Direction of gaze, 235–240
Discrimination-training procedures, 300
Discriminative stimulus, 357
Distal communicative acts, 335
Dizygotic twins, 226, 228–235
Dopamine, 212, 214, 215
Dopamine-β-hydroxylase, 216
Dopaminergic systems, 184
Down syndrome, 94, 107
Drug treatment, 386–404
DSM-III, 5, 8, 176, 177, 263, 264
DSM-IIIR, 264
Dual-process model, 17
Dyad studies, 331
Dysarthria, 139
Dysphasia, 153, 154

E

Eating behavior, 137–140
Echolalic speech
  communication enhancement, 300
  diagnostic boundaries, 269
  and gestalt language learning, 287, 288
  grammatical development, 101
  intentionality, 301, 302
  and social familiarity, 59

Educational curricula, 382
Educational methods, 6
EEG (electroencephalography)
  and arousal, 54, 55
  attention model, 162
  evaluation, 178, 179
  homeostatic model, 55
  laterality tests, 147–150, 178–180
  vitamin B_6 effect, 398
Electrodermal responses, 53, 54, 159–161
Electroencephalography (*see* EEG)
Emerging skills, 371
Emotional cues, 85
Emotional development, 57–62
Emotional surveillance, 189
Emotions (*see also* Affect)
  biological bases, 24, 25
  development, 24–26, 59–62
  lateralization, 189, 190
  nonverbal behavior, 24, 25
  primary deficits, 85–89
  recognition of, 33, 34
  right-hemisphere overactivation, 165, 166
  and self-recognition, 10–12
  socialization of, arousal, 59–62
  theoretical focus, 4
Empathy, 85–89
Employment programs, 302, 375
Encephalitis lethargica, 184
Endorphins, 217
Enkephalins, 217
Entorhinal cortex, 195
Environmental perspective, 4
Epinephrine, 212
Etiology, fuzzy boundaries, 266, 267
Event-related potentials (*see also* P3 wave)
  evaluation, 178–181
  and language, 150–154
  laterality tests, 147–150, 178–181
  neural model, attention, 162, 163
  nonspecific factors, 180, 181
  novel stimuli, 54, 162, 163, 178–181
  vitamin B_6 effect, 398
Eye contact
  communicative intent, 337–339
  imitation effect, 354
  inferior parietal lobule, 188
  qualitative differences, 14
  right-hemisphere lesions, 190
  superior colliculus, 196, 197
Eye movements, 183, 196

F

Facial expression
  and affect, 32
  blends, 61
  maternal imitation paradigm, 60, 61
  mirror self-recognition technique, 10–12
  recognition, of, 33, 34
  right-hemisphere activation, 166
  and social deficits, 9, 10
Facial recognition
  deficit, 33, 34, 83
  early development, 83
  hemispheric specialization, 189
Facilitative style, 298, 299
Familial transmission, 227
Familiarity
  and responsiveness, 65–69
  and social behavior, 58, 59, 329–332
Family burden, 381
Family support services, 378, 381
Fantasy play, 352
Fastigial nucleus, 124, 138, 139
Feingold diet, 399
Fenfluramine, 213, 389–395
Fixation cells, 164
Flexor–extensor dominance, 183
Folate, 398, 399
Formulaic language, 102, 108, 251
Fragile X syndrome
  autism association, 229
  diagnostic boundaries, 266, 267, 271
  folate treatment, 398, 399
Free-play, 80, 81
Frontal eye fields
  and attention, 196, 197
  sensory pathways, 191, 192
Frontal lobe syndromes, 189
Functional communication, 313
Functionalistic approach, 290, 296
Fuzzy set, 265, 270

G

Game play, 352
Gating, 182, 193
Gaze behavior
  arousal modulation, 50
  communication intent, 335–339
  frequency versus duration, 67
  imitation strategies, 62–65
  inferior parietal lobule, 188
  superior colliculus, 196
Gaze couplings, 95
Generalization
  facilitation, 356, 359
  multiple exemplars, 316, 317
  naturalistic teaching, 316, 319, 320
  peer training, 332, 358, 359
  social skills training, 356, 359
Generalized imitation, 353, 354
Genetics, 225–259
  cerebellar hypoplasia, 136, 137
  and metalinguistics, 225–229
  sibling studies, 229–259
  twin studies, 228, 229
Geometrical–technical perception, 28
George Peabody College program, 359
Gestalt style
  individual variation, 287, 288
  language acquisition, 108, 303
Gestural imitation, 81, 82
Gesture
  affective deficits, 15, 32
  communication enhancement, 294
  communication intent, 335–339
  frequency of, 330
  and social deficits, 9, 10, 12, 13
Glass theory, 236
Grammar, 101–104, 106
Grammaticality judgments, 237, 240, 244–249
Granule cells, 121–128, 133–140
Group homes, 375
Group training, 377

H

Habituation
  attention abnormalities, 53, 54
  brain systems, 163
  fenfluramine effects, 393
  novel stimuli, 159, 161, 163
Haloperidol, 388
Heart rate
  autonomic factors, 159–161
  cerebellar lesions, 138
  homeostatic model, 55
  and imitation, interventions, 63
  novel stimuli, 53, 54, 159–161
  two-component attention model, 51–56
5-HIAA (5-hydroxyindoleacetic acid), 210–213
High-functioning autistic children, 267, 268
Hippocampus
  attention model, 162
  cerebellar connections, 139
  directed attention, 188, 193–195
  limbic connections, 194, 195
  theta rhythm, 193, 194
Histidinemia, 219
Homeostatic model, 52, 55
Homocystinuria, 219
Homovanillic acid, 214, 215, 398
Horizontal communication development, 293, 294
Hovering score, 338
5-HT (*see* Serotonin levels)
5-HTP (5-hydroxytryptophan), 211
5-Hydroxyindoleacetic acid (*see* 5-HIAA)
5-Hydroxytryptophan (*see* 5-HTP)
Hyperlexia, 268
Hyperserotonemia, 210
Hypnotic drugs, 387

I

ICD-9, 264
Ideational abstraction, 27
Illinois Test of Psycholinguistic Ability, 244
Imagery, 358
Imipramine, 389
Imitation (*see also* Maternal imitation)
  communication training, 295
  early development, 81, 82
  and emotion recognition, 34
  intervention struggles, 62–64

Imitation (*continued*)
  and language level, 286
  versus object permanence, 82
  primary deficits, 85–89
  and social responsiveness, 7, 8, 81, 82, 85–89
  social skills training, 353
Imitative play
  intervention study, 64–70
  and social attention, 62–64
  social skills training, 353, 354
Incidental-teaching techniques, 319, 320
Independence skills, 376
Indicating behaviors, 12–16
Individual Education Plans, 372, 373
Individual Habitation Plan, 372, 373
Individual variation, 287, 288
Inferior parietal lobule
  directed attention, 186–199
  functions, 186, 187
  gaze behavior, 188
  intentional motor behavior, 195–198
  sensory pathways, 191, 192, 194
Information processing
  hippocampal theta rhythm, 193, 194
  and optimal arousal, 56, 57, 160, 161
  right-hemisphere overactivation, 165, 166
  sensory processing interface, 174–199
Information subtest, WISC, 39
Initiative
  communication enhancement, 298
  definition, 333–336
  language teaching techniques, 320
  peer interactions, 331–339
  quality of, 335–339
Instrumental gestures, 330
Intelligence (*see* IQ)
Intensionality, 25, 25n, 29–32, 38
Intentional communication
  and communication enhancement, 293, 296–300
  definition, 333–336
  development, 96, 106, 107
  echolalia understanding, 301, 302
  and initiative, 333–344
Intentional motor behavior, 187, 188, 195–198
Intentionality, 25, 25n
Interactionist approach, 290
International Classification of Diseases, 9th edition (*see* ICD-9)

Interpersonal relations (*see* Social interactions)
Interpositus nucleus, 138
Interruption strategy, 313, 318
Intonation, 97, 98, 190
Intonation–word learning, 287
Intralaminar thalamic nuclei, 192
Intrauterine hormones, 155
IQ
  autism subgroups, 275
  and diagnostic boundaries, 267, 268
  fenfluramine effect, 393
Irradiation, cerebellar hypoplasia, 133–136
Isolate toys, 353
Isolated play, 352
Isolation syndromes, 17

J

Jay Nolan Center, 376–378
Joint attention
  early development, 83, 84, 87
  and preverbal communication, 96
  primary deficits, 12–14, 87
  social interactions, 333
Joke interpretation, 239
Jowonio: The Learning Place, 360

K

Kanner, L., 3, 263, 270
Kanner syndrome, 123
Knowledge of persons, 34, 35, 82–85
Knowledge of self, 82–85

L

Language (*see also* Language development)
  enhancement of, 282–309
  hemispheric asymmetry, 150–156, 165, 166
  and motivation, 310–325
  nature of, 93, 94
  reinforcement techniques, 314, 315
Language adjustments, 299

Language comprehension, 288, 289
Language deficits (*see also* Language training)
  asynchrony, 106
  diagnostic boundaries, 269
  and fenfluramine, 393
  genetic influences, 231–235
  hemispheric asymmetry, 150–154, 165, 166
  right-hemisphere overactivation, 165, 166
  and sensory processing theory, 174
  social cognition relationship, 286, 287, 294, 295
  and social deficits, 39–43, 108, 109
Language development
  asynchrony, 105–108
  characteristics, 39–42
  interpersonal context, 29–32
  psycholinguistics, 92–115
  and social cognition, 286, 287, 294, 295
  and social–emotional development, 108, 109
  social impairment relationship, 39–43, 108, 109
  theories of, 283–289
Language production, 288, 289
Language training
  and motivation, 310–355
  reinforcement, 314, 315
  theoretical basis, 282–309
  treatment program, 374
Laterality (*see also* Left hemisphere; Reversed asymmetry; Right hemisphere)
  brain systems, 164–168
  and language ability, 150–154, 288
  normal development, 146
  phonology, 98
  tests, 146–156, 178–181
LEAP program, 361, 362
Learned helplessness, 314
Learning Accomplishment Profile, 361
Learning disabilities, 232
Learning Experiences . . . An Alternative Program for Preschoolers and Parents (*see* LEAP program)
Learning theory, 284
Left hemisphere
  cognitive tests, 146
  facial recognition, 189n
  right-hemisphere interactions, 167, 190n
Leisure skills, 375
Length complexity index, 152

Lexical development, 98–101, 106
Librium, 387
Limbic contingency, 187, 195
Limbic system
  afferents and efferents, 194, 195
  directed attention, 190–199
  reticular connections, 192, 193
  and signal properties, 42
Locomotion
  brain stem influence, 183
  hippocampal theta rhythm, 194
Locus ceruleus, 192, 193
Loose teaching, 357

M

Magnesium, 397, 398
Magnetic resonance imaging, 123, 129–132
Maternal imitation
  emotional development, 60, 61
  intervention study, 64–70
Mean length of utterance
  development, 101, 102, 108
  hemispheric asymmetry, 152
Means–ends behavior, 286
Median raphe reticular formation, 184
Megavitamin therapy, 396–398
Memory, 137–140
Mental age, 8
Mental retardation
  autism subgroups, 275
  diagnostic boundaries, 267, 268
Mesencephalic reticular formation, 184, 185
Metalinguistics, 225–259
Metaphor
  capacity for, 36, 37
  language development, 99
Metarepresentational capacity, 31
Metenkephalin, 217
3-Methoxy-4-hydroxyphenylglycol (*see* MHPG)
Methylphenidate, 387, 388
MHPG (3-methoxy-4-hydroxyphenylglycol), 216
Microscopic analysis, 277
Midbrain reticular formation, 192
Midtrimester bleeding, 271
Mirror self-recognition procedures, 10–12
Monoamine oxidase, 210–213

Monozygotic twins, 226, 228–235
Morphemes, 102–104
Mother–child interaction (*see also* Maternal imitation)
  language development, 95
Motility, brain stem, 183
Motivation
  cerebellar hypoplasia, 137–140
  communication enhancement, 297–300
  and intentional communication, 341, 342
  language use, 310–325
  and limbic system, 195–198
  reinforcement techniques, 314, 315
Motor behavior
  and abstract ability, 27, 28
  cerebellar hypoplasia, 137–140
  direct attention, 186–188
  early development, 177
Motor contingency, 187
Motor intention, 187, 188, 195–198
Motor stereotypes (*see* Stereotyped behavior)
Multifactorial transmission, 227
Multiple exemplars, 316, 317
Musical skills, 302

N

N1 wave
  evaluation, 178–181
  hemispheric asymmetry, 150–152, 155, 178–181
Naltrexone, 395, 396
Naming ability, 99
Natural language-teaching paradigm, 311–321
Natural reinforcement, 356, 357
Natural settings, treatment, 377–379
Naturalistic play interactions, 295
N_d wave, 181
Negation, study of, 105–107
Negative reinforcement, 376
Neglect syndromes, 184–188
Neocerebellar vermis, 129–140
Nervous mutations, 137
Neuroleptics, 388, 389
Neurological deficit (*see* Biological hypothesis)
Neuronal gating, 182, 193, 197

Nominal–pronominal strategies, 287
Nonverbal communication
  and affect, 14–16, 24, 25
  frequency, 330
  social deficits, 12–14
Noradrenergic system, 193
Norepinephrine, 215–217
Normalization principle, 377–379
Northwestern Syntax Screening Test, 152
Noun phrases, 102
Nouns, 99, 100
Novel stimuli
  autonomic response, 159–161
  neural model, 161, 162
  orienting response, 53–56, 159
  right-hemisphere overactivation, 164, 165
Nucleus accumbens
  limbic pathways, 194
  motor intention, 188
Nutrition, 396–399

O

Object concepts, 78, 79, 82
Object manipulation, imitation, 354
Object-sorting, 79
Object words, 311
Observational techniques, 370–373
Observer play, 352
Off–on mechanism, 273
Olivopontocerebellar degeneration, 128, 132
One-to-one training, 377
Operant reinforcement, 376
Opiate antagonists, 395, 396
Opioids, 217
Optimal stimulation
  and arousal, 52, 53
  and social relationships, 59–62
Orienting response
  attention model, 51, 52
  novel stimuli, 53, 54, 159–161
  physiology, 51–56, 159–161
Outcome, 271
Overactivation hypothesis, 153, 155, 156

P

P2 response amplitude, 180
P3 wave
  auditory and visual stimuli, 156–158, 180
  and neural systems, 158, 163
  nonspecific factors, 180, 181
  novel stimuli, 54, 163, 180, 181
  overactivation theory, 163
Parallel play, 352
Parent training
  language learning, 320, 321
  social skills, 360
Parietal efferents, 195–198
Parietal neglect, 185
Parieto-occipital width, 179
Passive interaction, 274, 275
Passive person–active environment model, 289,
    290
Past tense, 103
Peabody Picture Vocabulary Test, 39, 151, 152
"Peekaboo" game, 84
Peer interactions
  frequency of, 327–330
  methodological issues, 6n, 326–343
  responses to, 339–341, 352, 353
  theoretical issues, 326–343
Peer training
  generalization, 358
  research importance, 6n
  social interaction frequency, 333
  social responsiveness, 6, 352, 353
  social skills, 358, 360
Peptides, 217, 218
Perception of emotion, 33, 34
Performance scale, WISC, 225, 226, 231
Perinatal events, 271
Peripheral blood flow, 160, 161
Perseveration, 189
Personal relatedness (*see also* Social interactions)
  and emotions, 26
  primary deficits, 87
Pervasive developmental disorder, 269, 270
PG area
  directed attention, 186–190, 195, 196
  functions, 186, 187
  neuroanatomy, pathways, 190, 191, 195, 196

Pharmacological treatment, 386–404
Phenylketonuria, 219, 226
Phoneme segmentation, 244–249
Phoneme synthesis, 244–249
Phonology
  development, 96–98
  metalinguistics, 240, 244–249
Photographed facial expression, 33, 34
Physical restraint, 376
Physiognomic perception, 28
Piaget's theory
  imitation, 81
  language, 289, 290
  object constancy, 78
Pictorial communication, 302
Picture Arrangement subtest, WISC, 39
Picture cards, 374
Picture schedules, 302
Picture-sorting task, 33
Platelet serotonin, 212, 213
Play (*see also* Symbolic play)
  communication training, 295
  imitation strategies, 62–64
  peer-mediated interactions, 6
  social skills training, 352
Polygenic transmission, 227
Pontine reticular formation, 184, 185
Porges's attention model, 51, 52
Positive reinforcement, 376
Posterior parietal cortex, 186–188
Posterior vermis, 129–140
Posture, 9, 10
Pragmatic language
  in communication training, 297–300
  definition, 93, 94
  development of, deficits, 105–108
  language theories, 284, 285
  and social development, 32, 42
Predictability (*see* Stimulus predictability)
Predictive syntagms, 30
Premack principle, 314
Prepositus hypoglossi, 138
Preschool intervention, 382
Preverbal period, 293, 294
Primary deficits, 75–88
  versus ability theories, 291
  criteria, 76, 77
  definition, 75

Primary deficits (*continued*)
  early development research, 75–88
  identification of, 76–78
  versus secondary deficits, 75, 76
  theoretical approaches, 290, 291
Primate isolation syndrome, 16, 17
Problem behavior, 351, 352
Problem-solving skills, 79
Prompting, 354
Pronoun reversals, 288
Prosodic envelopes, 97
Prosody, 97, 98
  and diagnostic boundaries, 269
  overview, 97, 98
  right hemisphere, 184–186, 190
Proto-communicative signals, 30
Protodeclaratives, 96
Protoimperatives, 96
Proximal communication, 335
Psychoeducational Profile, 370
Psycholinguistics, 92–115, 284
Punishment, 376
Purkinje cells
  anatomy and development, 121–124
  and cerebellar hypoplasia, 133–140
  degeneration, 137
  genetic mutations, 137
  irradiation effects, 133–135
Pyridoxine, 397, 398

R

Raphe nuclei, 192
Rating scales, 369, 370
Reaction times, 164
Readiness models, 286
Reading disability, 232
Reciprocal relationships, 26
  communication enhancement, 298, 317
  development, 26, 84, 85
  primary deficit, 85–88
  versus self-recognition, 84
  social skills training, 353
Recognition, 33, 34
Recreational skills, 375
Referential–expressive development, 287

Referential looking behavior, 13
Referential word meaning, 41
Reinforcement
  language teaching program, 312
  social skills training, 356
  treatment strategies, 376
Relational meanings, 100, 101
Relaxation techniques, 358
REM bursts, 182, 183
REM sleep, 182, 183
Representational thinking (*see* Symbolic/representational thinking)
Residential living, 378–380
Resonate emotionally, ability to, 15, 16, 60
Response generalization, 356
Response interruption strategy, 313, 318
Restraint techniques, 376
Reticular formation, 162–168
Reticular neglect, 185
Reversed asymmetry
  current hypotheses, 154–156
  language ability, 150–153
  tests of, 147–150
Riddle interpretation, 239, 243–249
Right hemisphere
  directed attention, 189
  electrophysiology, 147–150
  facial recognition, 189, 189n
  language function, 150–155, 190
  left-hemisphere interactions, 167, 190n
  lesion effects, 190
  neglect syndromes, 184–186
  overactivation, 153, 164–168
Ritalin, 387, 388
Ritualistic behavior, 374, 375
Ritvo–Freeman Real-Life Rating Scale, 390
Role playing, 299
Rote memory, 295
Rubella, 209, 226

S

Saccades, 196
Schizophrenia, 265
SCIPPY program, 359
Sedatives, 387

Seizure disorders, 128, 132
Selective attention, 187
Self-control, 357, 358
Self-injurious behavior, 375
Self–other differentiation, 82–85
Self-recognition
    affective response, 10–12
    early development, 82–85
Self-stimulation
    and social familiarity, 59
    and social skills, 351
Semantics
    brain asymmetry, 152
    differential impairment, 41
    metalinguistics, 237
    word meaning deficits, 99, 100
Sensory contingency, 187
Sensory gating, 182, 193, 197
Sensory–motor period
    object concepts, 78, 79
    self–other differentiation, 82–85
    symbolic play, 80, 81
Sensory processing, 174–199
Sentence length, 101
Sentence meaning, 237, 244
Separations, attachment behavior, 7
Serotonergic system
    cerebellar hypoplasia, 139, 140
    directed attention, 193
Serotonin (5-hydroxytryptamine, 5-HT) levels
    fenfluramine effect, 389–395
    research studies, 210–214
Sex differences, 228
Sex education, 382
Sexual development, 381
Shaping, 315
Shared control, 317–319
Shared emotional experience, 29–32
Siblings, 229–235
    autism rate, 229–231
    cognitive impairments, 231–235
    limitations, 233–235
    metalinguistics, 240–252
Sign language, 374
Signal properties, 34
Similarities subtest, WISC, 39, 40
Skin conductance, 53, 54, 159–161
Sleep spindles, 182

Smiling, 335, 340
Social aloofness
    classification, 274–276
    and fuzzy boundaries, 266, 267, 271
Social attention (*see* Attention)
Social avoidance behavior, 318, 319
Social behavior (*see also* Social impairment)
    classification, 274, 275
    frequency, 330
Social cognition
    autism theories, 291, 303
    development, 286, 287
    and language acquisition, 286, 287, 294, 295
Social Competence Intervention Package for
        Preschool Youngsters (*see* SCIPPY pro-
        gram)
Social cues, 348, 349
Social development
    and arousal, 57–62
    foundations of, affect, 24–32
    Kanner's insight, 3
    language relationship, 108, 109
    and social skills, 347, 348
    theoretical focus, 4
Social impairment
    abstract thinking deficits, 37, 38
    additivity model, 268
    and affect, 9–12
    attention and arousal relationship, 56–70
    autism theory, 42, 43, 85–89
    biological hypothesis, 16, 17
    classification, 274, 275
    definition, 9–17
    developmental changes, 5
    and diagnostic boundaries, 267–270
    epidemiological study, 274, 275
    and language disorders, 39–42
    limitations of, theory, 267–270, 274–276
    primary deficits, 85–89
    research trends, 264
    right-hemisphere dysfunction, 190
Social interactions (*see also* Peer interactions)
    and affect, coordination, 59–62
    and cognitive impairment, 37–43
    and familiarity, 58, 59
    frequency of, 330–333
    responsiveness, 5, 6
    structure effects, 332, 333

Social interactions (*continued*)
  and symbolic thinking, 28–32
  understanding of, 35
Social isolation
  and biological hypothesis, 17
  time-out technique, 376
Social learning, 6
Social reciprocity (*see* Reciprocal relationships)
Social reinforcement
  natural settings, 354
  treatment strategies, 376
Social responsiveness
  peers, 339–341, 352, 353
  retrospective data, 8
  right-hemisphere overactivation, 165–167
  structured interactions, 5, 6
  young autistic child, 6–9
Social routines, 355
Social skills, 346–366
  component behaviors, 355, 356
  definition, 346, 347
  developmental principles, 347, 348
  environmental factors, 349
  and peer interaction frequency, 330
  peer training, 358–360
  preschool curriculum, 346–366
  programs, 358–362, 379
  targets for, 351–356
Social stimulation, 59–64 (*see also* Optimal stimulation)
Social toys, 353
Social withdrawal
  and familiarity, 58, 59
  right-hemisphere overactivation, 165–167
Sokolov's model, 162–164
Sound blending, 244
Sound reactivity, 176
Spatial tests, 145, 146
Speech acquisition, 284
Speech disorders
  cerebellar hypoplasia, 139, 140
  diagnostic boundaries, 268, 269
  family history, 232
  hemispheric asymmetry, 150–156
Splinter skills, 295
Spontaneous social initiative, 333–342
Spontaneous speech, 100
Startle response, 138

Stereotyped behavior
  EEG, 54
  and optimal stimulation, 52, 54, 55
  and play, 38, 39
  social-affective roots, 39
  stimulant drugs, 388
Stimulants, 387, 388
Stimulus generalization, 356
Stimulus overselectivity, 348, 349
Stimulus predictability
  imitation study, 64–70
  and social behavior, 8, 56–59
Stress, family, 381
Striatal neglect, 185
Striatum, 191, 197
Structured play, 80, 81
Substantia nigra, 183
Superior colliculus, 191–97
Superior posterior vermis, 129–140
Support services, 379–381
Sustained attention
  heart rate, 52, 54
  neurophysiology, 189
Symbolic play
  early development, 80, 81
  and language level, 286
  primary deficits, 85–89
  and social impairment, 38, 39, 85–89
Symbolic/representational thinking
  autism subgroups, 275
  capacity for, 35–42
  emergence of, 28–32, 35–42
  and indicating skills, 14, 15
  interpersonal context, 28–32
  and social impairment, 37–43
Synonymy judgments, 237, 240, 248
Syntax, 101–108, 237

T

Tardive dyskinesia, 389
Task variation, 315–319
TEACCH program, 369–372
Teacher-antecedent conditions, 334
Teacher behavior, and play, 353
Teaching loosely, 357
Tegretol, 399, 400

Telegraphic speech, 93, 101
Thalamic neglect, 185
Thalamic reticular formation, 185, 192
Thalamus, 162
Theory of mind, 106, 109
Theta rhythm, 193, 194
Thorazine, 388
Threshold point, heredity, 227
Thyroid hormone, 218
Time-out, 376
Tofranil, 389
Toys
  exploratory behavior, 66, 67
  imitation study, 64–70
  and predictability, 57
  social skills training, 352, 353
Transactional model, 290
Treatment, 367–385
  attention strategies, 62–70
  community resources, 379–381
  imitative play, 62–70
  normalization principle, 377–379
Treatment and Education of Autistic and Related Communication Handicapped Children (*see* TEACCH program)
Tricyclic antidepressants, 389
Tryptophan, 210
Tryptophan hydroxylase, 211
Turn-taking format, 318
Twins, 226–235

U

UCLA program, 360, 361
Uzgiris–Hunt Gestural Imitation Scale, 34

V

Valium, 387
Vanderbilt University program, 359
Vanillylmandelic acid (VMA), 216
Ventricular asymmetry, 179
Verb phrases, 102, 103

Verbal ability
  and metalinguistics, 225, 226
  social impairment relationship, 39–42
Verbal riddle, 239, 243–249
Verbal scale, WISC, 225, 226, 231–233
Verbs, 100
Vertical communication development, 293
Videotape-and-picture technique, 33
Videotaped faces/vocalization, 34
Vigilance, 186, 187 (*see also* Directed attention)
Visual–spatial ability
  differential performance, 145, 146
  self-recognition, 82–85
  training programs, 302
Visual stimuli, P3 wave, 156–158
Visual–vestibular interactions, 182
Vitamin B$_6$, 215, 397, 398
Vitamins, 396–399
Vocabulary subtest, WISC, 39, 40, 145, 146, 152
Vocal imitation, 81, 82
Vocalizations, 32, 184
Vocational rehabilitation, 375, 378, 379
Vocational settings, 302, 303
Vocational skills, 375–379
Voluntary attention, 162–165

W

Werner's concepts, 27, 28
Whole-body movement, 335
Wide Range Achievement Test, 232
WISC (Wechsler Intelligence Scale for Children)
  differential performance, 39, 40, 145, 146, 231
  genetic studies, 231–235
Word acquisition, 98–101
Word card systems, 374
Word consciousness, 243–249
Word meaning, metalinguistics, 237, 240, 243–249
Word order violations, 244
Written words, 302

Y

Young Autism Project, 360, 361